The
Occupational
Therapy
# MANAGER

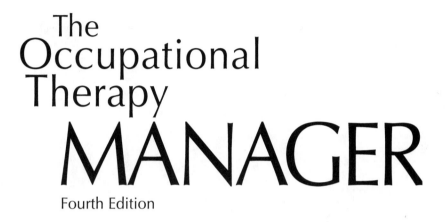

# The
# Occupational
# Therapy
# MANAGER

Fourth Edition

*Guy L. McCormack, PhD, OTR/L, FAOTA*
*Evelyn G. Jaffe, MPH, OTR, FAOTA*
*Marcia Goodman-Lavey, JD, OTR/L*

EDITORS

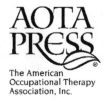

AOTA
PRESS

The American
Occupational Therapy
Association, Inc.

**Mission Statement**

The American Occupational Therapy Association advances the quality, availability, use, and support of occupational therapy through standard-setting, advocacy, education, and research on behalf of its members and the public.

*AOTA Staff*

Joseph C. Isaacs, CAE, Executive Director
Karen C. Carey, CAE, Associate Executive Director, Membership, Marketing, and Communications

Chris Davis, Managing Editor, AOTA Press
Suzanne Seitz, Production Editor
Barbara Dickson, Editorial Assistant

Robert A. Sacheli, Manager, Creative Services
Sarah E. Ely, Book Production Coordinator

The American Occupational Therapy Association, Inc.
4720 Montgomery Lane
PO Box 31220
Bethesda, MD 20824-1220
Phone: 301-652-AOTA (2682)
TDD: 800-377-8555
Fax: 301-652-7711
www.aota.org
To order: 1-877-404-AOTA (2682)

**Disclaimers**

This publication is designed to provide accurate and authoritative information in regard to the subject matter covered. It is sold or distributed with the understanding that the publisher is not engaged in rendering legal, accounting, or other professional service. If legal advice or other expert assistance is required, the services of a competent professional person should be sought.
—*From the Declaration of Principles jointly adopted by the American Bar Association and a Committee of Publishers and Associations*

It is the objective of The American Occupational Therapy Association to be a forum for free expression and interchange of ideas. The opinions expressed by the contributors to this work are their own and not necessarily those of either the editors or The American Occupational Therapy Association.

ISBN: 1-56900-178-2

Library of Congress Control Number: 2003104380

Design by Sarah E. Ely
Composition by Circle Graphics, Columbia, MD
Printed by Boyd Printing Company, Inc., Albany, NY

Cover art: Paul Klee, After a sketch from Zurick/Nach einer Skizze aus Zuerich, 1914, 123 water-color on paper; 13 × 10,3 cm; The Barnes Foundation Merion
© 2003 Artists Rights Society (ARS), New York / VG Bild-Kunst, Bonn

# Contents

# IV Leading and Organizing

**Chapter 11: Communication in the Workplace**
*Catherine Nielson, MPH, OTR/L, FAOTA*

**Chapter 12: Personnel Management: Measuring Performance,**
**Creating Success**
*Christine M. MacDonell, BS, OTR*

**Chapter 13: Motivating Employees**
*Kate Hayner, EdD, OTR*
*Evelyn G. Jaffe, MPH, OTR, FAOTA*

**Chapter 14: From Management to Leadership**
*Ann P. Grady, PhD, OTR, FAOTA*

# List of Tables, Figures, Exhibits, and Chapter Appendixes

# List of Abbreviations
and Acronyms

| | |
|---|---|
| ACAAI | American College of Allergy, Asthma, and Immunology |
| ACP | American College of Physicians |
| ACOTE | Accreditation Council for Occupational Therapy Education |
| ADA | American with Disabilities Act of 1990 |
| ADL | activities of daily living |
| AFC | academic fieldwork coordinator |
| AHA | American Hospital Association |
| ALJ | administrative law judge |
| AMA | American Medical Association |
| AOTA | American Occupational Therapy Association |
| AOTCB | American Occupational Therapy Certification Board |
| AOTPAC | American Occupational Therapy Political Action Committee |
| APC | Ambulatory Payment Classification |
| APHA | American Public Health Association |
| ASPA | Association of Specialized and Professional Accreditors |
| | |
| BBA | Balanced Budget Act of 1997 |
| BBRA | Balanced Budget Refinement Act |
| BCBS | Blue Cross/Blue Shield |
| BIA | Brain Injury Association |
| BIPA | Benefits Improvement and Protection Act |
| | |
| CABG | coronary artery bypass grafting |
| CAHEA | AMA's Committee on Allied Health Education & Accreditation |
| CAI | Cooperative Accreditation Initiative |
| CAM | complementary/alternative medicine |
| CARF | Commission on Accreditation of Rehabilitation Facilities |
| CDC | Centers for Disease Control and Prevention |
| CEU | continuing education unit |

CFO        chief financial officer
CHAP       Community Health Accreditation Program
CHEA       Council for Higher Education
CHOICE     Center for Humane Options in Child Birth Experiences
CMG        case mix group
CMS        Centers for Medicare and Medicaid
COPA       Council on Post-Secondary Education
CORF       comprehensive outpatient rehabilitation facility
COTA       certified occupational therapy assistant
CQAIE      Center for Quality Assurance in International Education
CQI        continuous quality improvement
CPI        Consumer Price Index
CPT        *Current Procedural Terminology*
CRT        controlled randomized trial

DAB        department appeals board
DHHS       U.S. Department of Health and Human Services
DME        durable medical equipment
DMEPOS     durable medical equipment, prosthetics, orthotics, and supplies
DMERC      durable medical equipment regional carrier
DNR        do not resuscitate
DOD        U.S. Department of Defense
DRG        diagnosis-related group
DSC        disease-specific care
DSM-IV     *Diagnostic and Statistical Manual of Mental Disorders, Fourth Edition*

EBP        evidence-based practice
EDSIS      AOTA's special interest section for education
EPA        Environmental Protection Agency
EPSDT      early and periodic screening, diagnosis, and treatment
ERC        ethically responsible creativity
ERISA      Employee Retirement Income Security Act

FEC        Federal Election Commission
FEHB       Federal Employees Health Benefits
FI         fiscal intermediary
FTE        full-time equivalent

GDP        gross domestic product
GEHA       Government Employees Hospital Association
GNP        gross national product
GRD        Government Relations Department

| | |
|---|---|
| HCFA | Health Care Financing Administration |
| HCPAC | Health Care Professionals Advisory Committee |
| HCPCS | Healthcare Common Procedure Coding System |
| HHA | home health agency |
| HIPPA | Health Insurance Portability and Accountability Act |
| HIV/AIDS | human immunodeficiency virus/acquired immune deficiency syndrome |
| HMO | health maintenance organization |
| HO | hearing officer |
| HPPD | hours per patient day |
| | |
| IADL | instrumental activities of daily living |
| ICD | *International Classification of Diseases* |
| IDEA | Individuals with Disabilities Education Act |
| IDN | integrated delivery network |
| IEP | individualized education plan |
| IRF | inpatient rehabilitation facility |
| IRR | internal rate of return |
| | |
| JCAHO | Joint Commission on Accreditation of Healthcare Organizations |
| JCI | Joint Commission International |
| JCR | Joint Commission Resources |
| | |
| LLC | limited liability company |
| LMRP | local medical review policy |
| | |
| MDS | Minimum Data Set |
| MOT | master's of occupational therapy |
| MPFS | Medicare Physician Fee Schedule |
| MR | medical review |
| | |
| NBCOT | National Board for Certification in Occupational Therapy |
| NIDRR | National Institute on Disability and Rehabilitation Research |
| | |
| OASIS | Outcome and Assessment Information Set |
| OPPS | outpatient prospective payment system |
| OT | occupational therapist, occupational therapy |
| OTA | occupational therapy assistant |
| OTPP | occupational therapist in private practice |
| OTR | occupational therapist registered |

PAC          political action committee
PACE         Program of All-Inclusive Care for the Elderly
PADL         personal activities of daily living
PAI          patient assessment instrument
PDU          professional development unit
PHI          protected health information
POS          point-of-service plan
PPO          preferred provider organization
PPS          prospective payment system
PT           physical therapy
PTAC         professional and technical advisory committee

QIP          quality improvement plan

RAI          resident assessment instrument
RAP          resident assessment protocols
RBRVS        Resource-Based Relative Value Scale
RCF          residential care facility
RCT          randomized controlled trial
RHHI         regional home health intermediaries
ROI          return on investment
RUG          resource utilization group
RT           rehabilitation therapy
RVU          relative value unit

SBA          Small Business Administration
SCHIP        State Children's Health Insurance Program
SIDS         sudden infant death syndrome
SLP          speech-language pathology
SNF          skilled nursing facility
SOAP         Society for Obstetric Anesthesia and Perinatology
SWOT         strengths, weaknesses, opportunities, and threats (analysis)

TBI          traumatic brain injury

USDE         U.S. Department of Education
USTF         Uniformed Services Treatment Facility

VA           Veterans Administration

WFOT         World Federation of Occupational Therapists
WHO          World Health Organization

# Preface

*"Each for himself, and God for us all, as the elephant
said when he danced among the chickens"*

JOHN McCAIN (*Time Magazine,* December 12, 1979, p. 16 )

This quote may appear peculiar, but it has significance for occupational therapy managers. First, managers must never lose site of their respect and responsibility for the people they serve. Second, managers are not above everyone else like a dancing elephant among the chickens. After all, it is the chickens that have the responsibility to lay the eggs, not the managers.

The first edition of *The Occupational Therapy Manager* was published in 1985. This fourth edition, the culmination of diligent work by many authors, is also a forward-thinking exploration into the various facets of management in a constantly changing health care environment. The book has been organized with the American Occupational Therapy Association's (AOTA's) *Occupational Therapy Practice Framework: Domain and Process* in mind; for example, it addresses the *domain* of occupational therapy, defined as those areas of human experience in which practitioners of the profession offer assistance to others. In other words, the domain includes performance in areas of occupation such as work to engage people in activities they find meaningful and purposeful.

Chapter 1 explores the historical development of management strategies from the classical to current trends. Management has not changed much over time; it still requires the ability to get ordinary people to perform extraordinary tasks. This book takes into account the *activity demands* and *performance requirements* needed to accomplish work-related tasks. Chapter 2 provides readers with a closer look at the skill sets or *performance skills* that are unique to managers and the similarities of the *performance patterns* of practitioners. Karen Jacobs reminds us of the importance of emerging practices and diversification.

Many new chapters have been added in this edition to address the changing role of occupational therapy managers and also the *Occupational Therapy Framework*. For example, William Frey outlines the importance of cultural competency and of universal systems of health care, which address the concept of *context*.

The *Occupational Therapy Practice Framework* also includes elements of *process* such as *evaluation, intervention,* and *outcomes*. Jane Acquaviva provides practical evaluation principles in her chapter on documentation. Catherine Nielson emphasizes the importance of communication. Christine MacDonell provides guidelines on performance appraisal, while Kate Hayner and Evelyn Jaffe describe the manager's role as a motivator. Along the same line, Ann Grady eloquently provides a careful analysis of styles of leadership.

In respect to intervention, Cynthia Epstein and Evelyn Jaffe address consultation as a role of managers. Outcomes are discussed by Randy Strickland, who outlines the strategic planning process. Janet Jabri provides an excellent overview of financial planning. Tammy Richmond adds a new chapter on marketing. Gordon Giles provides guidelines on how to write a plan for starting up a new business or practice. Sara Pazell and Evelyn Jaffe lay out the elements of entrepreneurial ventures. Beatriz Abreu provides an excellent chapter on evidence-based practice.

In respect to the intervention process, V. Judith Thomas adds one of the most comprehensive chapters on reimbursement one will find anywhere in the occupational therapy literature.

*The Occupational Therapy Manager* is also a rich resource on accrediting organizations and special issues encountered in fieldwork supervision. This edition also includes chapters on public policy, advocacy, and state regulations. Continuing competency is covered thoroughly by Penelope Moyers and Jim Hinojosa.

The original planning and development of this book could not have taken place without the efforts of Krishni Patrick, former editor of AOTA Press. Coeditors Evelyn Jaffe and Marcia Goodman-Lavey provided both detailed oversight and insightful suggestions concerning the content of the chapters. Special thanks go to Suzanne Seitz, Jeff Finn, Amy Eutsey, and Chris Davis for their organizational skills and for reminding us when to let go of the "lovies" and keep what is essential.

—Guy L. McCormack, PhD, OTR/L, FAOTA

# Defining and Rethinking Management

# Historical and Current Perspectives of Management

Guy L. McCormack, PhD, OTR/L, FAOTA

*"The manager has the task of creating a true whole that is larger than the sum of its parts, a productive entity that turns out more than the sum of the resources put into it."*

PETER DRUCKER

**Guy L. McCormack, PhD, OTR/L, FAOTA,** has been an educator, researcher, and author for 25 years. He is the founder and chairman of the Master of Occupational Therapy Program at Samuel Merritt College in Oakland, CA. He is currently working as a home health practitioner with the Sutter Visiting Nurses Association and Hospice in Emeryville, CA. In addition to his doctorate in human science, he has received extensive training in traditional Chinese medicine and has many certificates in alternative/complementary forms of intervention.

# Key Terms and Concepts

**Alderfer's ERG theory.** A motivation theory that categorizes needs in terms of existence (E), relatedness (R), or growth (G) aspects.

**Benchmarking.** A method of setting standards of performance based on the characteristics of organizations that have a high degree of success.

**Bureaucracy.** A system of classical management organizational design that promoted highly specialized jobs, a consistent system of rules, hierarchical structure, impersonal superior/subordinate relationships, and excessive red tape.

**Globalization.** A general term used to describe worldwide competition among large organizations for multi-national markets. The marketplace has undergone globalization due to computer technology, improved transportation, economic growth, communication, and changing consumer needs.

**Groupthink.** A group defense reaction that impairs the quality of group decisions.

**Hawthorne studies.** Famous studies conducted between 1924 and 1933 at the Western Electric Company to explore the effects of work conditions and environment on productivity. The study suggested that group dynamics and special attention paid to workers had a greater effect on productivity than extraneous variables such as room illumination.

**Henri Fayol (1841–1925).** A French industrialist known as the father of modern management. He developed widely used functions and principles of management.

**Herzberg's two-factor theory.** A theory of motivation that proposed some types of needs were motivational while others were not. This theory examined the influences of content, the experiences on the job and the context, and the feelings that surround the job.

**Human relations movement.** A movement in management in the 1920s that emphasized the human aspects of organizations. This movement grew out of a reaction to the shortcomings of classical scientific management.

**Learning organizations.** An organizational approach based on systems thinking and the belief that humans' natural motivation for learning should be integrated in management and organizations.

**Maslow's need hierarchy.** Motivational theory that postulates that people in the workplace are motivated by a desire to satisfy a set of internal needs.

**McGregor's theory X, theory Y.** Early motivational theory that stereotyped workers as either being lazy and needing to be controlled or as motivated self-starters who sought out responsibility.

**Organizational behavior.** The study of human behavior, attitude, expectations, and performance in the workplace.

**Scientific management.** Classical system of management attributed to Fredrick W. Taylor (1856–1915) that used time and motion studies and the piece rate to improve worker productivity.

**Virtual organizations.** An organization that is formed through airways, computers, or teleconferencing to conduct work in the absence of physical contact.

# Learning Objectives

After completing this chapter, you should be able to do the following:

- Identify the primary characteristics of scientific management.
- Describe the strengths and weaknesses of bureaucracy.
- Identify the major characteristics of the human relations movement.
- Compare and contrast scientific management with the human relations movement.
- Explain how McGregor's theory X, theory Y is useful for managers to understand.
- Compare and contrast Maslow's need hierarchy, Herzberg's two-factor theory, and Alderfer's ERG theory.
- Identify the primary lessons learned from the Hawthorne studies.
- Describe the main concepts that Henri Fayol contributed to management theory.
- Identify features of organizational philosophy that are prevalent today.
- Identify traits that are desirable for effective managers.
- Describe a historical perspective on management development.

According to traditional thinking, the role of a manager can be boiled down to four functions: planning, organizing, coordinating, and controlling. These four terms were first introduced by French industrialist Henri Fayol in 1916 and have dominated management vocabulary ever since the Industrial Revolution (Bovee, Thill, Wood, & Dovel, 1993).

However, times have changed. Today's occupational therapy manager is more like a juggler with many balls in the air. He or she faces different challenges than the typical manager confronted in the past. Today's manager needs to be politically correct, must have good interpersonal skills, and must demonstrate an ability to deal with a culturally diverse population. He or she must have systems in place to be informed on a day-to-day or minute-by-minute basis. The occupational therapy manager is obligated to disseminate information to staff and colleagues. This person must embrace change, possess technical knowledge, and be the voice for the department or unit. Managers are not always popular. They must play a decision-making role in the allocation of resources, handle confidential information, negotiate, lead, be an entrepreneur and, if that is not enough, be a source of inspiration.

The occupational therapy manager will find that time is the most difficult commodity to control. Time is a scarce and valued resource. The manager must have a vision that goes beyond issues of time and serves as a guide for the greater good of the organization. Above all else, he or she needs to be flexible and must learn to live with ambiguity.

This chapter reviews the historical roots of management and identifies current perspectives on management as it is practiced today. As we plan for the future, we can avoid mistakes of previous managers by looking at the past. A review of history allows one to stand back and see the influences that have left a lasting imprint on today's practices. This process allows the occupational therapy manager to sort out what works and what does not work in today's health care industry.

Historically, systems of management were developed and refined from techniques used in ancient civilizations. Early systems of management can be traced back to China, Egypt, Greece, Rome, and Java (Schermerborn, Hunt, & Asborn, 1994). Basically, management systems were created for very practical purposes: to protect society; to create better systems to plant and gather crops; to practice religion; to expand territory; and most important, to keep peace. In ancient civilizations, the need for management systems addressed basic needs and had survival value.

Ancient history has provided us with a clear lesson: Management systems are created to meet the needs of society. Albeit, the needs of society are not always virtuous. The Roman army used complex systems of management to mount military campaigns. The Chinese people needed a system to manage large populations on public projects such as building the Great Wall; thus, they invented written exams to systematically select individuals for jobs in public administration and to promote them by merit.

During the same era, the Europeans were managing a feudal system in which the selection for a job or position was based on birthright.

In today's health care industry, management systems are designed to meet the required best practices for efficiency; safety; appropriate staffing and supervision; effective use of supplies; and most important, cost containment (Mondy, Holmes, & Flippo, 1995). The occupational therapy manager should be familiar with the history of management and the theories that set the stage for the systems used today.

In the late 1800s, the United States and Europe took different paths to management. The United States was recovering from the post–Civil War era. This period was the dawn of the Industrial Revolution. The industrial might of the United States rested on basic industries such as steel production. The United States had vast natural resources; it also had the need to build railroads, bridges, ships, and large plants and to expand into the Western territories. While Europe was concerned mainly about better methods of administrating people and work, the central concern in the United States was directed toward individual tasks and fitting the best workers to those tasks (Davis, Hellervik, Skull, Gebelein, & Sheard, 1992). As a result of the diverging paths, the United States focused on a management system known as *scientific management,* whereas Europe focused on the science of *administration* (Bovee et al., 1993).

## Scientific Management

Scientific management was an outgrowth of the effects of industrialization and represents the classical management perspective. Frederick W. Taylor (1856–1915), who was a machinist and industrial engineer from Philadelphia, became known as the "father of scientific management" (Schermerborn et al., 1994). While working at Midvale Steel Company, Taylor observed that employees worked at less than their full capacity because they were concerned about being laid off when the job was completed. Taylor also observed that management did not clearly delineate tasks and paid little attention to matching the skills of employees with their assigned tasks. As a result, Taylor advocated scientific analysis of tasks as well as time and motion studies that examined the physical movements and time it took to complete a particular work task. Taylor showed in various studies that he could systematically increase a worker's productivity through better body mechanics, economy of motion, and monetary incentives. The analysis of jobs gave rise to the task concept, that is, what is to be done, how it is to be done, and exactly when it is to be completed. Work incentives were based on coercion and financial rewards for high output (Hodgetts, 1992; Taylor, 1911).

Taylor was very pragmatic. In industry, many of the practices he developed continue to be used today. He did not believe that gainful occupations should be based on tradition, rule of thumb, personal opinion, and guesswork. Taylor believed in proven fact. He found that standardized tools and procedures improved work performance and prevented injury. The same principle is accepted today in the science of human engineering called *ergonomics* (Bovee et al., 1993).

A task, according to Taylor, had to do with the amount of work to be performed, which was determined through time and motion studies. Taylor found that periods of rest are necessary for increased productivity. Therefore, he advocated establishing an assigned quota, which is similar to what is called a work *goal* today. Taylor also believed that money was a significant incentive to workers. In his famous pig iron study, Taylor matched workers with the right abilities to a task: to load by hand 92-pound blocks of iron, called "pigs," on freight cars. On the average, workers loaded 12.5 tons of these pigs for $1.15 a day. After conducting a time and motion study on the task, Taylor set up an incentive system in which a worker could earn $1.85 per day and take frequent rest periods. As a result of scientific management, "the first-class worker" could consistently load an average of 47.5 tons of pig iron per day (Schermerborn et al., 1994; Taylor, 1911).

A husband-and-wife team, Frank Bunker Gilbreth (1868–1924) and Lillian Moller Gilbreth (1878–1972), demonstrated that scientific management could be practiced in both the home and workplace. In his early years, Frank Gilbreth turned down an opportunity to attend college and instead became a bricklayer (Bovee et al., 1993; Pearce & Robinson, 1994). Gilbreth observed that the bricklayers who were training him used a variety of motions to complete their tasks. Using time and motion studies to analyze the most efficient method to lay bricks, Gilbreth was able to eliminate 16 motions from the process of brick laying. In addition, he invented an adjustable stand (adaptive device) to hold bricks so the workers would not have to bend over so often to pick up the bricks.

Gilbreth conducted several other studies on construction tasks using a hand-cranked movie camera and timing device (microchronometer) to shave off the time it took to perform specific work tasks. Together with Lillian, who had a background in psychology and management, the couple provided consultation to a variety of organizations to analyze work tasks. The Gilbreths had 12 children and claimed to have used scientific management to efficiently organize tasks in their own home such as preparing dinner, folding laundry, and cleaning the house (Bovee et al., 1993).

Over the years, scientific management has been criticized, expanded, and modified. Critics have argued that scientific management lacked the humanistic element; it emphasized the job task rather than the individual. Furthermore, scientific management did not address the benefits of work groups or teams in the workplace. Today, unions bargain for common wages, working conditions, and work rules for all employees rather than set up reward systems for a few selected workers.

Taylor made some assumptions about how workers needed to be organized, supervised, and structured to get the best production out of them. Taylor thought that studies and designs alone could maximize the worker's efficiency on the job. To his credit, he developed the piece-rate system and a process for scientific selection of best workers (Nadler & Nadler, 1998; Szelagyi & Wallace, 1990). The piece-rate system was based on a set pay rate for the number of products (pieces) the worker assembled in a work day. Some of these methods continue to be used today in a modified format. For instance, occupational therapists use some of the principles developed by Taylor when conducting an activity analysis. An activity analysis (a) breaks down a task or purposeful activity into the elements of motor skills, sensory awareness, and degree of difficulty; and (b) considers gradation, endurance, coordination, cognitive demands, and psychological benefits.

Compared with a time and motion study, an activity analysis is much more holistic and takes into account the significance and meaning the activity has to the client (Christiansen & Baum, 1997). The purpose of the activity analysis is to set up an occupation that is goal directed, purposeful, restorative, or designed to prevent or reverse dysfunction. The purpose of a time and motion study is to break down work into its constituent elements, or motions, to eliminate inefficiencies and wasted effort.

Occupational therapists also teach work simplification and use the principles of ergonomics to make adaptations that improve the place of work. Occupational therapists working in sheltered workshops often perform time and motion studies on small assembly jobs to be performed by individuals with physical or mental disabilities. These work environments commonly use a piece-rate system as an incentive for a person who has a developmental disability. However, in this context, the piece-rate system is presumably a behavioral management strategy to promote activity or habituate the individual to a productive and independent lifestyle.

## Administrative Management

While classical management focused on finding "one best way" to get work done on the factory floor, administrative management emphasized the flow of information and how organizations operate. Henri Fayol, known as the "father of modern management," believed that people are born with a talent to manage. He also believed that management skills could be learned, so he developed 5 functions and 14 principles of management that are commonly used today (Miles, 1975).

### Henri Fayol and the Concept of Modern Management

Henri Fayol (1841–1925), a French engineer who was influential throughout Europe, developed a systematic method of management that examined the organization from the top down (Bovee et al., 1993; Turban & Meredith, 1991). Fayol stressed the functional aspects of the organizational structure. According to Fayol (1929), business activities are composed of basic functions: technical activities, including production and manufacturing; commercial activities, such as buying and selling or exchanging; and financial, security, accounting, and managerial activities. All these activities were broken down into discrete functions.

Fayol also identified 5 important management components:
- Planning (developing a course of action)
- Organizing (mobilizing human resources and materials)
- Commanding (directing employees)
- Coordinating (integrating activities toward a common goal)
- Controlling (following up to make sure the goals are carried out).

In addition, he formulated 14 management principles derived from his own management experience. Of these, 6 of the most enduring follow (Szelagyi & Wallace, 1990):

- *Division of labor*—The breaking down of activities into smaller assemblies or subcomponents to produce better products with less effort.
- *Unity of command*—The principle that each person is to receive orders from only one person.
- *Chain of command*—The line of authority starting at the top and running to the bottom of the firm (strongly enforced in the military today).
- *Authority*—The right of managers to give orders and to establish a degree of responsibility.
- *Initiative*—The responsibility of managers to develop a clear plan and carry it out.
- *Esprit de corps*—The responsibility of managers to promote harmony and motivation among all members of the organization.

Fayol stressed that the individual interests of the manager and employees should be subordinate to the overall interests of the organization. This concept is prevalent in Japanese industry today (Szelagyi & Wallace, 1990). Additionally, Fayol emphasized that management skills become progressively more important as one moves up the ranks of the organization.

Fayol contributed to the formal organizational structure and communication processes in the workplace. Many of his principles are used today in the corporate world. However, the relationships between managers and people who are subordinate to them are less formal today. Today's manager can ill afford to operate without considering the impact of interpersonal relationships.

## Max Weber and the Concept of Bureaucracy

Max Weber (1864–1920) was a German sociologist who conducted a systematic study of the social changes brought on by the Industrial Revolution (Bovee et al., 1993). Weber observed that large-scale organizations were on the rise throughout society and that the business world was moving away from charismatic leaders and family-based systems to macrocosmic organizations. His observations led to a vision in which he outlined what he saw as an ideal type of organization. Weber believed in a theory of bureaucracy, a rigid management approach characterized by an organizational structure in which offices and management positions are arranged in a hierarchy of authority. Explicit policies and rules define lines of authority. According to Weber (1947), the authority to manage was implicit to the position held by the person, not by the person who holds the position. Bureaucracy was even more rigid than scientific management. It formed a management system that encouraged compartmentalization. Thus, work tasks were divided into specialized jobs that emphasized mastery of a narrow job skill. Bureaucracy gave rise to a strict hierarchical system and organizational structure with a very formal chain of command.

Critics of bureaucracy have labeled it "red tape" and find fault with its forcing a worker to progress through layers of authority to accomplish a simple task (Gabarra, 1992). The formal organizational structure created inflexibility and an impersonal work environment. For instance, senior workers or managers were encouraged to maintain an impersonal and formal relationship with subordinates. Job promotions were decided by a strict merit system. Policy and procedure dictated one best way to perform a job or task. The bureaucratic system favored managers because it emphasized position protection, politics, and preservation of authority (Pearce & Robinson, 1994).

As an organization, a bureaucracy forms a closed system of management, focusing on the internal workings of the organization rather than the outside influences created by the surrounding environment. This kind of system does not tend to be readily responsive to change. Within the bureaucratic organization, strict rules become ends in themselves. Strict rules can limit productivity and cause trained incapacity because rules specify only minimum requirements. On the positive side, bureaucracies do define rational networks of authority and activity that help to achieve the goals of the organization. Successful bureaucracies also provide economies of scale in obtaining the resources to elicit greater effectiveness (Pearce & Robinson, 1994).

## The Human Relations Movement and Motivational Theory

By the 1920s, many large organizations had adopted the notions of classical scientific management. For example, Henry Ford (1893–1947) had altered the industrial landscape with the introduction of the assembly line. Even hospital organizations were studied to improve workflow and efficiency. For example, to save critical time during surgery, Pamela B. Blake, the manager of a central sterile supply department in a large hospital in New York City, studied the operating-room preparatory area to determine how long employees took to set up for a medical procedure.

Hugo Munsterberg (1863–1916), the founder of industrial psychology, took a different path and made recommendations for motivating employees, for finding the best person for the job through psychological testing, and for creating better psychological conditions for the worker (Schermerborn et al., 1994). During this period, the humanistic movement was taking place, and occupational therapy became an official profession (in 1917). In addition, huge institutions were built to care for people with mental illness and infectious diseases (Quiroga, 1995).

Around the same time, Mary Parker Follett (1868–1933), a theorist whose ideas helped to move management more rapidly toward an era of humanistic perspectives, suggested that no individual could become whole without being a member of a group. The behavioral management movement began and gained momentum in the late 1920s. The focus shifted from considering the total organization and the specific effect managers had on employees to the study of behavior and humanistic management in the workplace.

## The Hawthorne Studies

Between 1924 and 1927, a series of studies was conducted to investigate the effects that work environment had on productivity. The most famous of these studies were the illumination studies, designed to see whether better lighting had an effect on the productivity of workers. Elton Mayo (1880–1949), who had joined the faculty at Harvard University in 1926, was invited to consult on the illumination project, which was already under way in Chicago at the Hawthorne Plant of Western Electric.

The study used a control group and an experimental group of women who assembled telephone relay equipment. The women in the experimental group were exposed to increases and decreases in illumination as they assembled equipment. The control group performed the same job, but the source of lighting was constant. The researchers were surprised to discover that, when they increased the lighting in the experimental group workroom, the output of both the experimental and control groups increased. Conversely, when the researchers lowered the lighting to a level described as "moonlight," both groups continued to improve their productivity (Mondy et al., 1995). The researchers were disappointed; they believed that they had failed to find any relationship between illumination and productivity.

A second set of studies was conducted on worker fatigue as the employees assembled relays in a controlled work environment. The researchers once again found that productivity rose without a clear correlation to the physical conditions that were being altered to influence the variable of productivity. Mayo and his colleagues concluded that the "social relationship" accounted for the increase in productivity. The most accepted explanation proposed thus far is the possibility that, when employees receive attention or are treated in a special way, they will improve their performance regardless of subtle changes in the environment. Today, this phenomenon is known as the *Hawthorne effect* (Pearce & Robinson, 1994).

These classic studies shifted the attention of managers away from planning physical work and monetary incentives and toward studying the significance of the social setting in the workplace. In addition, these studies gave impetus to the human relations movement, which is characterized by the concern for good human relationships between managers and subordinates. The human relations movement suggested that managers should act more collaboratively with subordinates, which requires good social skills in addition to the technical knowledge of the job (Bovee et al., 1993; Schermerborn et al., 1994).

## Maslow's Need Hierarchy

Abraham Maslow (1908–1970) was an educator, a plant manager, and a psychologist during his prolific career (Turban & Meredith, 1991). Maslow was interested in what motivates workers and proposed the hierarchy of needs theory. This famous theory put forth the notion that people are motivated by the need to satisfy a sequence of basic human needs, including physiological, safety, social, esteem, and self-actualization needs (Maslow, 1954). According to this theory, once a person satisfies his or her more basic needs, he or she will progress up the ladder to more advanced needs such as self-actualization. Maslow's contribution to the human relations movement was significant because he clarified the importance of intrinsic factors rather than financial incentives as sources of motivation. Other theorists and researchers followed in Maslow's footsteps, discovering many other factors that are believed to contribute to increases and decreases in motivation.

## Herzberg's Two-Factor Theory

In 1968, Fredrick Herzberg introduced a theory of motivation that was similar to Maslow's need theory (Szelagyi & Wallace, 1990). This theory has been called the *two-factor,* or *motivation–hygiene, theory* and has been widely applied by managers interested in motivation. Herzberg's research was conducted by using interview responses to questions concerning the content or experiences of the job and the context of those factors surrounding the job, for example, salary and working conditions. In essence, the research revealed two distinct types of motivational factors: satisfiers, or motivators, and dissatisfiers, or hygiene factors (Herzberg, Manser, & Snyderman, 1959).

Herzberg's theory evoked considerable controversy because of the qualitative research methods used to develop his instrument. Organizational behavior researchers place more emphasis on internal validity and reliability of an instrument before it is widely administered. Herzberg's approach provided a method of putting weighted value on a context of the job such as salary, company policies, and fringe benefits. He also looked at the intrinsic job conditions that help to build satisfaction, including achievement, the work itself, level of responsibility, and personal growth and development (Schermerborn et al., 1994; Szelagyi & Wallace, 1990).

## Alderfer's ERG Theory

Clayton Alderfer introduced another more recent theory on motivation that involves three categories: existence (E), relatedness (R), and growth (G) (Szelagyi & Wallace, 1990). Existence needs are the basic physiological and material needs such as thirst, hunger, and shelter. Included in this category would be working conditions, pay, and benefits. Relatedness needs are connected to interpersonal relations with others in the workplace. This category is similar to Maslow's safety, social, and ego–esteem needs. Growth needs relate to the efforts toward personal growth and creative needs. This category involves the engagement of tasks that require the full use of the person's capabilities to achieve the goal. Alderfer incorporated a satisfaction–progression component, which describes the situation in which a need is met and focus shifts to higher level needs, and a frustration–regression component, which describes the situation in which a higher order need remains unfulfilled or frustrated (Szelagyi & Wallace, 1990).

## McGregor's Theory X and Theory Y

Douglas M. McGregor (1906–1964) was a professor, a college president, and a consultant who specialized in psychology. Using a social science perspective, McGregor developed theory X and theory Y to depict two extreme examples of ways managers can relate to employees. Theory X represents the traditional view that employees are lazy and dislike work; thus, they must be coerced, controlled, directed, or threatened with punishment to get them to put forth effort. The theory describes the average human being as wanting to be directed, avoiding responsibility, and having little ambition. In short, theory X suggests that human beings naturally resist change (McGregor, 1960).

In contrast, theory Y is based on an entirely different set of assumptions. This theory proposes that work is as natural as rest and play—a concept that is similar to the founding philosophy of occupational therapy. In addition, theory Y suggests that people do not inherently dislike work and that employees can be creative in solving problems and in achieving organizational goals. Theory Y describes employees as willing to seek out responsibility and as having the capacity to exercise a relatively high degree of imagination, ingenuity, and creativity in a solution. Furthermore, people will exercise self-direction and self-control in the service of objectives to which they are committed. Theory Y states that the intellectual capacity of the average human being is only partially used (McGregor, 1960).

Theory X and theory Y uncovered diametrically opposing philosophies of management. Theory X was widely accepted by classical scientific managers before the human relations movement produced research that found the assumptions to be unacceptable. Today, most managers accept the theory Y tenets of collaboration, participation, and concern for worker morale.

## Summary of the Human Relations Movement and Motivational Theory

The human relations movement brought the human aspects of management back to the forefront. Yet, critics have argued that the human relations movement was based on qualitative evidence rather than pragmatic scientific evidence (Szelagyi & Wallace, 1990). Many of the ideas generated from the human relations movement were more theoretical than practical in the workplace. Surprisingly, subsequent studies investigating human relationships have found that job satisfaction does not necessarily lead to increased productivity.

## The Behavioral Science Movement

In the 1950s, the human relations movement ran out of steam because it did not produce empirical evidence that work productivity and job satisfaction were strongly correlated (O'Donnell, 1997). The behavioral science movement, the scientific study of human behavior in organizations to help managers function more effectively, began because organizations desired more empirical evidence to understand work performance (Mondy et al., 1995). Although better research methodology is available to a variety of disciplines that study organizational behavior, few hard-and-fast rules or ironclad theories for managing people have been discovered. The fact remains that people in organizations continue to act in unpredictable ways.

Current thinking in organizational behavior suggests that job satisfaction is related more closely to recognition of the individual than to the job itself. Employees today need a broader range of participation in the decision-making process. Maintaining a bidirectional flow of communication between the manager and the subordinate is essential, and redesigning routine jobs to allow a broader range of roles for employees is often beneficial. The manager must also be aware of the culture of an organization and, thus, should recognize the significance of the work setting's formal and informal communication systems to stay in touch with employee relationships.

## The Learning Organization

The learning organization is a current organizational theory based on systems thinking, the study of natural biological systems for learning (Crist, 1996). (Please see chapter 4 for a more detailed description of the systems theory.) According to advocates of the learning organization, the world is a holistic, dynamic, inextricably connected system where everything seems to affect everything else. The management theory is based on observations of how these systems continue to grow, evolve, and learn as well as how these observations can apply to human-made organizations. Understanding the learning organization requires a mental shift away from the linear and sequential clockwork system to a more complex, adaptive system. The learning organization is seen as an ideal working environment that is fluid, organic, and biological in nature. It disputes cause-and-effect relations in the workplace. Like the concept of holism, the concept of the learning organization agrees with the notion that all the parts of an organization influence the behavior of the whole organization. According to the learning organization concept, humans crave connectedness and meaning. Unlike Taylor's perception of classical management, employees in the learning organization are seen as seeking lasting and deep relationships in the working environment (Hesselbein, Goldsmith, & Bechard, 1997; Nadler & Nadler, 1998).

Implicit in the assumptions of the learning organization is the belief that employees grow by sharing information. In competitive markets, organizations are unlikely to share successful ideas. Therefore, trust is essential for employees to feel safe and to share knowledge within the organization itself. Ideally, a learning organization emphasizes a continuous exchange of and generation of new ideas. Work relationships are analogous to the neural network in the brain that uses redundancy, overlapping, and continuous transformation of information. The learning organization is an egalitarian model. That is, all members of the learning community are treated as equals and are seen as having something to offer to the organization. The learning organization views employees as highly capable entities with untapped resources (Large, 1999).

The organizational design of the learning community is a flat structure rather than a top-to-bottom, hierarchical chain of command. Lines of communication are porous; that is, a subordinate is able to directly contact managers in higher positions without going through specified channels (Crist, 1996; Hesselbein et al., 1997).

## Emerging Trends in Management

The role of the manager has changed in recent years. As previously mentioned, the occupational therapy manager should be aware of the formal organization and the informal organization. The formal organization usually has an organizational structure with published rules and policies. The policies help the manager make decisions and deal with issues that require routine answers. The informal system was revealed in the Hawthorne studies when the researchers found that the workers form groups with informal rules concerning work behavior. Also, according to the Hawthorne studies, workers respond positively to interest and attention.

Mayo and his colleagues discovered what they called a "social setting" that exists to bring meaning to work. The social relationship of employees influences quotas and productivity. For instance, Mayo found that "overproducers" were called "rate busters," and "underproducers" were labeled "rate chiselers" (Bovee et al., 1993; Hall, 2000). The penalty for violating the informal rules or norms of productivity were enforced through peer pressure, including sarcasm, ridicule, or a blow on the arm.

The informal system is also prevalent in the health care industry. Practitioners within the managed care system who are working in organizations such as rehabilitation and skilled nursing facilities work under strict payment and reimbursement systems. These systems apply a payment cap on the amount of services that can be provided for specific diagnoses and an expectation of how many clients or patients the practitioner must treat in a day. The practitioner must devote time to documentation, in-services, rounds, and interactions with family members. Over time, practitioners settle into a norm of work behavior that is acceptable to the setting. The occupational therapy manager is challenged to maintain morale, improve efficiency, and treat the practitioner as a whole person having needs and wants that demand satisfaction.

Researchers have learned that elements contained in the work or occupation itself are important factors in productivity. The following factors appear to improve motivation (Gabarra, 1992):

- Recognition from peers
- The sense of achievement that goes with successful completion of a job
- Advancement or promotion
- Status
- Supervision by a competent manager
- The job itself
- Coworker interpersonal relationships
- Opportunities for personal development
- Fringe benefits
- A safe and attractive work environment.

History has shown that coercion and punishment do not work as motivators for productivity (Szelagyi & Wallace, 1990).

Future occupational therapy managers will be more concerned with the accomplishment of objectives through the use of resources and the efforts of people working in groups. Classical theorists believed in applied time and motion studies, incentive wage systems, and a paternal relationship with the subordinate. Clearly, the role of the occupational therapy manager has been influenced by outside forces such as changes in state and federal legislation. Occupational therapy managers are often "formula driven" by factors such as staffing needs, fee-for-service regulations, prospective payment systems, or capitated contracts. Rigid systems can dampen the motivation for planning, organizing, coordinating, and controlling because the system does not allow the flexibility for the application of modern management theory.

Large-scale, conglomerate health care organizations are increasing in numbers because small, private, stand-alone organizations can no longer provide comprehensive services and compete financially. Although health care organizations are merging and becoming more like large business corporations, the days of the large occupational therapy department may be a thing of the past. Occupational therapy managers may work in smaller, community-based clinics in which interdisciplinary teams work in specialized units or groups. As health care organizations downsize or merge with larger consortiums, middle management positions are often eliminated. The occupational therapy manager will be challenged to make his or her services an essential component of the changing health care industry. In particular, the occupational therapy manager will need to effectively handle workplace diversity, navigate a continually changing work environment, develop a customer focus, and plan strategically (McCormack, Lloreas, & Burton, 1991).

## Workplace Diversity

According to the Bureau of Labor Statistics (2002), the need for occupational therapy practitioners is expected to increase. Because of the changing shortages of qualified health professionals and the effects of globalization, managers must contend with greater diversity in the workplace. The occupational therapy manager will need to be skilled in clinical reasoning, occupation-based activity, cultural diversity, and life care management (Belice & McGovern-Denk, 2002; Parker & Heisner, 2002).

The workplace will have "generation gaps": More occupational therapy practitioners will serve children in school-based settings, and the 76 million baby boomers (born between 1946 and 1964) will become the primary adult customers of occupational therapy services. Future student volunteers and new practitioners will come from either generation X (born between 1961 and 1981) or generation Y (born after 1981) age groups.

The new generations will pose different demands on the workplace. For example, occupational therapy practitioners who represent generation Y will rely on technology to get work done. The newer Y generation represents approximately 75 million people (Merritt, 2001). They are likely to be more skilled than their managers in the use of technology. As a group, the Y generation, also called the "millennials," are characterized as being "doers" and "achievers" (Beck, 1997). More of the Y generation are getting a jump on college by getting early tutoring and preparation on the SAT examination (Fitzgerald, 2001). They will be avid consumers of products; surveys show that 66% have savings accounts, 22% have checking accounts, 18% have stocks and bonds, and 8% have mutual funds (Chapman, 1997; Teenage Research Unlimited, 2001).

As a group, the Y generation will be more culturally diverse. Although the current demographics suggest that the majority of occupational therapists are White women, the cultural composition of occupational therapy students in public institutions, especially in California, is changing dramatically. Another unique feature of the Y generation is they tend to live at home for a longer period of time and continue to maintain good relationships with their parents and family (Strauss & Howe, 2000). The surveys suggest that the Y generation will be willing to work hard but not at the expense of his or her personal life.

Therefore, the occupational therapy manager will need to recognize the influence of both generational and organizational cultures as well as the consumer's greater influence on the delivery of services. Because members of generation Y are characterized as doers and achievers, they will be more service oriented. As future employees, generation Y will require more support from human resources, seeking out opportunities for personal growth and expecting seamless administrative services, accelerated opportunities for advancement, and mentoring and coaching relationships with their managers (Somer, 2001; Strauss & Howe, 2000). This last expectation in particular will present a challenge in the current fast-paced workplace, where time for mentoring and coaching relationships is scarce.

## Continual Change in Workplace Environment
Given the continuous changes in economic and political forces, the occupational therapy manager must adapt, use innovation, and instill tolerance for change. Many forces

come to bear on the workplace. For example, after September 11, 2001, no one can guarantee that the work environment will be safe and secure. Changes in cultural diversity in the workplace and reimbursement influences brought on by federal legislation will continually transform the work environment. Job security cannot be counted on in this dynamic work context. The manager has to accept the fact that change is the only constant in the work environment. He or she must plan for change because it is inevitable. In this changing environment, products, services, and job descriptions will have a shorter life span, and the marketplace will continually alter the reimbursement process for durable medical equipment, prosthetics, and orthotics.

## Customer Focus

In the near future, patients or clients will be viewed and treated more like customers. There will be a greater focus on links to customers, continuous quality assurance, and efficiency of services (Holland & Kerrigan, 1996).

The occupational therapy manager will likely be asking questions such as Who is our customer? Are clients and patients the only customers? What does our customer value? The formal role of wearing a white lab coat and prescribing for the patient will become passé. The distance between the health care professional and the customer will become minimized. Therapeutic relationships will evolve to become more like a partnership, allowing the consumer to make decisions about the course of action.

## Emphasis on Planning

The occupational therapy manager will place a greater emphasis on strategic planning, mission, and goals for the greater good of the organization. He or she will need to refine and alter his or her mission and core values to meet the changing demands of the environment. To deal with change, managers will need to be skilled in engaging staff members in a participatory process of redesigning and carrying out the goals to be accomplished.

The occupational therapy manager will need to be skilled with group decision strategies and aware of the phenomenon described as "groupthink" (Janis, 1971, 1972). According to Janis, several fiascoes have occurred in the group decision-making process when the thinking process of a group becomes too homologous or homogenous. Groups may develop an illusion of invulnerability and ignore threats as well as opportunities in the immediate environment. Groups can begin to believe that they have the only answer and begin to cast absolute or moralistic judgment on groups that have a diverging opinion. Groupthink can lead groups to engage in stereotypical perceptions and fall prey to (a) group pressure for compliance, (b) self-censorship for which one regrets not expressing his or her opinion in a meeting, or (c) what Janis has called "unanimity" (the false assumption that if someone remains silent, they are in agreement with the group's decision). Perhaps the most destructive outcome of groupthink is when group members appoint themselves to the duty of protecting the leader or key members of the group from new information that might shatter the complacency of the group. In effective groups, members inform the group of the best available data, even if it is not what the group wants to hear.

The occupational therapy manager will be an advocate of continuing education and continuing competency to maintain licensed and certified practitioners in the workplace. In addition, the manager should be capable in some settings of seeking out grants and other sources of funding for practitioner training and retraining as deemed necessary.

## The New Health Care Organization

The health care industry is likely to follow the trends of the corporate world, a prediction that suggests many changes may be on the horizon. In particular, technology will play an increasing role. The occupational therapy manager will participate in virtual organizations, where staff members may work in various locations using e-mail, fax, video conferencing, and conference calls to conduct business. Some practitioners may engage in telecommunication whereby the practitioner and the patient or client would consult directly, viewing each other on a monitor to carry out and follow up on treatment plans. Grand rounds may be viewed on a monitor from several hundred miles away (Hesselbein et al., 1997).

In addition, the occupational therapy manager will coordinate more open organizational systems that are more nimble and able to react quickly to changing trends. Some authors have referred to the organizations that can change rapidly and remain ultimately adaptable to new landscapes as "chameleon" organizations (Cross, Feather, & Lynch, 1994). Change, however, will not come easily, because the medical model has encouraged a hierarchical system. Physicians and administrators have enjoyed unquestionable authority. Nevertheless, current organizational systems downplay the concepts of job obedience, allegiance, and diligence. Employees expect to be managed with a participatory approach to the decision-making process. Now, we find an emphasis on the greater good and on a buy-in to the values and culture of the organization.

Like the corporate world, new organizations also will depend on alliances with other organizations. Every member of the organization will be expected to have knowledge about networking, that is, knowledge of the marketplace within and beyond the boundaries of the organization. Viable health care organizations will need to demonstrate flexibility, superior use of teams, strong core values, evidence-based competencies, acceptance for diversity, and a commitment to the individual (Manning & Haddock, 1995). Trust will be essential because intellectual property will be shared and protected.

New health care organizations also will allow "intrapreneurial" opportunities, that is, the support of opportunities for reasonably autonomous enterprises to operate within the larger corporate structure (Hesselbein et al., 1997; Mitchell & Burick, 1985). Employees will be able to run a business within the larger organization where they work. Organizations will continue to use benchmarking to determine the employee's strength and weaknesses, but the workplace will need to allow for the balance of work life and leisure to recruit valued employees from generation X and Y.

Theoretically, the occupational therapy manager will see a paradigmatic shift from a mechanical or Newtonian information model, in which forms and policies could be manually stored in a file cabinet, to a quantum physics model, in which computer information systems and technology will prevail. Most certainly, the occupational therapy manager will need to be interested in managing for a changing society.

## Conclusion

History has shown that organizations and styles of management reflect the needs of the day. Today, a new image of a more vibrant manager and organization has emerged in response to an ever-changing world. The new organization defines itself as an open system. The organization is seen as having "sensors" that monitor all parts of the system. New organizations have a strong sense of mission, purpose, and core values. New organizations are driven by information. This information is shared, and best practices are encouraged. The new organization will support the individual and will be open to candid communication. Although new organizations retain a sense of efficiency, quality output, and security, they also tolerate ambiguity. Finally, the new organization is said to have a "soul." That is, it has "attractors" that give meaning, point, and purpose for people to join the workplace (Hesselbein et al., 1997; Nadler & Nadler, 1998).

The contemporary occupational therapy manager must be a champion of change. He or she will be characterized as a person who will be able to articulate a compelling vision that excites and captures the imagination of others. This person must exhibit a sense of confidence and express confidence in others. The occupational therapy manager will remain a practitioner at heart so he or she can enable others to grow, to see the alternatives, and to overcome barriers. The manager should set high standards and expectations for him- or herself and be an energizing force who demonstrates a personal zest for life, shares a passion for the profession, and influences others to find excitement in their own success.

## References

Beck, M. (1997, February 3). The next big population bulge: Generation Y shows its might. *Wall Street Journal,* pp. 4–7.

Belice, P. J., & McGovern-Denk, M. (2002). Reframing occupational therapy in acute care. *OT Practice,* 7(8), 21–27.

Bovee, C. L., Thill, J. V., Wood, M. B., & Dovel, G. P. (1993). *Management.* New York: McGraw-Hill.

Bureau of Labor Statistics. (2002). Retrieved August 8, 2002, from http://www.bls.gov./clata/home.htm.

Chapman, B. (1997, December 12). The new generations are the best news yet. *Seattle Post-Intelligencer,* p. 8.

Christiansen, C., & Baum, C. (1997). *Occupational therapy: Enabling function and well-being.* Thorofare, NJ: Slack.

Crist, P. (1996). Organizational effectiveness. In M. C. Fish & M. Johnson (Eds.), *The occupational therapy manager* (rev. ed., pp. 163–190). Bethesda, MD: American Occupational Therapy Association.

Cross, A. F., Feather, J. J., & Lynch, R. L. (1994). *Corporate renaissance: The art of reengineering.* Cambridge, MA: Blackwell.

Davis, B. L., Hellervik, L. W., Skull, C. J., Gebelein, S. H., & Sheard, J. L. (1992). *Thinking strategically.* Minneapolis, MN: Personnel Decisions.

Fayol, H. (1929). *General and industrial management* (J. A. Conbrough, Trans.). Geneva: International Management Institution.

Fitzgerald, M. (2001, June 11). More are getting a jump on college. *Philadelphia Inquirer,* pp. 21–23.

Gabarra, J. J. (1992). *Managing people and organizations.* Boston, MA: Harvard Business School.

Hall, S. (2000, June 4). The smart set. *New York Times Magazine,* pp. 24–27.

Herzberg, F., Manser, B., & Snyderman, B. (1959). *The motivation to work* (2nd ed.). New York: Wiley.

Hesselbein, F., Goldsmith, M., & Bechard, R. (1997). *The organization of the future.* San Francisco, CA: Jossey-Bass.

Hodgetts, R. M. (1992). *Organizational behavior: Theory and practice.* New York: MacMillan.

Holland, B., & Kerrigan, S. (1996). An assessment model for service learning. *Journal of Community Service, 5,* 32–47.

Janis, I. L. (1971, November). Groupthink. *Psychology Today,* pp. 14–17.

Janis, J. L. (1972). *Victims of groupthink.* Boston: Houghton-Mifflin.

Large, E. (1999, January 12). Boomers, move over: It's time for the millennials. *Baltimore Sun,* pp. 215–232.

Manning, M., & Haddock, P. (1995). *Leadership skills for women.* Menlo Park, CA: Crisp Publications.

Maslow, A. H. (1954). *Motivation and personality.* New York: Harper & Row.

McCormack, G., Lloreas, L., & Burton, G. (1991). Culturally diverse elders. In M. Kiernat (Ed.), *Occupational therapy and the older adult* (pp. 11–25). Gaithersburg, MD: Aspen.

McGregor, D. (1960). *The human side of enterprise.* New York: McGraw-Hill.

Merritt, S. R. (2001). *Generation Y: A perspective on America's next generation and their impact on higher education.* Paper presented at the annual conference of the American Occupational Therapy Association, Philadelphia, PA.

Miles, R. E. (1975). *Theories of management: Implications for organizational behavior and development.* Philadelphia: McGraw-Hill.

Mitchell, C., & Burick, T. (1985). The right moves: Succeeding in a man's world without a Harvard MBA. *Harvard Business Review, 75,* 43–47.

Mondy, W., Holmes, R. E., & Flippo, E. B. (1995). *Management concepts and practices.* Boston, MA: Allyn & Bacon.

Nadler, D. A., & Nadler, M. B. (1998). *Champions of change.* San Francisco, CA: Jossey-Bass.

O'Donnell, M. (1997). Health impact of workplace health promotion programs and methodological quality of the research literature. *Articles on Health Promotion, 1,* 1–8.

Parker, S., & Heisner, C. (2002). Life care management and OT: A perfect match. *OT Practice, 7*(8), 28–31.

Pearce, J. A., & Robinson, R. B. (1994). *Strategic management: Formation, implementation and control.* Burr Ridge, IL: Irwin.

Quiroga, V. A. M. (1995). *Occupational therapy: The first 30 years.* Bethesda, MD: American Occupational Therapy Association.

Schermerborn, J. R., Hunt, F. G., & Asborn, R. N. (1994). *Managing organizational behavior* (5th ed.). New York: Wiley.

Somer, A. (2001, June 25). What are America's youngest citizens all about? *Advance for Occupational Therapy Practitioners,* pp. 13–14.

Strauss, W., & Howe, N. (2000). *Millenials rising: The next great generation.* New York: Vintage Books.

Szelagyi, A. D., & Wallace, M. J. (1990). *Organizational behavior and performance.* New York: HarperCollins.

Taylor, F. W. (1911). *The principles of scientific management.* New York: Harper & Row.

Teenage Research Unlimited. (2001, January 25). WWWTeens spend $155 billion in 2000. *San Jose Mercury News,* p. 4.

Turban, E., & Meredith, J. R. (1991). *Management science* (5th ed.). Boston, MA: Irwin.

Weber, M. (1947). *The theory of social and economic organization.* New York: Free Press.

# Occupational Therapy Skills and Management Skills

Guy L. McCormack, PhD, OTR/L, FAOTA

*"Life must be lived forwards, but can only be understood backwards."*

V. KIERKEGAARD IN QUIROGA

**Guy L. McCormack, PhD, OTR/L, FAOTA,** has been an educator, researcher, and author for 25 years. He is the founder and chairman of the Master of Occupational Therapy Program at Samuel Merritt College in Oakland, CA. He is currently working as a home health practitioner with the Sutter Visiting Nurses Association and Hospice in Emeryville, CA. In addition to his doctorate in human science, he has received extensive training in traditional Chinese medicine and has many certificates in alternative/complementary forms of intervention.

## Key Ideas and Concepts

**Hard data.** Aggregated data or information that is acquired through valid, reliable, measurable, and objective standards.

**Interactive management.** A management style that promotes open communication, feedback, and collaboration among all members of the organization.

**Multi-tasking.** A term to describe the ability to perform several tasks at the same time. It usually involves technology and good organization skills.

**Role delineation.** An organizational strategy that defines specific skills and tasks to be performed and also educational qualifications of the job description.

**Soft data.** Information that is based on faith, intuition, and subjective observations. Soft data is difficult to measure objectively with mathematical standards.

**Transformational management.** A style of management that is more contingent on relationship than compliance. Transformational managers involve employees in a relationship that causes shifts in belief systems, values, and the needs of the employee.

## Learning Objectives

After completing this chapter you should be able to do the following:

- Compare and contrast the skill sets of the occupational therapist and the occupational therapy manager.
- Recognize common images of the role of an occupational therapist.
- Describe the role of an occupational therapy manager in relationship to clinical practice.
- Identify common myths concerning the role of a manager.
- Describe the characteristics of interactive and transformational management styles.
- Describe how context influences the meaning of skill sets.

ll occupational therapists are managers to some degree. In addition, all occupational therapy managers use some degree of clinical practice skills that apply to both the positions of management and clinical practice. This chapter will identify the *skill sets*—the behaviors, manual skills, management skills, clinical skills, and psychological skills—that are typically associated with the role of an accomplished therapist and that of a manager. These skills sets will then be used to compare and contrast the role of being an occupational therapist with the role of an occupational therapy manager. In addition, the chapter will also discuss myths and stereotypes associated with gender and the role of being a manager.

The skill sets associated with the occupational therapy manager and the occupational therapist are very similar. Both the therapist and the manager are experts in multi-tasking; that is, they must perform a number of roles and tasks simultaneously to be effective on their respective jobs. The occupational therapist must manage his or her time each day to treat clients, maintain records, document treatment and other actions, and attend meetings and lectures. The occupational therapy manager must plan for staffing; coordinate services; organize supplies, materials, and equipment; monitor expenditures; examine billing codes; and coordinate with other disciplines. Additionally, the occupational therapy manager must control factors such as the use of resources, clinical materials, and equipment and must allot considerable time for documentation of measurable outcomes. Both the therapist and manager must engage in some degree of planning, organizing, coordinating, controlling resources, and assuming leadership initiatives. Although the job descriptions for the manager and the therapist are different, certain skills overlap considerably.

## The Vision of Becoming an Occupational Therapist

Many occupational therapy students enter the professional course of study with preconceived images and expectations about the role of being a therapist. Many students have asked instructors why they need to take management courses because all they plan to do is become an occupational therapist. Most students visualize themselves in a therapeutic role in which they spend the entire day involved in relationships that help or heal. This vision is consistent with the role defined in textbooks, which describe the occupational therapist as one who enables people to perform the day-to-day activities that are important to them (Christiansen & Baum, 1997). The roles and skill sets of the therapist are focused on enabling clients to gain independence "despite impairments, activity limitations, or participation restrictions, or despite risks for these problems" (Neistadt & Crepeau, 1997, p. 6).

The occupational therapist is characterized by helping others with physical, mental, or psychosocial limitations to overcome obstacles and to gain independence. This characterization sounds like a wonderful way to earn a living. Occupational therapy is a career that is both intrinsically rewarding and personally gratifying. In addition, the role of an occupational therapist is considered to be a steady, well-paying profession with relatively consistent demands and responsibilities. The practice of occupational therapy is seen as a profession that allows one to balance work, play, and leisure. Many occupational therapists are able to work and raise a family. Finally, according to the Bureau of Labor Statistics, occupational therapists will be in demand in the next decade, which suggests job security, job satisfaction, and independence in the choice of workplace.

## Importance of Management in Occupational Therapy Practice Skills

Many of these visions of the occupational therapist are true and can be realized. In addition, the basic skill sets that are required to become a competent therapist are similar to those required for the role of a manager because a therapist must possess an ability to manage people, to engage in planning, to control resources, and to organize time. The occupational therapist who does not have these skill sets will have difficulty surviving the rigors of today's health care environment. The manager is seen as a facilitator who must plan, organize, coordinate, and take control. The skill set of the occupational therapy manager involves the ability to endure long hours, enforce regulations, set policies, undergo high stress, and pay constant attention to detail. The occupational therapy manager has little time for the things that brought the person into the field of occupational therapy in the first place. Although these descriptions of the occupational therapist and the occupational therapy manager are stereotypical, they highlight the overlap between the two roles.

The occupational therapist performs several skills that require management ability. Throughout the course of the day, the therapist must engage in planning to accomplish the daily role of performing therapy. Planning may take the form of ordering the right equipment, working out the logistics of treating patients in different locations, collaborating with other disciplines, attending meetings, and allowing time for documentation. Therapists set goals, manage time, oversee assistants and coworkers, make important clinical decisions, and control outcomes. These roles are implicitly and explicitly managerial in nature.

## Management Myths

In 1916, Henri Fayol introduced the classical terms (planning, organizing, coordinating, and controlling) that are associated with the essential functions of management (Szelagyi & Wallace, 1990). In the current health care environment, the occupational therapy manager would be hard-pressed for time to accomplish these essential tasks on a daily basis. The four terms imply that the manager has the time to be thoughtful and reflective. Indeed, it is good practice to plan ahead and be concerned with objectives that can be accomplished through the efforts of other people. However, Fayol developed his principles of management in a different era. He could not have envisioned the pace of the 21st century. For example, the rate at which information is disseminated today would be a blur when compared to the pace of past centuries.

Mintzberg (1977) studied the role of the manager by collecting qualitative data from detailed diaries, performance records, ethnographic observations, and interviews. His findings suggest that the daily activities of the manager are anything but systematic and routine. According to Mintzberg, the role of the manager is fraught with myths and misunderstandings. For instance, the traditional view that managers are reflective and systematic planners is highly debated. The findings of Mintzberg's study revealed an entirely different picture of the manager's role.

Studies have shown (Davis & Cosenza, 1993) that managers work at an unrelenting pace, and their daily activities are characterized by spontaneity, brevity, interruptions, multi-tasking, and discontinuity. In fact, managers are oriented more toward action than reflection. This finding does not suggest that managers do not think things through and ponder before making decisions. It simply suggests that managers are responding to the pressures of the job. Because of time constraints, managers tend to be doers, and planning is often done in real time as the job demands are being addressed. Therefore, for many managers, planning is done in the context of their daily activities during which decisions are made based on experience in the position.

Another age-old myth is that managers rely on formal reports, statistical data, and aggregated information to perform effectively. On the contrary, says Mintzberg, as his studies of managers have shown, most managers prefer verbal media, meetings, and telephone calls over written documents. According to some estimates, managers spend an average of 66%–80% of their time engaging in oral communication (Solomon, 1988). The challenge for the occupational therapy manager is to focus less on simple cause-and-effect relationships and shift to more intuitive and associative forms of reasoning in which recognition of significant patterns in the workplace becomes an important source of information (Sanders, 2002).

E-mail has also given the manager a quick method of communicating with staff members and obtaining immediate feedback and follow-up information. Formal typed memos are becoming a thing of the past. The so-called "snail-mail," or use of regular postal services, has become burdensome for many managers. Administrative assistants are assigned the task of sorting the mail into categories of junk mail and mail that needs a response or immediate action. Some estimates suggest that only 13% of mail received by managers provides them with current information that is relevant to their job. Mintzberg found that managers often rely on "soft data" such as word of mouth and "hard data" drawn from inferential statistics to obtain information. E-mail is a much more efficient way to obtain this quick and direct information.

Another common myth is that managers do not have regular duties to perform (Mintzberg, 1977). Much has been written about the art of delegation, spending less time with customers so managers can free up time for planning. However, an important part of the manager's role is to perform public relations, attend ceremonies, and examine informal systems to keep in touch with what is going on in the surrounding environment. In fact, managers do perform regular duties and, in addition, participate in rituals, attend ceremonies, and take on routine negotiations.

## Gender Stereotypes and Management Roles

According to the American Occupational Therapy Association (AOTA, 2001) compensation survey, 94% of occupational therapists are women. It is difficult to determine how many occupational therapists are assigned middle- and upper-management roles. Unquestionably, women are well suited for management roles. Women perform effectively as managers in health care settings without adopting the "command and control" style that is commonly associated with men (Manning & Haddock, 1995). Qualitative studies show that women use nontraditional leadership styles and are more likely to practice "interactive or transformational leadership" (Rosener, 1991). Typically, men are more likely to be characterized by transactional leadership in which the job performance is perceived as a series of transactions with subordinates, using rewards for services rendered and punishment for performance deemed inadequate (Bass, 1985).

According to Rosener (1991), surveys comparing men and women show that women prefer interactive management styles that are characterized by working actively to form positive relationships with subordinates. Women managers encourage more inclusion and participation in the working relationship than do most men. The advantage of an interactive management style is that it gains better support from employees for implementing decisions. By having more people involved in the decision-making process, the interactive managers find they are more likely to be supported when backup systems need to be configured during periods when staff members are ill or absent from work.

Interactive, or participatory, management has some disadvantages in that it takes more time to solicit ideas from staff members. Interactive management also requires that the manager must give up some control. Managers who share power and information may be perceived as in need of approval or wanting to be liked by subordinates. In allowing more people to be involved in the decision-making process, turf conflicts may arise if employees disagree. In some organizations or departments, not everyone wants to participate in decision making. In health care settings, some staff members are limited in decision-making roles by licensure, the scope of practice parameters, their professional credentials, or their level of work experience.

However, the advantages of participatory management outweigh the disadvantages. The process involving the sharing of power and information can create loyalty by sending a message that the employees are trusted and their ideas are respected. Sharing power and information gives employees and coworkers the ability to reach decisions, solve problems, and see the value of their own decisions. These benefits are worth the risk that, by sharing power, people may reject or openly disagree with what the manager decides or may challenge his or her authority.

Women in management positions more often than men enable their employees to feel important when information is shared and participation is encouraged (Rosener, 1991). This approach, known as *transformational leadership,* is the process of motivating people by transforming their self-interest into the goals of the organization. Transformational managers often get others excited about their work and help them recognize the value of their services. According to Manning and Haddock (1995), women are more likely to generate power based on their charisma, personal contacts, and a good solid work record. In contrast, men tend to rely on their organizational position, title, and the ability to use the power of reward and punishment.

## Comparing and Contrasting the Roles of Occupational Therapist and Occupational Therapy Manager

The comparison and contrast of the role of therapist and manager presented here is based on a systematic analysis of the following occupational therapy textbooks and official documents: *Occupational Therapy Practice Framework: Domain and Process* (AOTA, 2002); *Glossary: Standards for an Accredited Program for the Occupational Therapist and for the Occupational Therapy Assistant* (American Council for Occupational Therapy Education, 1999); *The Guide to Occupational Therapy Practice* (Moyers, 1999); *Standards of Practice for Occupational Therapy* (AOTA, 1998); and *Occupational Therapy: Enabling Function and Well-Being* (Christiansen & Baum, 1997). These documents and textbooks provide guidelines for entry-level competencies for occupational therapists. Additionally, these documents and textbooks provide descriptive terms that are commonly used to define the skill sets of occupational therapy managers and therapists.

Table 2.1 lists in alphabetical order the descriptive terms or skill sets associated with occupational therapy. The second column of the table indicates which of these skill sets apply to the occupational therapist, and the third column indicates those for the occupational therapy manager. Readers may not agree with the placement of the checks in the columns; each occupational therapist and occupational therapy manager may work in an environment where the context of the skill set is different.

The most interesting finding about the list is that the meaning of a specific skill set may change when it is viewed in the context of the therapist or the manager. For example, the term *caregiver* is associated with the clinical role, but managers in the healing professions may assume clinical duties and continue to see themselves in the caregiver role. Clearly, skill sets such as therapeutic use of self, activity analysis, and therapeutic use of occupations fall within the realm of the occupational therapist; the term *administration* is clearly linked to the occupational therapy manager. However, it became evident that both the occupational therapist and the occupational therapy manager perform the majority of the skill sets in some capacity. The term *coach,* for

**Table 2.1 Occupational Therapy Skill Sets.**

| Skill Sets | OT Practitioner | OT Manager | Skill Sets | OT Practitioner | OT Manager |
|---|---|---|---|---|---|
| Accommodations | √ | √ | Clinical reasoning | √ | |
| Accountability | √ | √ | Coach | √ | √ |
| Acknowledging strengths | √ | √ | Code of ethics | √ | √ |
| Actions plans | √ | √ | Cognitive restructuring | √ | |
| Activities of daily living (ADL) | √ | | Collaboration | √ | √ |
| Activity analysis | √ | | Collecting data | √ | √ |
| Activity demands | √ | | Communication | √ | √ |
| Adaptation (outcomes) | √ | √ | Compassion | √ | √ |
| Adaptation of environment | √ | √ | Compensation | √ | |
| Adaptation of performance skills | √ | √ | Computer skills | √ | √ |
| Adjunctive methods | √ | | Conflict resolution | | √ |
| Administration | | √ | Consultation | √ | √ |
| Advocacy (political) | √ | √ | Consumer advocacy | √ | √ |
| Aligning goals with mission statement | √ | √ | Context (cultural) | √ | √ |
| Allocation of resources | √ | √ | Continuing competence | √ | √ |
| Analytical problem solver | √ | √ | Continuous quality improvement | √ | √ |
| Annual performance assessment | √ | √ | Core values | √ | √ |
| Appeal for reimbursement | √ | √ | Cost containment | √ | √ |
| Application of PAMS | √ | | Course of treatment | √ | |
| Assertiveness | √ | √ | Crafts person | √ | |
| Assessment | √ | √ | Critique of research studies | √ | √ |
| Assistive technology | √ | √ | Cultural competency | √ | √ |
| Attends rounds & meetings | √ | √ | Current policy awareness | √ | √ |
| Author | √ | √ | Decision making | √ | √ |
| Baseline assessment | √ | | Delegation | ? | √ |
| Basic life skills manager | √ | √ | Delivery of services | √ | √ |
| Behavior manager | √ | √ | Descriptive research | √ | √ |
| Budget manager | √ | √ | Designing | √ | √ |
| Caregiver | √ | | Diagnosis | √ | |
| Client-centered approach | √ | √ | Directing | √ | √ |
| Charismatic leader | √ | √ | Discharge planning | √ | |
| Charting | √ | | Discontinuation reports | √ | ? |
| Clinical judgment | √ | √ | Discrimination (sensory) | √ | |
| | | | Disease/disability prevention | √ | √ |
| | | | Dispute resolution | ? | √ |
| | | | Documentation | √ | √ |
| | | | Domestic violence | √ | |
| | | | Dressing skills | √ | |
| | | | Driving (adaptive) | √ | |
| | | | Early intervention | √ | |
| | | | Educational activity | √ | √ |

(continued)

| Skill Sets | OT Practitioner | OT Manager | Skill Sets | OT Practitioner | OT Manager |
|---|:---:|:---:|---|:---:|:---:|
| Educator | √ | √ | Interdisciplinary | √ | √ |
| Empathetic | √ | √ | Interpersonal skills | √ | √ |
| Enabling activity | √ |  | Interventions | √ | √ |
| Engagement in occupation | √ | √ | Interviewing | √ | √ |
| Endurance | √ | √ | Instrumental activities of daily living | √ | √ |
| Energy conservation | √ | √ | Job analysis | √ | √ |
| Enthusiasm | √ | √ | Job description | √ | √ |
| Entrepreneur | √ | √ | Judgment (clinical) | √ | √ |
| Environmental context | √ | √ | Knowledge | √ | √ |
| Environmental factors | √ | √ | Language | √ | √ |
| Environmental modification | √ | √ | Leadership | √ | √ |
| Ergonomics | √ | √ | Learning styles |  | √ |
| Ethics | √ | √ | Legislation awareness | √ | √ |
| Evaluation | √ | √ | Leisure | √ | √ |
| Evidence-based practice | √ | √ | Life balance | √ | √ |
| Explanation of services | √ | √ | Life style redesign | √ |  |
| Feedback | √ | √ | Long term plan | √ | √ |
| Feeding and swallowing | √ |  | Maintains records | √ | √ |
| Fieldwork educator | √ | √ | Managed care | √ | √ |
| Fiscal planning | √ | √ | Management | √ | √ |
| Flexible | √ | √ | Marketing | √ | √ |
| Focus group | √ | √ | Measurement | √ | √ |
| Follow up | √ | √ | Meetings (attends/conducts) | √ | √ |
| Frames of reference | √ | √ | Mentoring | √ | √ |
| Functional activities | √ |  | Models behavior | √ | √ |
| Grading activities | √ |  | Monitors | √ | √ |
| Grant writing | √ | √ | Narrative reasoning | √ | √ |
| Group process | √ | √ | Normative ethics | √ | √ |
| Guidance | √ | √ | Observation | √ | √ |
| Habit training | √ |  | Occupational performance | √ | √ |
| Health educator | √ | √ | Occupational profile | √ |  |
| Health promotion | √ | √ | Occupational science | √ | √ |
| Health care professional | √ | √ | Orientation | √ | √ |
| Home health | √ |  | Outcome studies | √ | √ |
| Improvement measures | √ | √ | Passive range of motion | √ |  |
| Independence | √ |  | Peer review | √ | √ |
| Information retrieval | √ | √ | Performance patterns | √ | √ |
|  |  |  | Performance skills | √ |  |
|  |  |  | Play | √ | √ |

(*continued*)

**Table 2.1**  (*Continued*)

| Skill Sets | OT Practitioner | OT Manager | Skill Sets | OT Practitioner | OT Manager |
|---|---|---|---|---|---|
| Physical capacity evaluation | √ | √ | Staff development | √ | √ |
| | | | Staffing | | √ |
| Policy management | √ | √ | Strategic planning | √ | √ |
| Politician | √ | √√ | Stress management | √ | √ |
| Pragmatic reasoning | √ | √ | Substance abuse management | √ | √ |
| Prevention | √ | √ | | | |
| Process skills | √ | | Supervision | √ | √ |
| Problem solving | √ | √ | Task analysis | √ | √ |
| Productivity | √ | √ | Task groups | √ | √ |
| Progressive discipline | ? | √ | Teacher | √ | √ |
| Public policy | √ | √ | Test giver | √ | √ |
| Qualitative research | √ | √ | Therapeutic relationship | √ | ? |
| Quality assurance | √ | √ | | | |
| Questioning | √ | √ | Time management | √ | √ |
| Reevaluation | √ | √ | Tolerance for diversity | √ | √ |
| Reasoning | √ | √ | Trainer | √ | √ |
| Referral management | √ | √ | Values clarification | √ | √ |
| Remediation | √ | | Virtual (computers) | √ | √ |
| Risk taking | √ | √ | Vocational exploration | √ | √ |
| Safety management | √ | √ | Wellness | √ | √ |
| Satisfaction, consumer | √ | √ | Work conditioning | √ | √ |
| Scheduling | √ | √ | Work performance evaluation | √ | √ |
| Selection process | √ | √ | | | |
| Self-assessment | √ | √ | Work simplification | √ | √ |
| Self-efficacy | √ | √ | Worker's compensation | √ | √ |

A check (√) indicates that the skill set falls into either the manager's role or the practitioner's role. Double check (√√) indicates the skill set falls into both the manager's and practitioner's role. A question mark (?) indicates that it is uncertain if the skill set falls into the manager's role or the practitioner's role; it could be either.

example, is used in management to build morale and provide guidance for accomplishing new skills. The therapist coaches patients to relearn an occupation-based activity. Both the therapist and the manager carry out roles of coaching with either patients or employees. Out of 206 skill sets identified, only 23 are what might be described exclusively as roles performed by occupational therapists. Conversely, only 4 can be exclusively associated with the role of the occupational therapy manager.

## Conclusion

One could argue that the skill sets described in Table 2.1 do not reflect all of the skill sets required to perform the roles of therapist and manager. Nevertheless, the argument remains strong that the roles overlap considerably. In the final analysis, occupational therapists and occupational therapy managers have roles that involve working closely with people to enable them to engage in purposeful activity. Inherent in both positions is the need to be a decision maker. Both the therapist and manager have to make informed decisions, but at the same time, both should encourage clients or subordinates to participate in the decision-making process. Both the occupational therapist and occupational therapy manager are concerned with the accomplishment of objectives, often through the efforts of other people. To accomplish objectives, both should be good listeners and good communicators. In either position, the therapists and managers must often be peacemakers, visionaries, self-critics, and team captains. Whether the person is a therapist or a manager, he or she must enjoy and appreciate people; exhibit trust; and possess modesty, patience, and sensitivity.

Nevertheless, we must recognize that the context in which the skill set is performed can change the meaning and purpose of activity. Both the occupational therapist and manager work within a context that influences their perceptions of the skill set, but it also can influence the perception of the client or subordinate. Finally, although their roles have many similarities, the occupational therapist and the occupational therapy manager do perform different functions and make contributions that are distinctly different. Not all occupational therapists can become effective administrative managers.

# References

Accreditation Council for Occupational Therapy Education. (1999). Glossary: Standards for an accredited program for the occupational therapist and for the occupational therapy assistant. *American Journal of Occupational Therapy, 53*(6), 590–591.

American Occupational Therapy Association. (1998). Standards of practice for occupational therapy. *American Journal of Occupational Therapy, 52*(10), 866–869.

American Occupational Therapy Association. (2000). *AOTA 2000 member compensation survey.* Bethesda, MD: Author.

American Occupational Therapy Association. (2002, February). *Occupational therapy practice framework: Domain and process.* Bethesda, MD: Author.

Bass, B. M. (1985). *Leadership and performance based expectations.* New York: Free Press.

Christiansen, C., & Baum, C. (1997). *Occupational therapy: Enabling function and well-being.* Thorofare, NJ: Slack.

Davis, D., & Cosenza, R. M. (1993). *Business research for decision making.* Belmont, CA: Wadsworth.

Manning, M., & Haddock, P. (1995). *Leadership skills for women.* Menlo Park, CA: Crisp.

Mintzberg, M. (1977). Folklore and fact. *Harvard Business Review, 66,* 32–35.

Moyers, P. A. (1999). The guide to occupational therapy practice. *American Journal of Occupational Therapy, 53*(3), pp. 4–12.

Neistadt, M. E., & Crepeau, E. B. (Eds.). (1997). *Willard & Spackman's occupational therapy* (9th ed.). Philadelphia: Lippincott.

Rosener, J. B. (1991). Ways women lead. *Harvard Business Review, 66,* 115–125.

Sanders, T. I. (2002). In fighting terror, we can't think straight. *Viewpoint*. Retrieved May 12, 2002, from http://www.insidebayarea.com or triblet@angnewspapers.com.

Solomon, T. (1988). Value profiles of male and female entrepreneurs. *International Small Business Journal, 6*(3), 24–33.

Szelagyi, A. D., & Wallace, M. J. (1990). *Organizational behavior and performance*. Philadelphia: HarperCollins.

**Additional Resources**

American Occupational Therapy Association. (1991). Essentials and guidelines for an accredited educational program for the occupational therapist. *American Journal of Occupational Therapy, 45*(12), 1077–1084.

Fisk, M. C., & Johnson, M. (Eds.). (1996). *The occupational therapy manager* (rev. ed.). Bethesda, MD: American Occupational Therapy Association.

# Evolution of Occupational Therapy Delivery Systems: The Medical Model and Beyond

Karen Jacobs, EdD, OTR/L, CPE, FAOTA

*"Change happens . . . they keep moving the cheese."*

SPENCER JOHNSON

**Karen Jacobs, EdD, OTR/L, CPE, FAOTA,** is a clinical associate professor in the Department of Occupational Therapy at Boston University and the immediate past-president of AOTA. She is the founding editor of the interdisciplinary and inter-national journal *WORK: A Journal of Prevention, Assessment, and Rehabili-tation* (IOS Press, The Netherlands). Her doctor-ate is from the University of Massachusetts at Lowell.

## Key Terms and Concepts

**Capitation.** A fixed amount periodically paid to a provider for delivery of services for each person covered under a contract or a policy.

**Entitlements.** Government payments that are made through legislatively specified programs to individuals having certain designated characteristics and circumstances, such as age or need (Legislative Indexing Vocabulary, http://www.loc.gov/lexico/servlet/lexico).

**Health maintenance organization (HMO).** "A prepaid organized delivery system where the organization and the primary care physicians assume some financial risk for the care provided to its enrolled members" (Weiner & de Lissovoy, 1993, p. 96).

**Indemnity.** The standard fee-for-service insurance policies provided by employers, organizations, or individuals. Usually the most expensive type, this insurance covers service from any provider.

**Managed care.** A synonym for all kinds of integrated delivery systems, in contrast with unmanaged, fee-for-service care. Also, "the entire range of utilization control tools that are applied to manage the practices of physicians and others, regardless of the setting in which they practice" (Weiner & de Lissovoy, 1993, p. 97).

**Medigap insurance.** Medicare supplemental insurance policies that are available through private companies.

**Point of service plan (POS).** An open-access plan similar to an HMO that provides limited coverage for self-referral outside the network (Andersen, Rice, & Kominski, 2001).

**Preferred provider organization (PPO).** An entity that "acts as a broker between the purchaser of care and the provider. . . . Consumers have the option of using the 'preferred' providers available within the plan, or not" (Weiner & de Lissovoy, 1993, p. 99).

## Learning Objectives

After completing this chapter, you should be able to do the following:

■   Describe how health care is delivered in the United States.

■   Describe the evolution of occupational therapy in the U.S. health care system.

■   List three basic models of integrated delivery systems.

■   List two health care cost containment strategies used since the 1980s.

■   Discuss two strategies to assist in the recognition of occupational therapy in health.

Occupational therapy has been practiced in the U.S. health care system since the early 1900s. Occupational therapy services are affected by the health care system's vulnerabilities and its strengths. This system has shifted from a provider-driven industry to a payer-driven industry and, eventually, will become a consumer-driven industry (DeJong & Sutton, 1994). Health care costs rose from $27.1 billion in 1960 to $1.3 trillion in 2000 (http://www.hcfa.gov/stats/nhe-oact/tables/t1.htm; http://www.hcfa.gov/stats/nhe-oact/tables/chart.htm; Table 3.1 and Figures 3.1a and 3.1b provide details). Because of the health care industry's rising costs, its growing emphasis on outcomes and accountability, its lack of services to meet specific needs, the imbalance of health care services for different populations of the society, and advances in medical technology, the government and the public have begun to scrutinize its practices. The public expects accessible and affordable health care, viewing that care as a right that is grouped in the same category with education, police protection, and fire protection—public services supported by a general tax base and offered by public servants. In contrast, health care moneys are generated by business and industry, third-party payers, government subsidies, private fundraising, and individuals. Moreover, providers of care are independent, licensed practitioners. This chapter explores various aspects of the U.S. health care system and its effect on the evolution of the occupational therapy delivery system.

## The Right-to-Health Concept and Ethics

The basis for much of the government's involvement in health care is the concept of the right to health. Although the *Congressional Record* refers to this concept as early as 1796 (Baum, 1992), it came to full attention in 1944 in President Franklin D. Roosevelt's Economic Bill of Rights in which he proclaimed "the right to adequate needed care and the opportunity to achieve and enjoy good health," equating the right to health care with the most fundamental social and political rights guaranteed to every citizen (Chapman & Talmedge, 1971, p. 35).

Very few political leaders would publicly declare that they do not support a right to health care. However, many politicians debate this right on a daily basis as the government struggles to balance the budget. The right, which would guarantee equal access to "basic and adequate health care"—(Chapman, 1993, p. vi) a standard package including preventive, primary, reproductive, and long-term care; most types of acute care; and mental health services (p. vi)—would demand huge financial resources.

---

This chapter is based in part on "The Evolution of the U.S. Health Care System," by C. M. Baum, 1992, in J. Bair and M. Gray (Eds.), *The Occupational Therapy Manager* (rev. ed., pp. 1–25). Copyright © 1992 by the American Occupational Therapy Association. The graduate occupational therapy students who attended the Professional Service Management course in spring 2002 at Boston University, Sargent College of Health and Rehabilitation Sciences, Programs in Occupational Therapy obtained much of the research material for the chapter. The author expresses great appreciation to these colleagues for their efforts.

**Table 3.1 National Health Expenditures, 1960–2000.**

| | | Total | | | Private Funds | | | Government Funds | | |
|---|---|---|---|---|---|---|---|---|---|---|
| Year | GDP (in $ billions) | Amount (in $ billions) | Per Capita | % of GNP | Amount (in $ billions) | Per Capita | % of Total | Amount (in $ billions) | Per Capita | % of Total |
| 2000 | 9,873 | 1,299.5 | 4,637 | 13.2 | 712.3 | 2,542 | 54.8 | 587.2 | 2,096 | 45.2 |
| 1999 | 9,269 | 1,215.6 | 4,377 | 13.1 | 666.5 | 2,400 | 54.8 | 549.0 | 1,977 | 45.2 |
| 1998 | 8,782 | 1,149.8 | 4,177 | 13.1 | 628.8 | 2,285 | 54.7 | 520.9 | 1,893 | 45.3 |
| 1997 | 8,318 | 1,091.2 | 4,001 | 13.1 | 588.8 | 2,159 | 54.0 | 502.4 | 1,842 | 46.0 |
| 1996 | 7,813 | 1,040.0 | 3,849 | 13.3 | 558.2 | 2,066 | 53.7 | 481.8 | 1,783 | 46.3 |
| 1995 | 7,400 | 990.3 | 3,698 | 13.4 | 534.1 | 1,994 | 53.9 | 456.2 | 1,704 | 46.1 |
| 1994 | 6,735 | 938.3 | 3,463 | 13.9 | 518.1 | 1,912 | 55.2 | 420.2 | 1,551 | 44.8 |
| 1993 | 6,343 | 884.2 | 3,299 | 13.9 | 496.4 | 1,852 | 56.1 | 387.8 | 1,447 | 43.9 |
| 1992 | 6,020 | 820.3 | 3,094 | 13.6 | 462.9 | 1,746 | 56.4 | 357.5 | 1,348 | 43.6 |
| 1991 | 5,725 | 755.6 | 2,882 | 13.2 | 432.9 | 1,651 | 57.3 | 322.6 | 1,230 | 42.7 |
| 1990 | 5,546 | 696.6 | 2,686 | 12.6 | 410.0 | 1,581 | 58.9 | 286.5 | 1,105 | 41.1 |
| 1989 | 5,251 | 623.9 | 2,433 | 11.9 | 370.7 | 1,446 | 59.4 | 253.2 | 987 | 40.6 |
| 1987 | 4,540 | 506.2 | 2,013 | 11.1 | 298.6 | 1,187 | 59.0 | 207.6 | 825 | 41.0 |
| 1985 | 4,039 | 434.5 | 1,761 | 10.8 | 259.4 | 1,051 | 59.7 | 175.1 | 709 | 40.3 |
| 1980 | 2,708 | 251.1 | 1,068 | 9.3 | 145.8 | 620 | 58.1 | 105.3 | 448 | 41.9 |
| 1970 | 1,011 | 74.3 | 346 | 7.4 | 46.6 | 217 | 62.7 | 27.7 | 129 | 37.3 |
| 1960 | 513 | 27.1 | 143 | 5.3 | 20.5 | 108 | 75.5 | 6.7 | 35 | 24.5 |

*Note.* Per capita amounts are based on July 1 Social Security area population estimates for 1960–1990, estimated by the Health Care Financing Administration for 1991–1994. GDP= gross domestic product. GNP= gross national product.

From "National Health Expenditure Projections, 1994–2005 [DataView]" (pp. 234–235), by S. T. Burner and D. R. Waldo, 1995, Summer, *Health Care Financing Review, 16*(4); and "National Health Expenditures, 1993" (p. 280), by K. R. Levit, A. L. Sensenig, C. A. Cowan, H. C. Lazenby, P. A. McDonnell, D. K. Won, et al., 1994 (Fall), *Health Care Financing Review, 16*(1). Data from 1995–2000 retrieved from the Health Care Financing Administration Web site: http://www.hcfa.gov/stats/nhe-oact/tables/t1.htm.

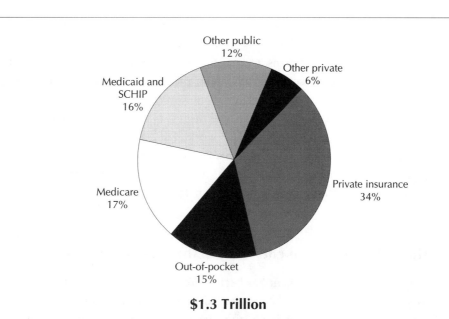

**$1.3 Trillion**

### Figure 3.1a  Where the Nation's Health Dollars Came From in 2000.

*Note.* The category labeled "Other public" represents money from programs such as workers' compensation, public health activity, Department of Defense, Department of Veterans Affairs, Indian Health Service, and state and local government hospital subsidy and school health. The category labeled "Other private" represents money from industrial in-plant, privately funded construction, and nonpatient revenues, including philanthropy.

*Source.* Centers for Medicare & Medicaid Services, Office of the Actuary, National Health Statistics Group; retrieved in 2001 from the Health Care Financing Administration Web site: http://www.hcfa.gov/stats/nhe-oact/tables/chart.htm.

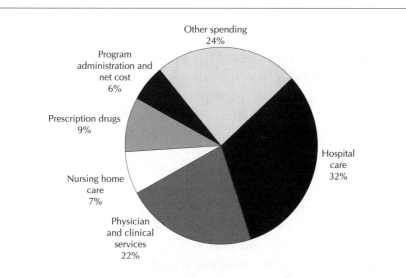

**$1.3 Trillion**

### Figure 3.1b  Where the Nation's Health Dollars Went in 2000.

*Note.* The label "Other spending" includes dentist services, other professional services, home health, durable medical products, over-the-counter medicines and sundries, public health, research, and construction.

*Source.* Centers for Medicare & Medicaid Services, Office of the Actuary, National Health Statistics Group; retrieved in 2001 from the Health Care Financing Administration Web site: http://www.hcfa.gov/stats/nhe-oact/tables/chart.htm.

Related to the right-to-health concept is the matter of ethics (see Chapter 21, Ethical Dimensions of Occupational Therapy, for a more complete discussion of this topic). Society, through its laws and systems, tries to clarify moral values in relation to health care. As ethical issues are raised, especially about the technology available to create, maintain, and prolong human life, limits increasingly may be placed on health services for moral and economic reasons. Occupational therapists who enter management are likely to encounter ethical dilemmas in their work. They need to develop an understanding of potential conflicts and ways of maintaining their personal ethics while successfully carrying out their roles. Goals such as independence, self-determination, and competency—all seen in the practice of occupational therapy—are based on values and morals (Bloom, 1994).

## The Federal Government's Role in the Health Care System

Historically, the federal government has been locked into the role of providing assistance, not control. Since the mid-1940s, the federal government has made many significant contributions to the evolving health care system. The following summary of major historical events offers a perspective on these contributions.

### Construction of Health Care Facilities

Minimal hospital construction occurred in the United States during the Depression and World War II. In 1944, the American Hospital Association (AHA) and the U.S. Public Health Service organized a commission on hospital care to determine the need for new hospital facilities. The work of the commission was reflected in the Hospital Survey and Construction Act of 1946, Title VI of the Public Health Service Act. Popularly known as the Hill–Burton Act, this legislation assisted the states in determining their need for hospitals and other health care facilities. Also, it provided grants to states for construction projects. Over the next two decades, Congress extended and amended the Hill–Burton Act frequently, expanding its programs to cover diagnostic and treatment centers, chronic disease hospitals, rehabilitation facilities, and nursing homes. In 1964 and again in 1970, Congress earmarked funds for modernization of these health care facilities.

In 1963, the Mental Retardation Facilities Construction Act and the Community Mental Health Centers Act (P.L. 88–164) were passed to provide funding for the construction of facilities for people with mental retardation and for the construction of community-based mental health centers. Extensions and amendments to this federal legislation continued into the early 1980s.

The Hill–Burton Act was greatly modified in the National Health Planning and Resources Development Act of 1974. This legislation was especially critical in modernizing health care facilities. Many of the facilities built between 1946 and 1974 were struggling to survive, and their struggle was having a major effect on the total cost of health care. By the mid-1960s, new facilities were operational, but too few health professionals were available to staff them. Also, some health facilities were obsolete, requiring nearly $20 billion a year for modernization. Construction costs of facilities increased from $470 million in 1968 to $712 million in 1971. By the early 1970s, the federal government began to recognize the need for systems to control and establish meaningful plans for future construction.

## Human Resources Legislation

Since the mid-1950s, the federal government has had an important role in financing human resources for health. Its first peacetime legislation to support training of health care professionals was the Health Amendments Act of 1956, benefiting public health personnel and professional and practical nurses. In 1958, Congress established a program of formula grants to schools of public health. Soon to follow was a program of project grants for these and other schools training public health personnel.

The first construction grants for teaching facilities came in 1963, in the Health Professions Educational Assistance Act. Schools of medicine, dentistry, pharmacy, podiatry, nursing, and public health were the eligible recipients. This act also made student loan funds available in medicine, osteopathy, and dentistry. In 1964, the Nurse Training Act provided separate funds for nursing school construction, set aside funds to expand educational training programs in nursing, and established nursing student loan programs. The Health Professions Educational Assistance Act Amendments of 1965 authorized grants to improve the quality of schools of medicine, dentistry, osteopathy, optometry, and podiatry. The amendments also made scholarship funds available to those schools and to schools of pharmacy.

The first federal funds for support of occupational therapy education came in 1966, with the Allied Health Professions Personnel Training Act. This legislation authorized the award of construction and improvement grants to training centers for allied health professions. It also made advanced traineeships available to allied health professionals. The Health Manpower Act of 1968 extended most of the programs for health and allied health professionals, including those for occupational therapy personnel.

Legislation supporting training in various ways continued into the 1970s (e.g., the Health Training Improvement Act of 1970, the Comprehensive Health Manpower Training Act of 1971, the Nurse Training Act of 1975). In the 1970s and the 1980s, however, the federal government began to limit moneys for traineeships. In 1980, the training money for the Allied Health Professions Personnel Training Act was eliminated from the federal budget. From the late 1980s to the early 1990s, the government published several reports that documented a shortage of allied health professionals. In 1990, moneys for the Allied Health Professions Personnel Training Act were returned to the federal budget (Elwood, 1991).

## Health Planning

By the early 1970s, the federal government was acutely aware of the need to control health care costs. Several major pieces of legislation addressed that need. A 1972 amendment to the Social Security Act created professional standards review organizations. Under this plan, associations of physicians in a geographic area reviewed professionals' activities and institutions' services to monitor and control both cost and quality of care. The law made it possible to give hospital utilization review committees the responsibility of carrying out these functions. Also in 1972, Congress enacted legislation giving the secretary of state the authority to establish limitations on Medicare reimbursements for routine services provided under Part A of Medicare (Hospital Insurance).

Two years later, Congress passed the National Health Planning and Resources Development Act to ensure the development of both a national health policy and effective state and area programs for health planning and for resource allocation. Under the provisions of this act, each state is divided into health service areas, and health systems agencies are designated to administer them. The agencies have three purposes:

- To improve the health of area residents
- To increase the accessibility, the acceptability, the continuity, and the quality of health services
- To restrain costs and to prevent duplication of health services.

In 1982, Congress enacted the Tax Equity and Fiscal Responsibility Act, which, among other provisions, extended the 1972 limits on reimbursements under Medicare to cover ancillary and rehabilitation services. Occupational therapy services are included under this provision.

In April 1983, President Ronald Reagan signed the Social Security Amendments into law, amendments that contained a congressional mandate to alter the way in which health care was subsidized and delivered. The intent of the legislation was to impose further constraints on the level of federal spending for Medicare benefits, particularly for inpatient hospital care. The law fundamentally changed the formula for disbursing health care dollars. For decades, health care had relied almost exclusively on a hospital-based delivery system: On the basis of a financial formula, the payer (the federal government, an insurance company, or an individual) reimbursed hospitals for the cost of the services provided. Under the Medicare prospective payment system (PPS) created by the Social Security Amendments of 1983, the Health Care Financing Administration (HCFA) established a nationwide schedule defining the payment that the government would make for each inpatient stay by a Medicare beneficiary. The level of payment per case is determined by about 500 descriptive categories called *diagnosis-related groups* (DRGs; *DRG Handbook,* 1994).

The PPS has had a profound effect on the development of the health care industry. It has reduced emphasis on inpatient services and expanded outpatient and community programs. Changes have occurred within both Medicare Part A (Hospital Insurance) and Medicare Part B (Supplementary Medical Insurance), some of which directly affect occupational therapy. In 1986, Congress enacted legislation expanding Medicare coverage of occupational therapy services under Part B to include "services furnished in a skilled-nursing facility (when Part A coverage has been exhausted), in a clinic, [in a] rehabilitation agency, [in a] public health agency, or by an independently practicing therapist" (Social Security Administration, 1994, p. 94). The effect of the PPS on reimbursement for rehabilitation services becomes very apparent in a comparison of Medicare Part A payments to inpatient hospitals, home health agencies, and skilled nursing facilities before and after introduction of the PPS. "During the 1980s, Medicare costs rose in real terms at more than seven percent and Medicaid expenses at about six percent a year" (Nichols, 1999). In 1983, Medicare paid inpatient hospitals $34.3 billion, home health agencies $1.3 billion, and skilled nursing facilities $0.5 billion. In 2000, it paid inpatient hospitals $125.7 billion (about 3 times the 1983 figure), home health agencies $9.2 billion (about 7 times the 1983 figure), and skilled nursing facilities $9.5 billion (about 19 times the 1983 figure; Social Security Administration, 1994; www.hcfa.gov/stats/nhe-oact/tables/t10.htm).

In 1993, following up on a campaign promise, President Bill Clinton formally introduced a health care reform bill. After many debates, however, the 103rd Congress failed to approve any health care reform bills (Rubin, 1994a, 1994b). In addition, later legislation in 1997 had little effect on health care reform:

> The 1997 Balanced Budget Act achieved some Medicare savings and, to a much lesser extent, reduced Medicaid spending, but the budget agreement did little to address the long-term demographic problem that threatens the adequacy of Medicare funding: the decline in the worker/beneficiary ratio from the current three-to-one to two-to-one by the time the last baby boomers are retired. As a result, many inside and outside of Congress are proposing long-term structural changes to both programs that will institutionalize cost containment incentives. Managed care and the increased health plan competition that managed care makes possible are central to these structural proposals. (Nichols, 1999)

Although comprehensive reform seems unlikely, a new bill under review in the House of Representatives of the 107th Congress proposes to enact legislation by October 2004 that provides access to comprehensive health care for all Americans that is affordable, cost-efficient, and able to ensure continuity of coverage and care (http://thomas.loc.gov). Comprehensive reform at this time, however, is unlikely. Instead, change will probably come under the rubric of insurance reform because of the fallout related to managed care.

### Summary of Federal Government's Role in Health Care

Tracing the federal government's role in the evolution of health care shows the current situation in perspective:

- The government built the facilities.
- The government supported training of the human resources.
- The government pays a large portion of health care costs.
- The government supports research.
- The government has been unsuccessful in controlling costs.
- The government is responsible for providing care when people do not have access to health insurance.

## Organizations Providing Care

When people think of the hospital today, they envision a sophisticated facility providing technically advanced procedures to support life and a healthful status. Hospitals, however, were not medically oriented until after the turn of the century. Initially, they were facilities for people who were indigent, and the majority of health care was delivered at home. From the early 1900s until the early 1970s, most health care was provided and delivered in two facilities, the physician's office and the hospital. Nursing homes were mostly for custodial management, and today's concept of home health care was in its early development.

Modern health care organizations are the result of scientific developments and changes in society. Other facilities are now becoming basic to providing health services to U.S. citizens (Shepp, 1980). The system includes government, nonprofit, and for-profit facilities (Table 3.2).

### Vertically Organized Hospitals

Methods of delivering health care services at less cost than that associated with hospitals have existed for years. Hospitals have been reluctant to support these systems because, under the former payment structure, they were paid for the services that they provided to hospitalized people. The set fees under the PPS now make it economically advantageous for hospitals to move patients with long-term problems out of acute care beds into another type of health care setting as quickly as feasible. Instead of staying in the hospital, patients go to home health care, nursing facilities, hospices, designated subacute care beds, designated rehabilitation beds, designated psychiatric beds, wellness or fitness programs, outpatient surgery, day treatment for elderly people, or outpatient programs. This system has expanded both the importance and the use of the rehabilitation fields and has allowed the hospital to support these fields. Thus, most hospitals are now organized in a vertical system as illustrated in Figure 3.2.

The vertical organization serves the hospital system well. Patients can be readmitted for necessary procedures, and the hospital is able to keep patients in its market by placing them in affiliated systems. This very skillful economic strategy has also created the greatest opportunity in history for rehabilitation. For nearly every one of a hospital's

**Table 3.2 Health Care Organizations.**

| Type of Organization | General Description |
| --- | --- |
| Federal government | Hospitals serving disabled veterans |
| | Hospitals serving the armed forces and the Coast Guard |
| | Indian Health Service |
| | Public Health Service hospitals and clinics (including a leprosarium) |
| | Medical facilities associated with prisons |
| State government | Infirmaries associated with prisons and reformatories |
| | Hospitals for people with mental illness |
| | State medical school hospitals and clinics |
| Local government | City hospitals and clinics |
| | County hospitals and public health clinics |
| | Rehabilitation facilities |
| Nonprofit organization | Charity hospitals |
| | Community hospitals |
| | Health maintenance organizations (HMOs) |
| | Home health facilities |
| | Hospices |
| | Industrial hospitals and clinics |
| | Preferred provider organizations (PPOs) |
| | Private teaching hospitals |
| | Religious hospitals |
| | Specialty hospitals |
| | Surgical centers |
| | Wellness centers |
| For-profit organization | Facilities owned by individuals or groups for the care of their own patients or clients |
| | Investor-owned facilities (hospitals, laboratories, nursing homes, surgical centers, rehabilitation facilities, home health facilities, HMOs, PPOs, and hospices), including corporations and management corporations |
| | Walk-in medical clinics |

*Note.* Adapted from *Health Services in the United States* (2nd rev. ed., pp. 8–16), by F. A. Wilson and D. Neuhauser, 1985, Cambridge, MA: Ballinger; and *A Guide to Health Care Facilities: Personnel and Management* (3rd ed., pp. 16–23), by R. Sloane, 1992, Ann Arbor, MI: Health Administration Press.

vertical programs to be effective, the programs require the rehabilitation profession's skills. The challenge to the profession is to provide the human resources to staff the programs. Should occupational therapy not have enough personnel, other professions will expand their roles to fill the needs.

## Health Networks

In today's changing society and economy, the free-standing hospital has become financially vulnerable. Concern about this vulnerability has led to the formation of large

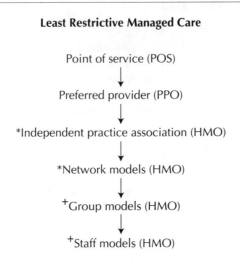

**Least Restrictive Managed Care**

Point of service (POS)

Preferred provider (PPO)

*Independent practice association (HMO)

*Network models (HMO)

+Group models (HMO)

+Staff models (HMO)

**Most Restrictive Managed Care**

**Figure 3.2  Degree of Restriction in Managed Care.**
*Note:* * = Open panel (access); coverage for self-referral outside the network. + = Closed panel (access); no coverage for self-referral outside the network.

health networks linking individual facilities that represent only one of several related corporate activities. Either a multi-hospital system or a diversified, single-hospital system is created when two or more hospitals are owned, leased, sponsored, or contract managed by a central organization. A network is created when some combination of hospitals, physicians, other providers, insurers, and community agencies work together to coordinate and deliver services (http://www.aha.org). This phenomenon is evident in the public sector and in the private sector. Since the 1970s, many types of multi-institutional systems have developed, each with distinct ownership and governance. They have six features in common:

- Strong financial and organizational management
- A well-developed market strategy
- Built-in referral strategies to keep their use high
- A broad geographical approach
- An expansive model of service delivery, from primary to restorative care, including home health services, ambulatory services, and skilled nursing facilities
- Shared services for purchasing, billing, maintenance, and marketing.

The trend toward large corporate systems taking over facilities with fewer than 100 beds continues in the 21st century. In a 1993 survey, the AHA (1994) found that 50% of all hospital systems were owned by for-profit, multi-institutional systems. In 2001, the AHA found that 3,544 (61%) of the 5,810 hospitals in the United States were part of either a system or a network (http://www.aha.org).

## Alternative or Integrated Delivery Systems

Along with vertically organized hospitals and large health networks have come alternative delivery systems, more appropriately called "integrated delivery systems" because they "usually involve a significant degree of integration between payer and providers" (Weiner & de Lissovoy, 1993, p. 94). They also depend on managed care systems. Some people use the term *managed care* as a synonym for all kinds of integrated delivery systems, contrasting these systems with unmanaged, fee-for-service care. More recently, however, the term frequently has denoted "the entire range of utilization control tools that are applied to manage the practices of physicians and others, regardless of the setting in which they practice" (p. 97). Thus, traditional insurers who have introduced various utilization controls are practicing managed care. The types of controls used to manage care include "preadmission certification, mandatory second opinion before surgery, certification of treatment plans for discretionary nonemergency services (such as mental health care), primary care physician gatekeepers, and nonphysician case managers to monitor the care of particular patients" (p. 97).

The concept of managed care has proved so successful in containing costs that many variants of managed care have evolved as large health care organizations and insurance companies compete in the marketplace for new members. Enrollment in traditional health insurance plans of the managed indemnity or indemnity type has been steadily falling (Loomis, 1994). *Indemnity,* generally meaning security against loss, refers to the standard fee-for-service insurance policies carried by many employers, organizations, and individuals. Usually, the most expensive type, this insurance covers service from any provider.

The three major types of integrated delivery systems operating in today's health care market are health maintenance organizations (HMOs), preferred provider organizations (PPOs), and point of service (POS) plans. It is important for these delivery services to have good prices and high-quality services oriented to wellness and low costs. Occupational therapy products offered in HMOs, PPOs, and POS plans include developmental screenings, training in stress management, arthritis programs, ergonomic consultations, functional capacity evaluations, and hand-related services. Some integrated delivery services require home health rehabilitation services. Many are eager to develop contractual relationships for a full scope of rehabilitation services. In HMOs, which require referrals, physicians, nurse-practitioners, and social workers are becoming more oriented to occupational therapy's capacity to help them save money and promote health. A rehabilitation organization can develop a business arrangement with an HMO to receive a set amount per month per enrollee.

Individual physicians and practices have taken advantage of the financial benefits of participating in a prepaid group practice, which enables a more efficient delivery of health care services. HMOs began to multiply in 1973 when the federal government, faced with spiraling health care costs, passed the Health Maintenance Organization Act to foster HMOs through loans and grants. In 1971, there were 39 HMOs (*HMO Fact Sheet*, 1985). In 1987, the number peaked at 662, with an enrollment of more than 28.5 million people. By 1995, the number of HMOs had decreased to 550; the enrollment, however, had increased to nearly 46.2 million people, or 19.4% of the U.S. population (U.S. Bureau of the Census, 2001). In 2000, HMO membership exceeded more than 80 million in 568 HMOs (U.S. Bureau of the Census, 2001). The following sections provide specific explanations of the three main integrated delivery systems.

### HMOs

An *HMO* is "a prepaid organized delivery system where the organization and the primary care physicians assume some financial risk for the care provided to its enrolled members" (Weiner & de Lissovoy, 1993, p. 96). Often, the physicians in an HMO are periodically paid a capitation, that is, a fixed amount for each person covered. HMOs are a "traditional form of managed care" (Andersen, Rice, & Kominski, 2001, p. 390) and typically require patients to contact a primary care physician to receive a referral before obtaining specialty care (pp. 390–391). The physicians can contract with an HMO in several ways. In a closed-panel HMO, physicians are allowed to treat only patients who are subscribers to the HMO. The closed-panel HMO can contract exclusively with a single group practice (group model) or can employ individual physicians (staff model). These plans are often viewed as restrictive because clients are not permitted to choose a doctor outside of the HMO. In contrast, open-panel HMOs avoid these restrictions. In open-panel HMOs, network association and independent practice association models permit HMOs to contract with multiple medical groups or individual physicians, respectively. In these cases, physicians also are permitted to contract with more than one HMO and may treat patients who are not enrolled in the HMO. HMOs contribute significantly to lower health care costs because they provide services at little or no charge above the fixed enrollment fee that members pay.

### PPOs

PPOs are less restrictive than traditional HMOs because subscribers can self-refer to specialists and are not required to consult with a primary care physician before receiving specialty care (Andersen et al., 2001). Consumers can either use the "preferred" providers available within the plan or use other providers (Weiner & de Lissovoy, 1993). PPOs contract with physicians and groups, although clients are not required to use the doctors within the group. The physicians in a PPO agree to follow "utilization management guidelines" (Andersen et al., 2001, pp. 391) and receive a discounted fee for services. Clients receive financial incentives to use physicians within the PPO network, although they generally receive coverage for services provided by physicians who are not in the PPO. According to the American Managed

Care and Review Association surveys, the number of PPOs in the United States increased from 571 to 1,037 between 1990 and 1998. By 2001, 98.4 million Americans were enrolled in PPOs (PPO Directory and Performance Report, 2.0).

## POS Plans

POS plans, developed in the 1980s, are similar to open-panel HMOs, but these plans permit limited coverage on a self-referral basis for services by physicians outside the network (Andersen et al., 2001). POS plans can have a varied billing system in which clients who work through a primary care physician pay the lowest copayments, whereas these payments increase when the client self-refers within the network or receives services from a physician outside of the network. A POS plan "offers the consumer a choice of options at the time he or she seeks services (rather than at the time they [sic] choose to enroll in a health plan)" (Weiner & de Lissovoy, 1993, p. 99).

## Public Health Organizations

The medical–industrial complex does not provide all health care services. The American Public Health Association (APHA), a voluntary organization of public health professionals, is in its second century of service to the nation (http://www.apha.org). APHA actively serves the public, its members, and the public health profession through its scientific and practice programs, public health standards, publications, educational services, and advocacy efforts.

Members of the APHA work in public health systems at the local, state, national, and international levels. The backbone of these systems at the national level is the U.S. Public Health Service, the oldest agency of the U.S. Department of Health and Human Services. Established in 1798 as the Marine Hospital Service for the "'care and relief of sick and disabled seamen'" (U.S. Public Health Service, ca. 1988, p. 1), it was first concerned with attending to the health of merchant seamen and preventing epidemics of disease. In the late 19th century, its scope broadened to encompass biomedical research, regulation of biological products in interstate commerce, and studies of environmental hazards. In 1887, it initiated a research program called the Hygienic Laboratory, which became the National Institute (now Institutes) of Health in 1930. Under that institute's auspices, 13 specialty institutes have formed over the years. In 1889, Congress organized the Marine Hospital Service's professional personnel into a quasi-military corps of physicians under a surgeon general. The Marine Hospital Service took on the name U.S. Public Health Service in 1912. In 1946, the Communicable Disease Center, now the Centers for Disease Control and Prevention, was established. The Public Health Service now comprises five agencies: the Substance Abuse and Mental Health Services Administration, the Centers for Disease Control and Prevention, the Food and Drug Administration, the Health Resources and Services Administration, the National Institutes of Health, and the office of Public Health and Science.

For occupational therapists and support personnel, the public health system represents a critical link to people who, because of their location or inability to pay, do not use the private health system. Public health is primarily concerned with preventing disease by coordinating public programs, but increasingly, it is providing medical care to individual patients through neighborhood health centers. At the start of the 21st century, despite the prevalence of health insurance coverage, approximately 44 million Americans were without any kind of health insurance (Andersen et al., 2001). This group of uninsured people includes all ages, incomes, geographic settings, races, and ethnic groups; the young fare worse than the old, and the poor and the middle class worse than the well-to-do (U.S. Bureau of the Census, 2001).

The Public Health Service is responsible for several programs of great interest to occupational therapists (see Appendix 3.B). Voluntary organizations and foundations supplement these efforts with a multitude of programs and services (see Appendix 3.C).

## The Evolution of Occupational Therapy

Historians of occupational therapy have begun to document the evolution of its theories and concepts of occupation. Christiansen and Baum (1991), Hopkins and Smith (1994), and Quiroga (1995) offered an important complement to the contemporary picture of occupational therapy and should be studied in concert with this chapter.

Trends in the supply and the distribution of occupational therapists offer another historical perspective on occupational therapy. With respect to supply, the profession increased by 41,000 between 1970 and 1984. This increase represented "more than entered the profession in all its previous years combined" (American Occupational Therapy Association [AOTA], Ad Hoc Commission 1983–84, p. 17). During the 1970s, the growth rate was 9%–10% per year. In the mid-1980s, it slowed to 5%, apparently because of a stabilization of output from occupational therapy education programs.

The 1990s saw the growth rate rise to an average 7%, influenced by an increase in the number of occupational therapists trained outside the United States (Mindy Hecker, director, Membership Department, AOTA, personal communication, December 1995). Between 1991 and 1993, the number of graduating occupational therapists grew by 22%, and the number of graduating occupational therapy assistants, by 26%. In 1992, there were 3,000 new occupational therapists and 1,300 new occupational therapy assistants. In 1995, 48,736 registered occupational therapists and 13,087 certified occupational therapy assistants were documented (AOTA, 1995b). From 1995 to December 2001, 20,552 new occupational therapy assistants and 38,004 new occupational therapists obtained certification (J. Jennings, administrative assistant, Membership Department, AOTA, personal communication, February 12, 2002). As of 1999, there were 300 accredited programs, and by January 2002, that number had grown to 337. In addition, eight programs are currently under development and are accepting students (AOTA, 2002a).

The growth in the number of occupational therapists and occupational therapy assistants has been accompanied by some changes in the distribution of practitioners across practice settings. Table 3.3 presents data on the numbers and the percentages of occupational therapists and occupational therapy assistants in various employment settings at 4- or 5-year intervals from 1973 through 2000. Data were not available before 1973. In particular, the data on occupational therapists reveal a major increase in the percentage of occupational therapists working in the school system between 1997 and 2000. As of 2000, nearly a quarter of all occupational therapists were working in schools. This number most likely reflects increases in the school-age population and the enactment of the Individuals with Disabilities Education Act (IDEA; P.L. 105–17, June 1997), which mandates service delivery in the schools.

In addition, the data indicate an emergence of occupational therapists in the general hospital settings of neonatal intensive care units, early intervention centers, psychiatric units, and rehabilitation units as well as in physicians' offices and retirement or senior centers. HMOs maintained a relatively stable percentage of occupational therapists. However, moderate to major decreases occurred in the percentages of occupational therapists in college or university settings, community mental health centers, correctional institutions, day care centers and programs, psychiatric hospitals, rehabilitation hospitals and centers, residential care facilities, and vocational or prevocational programs.

Carr (1993) observed that occupational therapy assistants "were trained initially to work in psychiatric hospital practice settings and then in nursing homes and other general medical settings. Many still work in those facilities. The dispersion of certified occupational therapy assistants into nontraditional settings came about, not because of training, but because of federal legislation" (p. 26). Many similarities occur between distribution patterns of occupational therapists across practice settings and those of occupational therapy assistants:

- The percentage of occupational therapy assistants has increased in the same settings identified earlier for occupational therapists.
- Occupational therapy assistants have emerged in the same new settings as have occupational therapists.
- The percentage of occupational therapy assistants has decreased in most of the same settings (plus HMOs) as occupational therapists.

In 1995, 90% of occupational therapists and occupational therapy assistants were employed, and the future looked good for new graduates. Although federal legislation (e.g., the Balanced Budget Act, 1997, which tried to impose limits on reimbursement for therapy services) may adversely affect the job market for occupational therapists in the short term, it is projected that the demand for therapists should continue to increase as the number of individuals needing services continues to grow (U.S. Department of Labor, 2001).

Table 3.3  Primary Employment Settings of Occupational Therapists and Occupational Therapy Assistants, 1973–2000.

| Primary Employment Setting | % Registered Occupational Therapists | | | | | | | % Certified Occupational Therapy Assistants | | | | | | |
|---|---|---|---|---|---|---|---|---|---|---|---|---|---|---|
| | 1973 | 1977 | 1982 | 1986 | 1990 | 1997 | 2000 | 1973 | 1977 | 1982 | 1986 | 1990 | 1997 | 2000 |
| College, two-year | 1.4 | 1.2 | 0.8 | 0.7 | 0.6 | 0.8 | 0.9 | 0.8 | 0.9 | 0.6 | 0.8 | 0.9 | 1.9 | 2.5 |
| College/university, four-year | 5.6 | 4.9 | 4.1 | 3.1 | 3.4 | 3.3 | 5.6 | 0.7 | 0.6 | 0.9 | 0.3 | 0.3 | 0.0 | 0.0 |
| Community mental health center/program | 4.2 | 4.3 | 2.4 | 1.6 | 1.1 | 0.5 | 0.9 | 4.0 | 3.5 | 3.1 | 3.8 | 1.7 | 0.4 | 0.8 |
| Community residential care facility | — | — | — | — | — | 0.3 | 0.4 | — | — | — | — | — | 1.5 | 0.8 |
| Comprehensive out-patient rehab facility | — | — | — | — | — | 1.1 | 1.7 | — | — | — | — | — | 1.5 | 0.4 |
| Correctional institution | 0.2 | 0.2 | 0.1 | 0.1 | — | — | — | 0.3 | 0.2 | 0.1 | 0.2 | — | — | — |
| Day care center/program | 1.4 | 1.1 | 1.0 | 1.1 | 0.9 | — | — | 1.2 | 2.4 | 2.0 | 4.3 | 1.7 | — | — |
| Day care program—adult | — | — | — | — | — | 0.1 | 0.3 | — | — | — | — | — | 0.4 | 0.0 |
| Day care program—pediatric | — | — | — | — | — | 0.3 | 0.6 | — | — | — | — | — | 0.4 | 1.2 |
| Day treatment | — | — | — | — | — | 0.4 | 0.5 | — | — | — | — | — | 0.4 | 0.4 |
| Early intervention program | — | — | — | — | — | 2.2 | 3.7 | — | — | — | — | — | 1.1 | 2.5 |
| Freestanding—behavioral health | — | — | — | — | — | 1.1 | 1.0 | — | — | — | — | — | 1.5 | 2.1 |
| Freestanding—home health agency | 0.9 | 2.2 | 3.8 | 4.6 | 3.6 | 4.5 | 3.9 | 0.2 | 0.4 | 0.8 | 1.2 | 1.5 | 1.9 | 0.8 |
| Freestanding—interme-diate nursing facility | — | — | — | — | — | 1.1 | 0.3 | — | — | — | — | — | 1.5 | 1.2 |

(continued)

| | % Registered Occupational Therapists | | | | | | | Primary Employment Setting | % Certified Occupational Therapy Assistants | | | | | | |
|---|---|---|---|---|---|---|---|---|---|---|---|---|---|---|---|
| | 1973 | 1977 | 1982 | 1986 | 1990 | 1997 | 2000 | | 1973 | 1977 | 1982 | 1986 | 1990 | 1997 | 2000 |
| | — | — | — | — | — | 16.3 | 7.7 | Freestanding—skilled nursing facility | — | — | — | — | — | 34.7 | 25.2 |
| | — | — | — | — | — | 5.2 | 2.0 | Freestanding—subacute nursing facility | — | — | — | — | — | 6.8 | 7.0 |
| | — | — | 2.5 | 2.4 | 3.7 | — | — | Freestanding—outpatient clinic | — | — | 1.7 | 0.9 | 2.2 | — | — |
| | — | — | — | — | — | 3.9 | 3.8 | Freestanding—rehabilitation hospital | — | — | — | — | — | 2.3 | 1.7 |
| | — | — | — | — | — | 2.2 | 2.0 | Freestanding—rehabilitation hospital outpatient services/department | — | — | — | — | — | 0.4 | 0.0 |
| | — | — | — | — | — | 6.4 | 6.5 | General hospital—acute | — | — | — | — | — | 4.9 | 2.5 |
| | — | — | — | — | — | 2.3 | 2.2 | General hospital—behavioral health | — | — | — | — | — | 2.3 | 1.7 |
| | — | — | 0.0 | 0.1 | 0.0 | 0.0 | 0.1 | General hospital—hospice | — | — | — | — | — | 0.0 | 0.0 |
| | — | — | — | — | 0.7 | 0.9 | 0.4 | General hospital—neonatal intensive care unit | — | — | — | — | 0.1 | 0.0 | 0.0 |
| | — | — | — | — | — | 6.1 | 5.6 | General hospital—outpatient services | — | — | — | — | — | 2.3 | 2.5 |
| | — | — | — | — | — | 0.1 | 0.5 | General hospital—partial hospitalization unit | — | — | — | — | — | 0.0 | 0.4 |
| | — | — | — | — | — | 0.3 | 1.2 | General hospital—pediatric unit | — | — | — | — | — | 0.0 | 0.4 |
| | — | — | — | — | 3.5 | — | — | General hospital—psychiatric unit | — | — | — | — | 4.0 | — | — |

*(continued)*

**Table 3.3** (Continued)

| Primary Employment Setting | % Registered Occupational Therapists | | | | | | | % Certified Occupational Therapy Assistants | | | | | | |
|---|---|---|---|---|---|---|---|---|---|---|---|---|---|---|
| | 1973 | 1977 | 1982 | 1986 | 1990 | 1997 | 2000 | 1973 | 1977 | 1982 | 1986 | 1990 | 1997 | 2000 |
| General hospital—rehabilitation unit | — | — | — | 4.2 | 5.3 | 4.7 | 5.1 | — | — | — | 4.5 | 5.5 | 5.7 | 6.6 |
| General hospital—skilled nursing unit | — | — | — | — | — | 2.1 | 2.1 | — | — | — | — | — | 2.3 | 2.9 |
| General hospital—subacute unit | — | — | — | — | — | 1.1 | 0.8 | — | — | — | — | — | 3.9 | 2.1 |
| General hospital—all other | 20.5 | 19.8 | 25.3 | 22.0 | 15.9 | — | — | 15.1 | 12.7 | 17.8 | 14.1 | 9.4 | — | — |
| Group home | — | — | — | — | — | 1.1 | 0.2 | — | — | — | — | — | 0.8 | 0.4 |
| Hospital-based home health care | — | — | — | — | — | 2.7 | 1.6 | — | — | — | — | — | 0.8 | 0.8 |
| HMO (including PPO/IPA; staff model) | 0.3 | 0.2 | 0.2 | 0.3 | 0.4 | 0.2 | 0.2 | 0.7 | 0.3 | 0.3 | 0.2 | 0.1 | 0.0 | 0.2 |
| Independent living center | — | — | — | — | — | 0.2 | 0.3 | — | — | — | — | — | 0.0 | 0.4 |
| Industrial rehab/work programs | — | — | — | — | — | 0.6 | 1.0 | — | — | — | — | — | 0.0 | 0.8 |
| Mobile treatment team/home care | — | — | — | — | — | 0.2 | 1.1 | — | — | — | — | — | 0.0 | 0.0 |
| Partial hospitalization program (community-based, not outpatient) | — | — | — | — | — | 0.0 | 0.0 | — | — | — | — | — | 0.0 | 0.0 |

(continued)

| % Registered Occupational Therapists | | | | | | | Primary Employment Setting | % Certified Occupational Therapy Assistants | | | | | | |
|---|---|---|---|---|---|---|---|---|---|---|---|---|---|---|
| 1973 | 1977 | 1982 | 1986 | 1990 | 1997 | 2000 | | 1973 | 1977 | 1982 | 1986 | 1990 | 1997 | 2000 |
| 2.9 | 2.0 | 1.6 | 1.7 | 1.7 | — | — | Pediatric hospital | 1.5 | 1.2 | 0.8 | 0.4 | 0.7 | — | — |
| — | — | — | 1.1 | 1.2 | 0.5 | 0.8 | Physician's office | — | — | — | 0.2 | 0.3 | 0.0 | 0.4 |
| — | — | 0.7 | 0.5 | 0.8 | — | — | Private industry | 1.0 | 0.5 | 0.7 | — | — | — | — |
| 1.3 | 2.1 | 3.5 | 6.0 | 7.7 | 3.9 | 5.5 | Private practice (office-based) | 0.3 | 0.4 | 1.2 | 1.9 | 2.7 | 1.5 | 4.5 |
| 13.8 | 11.2 | 7.4 | 6.9 | 4.6 | — | — | Psychiatric hospital | 22.6 | 14.3 | 9.7 | 8.4 | 6.6 | — | — |
| 1.6 | 1.5 | 0.8 | 0.9 | 0.9 | 0.1 | 0.3 | Public health agency | 0.5 | 0.5 | 0.3 | 0.4 | 0.6 | 0.4 | 0.0 |
| — | — | — | — | — | 2.1 | 2.8 | Rehabilitation agency/ clinic | — | — | — | — | — | 1.1 | 2.1 |
| 13.4 | 10.9 | 8.9 | 10.5 | 11.4 | — | — | Rehabilitation hospital/ center | 9.5 | 11.0 | 8.4 | 8.4 | 10.9 | — | — |
| 0.3 | 0.3 | 0.4 | 0.2 | 0.2 | — | — | Research facility | 0.2 | 0.3 | 0.1 | 0.0 | 0.2 | — | — |
| — | 4.4 | 4.2 | 3.3 | 2.7 | — | — | Residential care facility, including group home, independent living center | — | 8.5 | 7.6 | 7.5 | 5.9 | — | — |
| — | — | — | — | — | 0.2 | 0.2 | Retirement/assisted living | — | — | — | — | — | 0.8 | 0.0 |
| — | — | — | 0.2 | 0.2 | — | — | Retirement or senior center | — | — | — | 1.1 | 0.8 | — | — |
| 11.0 | 14.0 | 18.3 | 17.0 | 18.6 | 18.1 | 24.9 | School system (including private schools) | 3.6 | 6.2 | 11.3 | 14.4 | 17.0 | 15.1 | 22.3 |
| — | — | — | — | — | 0.2 | 0.0 | Senior center | — | — | — | — | — | 0.4 | 0.0 |
| 0.7 | 0.7 | 0.7 | 0.4 | 0.4 | 0.1 | 0.0 | Sheltered workshop | 1.4 | 0.9 | 1.9 | 1.6 | 1.6 | 0.8 | 0.8 |

*(continued)*

**Table 3.3** (Continued)

| Primary Employment Setting | % Registered Occupational Therapists | | | | | | | % Certified Occupational Therapy Assistants | | | | | | |
|---|---|---|---|---|---|---|---|---|---|---|---|---|---|---|
| | 1973 | 1977 | 1982 | 1986 | 1990 | 1997 | 2000 | 1973 | 1977 | 1982 | 1986 | 1990 | 1997 | 2000 |
| Skilled nursing home/intermediate care facility | 6.2 | 7.9 | 6.0 | 5.8 | 6.4 | — | — | 22.8 | 26.1 | 22.5 | 20.1 | 20.1 | — | — |
| Supervised housing | — | — | — | — | — | 0.0 | 0.0 | — | — | — | — | — | 0.0 | 0.0 |
| Supported employment | — | — | — | — | — | 0.0 | 0.0 | — | — | — | — | — | 0.0 | 0.0 |
| Transitional program | — | — | — | — | — | 0.1 | 0.2 | — | — | — | — | — | 0.4 | 0.4 |
| Vocational or prevocational program | 0.7 | 0.5 | — | — | — | — | — | — | — | — | 1.6 | 0.8 | — | — |
| Voluntary agency (e.g., Easter Seals, United Cerebral Palsy) | — | 1.7 | 1.7 | 1.4 | 1.0 | 0.2 | 0.3 | — | 0.4 | 1.2 | 1.2 | 1.1 | 0.4 | 0.8 |
| Other | 14.2 | 9.4 | 5.4 | 3.2 | 2.5 | 1.3 | 1.7 | 14.7 | 9.3 | 6.7 | 2.3 | 2.3 | 0.8 | 1.7 |
| **Total** | **99.9** | **100.0** | **99.8** | **100.0** | **99.9** | — | — | **100.1** | **100.1** | **100.0** | **100.0** | **99.8** | — | — |

*Note.* Missing data are due to changing employment categories on the various administrations of the surveys. Recoding of additional settings from the "Other" category to existing alternatives may explain the decline in that category. For this reason, small differences in the percentages over time should be interpreted with care. The percentages contained in this report, with the exception of the demographic and educational information, represent only the individuals who responded to the AOTA Member Data Survey. They do not include the occupational therapy personnel who chose not to answer and return the survey. Adapted from *1990 Member Data Survey* and *2000 Member Data Survey* by American Occupational Therapy Association, Member Services, 1990 and 2000, Rockville (1990)/Bethesda (2000), MD: Author.

# The Future

The health care system is at a crossroads. The public and private sectors must deal with changing conditions. The public is demanding accountability for and outcomes from health care. Where do the system and occupational therapy go from here? The following sections describe current trends and projections of outcomes and provide opinions about roles and opportunities for occupational therapists and the support personnel relative to them. These trends can give the occupational therapy manager and occupational therapist a sense of the health care environment for strategic planning purposes.

## Economic Trends

Economists continue to influence the delivery of health care. They believe that the constant threat of competition and the daily struggle providers have to protect their programs may bring out the best in them. The health care industry has adopted the concepts and the practices basic to competition, and the government is stimulating competition to control costs. Government spending currently accounts for 45% of total health costs (Andersen et al., 2001). This level of government spending means that competitive programs will flourish and those not able to keep pace in the marketplace will fail. A competitive market can be described as a social arrangement whereby life is made difficult for providers so that consumers will have access to reasonably priced services. More mergers will occur as health networks are established, and there will be a much greater emphasis on HMOs, which try to limit costs by being paid on a capitation basis (Andersen et al., 2001).

Consumers themselves have a direct financial effect on health care, including occupational therapy services. Copayments require them to pay a portion of health care costs out-of-pocket. It will be very important to keep occupational therapy services defined in a way that consumers and third-party payers will be eager to purchase them.

## Cost Containment

Since the early 1980s, the costs of medical care items have risen fivefold, whereas the cost of other items in the Consumer Price Index (CPI) tripled. The disparity between the rise in medical care costs and the cost of other expenditures has decreased in the past few years. For example, between 1995 and 1998, medical prices rose 10%, only 3% more than the rise in the CPI as a whole (Andersen et al., 2001).

From 1960 to 1994, expenditures for health care rose from 5.3% of the gross domestic product to 13.9% (Burner & Waldo, 1995; Levit et al., 1994). However, from 1994 to 1997, the health care expenditures decreased to 13.5% (Andersen et al., 2001). The Centers for Medicare and Medicaid Services, formerly HCFA, has predicted that health care expenditures will increase to 16.2% in 2008. The spiraling costs generated proposals for health care reform and many containment practices, including

- Alternatives to inpatient care such as ambulatory or outpatient care;
- Self-insurance;
- Greater emphasis on utilization review (i.e., independent review of providers' performance to validate quality of care);
- Adherence to DRGs;
- Elimination of redundancy in services;
- Formation of medical service alliances;
- The merging of insurance providers, hospitals, and health care organizations; and
- The range of utilization control tools known as managed care.

Several of the proposals have already been implemented, and health care in the United States is in a state of change.

These cost-containment practices—managed care, in particular—are having a profound effect on organizational structures and, in turn, on clinical practice. To contain costs and compete successfully for managed care contracts, provider organizations are compressing their structures, cutting their staffs, and reorganizing their way of doing business. The following sections highlight the ramifications of these changes.

### Emphasis on Case Managers Who Control Services

Case managers emerged in the mid-1990s and have become a central force in the delivery of health care services. "Case management evolved in order to maximize health care expenditures by allocating resources to the most appropriate and effective care" (Fisher, 1995, p. 1). The external case manager, an employee of a managed care company, functions as a watchdog or a medical ombudsman, coordinating the care received by the company's members or policyholders—typically, the most expensive cases. External case managers are usually registered nurses or social workers (Weiner & de Lissovoy, 1993). They are expected to control the cost of services and the length of services, in the context of the most appropriate outcome (Fisher, 1995). The internal case manager functions as a liaison between clinical staff members and the external case manager. This person is usually a clinician and, frequently, a practitioner providing services to the patient whose case he or she is managing. Internal case managers rarely control the cost of services; their role is to explain the need for the services (Fisher, 1995).

External case managers, not physicians or clinicians, are deciding how much of a specific service a patient will receive. Occupational therapy managers and occupational therapists are finding themselves "negotiating, arguing, and justifying their services" to external case managers (Freda, 1995, p. 1). Moreover, these case managers are requiring frequent progress reports for their patients and, in many situations, will authorize only a few sessions at a time. Continuation of clinical services will depend on the actual progress of the patient toward the goals that the case manager feels are appropriate

(Freda, 1995). On any given case, the occupational therapy manager or occupational therapist must understand the external case manager's perspective and responsibility and collaborate with him or her to ensure that both parties achieve their objectives. In addition, occupational therapy managers and occupational therapists are also finding themselves (a) interacting with internal case managers where they must collaborate or (b) taking on the role themselves for which they must learn new skills.

### Shorter Lengths of Stay in Hospitals and More Delivery of Services Outside the Traditional Hospital

Alternative services are not just in outpatient facilities and homes but, of late, in day treatment programs and designated subacute care beds. As noted earlier, this shift represents an opportunity for occupational therapy and for the rehabilitation field in general.

### An Increase in Maximized Interventions

Health care organizations are overlapping several clients' treatments to maximize the number of interventions per hour. In addition, they are increasing the mix of group and individual treatment sessions (Freda, 1998).

### A Much Greater Use of Less Expensive Aides and Technicians in Occupational Therapy Departments

The number of professional staff members relative to the number of nonprofessional staff members is decreasing, and professional staff members are doing more supervising than before. To control costs, organizations are asking occupational therapy assistants to take on more responsibilities. In some settings, occupational therapists provide off-site supervision while an occupational therapy assistant carries out the intervention. Another cost-cutting measure is to have occupational therapists teach caregivers (e.g., family members) to carry out certain services that do not call for professional or paraprofessional skills. The more widespread use of aides and technicians is requiring managers and therapists to develop statements of appropriate competencies, improve the orientation given to new personnel, and plan as well as carry out in-service training for support personnel already on the job. "Clear, definitive boundaries and role delineation are needed to guarantee quality care" (Freda, 1995, p. 2). Moreover, all the models, old and new, call for careful collaboration among personnel and appropriate supervision by occupational therapists and occupational therapy assistants (AOTA, 1995a, 1995b).

### A Growing Need to Enhance Supervisory Skills

The increased reliance on aides and technicians requires therapists to enhance their competence in supervision, particularly, their ability to recognize when they should intervene in treatment or reassess a patient's condition. They must also enhance their competence in documentation.

### Increasingly Specific Expectations for Documentation

Documentation must "be timely, [be] integrated for multiple services, be functionally oriented, speak to specific goal attainment, give a specific plan and time line for goal attainment, [and] give a very accurate 'snapshot' of the patient" (Freda, 1995, p. 3). Critical pathways, or care maps, have thus become an essential type of record. They indicate the course of patient treatment on a timeline, with an outcome orientation and prompts for multidisciplinary staff members to perform certain interventions so that costs are contained and quality, as defined by the consumers, is assured (Underwood, 1995). The pathways, or maps, provide the opportunity to record variances from the expected course of treatment. "They also furnish managed care companies [with] very clear information on the product they are considering purchasing and what can be expected in a predetermined length of time" (Freda, 1995, p. 3).

### Increasing Demands on Occupational Therapy
### Managers and Occupational Therapists

All this change requires that occupational therapy managers in particular be aware of the many changes occurring in health care. They must organize staff members to respond with careful client evaluation, planning, and service delivery. The competitive market plan guarantees that costs will continue to be the topic of debate in health care delivery. On a daily basis, occupational therapy managers and occupational therapists must be cognizant of the cost considerations for patients as well as clients and employers. Consumers and insurers will continue to scrutinize the types of diagnoses rendered, the types of treatments and evaluations provided, to whom they are provided, the settings in which they are provided, the duration of treatments, and the effectiveness of treatments to bring about functional performance. They will be asking the question, What can be expected from this expenditure?

   To provide information on the importance of their services, occupational therapy managers and occupational therapists must integrate concepts about expectations for a patient's quality improvement into daily activities and must document program effectiveness. They must use standard and reliable measures to show functional changes in the occupational performance of patients and clients. In addition, occupational therapists should use current research to support their intervention strategies, and more occupational therapists should begin to conduct research studies within their practices. Mere generalizations about occupational performance will not demonstrate the necessity for services.

### More Adjustments to Occur in Professional Support Systems

Because of the heightened expectations for productivity, therapists are busier than they were before. To be successful, they need support from the various systems within the organization—for example, adequate space for the increased number of patients therapists must see at the same time and orientation for patients to the new models of service delivery (Freda, 1995).

*Increased Emphasis on Wellness*

With cost containment as a mandate for the health care industry, the philosophy of wellness is becoming increasingly important to all in the health care equation: consumers, providers, and the federal government. If people stay well, everyone benefits. This emphasis is consistent with occupational therapy's goal of optimal function in occupational performance areas.

## Inclusion of Occupational Therapy Services in Managed Care Plans

During the past two decades, the number of privately insured Americans covered by managed care plans has increased steadily. In 1992, HMOs and PPOs covered about 40% of the U.S. population (U.S. Bureau of the Census, 1994), and in 1993, HMOs, PPOs, and POS plans held 51% of the market among insured people (Health Insurance Association of America, 1994). Between 1990 and 1999, the number of people enrolled in HMOs increased by 145%. By 1997, 33% of employees received their health care benefits through HMOs, 40% received their benefits through PPOs, and 27% paid a fee for service (Andersen et al., 2001).

One of the major goals of managers in managed care organizations is to cut costs, and a strategy for reducing costs is utilization review. Utilization review involves the "evaluation of the necessity, appropriateness, and efficiency of the use of health care services, procedures, and facilities" (Pohly, 1997) and "has become the standard method by which payers monitor provider performance" (Foto & Swanson, 1993, p. 123).

In addition to utilization review, managed care systems cut costs by encouraging or requiring their enrollees to use selected providers. Unfortunately, some managed care organizations and health insurers attempt to save additional money by engaging in discriminatory practices that deny consumers rightful access to a variety of health professionals, including occupational therapists. Fortunately, some proposals for health care reform would broaden managed care coverage in both enrollment and service, and all reforms should prohibit arbitrary exclusion of entire classes or types of professionals from provider panels and networks. Reforms should also require managed care organizations to meet specific criteria to ensure a sufficient number, mix, and distribution of health care providers within their networks to meet the diverse needs of consumers and to give consumers the option of choosing certain specialists as their gatekeepers within the health plan (Somers & Browne, 1994, p. 3).

To provide improved managed care, insurance companies and health care providers have begun consolidating ("Blue Shield, Unihealth," 1993). Financial coverage from Medicare, Medicaid, HMOs, PPOs, and other private group insurance plans is accepted by major rehabilitation centers throughout the country. To manage catastrophic conditions such as head or spinal cord injuries, managed care industries are setting up their own rehabilitation programs. In the late 1990s, some of the major rehabilitation organizations have become linked contractually to the insurance industry or were replaced by facilities directly managed by the insurer.

Occupational therapists and other health care professionals are competing for a shrinking health care dollar. To fit with the current cost-cutting philosophy of managed care organizations, occupational therapy managers and occupational therapists must prove that their products are both essential and cost-effective to the hospital, the physician, the client, and business and industry. Improving function, which has long been the mission of occupational therapy, is now also being used by other professionals in the documentation they submit to receive third-party payment. Thus, occupational therapists must better explain what their profession involves and pinpoint their area of expertise so their services continue to be used. Otherwise, consumers may look to other, more cost-effective, but not necessarily better, sources of health care. Increasing the public's awareness of the varied services of occupational therapy will aid in marketing those services. Educating the government is equally important. One way to increase government awareness is to write to legislators explaining the mission of occupational therapy and the importance of including it in any comprehensive health care plan (Scott & Somers, 1992).

**Cross-Training Initiatives**
Providing health care requires a large number of personnel. As Appendix 3.A indicates, there are close to 200 occupations in health care, including many professions. New ones seem to appear continually because of innovative technology and advances in procedures that require additional specialized skills. The practice of cross-training is being used as one way manage the plethora of professions and skills. *Cross-training* is the preparation of a person in one profession to perform skills typically associated with another profession. A multi-skilled therapist from one profession has established competence in specific skills sets usually associated with another profession.

As indicated earlier, current workforce shortages and economic pressures have precipitated a growing movement by hospitals and other providers to use more aides and other noncredentialed personnel in the delivery of services. There are also efforts or proposals to develop cross-training programs, and state hospital associations and others are pressing state legislatures to deregulate practice acts, which apply to the health care professionals the industry employs. Initiatives along these lines could range from amendments to practice acts that would relax requirements for supervision of personnel to proposals for much broader modification of licensure laws—substituting some form of institutional licensure, or credentialing of a facility—that would allow the facility's administration to determine necessary staff qualifications and composition. These efforts would seriously threaten the legal framework that state associations and AOTA have constructed over the past two decades (Somers & Browne, 1994).

A white paper published by AOTA, *Occupational Therapy and Cross Training Initiatives,* responds to initiatives at institutional, local, state, and national levels. It proposes limiting the scope of cross-training to "(a) certified occupational therapy practitioners who are learning skills typically associated with other professions; and (b) certified [occupational therapy] practitioners who are teaching occupational therapy skills to others" (AOTA, Intercommission Council, 1995, p. 1).

## Additional Payment Sources

In the past, rehabilitation organizations and professionals expected payment from medical insurance providers. This practice will continue to be true for chronic medical problems causing disability. However, other disabling conditions are the result of work, home, and automobile accidents, which are covered by liability insurance. The insurance industry has recognized the cost–benefit potential of comprehensive models of rehabilitation that help a person acquire skills to function at a community level and become employed. This recognition has been the impetus for occupational therapists to move out of the medical model and provide their services in a variety of environments. The percentage of occupational therapists working in community-based settings is increasing, especially in settings such as home health agencies, outpatient clinics, private practice (self-employed), school systems, and skilled nursing and intermediate care facilities (Scaffa, 2001).

## Work-Related Health Care Trends

Work-related injuries in the United States have increased to epidemic proportions in the past decade. In the coming decade, business will spend billions of dollars on medical expenses, disability compensation, and lost productivity. Examples of growing work-related injuries include carpal tunnel syndrome and repetitive motion injury. Costs associated with these injuries can be controlled through the use of ergonomics and management strategies. "Ergonomics focuses on humans and their interactions with the environment" (Rice, 1999, p. 10). It is also "the study of work performance with an emphasis on worker safety and productivity" (p. 9). Occupational therapists use ergonomic principles to provide products such as educational programs and worksite analysis not only to rehabilitate workers with illness or injury but also to assist business and industry in organizing and designing the workplace to prevent costly accidents and illnesses. Occupational therapists have been active in designing and carrying out work injury prevention programs in collaboration with managers and employees. Outcomes measures from successful programs can be used as a marketing strategy to validate the efficacy of occupational therapy.

## Trends in the Application of Technology

The capability of advanced medical technology to save and extend the lives of people who have sustained injuries or illnesses such as stroke, traumatic brain injury (TBI), and spinal cord injury has changed the rehabilitation population that occupational therapists serve. To optimize the functional performance of people with disabilities, occupational therapists must be knowledgeable and proficient in using and integrating basic and complex technology (Burwell, 2001; Hammel, 1993).

The rehabilitation field is benefiting from major technological advances. For example, the use of interactive driving simulators that assess the driving abilities of people with impairments (e.g., from stroke, aging) together with adaptive driving equipment have become marketable. Other forms of technology are also being researched to determine which motions contribute to the development of cumulative trauma disorders. This information may prove invaluable for preventive health care in high-risk populations. The use of computer applications, environmental adaptations, and implanted computers to control motions and bodily functions has increased. For example, assistive devices such as an environmental control unit can improve quality of life for people with a high spinal-cord lesion. In addition, technological devices such as word prediction software and devices that produce digitized or synthesized speech can enhance a person's ability to communicate and interact with others (Burwell, 2001).

Occupational therapy managers and occupational therapists must stay informed about and be involved in research that links technology to occupational performance. One way to meet this obligation is to join AOTA's Technology Special Interest Section. For people who are interested in becoming certified as assistive technology practitioners, a professional certification program is offered through the Rehabilitation Engineering and Assistive Technology Society of North America (Burwell, 2001). Another avenue to stay informed is the Internet, for example, using the World Wide Web, e-mail, newsgroups, and mailing lists, to access resources and information from different organizations around the world (Lazzaro, 2001).

## Recognition for Occupational Therapy in Health Care

In a competitive environment, a successful strategy is to streamline efforts and direct them to doing the best job possible. For occupational therapists and occupational therapy assistants, this approach means helping patients and clients (a) to acquire the skills they need to function at their maximum level and (b) to return to a degree of independence with a choice of acceptable options in performing everyday activities. What occupational therapy does must be very visible and easily marketable (see chapter 7, Marketing). Occupational therapy will have to be described as products—for example, in terms of driving programs, work evaluations, seating and mobility clinics, and life skills programs. These labels will make the services easier to understand and will assist purchasers in understanding the results.

Society is demanding accountability for its dollars. The services that occupational therapists offer to the health care system are gaining increased recognition for many reasons, which are described in the following sections.

### More Acceptance of Disabling Conditions

The public is more accepting of the roughly 20% of Americans who have disabling conditions. AOTA and occupational therapists were pivotal in the passage and implementation of the 1990 Americans with Disabilities Act.

### Increasing Consequences of Chronic Disease

Chronic disease is responsible for the death of more than 1.7 million people in the United States. Cardiovascular disease and cancer are the leading killers, causing two-thirds of these deaths. Treatment of these diseases accounts for "70% of the $1 trillion spent on health care each year" (Centers for Disease Control and Prevention, 2000). In addition, 1 out of every 10 Americans may experience major limitations in everyday living as a consequence of chronic disabling conditions such as arthritis and diabetes.

### Increased Need for Intervention Related to TBI

TBI has become a social problem, and rehabilitation for TBI requires occupational therapy intervention. Each year, an estimated 1.5 million Americans sustain a TBI. Of these, 230,000 are hospitalized and survive; 80,000–90,000 experience a resulting long-term disability (Division of Acute Care, Rehabilitation Research, and Disability Prevention et al., 2001). The estimated annual cost of direct medical care (acute care and rehabilitation service) for all people in the United States who sustain a TBI is $48.3 billion (Agency for Health Care Policy and Research, 1998).

### Growing Elderly Population

As the current population ages, occupational therapists and occupational therapy assistants will continue providing programs to increase independence and maintain function in the elderly population, thus decreasing the costs of long-term health management. In 2000, people 65 years old or older constituted 12.4% of the nation's population. By 2020, it is estimated that 25% of the population will be older than age 60. (Centers for Disease Control and Prevention, 2000; U.S. Bureau of the Census, 2001).

### Increased Awareness of Needs Related to Atypical Cases

The change to a PPS has raised the consciousness of all providers to the fact that some people do not fit within the norm for care and that society has a responsibility to them.

### Increased Occurrence of Cumulative Trauma Disorders and Chronic Back Problems

Occupational therapists and occupational therapy assistants have become more active in the workplace because of the increased incidence of cumulative trauma disorders (e.g., carpal tunnel syndrome) and chronic back problems. The U.S. Department of Labor (2001) revealed that, in 1999, musculoskeletal problems accounted for more than 580,000 of the 1,700,000 cases in which employees missed from 1 to 30 or more days of work. The department also reported that repetitive motion was the source of many of these cases, with close to 30,000 workers diagnosed with carpal tunnel syndrome, 15,000 having tendonitis, and more than 50,000 citing soreness or pain as the reason they missed work. Overall productivity in the workplace is affected by this quantity of workers missing days of work.

*Increased Homeless Population*

Although the number of people experiencing homelessness in the United States is difficult to determine, Burt (2000), relying on data from the 1996 census, reported that at
least 2.3 million adults are likely to experience homelessness during the course of a year.
Recent data suggest that, with the current economic situation, homelessness and hunger
are on the rise (Lowe, Slater, Welfey, & Hardie, 2001). Occupational therapists and
occupational therapy assistants can help improve the quality of life of people who are
homeless by addressing areas such as self-care, social skills, money management, time
management, nutrition, leisure, and productivity (Westermeyer, 2001a).

*Growing Focus on Wellness*

The health care industry and the public are becoming more aware of the advantages
in health care approaches that are based on wellness. Health promotion, wellness, and
prevention are values inherent in the practice of occupational therapy.

## Opportunities in Occupational Therapy

The role of occupational therapy may imminently undergo even greater changes than
it has so far in its evolution. This time in our history is a very important one for occupational therapy. With the expansion of home health care organizations, the increased
role of skilled nursing facilities as rehabilitation settings for the elderly population, the
establishment of comprehensive outpatient rehabilitation facilities, and employers'
emphasis on returning people who have had injuries to gainful employment, the need
for occupational therapy services is expected to grow. Health care organizations need
occupational therapy services to increase and maintain their market share. The profession must respond with confidence that it is giving the people it serves the opportunity
to gain meaningful lives. The situation today is similar to that during the moral treatment movement when the founders of occupational therapy sought to bring human-
ness and a new morality to a system that did not place an acceptable level of effort on
supporting human potential.

Although occupational therapy's development has not been easy, the profession is
now ready to assume a responsible role in offering support and direction as the health
care system struggles to be effective. Occupational therapists and occupational therapy
assistants must understand why assuming this role is difficult, and they must realize
that, with specific knowledge and skills and with a strong commitment to the profession's potential contribution, patients and clients and society as a whole will benefit.

According to the AOTA (2002b), the top emerging practice areas include school
violence prevention, design and accessibility consultation and home modification,
driver rehabilitation training, ergonomics consultation, health and wellness consultation, low-vision services, and assistive technology. Occupational therapists are beginning to capitalize on trends in emerging practice areas by taking an idea and turning it
into a successful business.

According to AOTA's 2000 Member Compensation Survey, 19% of occupational therapists were self-employed in 2000. These are therapists who are paid either on a contractual basis or directly by their client or their client's agent. Of these therapists, 11% report that they are self-employed on a full-time basis and 8.7% on a part-time basis. According to the survey, "the percentage of OTs who are self-employed has remained relatively constant since 1997, ending the declines seen since 1990. The percentage of self-employed OTAs, however, has dropped noticeably since the 1997 survey, down to 7.4% from a peak of more than 11%" (AOTA, 2000b, p. 19).

Most (68.1%) of the self-employed occupational therapists classify themselves as independent contractors or solo practitioners. Those in the next largest group (17.8%) classify themselves as running a multispeciality group practice. Of all the self-employed occupational therapists, 56.1% described the legal structure of their practice as a sole proprietorship.

## Conclusion

The health care industry has become the subject of scrutiny by the government and the public for the following reasons:
- Rising costs
- A growing emphasis on evidence-based practice and accountability
- A lack of services to meet specific needs
- An imbalance of services for different populations of the society
- Advances in medical technology.

In the past, the health care system was described in terms of health problems. Today, health care is cast in economic terms.

The basis for much of the government's involvement in health care goes back to the concept of the right to health. Related to this concept is the matter of ethics. Increasingly, limits may be placed on health services for moral and economic reasons as ethical issues are raised about the technology available to create, maintain, and prolong life.

The federal government has made many significant contributions to health care since the mid-1940s through its support of construction of facilities, training of personnel, and planning of health systems. By the early 1970s, the government was acutely aware of the need to control costs, and several pieces of major legislation followed. A new system of payment for hospital services to Medicare beneficiaries was introduced that has had a profound effect on the health care field.

Organizations providing care have diversified greatly. The free-standing hospital has become vulnerable to financial loss. This situation has led to the formation of large health networks linking individual facilities that represent only one of several related corporate activities. Along with these phenomena have come integrated delivery systems, which "usually involve a significant degree of integration between payer and providers" (Weiner & de Lissovoy, 1993, p. 94). These delivery systems also involve managed care, which is not only a synonym for all kinds of integrated delivery systems but also a term used to denote "the entire range of utilization control tools that are applied to manage the practices of physicians and others, regardless of the setting in which they practice" (p. 97). The three major types of integrated delivery systems operating in today's health care market are HMOs, PPOs, and POS plans. In addition to these systems, public health programs are operating that are primarily concerned with preventing disease through public programs but, increasingly, are providing medical care to individual patients through neighborhood health centers.

The health care industry has adopted the concepts and the practices basic to competition, and the government is stimulating competition to control costs. Cost-containment practices—managed care, in particular—are having a profound effect on organizational structures and, in turn, on clinical practice.

Providing health care requires a large number of personnel. The industry now has close to 200 occupations, including many professions. Data on the supply and the distribution of occupational therapists and occupational therapy assistants indicate that the profession continues to expand. However, the growth has not kept pace with the demand. Shortages are evident in certain geographic areas and practice settings.

On a daily basis, occupational therapy managers and occupational therapists must be cognizant of cost considerations for patients, clients, and employers. To provide information on the importance of their services, occupational therapy managers and occupational therapists must integrate quality improvement concepts into daily activities and document program effectiveness. They must use standard and reliable measures to show functional changes in the occupational performance of patients and clients.

This time is a very important one for occupational therapy. The profession must respond with confidence that it is giving the people it serves the opportunity to gain meaningful lives. The profession is now ready to assume a responsible role in offering support and direction to the health care system.

## References

Agency for Health Care Policy and Research. (1998, December 2). Rehabilitation for traumatic brain injury: Summary, evidence report/technology assessment: Number 2. Retrieved March 13, 2002, from http://ww.ahcpr.gov/clinic/epcsums/tbisumm.htm

Allied Health Professions Personnel Training Act of 1966, Pub. L. No. 89–751, 80 Stat. 1222–1240.

American Hospital Association. (1994). *Guide to the health care field*. Chicago: Author.

American Occupational Therapy Association. (1995a). Guide for supervision of occupational therapy personnel. *American Journal of Occupational Therapy, 49,* 1027–1028.

American Occupational Therapy Association. (1995b). Use of occupational therapy aides in occupational therapy practice [Position paper]. *American Journal of Occupational Therapy, 49,* 1023–1025.

American Occupational Therapy Association. (2000a). *2000 member data survey.* Bethesda, MD: Author.

American Occupational Therapy Association. (2000b). *Member compensation survey: Final report.* Bethesda, MD: Author.

American Occupational Therapy Association. (2002a). ACOTE January 2002 accreditation action. Retrieved February 22, 2002, from http://www.aota.org/ nonmembers/area 13

American Occupational Therapy Association. (2002b). *Emerging practice areas.* Retrieved February 22, 2002, from http://www.aota.org/members/area7/index.asp?PLACE=/members/area7/index.asp

American Occupational Therapy Association, Ad Hoc Commission on Occupational Therapy Manpower. (1983–84). *Occupational therapy manpower: A plan for progress.* Rockville, MD: Author.

American Occupational Therapy Association, Intercommission Council. (1995). *White paper: Occupational therapy and cross training initiatives.* Bethesda, MD: Author.

Americans with Disabilities Act of 1990, Pub. L. No. 101–336, 42 U.S.C. § 12101.

Andersen, R. M., Rice, T. H., & Kominski, G. F. (2001). *Changing the U.S. health care system* (2nd ed.). San Francisco: Jossey-Bass.

Baum, C. M. (1992). The evolution of the U.S. health care system. In J. Bair & M. Gray (Eds.), *The occupational therapy manager* (pp. 1–25). Rockville, MD: American Occupational Therapy Association.

Bloom, G. (1994). Ethics. In K. Jacobs & M. Logigian (Eds.), *Functions of a manager in occupational therapy* (pp. 51–66). Thorofare, NJ: Slack.

Blue Shield, Unihealth plan giant merger. (1993, June 29). *Los Angeles Times,* p. A1.

Burner, S. T., & Waldo, D. R. (1995, Summer). National health expenditure projections, 1994–2005 [DataView]. *Health Care Financing Review, 16,* 221–242.

Burt, M. (2000, February 1). *America's homeless II: Populations and services.* Retrieved February 27, 2002, from http://www.urban.org/housing/homeless/numbers/sld002.htm

Burwell, C. (2001). The apprentice: A primer for assistive technology in the real world. Retrieved February 15, 2002, from http://www.geocities.com/ at_apprentice/index.html

Carr, S. (1993). The COTA heritage. In S. Ryan (Ed.), *The certified occupational therapy assistant* (2nd ed., pp. 21–32). Thorofare, NJ: Slack.

Centers for Disease Control and Prevention. (2000). *Unrealized prevention opportunities: Reducing the health and economic burden of chronic disease.* Retrieved February 26, 2002, from http://www.cdc.gov/nccdphp/upo/intro.htm

Centers for Medicare and Medicaid Services. Retrieved February 2, 2002 from http://www.hcfa.gov/stats/nhe-oact/tables/tl.htm and http://www.hcfa.gov/stats/nhe-oact/tables.chart.htm

Chapman, A. R. (1993). *Exploring a human rights approach to health care reform.* Washington, DC: American Association for the Advancement of Science.

Chapman, B., & Talmedge, J. (1971, January). The evolution of the right to health concept in the United States. *The Pharos,* pp. 30–51.

Christiansen, C., & Baum, C. (Eds.). (1991). *Occupational therapy: Overcoming human performance deficits.* Thorofare, NJ: Slack.

Community Mental Health Centers Act of 1963, Pub. L. No. 88–164, Title II, 77 Stat. 290.

Comprehensive Health Manpower Training Act of 1971, Pub. L. No. 92–157, Title I, §§ 101–110, 85 Stat. 431–461.

DeJong, G., & Sutton, J. (1994, November 23). *REHAB 2000: The evolution of medical rehabilitation in American health care.* Paper presented at the National Rehabilitation Hospital Research Center, Washington, DC.

Division of Acute Care, Rehabilitation Research, and Disability Prevention; National Center for Injury Prevention and Control; Centers for Disease Control and Prevention; & U.S. Department of Health and Human Services. (2001, December). *Traumatic brain injury in the United States: A report to Congress.* Retrieved February 27, 2002, from http://www.cdc.gov/ncipc/pub-res/tbicongress.htm
(Note: These TBI statistics were also listed at http://www.cdc.gov/ncipc/dacrrdp/tbi.htm with the request that they not be published elsewhere without the approval of the CDC.)

*The DRG handbook: Comparative clinical and financial standards.* (1994). Cleveland, OH: HCIA.

Elwood, T. (1991). A view from Washington. *Journal of Allied Health, 20,* 47–62.

Fisher, T. (1995). *The case manager in case management.* Unpublished manuscript, Columbia Healthcare.

Foto, M., & Swanson, G. (1993). Utilization review and managed care. *Rehab Management* (Marina del Ray, CA: CurAnt Communications), 6, 123–125.

Freda, M. (1995). *Managed care's impact on delivery of occupational therapy.* Unpublished manuscript.

Freda, M. (1998). Facility-based practice settings. In M. C. Neistadt & E. B. Crepeau (Eds.), *Willard and Spackman's occupational therapy* (9th ed., pp. 803–817). Philadelphia: Lippincott Williams & Wilkins.

Hammel, J. (1993). What should occupational therapy practitioners know about technology? *Technology Special Interest Section Newsletter, 3*(3), 1–2.

Health Amendments Act of 1956, Pub. L. No. 84–911, Ch. 871, 70 Stat. 923.

Health Insurance Association of America. (1994). *Source book of health insurance data.* Washington, DC: Author.

Health Maintenance Organization Act of 1973, Pub. L. No. 93–222, 87 Stat. 914.

Health Manpower Act of 1968, Pub. L. No. 90–490, 82 Stat. 773.

Health Professions Educational Assistance Act of 1963, Pub. L. No. 88–129, 77 Stat. 164.

Health Professions Educational Assistance Act Amendments of 1965, Pub. L. No. 89–290, 79 Stat. 1052.

Health Training Improvement Act of 1970, Pub. L. No. 91–519, 84 Stat. 1342.

*HMO fact sheet.* (1985, April). Bethesda, MD: U.S. Public Health Service, Office of Health Maintenance Organizations.

Hopkins, H. L., & Smith, H. D. (Eds.). (1994). *Willard and Spackman's occupational therapy* (8th ed.). Philadelphia: Lippincott.

Hospital Survey and Construction Act of 1946 (Hill–Burton Act), Pub. L. No. 79–725, Title VI of the Public Health Service Act, Ch. 958, 60 Stat. 1040.

Individuals with Disabilities Education Act of 1997, Pub. L. No. 105–17.

InterStudy Publications. (2001). *The PPO directory and performance report, 2.0.* St. Paul, MN: Author.

Lazzaro, J. J. (2001). *Adaptive technologies for learning and work environments.* (2nd ed.). Chicago: American Library Association.

*Legislative Indexing Vocabulary (LIV) Library of Congress Thesauri.* Retrieved February 2, 2002, from http://www.loc.gov/lexico/servlet/lexico

Levit, K. R., Sensenig, A. L., Cowan, C. A., Lazenby, H. C., McDonnell, P. A., Won, D. K. et al. (1994, Fall). National health expenditures, 1993. *Health Care Financing Review, 16,* 247–292.

Loomis, C. (1994, July 11). The real action in healthcare. *Fortune, 130,* 149.

Lowe, E. T., Slater, A., Welfey, J., & Hardie, D. (2001, December). *A status report on hunger and homelessness in America's cities 2001: A 27-city survey.* Retrieved February 27, 2002, from http://usmayors.org

Mental Retardation Facilities Construction Act and the Community Mental Health Centers Act of 1963, Pub. L. No. 88–164.

National Health Planning and Resources Development Act of 1974, Pub. L. No. 93–641, 88 Stat. 2225.

Nichols, L. (1999, January). What price health care quality? *USA Today.*

Nurse Training Act of 1964, Pub. L. No. 88–581, 78 Stat. 908.

Nurse Training Act of 1975, Pub. L. No. 92–158, 85 Stat. 465.

Pohly, P. (1997). *Pam Pohly's net guide: Glossary of terms in managed health care.* Retrieved February 13, 2002, from http://www.pohly.com/terms_u.html

Public Health Service Act of 1944, Pub. L. No. 78–410, Ch. 373, 58 Stat. 682.

Quiroga, V. A. M. (1995). *Occupational therapy: The first thirty years, 1900–1930.* Bethesda, MD: American Occupational Therapy Association.

Rice, V. (1999). Ergonomics: An introduction. In K. Jacobs & C. Bettencourt (Eds.), *Ergonomics for therapists* (pp. 3–12). Newton, MA: Butterworth-Heinemann.

Rubin, A. (1994a). Clinton's health-care bill. *Congressional Quarterly, 52,* 492–504.

Rubin, A. (1994b). Uncertainty, deep divisions cloud opening of debate. *Congressional Quarterly, 52,* 2344–2353.

Scaffa, M. (Ed.). (2001). *Occupational therapy in community-based practice settings.* Philadelphia: F. A. Davis.

Scott, S., & Somers, F. (1992). Orientation to payment. In J. D. Acquaviva (Ed.), *Effective documentation for occupational therapy* (pp. 5–22). Rockville, MD: American Occupational Therapy Association.

Social Security Administration. (1994). *Social Security bulletin, annual statistical supplement.* Washington, DC: U.S. Government Printing Office.

Social Security Act Amendments of 1972, Pub. L. No. 92–603, 86 Stat. 1329.

Social Security Act Amendments of 1983, Pub. L. No. 98–21, 97 Stat. 65.

Somers, F., & Browne, S. (1994). *Key health care reform issues for 1995 state legislative sessions.* Rockville, MD: American Occupational Therapy Association.

Tax Equity and Fiscal Responsibility Act of 1982, Pub. L. No. 97–248, 96 Stat. 324.

Underwood, R. (1995). *Critical pathways: The OT's role* [Disk version of on-line workshop]. Bethesda, MD: American Occupational Therapy Association.

U.S. Bureau of the Census. (1994, September). *Statistical abstract of the United States* (114th ed.). Washington, DC: U.S. Government Printing Office.

U.S. Bureau of the Census. (2001). *Statistical abstract of the United States* (121st ed.). Washington, DC: U.S. Government Printing Office.

U.S. Department of Labor, Bureau of Labor Statistics. (2001). Cases and demographic characteristics for work-related injuries and illnesses involving days away from work. Retrieved February 26, 2002, from http://stats.bls.gov/lif/oshwc/osh/case/ostb0911.pdf

U.S. Department of Labor, Bureau of Labor Statistics. (2002). *Occupational outlook handbook: 2002–03 edition.* Retrieved February 22, 2002, from http://www.bls.gov/oco/ocos078.htm

U.S. Public Health Service. (ca. 1988). *The Public Health Service: Some historical notes* [PHS Fact Sheet]. Bethesda, MD: Author.

Weiner, J. P., & de Lissovoy, G. (1993, Spring). Razing a tower of Babel: A taxonomy for managed care and health insurance plans. *Journal of Health Politics, Policy, and Law, 18,* 75–103.

Westermeyer, L. (2001a). Implications for OT practitioners. In *Occupational therapy and homelessness: A web based resource.* Retrieved February 27, 2002, from http://www.uic.edu/ahp/OT/occupational_therapy_and_homeles.htm

Westermeyer, L. (2001b). *Occupational therapy: A web-based resource.* Retrieved February 26, 2002, from http://www.uic.edu/ahp/ot/occupational-therapy-and-homeless.htm

## Appendix 3.A  Health Care Occupations.

| Field | Professional Title |
|---|---|
| Basic sciences in the health field | Biochemist |
| | Biological scientist |
| | Biologist |
| | Biophysicist |
| | Chemist |
| | Epidemiologist |
| | Medical scientist |
| | Microbiologist |
| | Physical scientist |
| | Physicist |
| | Wildlife biologist |
| | Zoologist |
| Biomedical engineering | Biomedical engineer |
| Chiropractic | Chiropractor |
| Dentistry and allied services | Dental assistant |
| | Dental hygienist |
| | Dentist |
| | Oral and maxillofacial surgeon |
| | Orthodontist |
| Dietetic and nutritional services | Dietetic technician |
| | Dietitian |
| | Nutritionist |
| Environmental sanitation | Environmental scientist and specialist |
| Food and drug protective services | Food science technician |
| | Food scientist |
| Health education | Health educator |
| Health information | Health Information technician |
| Health technology | Biological technician |
| | Cardiovascular technician |
| | Cardiovascular technologist |
| | Chemical technician |
| | Diagnostic medical stenographer |
| | Health technician |
| | Health technologist |
| | Occupational health and safety specialist |
| | Occupational health and safety technician |
| Medical and clinical laboratory services | Medical and clinical laboratory technician |
| | Medical and clinical laboratory technologist |
| Medical records | Medical records technician |

*(continued)*

**Appendix 3.A**  (*Continued*)

| Field | Professional Title |
| --- | --- |
| Medicine and osteopathy | Anesthesiologist |
| | Family and general practitioner |
| | Internist |
| | Obstetrician and gynecologist |
| | Pediatrician |
| | Physician |
| | Psychiatrist |
| | Surgeon |
| Nursing and related services | Attendant |
| | Home health aide |
| | Licensed practical nurse |
| | Licensed vocational nurse |
| | Nursing aide |
| | Orderly |
| | Registered nurse |
| Occupational therapy | Occupational therapist |
| | Occupational therapy aide |
| | Occupational therapy assistant |
| Opticianry | Optician, dispensing |
| Optometry | Optometrist |
| Orthotic and prosthetic technology | Orthotist |
| | Prosthetist |
| | Prosthodontist |
| Pharmacy | Pharmacist |
| | Pharmacy aide |
| | Pharmacy technician |
| Physical education and training | Athletic trainer |
| Physical therapy | Physical therapist |
| | Physical therapist aide |
| | Physical therapist assistant |
| Physician extenders | Physician assistant |
| | Surgeon technologist |
| Podiatric medicine | Podiatrist |
| Psychology and sociology | Clinical psychologist |
| | Counseling psychologist |
| | Educational psychologist |
| | School psychologist |
| | Psychologist |
| | Social science research assistant |
| | Sociologist |

(*continued*)

**Appendix 3.A** (*Continued*)

| Field | Professional Title |
|---|---|
| Radiologic technology | Nuclear medicine technician |
| | Nuclear medicine technologist |
| | Radiation therapist |
| | Radiologic technician |
| | Radiologic technologist |
| | Recreational therapist |
| Recreational therapy | Respiratory therapist |
| Respiratory therapy | Respiratory therapy technician |
| Social work | Child social worker |
| | Family social worker |
| | Medical and public health social worker |
| | Mental health and substance abuse social worker |
| | School social worker |
| | Social worker |
| Specialized rehabilitation and counseling services | Behavioral disorder counselor |
| | Community and social service specialist |
| | Educational counselor |
| | Marriage and family therapist |
| | Mental health counselor |
| | School counselor |
| | Social and human service assistant |
| | Substance abuse counselor |
| Speech pathology and audiology | Audiologist |
| | Speech and language pathologist |
| Veterinary medicine | Animal scientist |
| | Laboratory animal caretaker |
| | Veterinarian |
| | Veterinary assistant |
| | Veterinary technician |
| | Veterinary technologist |
| Vocational rehabilitation counseling | Rehabilitation counselor |
| | Vocational counselor |
| Miscellaneous health services | Emergency medical technician |
| | Health diagnosing and treating practitioner, all other |
| | Health care support worker |
| | Massage therapist |
| | Medical assistant |
| | Medical equipment preparers |
| | Paramedic |
| | Psychiatric aide |
| | Therapist, all other |

*Note.* Adapted from O*Net Online, 2001, retrieved February 20, 2002, from http://online.onetcenter.org/; and from *The Occupational Outlook Handbook* (2002–2003 ed.), retrieved February 20, 2002, from http://www.bls.gov/oco.

## Appendix 3.B  Selected Programs of the U.S. Public Health Service.

| Program | Function |
|---|---|
| **Substance Abuse and Mental Health Services Administration** | |
| National Institute of Mental Health | Conducts and supports research on mental health, funds training of new researchers, gives technical assistance, and disseminates information |
| National Institute on Alcohol Abuse and Alcoholism | Conducts and supports research on alcohol abuse, funds training of new researchers, gives technical assistance, and disseminates information |
| National Institute on Drug Abuse | Conducts and supports research on drug abuse, gives technical assistance, and disseminates information |
| **Centers for Disease Control and Prevention** | |
| National Center on Birth Defects and Developmental Disabilities | Improves the health and wellness of people with disabilities and offers leadership for prevention of developmental disabilities and birth defects |
| National Center for Chronic Disease Prevention and Health Promotion | Prevents death and disability from chronic disease and promotes healthy personal behaviors |
| National Center for Environmental Health | Prevents and controls death and disease secondary to interactions between people and their environment |
| National Center for Health Statistics | Monitors health of American people, effect of illness and disability, and factors affecting health and nation's health care system |
| National Center for HIV, STD, and TB Prevention | Prevents and controls vaccine-preventable diseases, HIV infection, sexually transmitted diseases, tuberculosis, dental diseases, and introduction of diseases from other countries |
| National Center for Infectious Diseases | Prevents sickness, disability, and death caused by infectious diseases, both around the world and in the United States |
| National Center for Injury Prevention and Control | Prevents and controls nonoccupational injuries |
| National Immunization Program | Prevents illness, disability, and death from vaccine-preventable diseases in adults and children |
| National Institute for Occupational Safety and Health | Prevents workplace-related injuries, illnesses, and premature death from occupational hazards |

*(continued)*

**Appendix 3.B** *(Continued)*

| Program | Function |
|---|---|
| **Food and Drug Administration** | |
| Center for Devices and Radiological Health | Ensures safety of medical devices |
| Center for Biologics Evaluation and Research | Enhances the public health through regulation of biological products: blood, vaccines, therapeutics, and related drugs and devices |
| Center for Drug Evaluation and Research | Assures that safe and effective drugs are available to the American people |
| Center for Food Safety and Applied Nutrition | Ensures the safety of food and color additives, dietary supplements, infant formulas, and medical foods; proper labeling of food and cosmetics; and development of international food standards |
| Center for Veterinary Medicine | Helps humans and other animals by ensuring safe and effective animal health products |
| National Center for Toxicological Research | Conducts peer-reviewed scientific research that supports and anticipates the FDA's current and future regulating needs |
| **Health Resources and Services Administration** | |
| Bureau of Health Professions | Helps to ensure access to quality health care professionals in all geographic areas and to all segments of society |
| Office of Special Programming | Provides leadership and direction in administering the Division of Facilities Compliance and Recovery, Division of Facilities and Loans, Division of Transplantation, State Planning Grants Program, and National Vaccine Injury Compensation Program |
| Federal Office of Rural Health Policy | Develops health care policy for rural America |
| HIV/AIDS Bureau | Provides federal funds for HIV/AIDS care for low-income as well as un- and underinsured individuals |
| Bureau of Primary Health Care | Ensures that underserved and vulnerable people get the health care they need |

*(continued)*

**Appendix 3.B** (*Continued*)

| Program | Function |
| --- | --- |
| Maternal and Child Health | Works in partnership with states, communities, and families to strengthen maternal and child health infrastructure, to ensure the availability and use of medical homes, and to build the knowledge and human resources that will ensure continued improvement in the health, safety, and well-being of the MCH population |
| **National Institutes of Health** | |
| National Library of Medicine | Maintains database on health care |
| 19 specialty institutes | Conduct and support programs of basic and clinical research |
| 7 specialty centers | Support and conduct scientific research |
| **Office of Public Health and Science** | |
| Healthy People 2010 | Challenges individuals, communities, and professionals to take specific steps to ensure that all people enjoy good health |

*Note.* Extracted from *Health Services in the United States* (2nd rev. ed., pp. 149–154), by F. A. Wilson and D. Neuhauser, 1985, Cambridge, MA: Ballinger; *CDC: Centers for Disease Control and Prevention* [Fact sheet], by CDC, 1994, May, Atlanta, GA: Author; and *Public Health Service Alcohol, Drug Abuse, and Mental Health Administration; Public Health Service Centers for Disease Control; Public Health Service Food and Drug Administration; Public Health Service Health Resources and Services Administration; Public Health Service National Institutes of Health;* and *The Public Health Service Today* [Fact sheets], by U.S. Public Health Service, ca. 1988, Bethesda, MD: Author. Fact sheets retrieved February 12, 2002, from the following sites:
— U.S. Department of Health and Human Services, Centers for Disease Control and Prevention, http://www.cdc.gov/aboutcdc.htm
— U.S. Department of Health and Human Services, National Institutes of Health, http://www.nih.gov/icd/
— U.S. Department of Health and Human Services, Office of Public Health and Science, http://www.hhs.gov/agencies/ophs.html/
— U.S. Department of Health and Human Services, Bureau of Health Professions, http://www.bhpr.hrsa.gov/
— U.S. Department of Health and Human Services, U.S. Food and Drug Administration, http://www.fda.gov

## Appendix 3.C  Public Health Programs.

| Focus | Organization and Web Site |
|---|---|
| AIDS/HIV | AIDS.ORG—www.aids.org |
| | AIDS Action—www.aidsaction.org |
| | AIDS Treatment Data Network—www.aidsinfonyc.org/network |
| | AIDS Action Committee—www.aac.org |
| | Children with AIDS Project—www.aidskids.org |
| | Center for AIDS Prevention Studies—www.caps.ucsf.edu |
| | HIV/AIDS Treatment Information Service—www.hivatic.org |
| Aging | Alliance for Aging Research—www.agingresearch.org |
| | American Association for Geriatric Psychiatry—www.aagpga.org |
| | National Institute on Aging—www.nia.nih.gov |
| | U.S. Administration on Aging—www.aoa.gov |
| Alcoholism | Alcoholics Anonymous—www.alcoholics-anonymous.org |
| | AL-ANON Family Group Headquarters—www.al-anon.org |
| | National Council on Alcoholism & Drug Dependency—www.ncadd.org |
| | National Institute on Alcohol Abuse & Alcoholism—www.niaaa.nih.gov |
| Alternative birth | American College of Nurse-Midwives—www.acnm.org |
| | American Nurses Association—www.nursingworld.org |
| | Center for Humane Options in Child Birth Experiences (CHOICE)—www.birthchoice.org |
| | National Association of Childbearing Centers—www.birthcenters.org |
| | Society for Obstetric Anesthesia and Perinatology (SOAP)—www.soap.org |
| Arthritis | Arthritis Foundation—www.arthritis.org |
| | National Center for Chronic Disease Prevention & Health Promotion—www.cdc.gov/nccdphp/ |
| | National Institute of Arthritis & Musculoskeletal & Skin Diseases—www.niams.nih.gov |
| Battered women | Abused Women's Aid in Crisis—www.awaic.org |
| | Family Violence Prevention Fund—www.fvpf.org |
| | National Organization for Women—www.now.org |
| | National Women's Health Information Center—www.4women.gov |
| | Violence Against Women—www.ojp.usdoj.gov/vawo/ |
| | Women in Transition—www.womenintransitioninc.org |
| Blindness, impaired vision | American Academy of Ophthalmology—www.aao.org |
| | American Foundation for the Blind—www.afb.org |
| | National Eye Institute—www.nei.nih.org |
| | National Federation of the Blind—www.nfb.org |
| | Prevent Blindness America—www.preventblindnessamerica.org |

*(continued)*

**Appendix 3.C** (*Continued*)

| Focus | Organization—Web Site |
| --- | --- |
| Burn injuries | American Burn Association—www.ameriburn.org |
| | International Society for Burn Injuries—www.worldburn.org |
| | Phoenix Society—www.phoenix-society.org |
| | Shriner's Hospital for Crippled Children—www.shrinershq.org |
| Cancer | American Association for Cancer Education—www.aaceonline.com |
| | American Cancer Society—www.cancer.org |
| | Breast Cancer Advisory Center—www.rkbcac.org |
| | National Alliance of Breast Cancer Organizations—www.nabco.org |
| | National Cancer Institute—www.nci.nhi.gov |
| Cystic fibrosis | Cystic Fibrosis Foundation—www.cff.org |
| | Cystic Fibrosis Research Inc.—www.cfri.org |
| Deafness, impaired hearing | Acoustical Society of America—www.asa.aip.org |
| | Council for Exceptional Children—www.cec.sped.org |
| | American Society for Deaf Children—www.deafchildren.org |
| | Hear Center—www.thehearcenter.com |
| | National Association of the Deaf—www.nad.org |
| | National Institute of Deafness and Other Communication Disorders—www.nidcd.nih.gov |
| Drug/tobacco abuse | Do It Now Foundation—www.doitnow.org |
| | Families Anonymous—www.familiesanonymous.org |
| | National Clearinghouse for Alcohol & Drug Information—www.health.org |
| | National Institute on Drug Abuse—www.drugabuse.gov/NIDAHome1.html |
| | Office of National Drug Control Policy—www.whitehousedrugpolicy.gov |
| | Office on Smoking and Health—www.cdc.gov/tobacco/ |
| Eye tissue for transplant | Eye Bank Association of America—www.restoresight.org |
| | Lions Club International—www.lionsclubs.org |
| Environmental quality | U.S. Environmental Protection Agency (EPA)—www.epa.gov |
| | National Center for Environmental Health, Centers for Disease Control and Prevention—www.cdc.gov/nceh/ncehhome.htm |
| | National Safety Council—www.nsc.org |
| Family planning | Advocates For Youth—www.advocatesforyouth.org |
| | Americans United for Life Choice—www.unitedforlife.org |
| | Choice—www.choiceusa.org |
| | Family Planning International Assistance—www.plannedparenthood.org/fpia/ |
| | National Abortion Federation—www.prochoice.org |
| | Planned Parenthood Federation of America—www.plannedparenthood.org |

(continued)

**Appendix 3.C** *(Continued)*

| Focus | Organization—Web Site |
| --- | --- |
| | National Family Planning and Reproductive Health Association—www.nfprha.org |
| | March of Dimes Birth Defects Foundation—www.modimes.org |
| | National Council on Family Relations—www.ncfr.org |
| | National Healthy Mothers, Healthy Babies Coalition—www.hmhb.org |
| Genetic services | Brittle Bone Society—www.brittlebone.org |
| | American (Medical Science) Genetics and Molecular Medicine—www.ama-assn.org |
| | National Arthrogryposis Foundation—faraino@bellsouth.net |
| | Learning Disabilities Association of America—www.ldanatl.org |
| | Muscular Dystrophy Association—www.mdausa.org |
| | Spina Bifida Association—www.sbaa.org |
| | Clinical Genetic Services—www.kumc.edu/gec/prof/kugenes.html |
| Hemophilia | American Association of Blood Banks—www.aabb.org |
| | National Hemophilia Foundation—www.hemophilia.org |
| Home health care | National Association for Home Care—www.nahc.org |
| | American Association for Home Care—www.aahomecare.org |
| Homelessness | Administration for Children and Families—www.www.acf.dhhs.gov |
| | Assistant Secretary for Planning and Evaluation—www.aspe.hhs.gov |
| | Freedom From Hunger—www.freefromhunger.org |
| | U.S. Department of Housing and Urban Development—www.hud.gov |
| Hospice care | American Association of Suicidology—www.suicidology.org |
| | Hospice Association of America—www.hospice-america.org |
| | National Hospice and Palliative Care Organization—www.nhpco.org |
| Immunology | American Academy of Allergy, Asthma and Immunology—www.aaaai.org |
| | American College of Allergy, Asthma and Immunology (ACAAI)—www.acaai.org |
| | Immunization Action Coalition—www.immunize.org |
| | National Immunization Program, Centers for Disease Control and Prevention—www.cdc.gov/nip/ |
| Injury and violence | National Youth Violence Prevention Resource Center—www.cdc.gov |
| | National Women's Health Information Center—www.4woman.gov |
| | Administration for Children and Families—www.acf.dhhs.gov |

*(continued)*

**Appendix 3.C** (*Continued*)

| Focus | Organization—Web Site |
|---|---|
| | National Center for Injury Prevention and Control—www.cdc.gov/ncipc/ |
| | National Crime Prevention Council—www.ncpc.org |
| Mental health | Academy of Psychosomatic Medicine—www.apm.org |
| | American Academy of Child and Adolescent Psychiatry—www.aacap.org |
| | American Psychiatric Association—www.psych.org |
| | National Mental Health Services Knowledge Exchange Network, Center for Mental Health Services—www.mentalhealth.org |
| | Center for Mental Health Services, Substance Abuse and Mental Health Services Administration—www.mentalhealth.org/cmhs/ |
| | National Institute of Mental Health, National Institutes of Health—www.nimh.nih.gov |
| Multiple sclerosis | American Red Cross—www.redcross.org |
| | National Multiple Sclerosis Society—www.nmss.org |
| Muscular dystrophy | Muscular Dystrophy Association—www.mdausa.org |
| | Myasthenia Gravis Foundation of America—www.myasthenia.org |
| | National Ataxia Foundation—www.ataxia.org |
| Overweight and obesity | American Obesity Association—www.obesity.org |
| | National Institute of Diabetes and Digestive and Kidney Diseases—www.niddk.nih.gov |
| Pain | American Academy of Pain Management—www.aapainmanage.org |
| | American Academy of Medical Acupuncture—www.medicalacupuncture.org |
| | International Council of Medical Acupuncture and Related Techniques—www.icmart.org |
| | American Chiropractic Association—www.amerchiro.org |
| | National Spinal Cord Injury Foundation—www.spinalcord.org |
| Physical activity | American Heart Association—www.americanheart.org |
| | International Food Information Council Foundation—www.ific.org |
| | National Heart, Lung, and Blood Institute—www.nhlbi.nih.gov |
| Preventive medicine | International Health Evaluation Association—www.ihea.net |
| | National Acupuncture and Oriental Medicine Alliance—www.acuall.org |
| | National Center for Complementary and Alternative Medicine—www.nccam.nih.gov |
| Rehabilitation | Brain Injury Association (BIA)—www.biausa.org |
| | American Academy of Physical Medicine & Rehabilitation—www.aapmr.org |
| | American Deafness and Rehabilitation Association—www.adara.org |

(*continued*)

**Appendix 3.C**  (*Continued*)

| Focus | Organization—Web Site |
| --- | --- |
| | American Occupational Therapy Association—www.aota.org |
| | American Physical Therapy Association—www.apta.org |
| | National Easter Seal Society—www.easter-seals.org |
| Sickle-cell anemia | Sickle Cell Anemia Research Foundation— www.scarf.qpg.com |
| | Sickle Cell Disease Association of America, Inc.— http://sicklecelldisease.org |
| | American Sickle Cell Anemia Association—www.ascaa.org |
| Smoking | American Cancer Society—www.cancer.org |
| | American Heart Association—www.americanheart.org |
| | American Lung Association—www.lungusa.org |
| | American Society of Clinical Oncology—www.asco.org |
| | National Cancer Institute, National Institutes of Health— www.nci.nih.gov |
| Spinal cord injury | American Paraplegia Society—www.apssci.org |
| | American Spinal Injury Association—www.asia-spinalinjury.org |
| | National Easter Seal Society—www.easter-seals.org |
| | National Spinal Cord Injury Association— www.spinalcord.org |
| Sports medicine | American Alliance for Health, Physical Education, Recreation, and Dance—www.aahperd.org |
| | American College of Sports Medicine—www.acsm.org |
| | National Association for Sport and Physical Education— www.aahperd.org/naspe/naspe-main.html |
| | Disabled Sports USA—www.dsusa.org |
| Stroke | American Stroke Association—www.strokeassociation.org |
| | National Stroke Association—www.stroke.org |
| | National Institute of Neurological Disorders and Stroke, National Institutes of Health—www.ninds.nih.gov |
| Sudden infant death syndrome | National Sudden Infant Death Syndrome Resource Center— www.sidscenter.org |
| | National SIDS & Infant Death Program Support Center— http://sids-id-psc.org |
| | SIDS Alliance—http://sidsalliance.org |
| | SIDS Network—http://sids-network.org |
| Traumatic brain injury | National Resource Center on Traumatic Brain Injury— www.neuro.pmr.vcu.edu |
| | Brain Injury Association Inc.—www.biausa.org |
| | Brain Injury Society—www.bisociety.org |

*Note.* Extracted from www.healthypeople.gov and an independent Internet search by the author.

# New Organizational Perspectives

Guy L. McCormack, PhD, OTR/L, FAOTA
Evelyn G. Jaffe, MPH, OTR, FAOTA
William Frey, BSOT, MEd, MHA, PhD

*"Man shapes himself through decisions that shape his environment."*

RENE DUBOS

**Guy L. McCormack, PhD, OTR/L, FAOTA,** has been an educator, researcher, and author for 25 years. He is the founder and chairman of the Master of Occupational Therapy Program at Samuel Merritt College in Oakland, CA. He is currently working as a home health practitioner with the Sutter Visiting Nurses Association and Hospice in Emeryville, CA. In addition to his doctorate in human science, he has received extensive training in traditional Chinese medicine and has many certificates in alternative/complementary forms of intervention.

**Evelyn G. Jaffe, MPH, OTR, FAOTA,** is an assistant professor at Samuel Merritt College. She has been a consultant in occupational therapy for over 35 years, specializing in community mental health, high-risk infants, school-age parents, and primary prevention in the workplace. She earned her master's degree from the School of Public Health at the University of Michigan.

**William Frey, BSOT, MEd, MHA, PhD,** is a professor in the Department of Health Services Administration at Saint Mary's College of California in Moraga. He has been a registered occupational therapist since 1971, is a senior fellow of the Quincy Foundation for Medical Research in San Francisco, and is a fellow of the American College of Healthcare Executives.

## Key Terms and Concepts

### Wellness Health Promotion and Complementary Therapies

**Complementary/alternative medicine (CAM).** Represents a group of diverse interventions and products designed to alleviate symptoms and conditions of dysfunction in conjunction with, or separate from, conventional medicine interventions.

**Disease orientation.** Represents one's perspective or a belief concerning the root cause of a disease.

**Dualism.** The theory that the mind is separate from the body.

**Habit training.** A treatment approach developed by Eleanor Clark Slagle for people with mental illness. It is based on the assumption that behavior is formed by "habit reactions" and that structured physical and mental occupations can overcome undesirable habits and develop socially acceptable behavior.

**Health.** A general condition of the body, mind, and spirit with reference to the fullness of life, a sense of well-being, vigor, vitality, and wholeness.

**Health promotion.** The art and science of helping people change their lifestyles to move toward a state of optimal health.

**Holism.** The view that everything is an integrated whole and has a reality independent of and greater than the sum of its parts. Holism views everything in terms of relationships, patterns of organization, inter-reactions, and processes that combine to form a unified whole.

**Pleasurable ease.** A term coined by Adoft Meyer to describe the state of well-being that is produced by being in harmony with the rhythms of life and through the occupations of work, play, rest, and sleep.

**Prevention.** A process designed to deter illness and disease through healthful actions.

**Reductionism.** The belief that entities of a particular kind are composed of combinations of smaller entities of a basic type. The belief that, to understand a system or organism, it must be broken down into its smallest components to examine how it works as a whole.

**Wellness.** The process of adopting patterns of behavior that lead to life satisfaction through improved physical, emotional, and spiritual well-being.

### Systems Theory in Occupational Therapy

**Closed system.** A system with impermeable boundaries; it does not exchange matter or energy with its environment.

**Dynamic systems theory.** An explanation of how patterns of stability and change emerge in human behavior and, especially, how they influence the dynamics of systems over time.

**Ecological systems theory.** A theory of systems that is based on dynamic interaction among all components of a society.

**Environment and systems analysis.** A form of systems analysis that considers the specific environmental influences on various systems. These influences can be generated by the following kinds of environments:

*Human environment*—individuals who may influence the outcome

*Macroenvironment*—forces in the larger environment

*Microenvironment*—forces close to the issues

*Natural environment*—the particular setting or settings

*Physical environment*—external factors or conditions.

**Feedback.** Information that results from the consequences of the system's output and that is subsequently returned to a system.

**General systems theory.** The construct that change in one part of the system causes inherent change in the total system (von Bertalanffy, 1968).

**Input.** The process by which matter, energy, and information enter the system from the environment.

**Open system.** A system whose organization is characterized by exchanges of energy with the environment.

**Open system theory.** The concept of the exchange of matter with its environment (von Bertalanffy, 1968).

**Output.** The action of the system on the environment as a result of the throughput transformation of input.

**Systems analysis.** The identification and determination of the state of the system; the study and evaluation of all internal and external environmental factors influencing the system.

**Throughput.** The process of transformation of input into another form passing through the organism or system.

## Cultural Perspectives in Occupational Therapy

**Cultural bias.** When beliefs and practices of a different culture are not valued by a dominant culture. A dominant culture makes assumptions about the abilities and motives of the minority culture.

**Cultural competence.** Culturally competent occupational therapists and occupational therapy assistants are aware of their own cultural beliefs and respect the differences that may be held by members of other cultures. Culturally competent occupational therapists and occupational therapy assistants actively challenge their assumptions about human behavior and are actively developing appropriate strategies to work more effectively with clients of different cultures.

**Cultural differences.** Integrated patterns of thoughts, communication, and actions that differ among social groups. Cultural differences do not equate with pathology or inferiority. Differences may be attributed to factors such as ethnicity, race, social class, gender, sexual orientation, religious orientation, age, or disability.

**Culture.** A set of beliefs, values, rules, and social practices that individuals use to construct meaning. This set of guidelines is complex, inherited and, at the same time, emerging.

**Globalization.** The fast-paced integration of markets, policies, technologies, and knowledge around the globe. This process of integration is causing value conflicts and raises questions about how we treat each other.

**World Federation of Occupational Therapists (WFOT).** An international forum for occupational therapists, students, and related organizations to exchange ideas to improve the practice of occupational therapy worldwide.

# Learning Objectives

After completing this chapter, you should be able to do the following:

## Wellness Health Promotion and Complementary Therapies

- Describe the results of national surveys concerning trends on the wellness–illness continuum.
- Discuss reasons for consumer-driven interest in complementary and alternative methods of treatment.
- Evaluate how managed care and federal legislation have altered health care delivery and caused consumers to become disenchanted with the current delivery systems.
- Discuss how occupational therapy has operated in managing services within both the medical model and the wellness health promotion model.
- Describe the health-related trends in the elderly population.
- Describe the *Healthy People 2010* document and how it may affect health promotion in the next decade.

■ Understand the value of documents produced by World Health Organization, the U.S. Department of Health and Human Services, and the Centers for Disease Control and Prevention.

## Systems Theory in Occupational Therapy

■ Describe the basic principles of general systems theory.

■ Describe the four components of a systems approach.

■ Identify concepts of systems theory and a systems approach to the development of occupational therapy services or programs.

■ Identify the characteristics of a systems approach as used by the occupational therapy manager, consultant, and entrepreneur.

■ Identify the components of an environment and systems analysis.

■ Describe an environment and systems analysis as an occupational therapy manager in an occupational therapy department.

■ Describe an environment and systems analysis in community-based facilities or agencies for the development of new programs or services.

## Cultural Perspectives in Occupational Therapy

■ Explain the evolving role of the occupational therapy manager in promoting a culturally sensitive practice environment.

■ Understand the value of cultural competence in occupational therapy practice.

■ Describe how an occupational therapist or occupational therapy assistant might incorporate cultural variables into occupational therapy goals and interventions.

■ Determine your own cultural biases and how they might affect your practice.

This chapter consists of three sections that reflect new organizational perspectives and trends in management. Styles of management are inherently influenced by outside forces and organizational perspectives or influences derived from the global environment. Therefore, it is important for managers to be aware of the larger picture.

## Wellness Health Promotion and Complementary Therapies

The health care industry has undergone more changes recently than it has in its past 300 years of existence. Health care expenditures have grown four to five times faster than the country's collective wealth. The United States spends a higher percentage of its gross national product on health than does any other country (Marmor & Mashaw, 1990). As managed care initiatives and federal legislation have attempted to control the escalating cost of health care, there have been some significant changes in the delivery of health care. Changes in Medicare and the proposed $1,500 cap on payment for services to the elderly population have driven many occupational therapists and occupational therapy assistants out of skilled nursing facilities to new endeavors in the community.

At the same time, there have been philosophical paradigm shifts taking place in health care. In the past, the medical model has influenced the disease orientation of the health care industry. This paradigm emphasized dualism, or the separation of mind and body. The medical model also promotes reductionism, the act of breaking things down to their smaller components to understand the whole. For example, practitioners who are highly trained in specialized fields of study treat mental and physical illnesses as separate conditions. The human body has been studied by dissection and by the examination of tissues and cells, the biochemical constituents of the body, and even the subatomic level to gain an understanding of the whole. In the final analysis, it is difficult to understand if we truly gain a better understanding by breaking things down into small parts or by standing back and examining the combined facets of context, relationships, inter-relations, processes, and patterns that make up the whole. Readers are encouraged to read the following sections and keep an open mind to the new organizational perspectives contained therein.

The American Occupational Therapy Association's *Member Compensation Survey* (AOTA, 2001) suggests that more occupational therapists are working outside of conventional medical settings and in the community health promotion and wellness programs. This transition to the community and the development of practices that follow nonmedical models provide a more natural role for occupational therapists and

---

Guy L. McCormack wrote the section "Wellness Health Promotion and Complementary Therapies," Evelyn G. Jaffe wrote the section "Systems Theory in Occupational Therapy," and William Frey wrote the section "Cultural Perspectives in Occupational Therapy."

occupational therapy assistants. Their role in the community is more natural because, there, occupational therapy is best described as a health discipline rather than as a medical profession that is interested in the effects of disease and injury (Christiansen & Baum, 1997).

Occupational therapy is grounded in humanistic values and in the philosophy of treating the whole person. The holistic philosophy of occupational therapy is simply not a good fit for the medical model, which is centered around medical diagnosis and depends on high technology, a reductionistic view of the human organism, and the separation of mind and body (Edelman & Mandle, 1998). The concept of holism is not new or unique to occupational therapy. The ancient Greeks believed that the process of healing (*hael*) was to make whole. In addition, the Greek term *holos* means entire, the completeness of a thing, or homogeneous (Thomas, 1989).

Occupational therapy practitioners are prepared to be holistic in the intervention planning process by using inductive reasoning to analyze patterns, themes, and categories as they emerge from activities of daily living. In addition, practitioners use observations and interactions within the context of real-life situations in which people live, work, and play (Fleming & Mattingly, 1994; Yerxa, 1991). This holistic perspective makes occupational therapy distinctive and separate from the medical model. The medical model is characterized by hypothetical–deductive reasoning (Mattingly, 1991). However, occupational therapists and practitioners assistants in the medical setting have struggled to apply holism within a medical model and have reverted to a simultaneous application of and have been compromised by simultaneously applying reductionistic and holistic practices (Finlay, 2000). The core mission of occupational therapy is to recover independence and function in activities of daily living (AOTA, 1995, pp. 1029–1031). In the context of the occupational therapy process, intervention includes remediation and restoration, compensation and adaptation, disability prevention, and wellness and health promotion (Moyers, 1999).

Many authors have credited Adolf Meyer for the original philosophy of occupational therapy (Christiansen & Baum, 1997; McCormack, 1994). Meyer, a psychiatrist toward the end of the 19th century who provided the philosophical foundation of occupational therapy, was influenced by Darwinian biology and saw individuals both holistically and as having the capacity to adapt to their environment. According to Meyer (1922), "Our conception of man is that of an organism that maintains and balances itself in the world of reality and actuality by being in active life and active use" (p. 6). Meyer and Eleanor Clark Slagle, one of the founders of the Society for the Promotion of Occupational Therapy (which became the AOTA) and the director of the Henry P. Favill School of Occupations in Chicago (which was the first formal school of occupational therapy in the United States), believed that people with mental illness were unable to function in their environment because of defective habits learned early in life. They believed that habit regimes diverted attention away from the illness and restored balance and healthful life styles (Quiroga, 1995). Meyer was among the early pioneers who described how work, play, rest, and sleep were embedded in the rhythms of life. He believed that engagement in purposeful activities or in the act of "doing" had therapeutic value. Meyer (1922) proclaimed that engagement in purposeful activities brought about a balance, or what he termed "pleasurable ease" (p. 5).

During the same period, Jan Smuts (1926), a prime minister of South Africa, wrote the book *Holism and Evolution* in which he described *holism* as a creative force that exists within each person and moves toward a synthesis. As humans grow and develop, they evolve into a new level of being—a new whole—and this whole is greater than the sum of the parts.

By definition, *occupational therapy* enables people to do the "day-to-day activities that are important to them despite impairments, activity limitations, or participation restrictions or despite risks of these problems" (Neistadt & Crepeau, 1998, p. 5). The role of occupational therapy in the community is not to make the person "get well"; rather, it is to help the person understand and be connected with what is happening to his or her body within the context of his or her environment and lifestyle (AOTA, 1995). In the carrying out of wellness programs and health promotion, occupational therapists and occupational therapy assistants can become experts in functional analysis and lifestyle redesign (Clark, Azen, & Zemke, 1997).

## Health and Health Promotion

The ancient Greeks believed that health was a condition of perfect equilibrium or unity among all aspects of the individual (Cohen, 1998). According to Jona (2000), *health* is a positive, balanced state of being that reflects the best achievable physical, psychological, emotional, social, spiritual, and intellectual levels of functioning at a given time (p. 15). O'Donnell (1989) defined *health promotion* as the science and art of helping people change their lifestyles to move toward a state of optimal health. *Optimal health* is defined as a balance of physical, emotional, social, spiritual, and intellectual health.

The World Health Organization (WHO) has done much to shape the thinking about health and health promotion (MacLachlan, 2001). In 1949, WHO defined health as "a complete state of physical, mental, and social well being, and not merely the absence of disease, and infirmity" (WHO, 1958, p. 459). In 1986, WHO defined health as "the extent to which an individual or group is able, on the one hand, to realize aspirations and satisfy needs, and on the other hand, to change or cope with the environment" (WHO, 1992, p. 74). Breslow (1997) cited the definition of health developed by the First International Conference on Health Promotion as a "state of optimum capacity for effective performance of valued tasks. . . . [P]ositive health is associated with capacity to enjoy life and to withstand challenges"(p. 253). These definitions resonate very well with the philosophy of occupational therapy.

Another benefit of health promotion is that, in the long run, it saves money on health care costs (Aladana, 2001). Numerous studies have shown that carrying out health promotion and disease management programs results in lower levels of absenteeism at work and reduced health care costs (Aladana, 2001; Golaszewski, 2001; Pelletier, 2002).

The definitions stated above suggest that health is multidimensional and that *health* is a relative term. In 1992, the WHO in Canada and the Ohawa Chapter on Health Promotion identified five key areas of focus:

1. Building health public policy
2. Creating supportive environments
3. Strengthening community action
4. Developing personal skills
5. Reorienting health services to primary and preventive health care.

However, the area of health and wellness has focused on many prominent themes. Today, more emphasis is being placed on prevention, risk reduction, and the illnesses–wellness continuum. The occupational therapy manager must grapple with the question of what constitutes health in his or her setting. Is health promotion a primary mission of the health care organization, or is the focus of the organization on the absence of disease and infirmity (physical weakness)? In the realm of occupational therapy, health has always been associated with wholeness, balance, and empowerment. Health promotion is simply the process of getting people to adhere to or align themselves with certain values related to health. The occupational therapy manager is in the position to make health promotion an agenda for his or her program.

### Wellness

So what is wellness? *Wellness* is a lifelong process of striving for a state of health and of adapting patterns of behavior to lead to improved physical, emotional, and spiritual health as well as to life satisfaction (Johnson, 1996). Wellness is a process through which one creates a better lifestyle by incorporating a good balance of health habits such as exercise, an adequate amount of sleep, positive thinking, and use of social resources (Swarbrich, 1997). Additionally, wellness can be described as a personal state of being or a journey toward a higher level of functioning. Dunn (1977) stated that wellness is an integrated method of functioning, which is oriented toward maximizing the individual's potential. Wellness requires that the individual maintain a state of balance and purposeful direction within the community where he or she must function effectively (p. 4).

### Culture

Many scholars have argued convincingly that health should be defined within the context of *culture* (MacLachlan, 2001), which can be a conduit for health. For health promotion to be effective, it must embrace cultural complexity by identifying appropriate goals from within the cultural context of the community. The term *community* originated from the idea of a sharing wall. A wall creates a psychological space that is common to those who share it, and they share a responsibility to live within the enclosure. Health promotion will be promoted by taking into account how people live their lives (Furnham & Vincent, 2001).

### Healthy People 2010

*Healthy People 2010* (U.S. Department of Health and Human Services [DHHS], 2001), sponsored by the Institute of Medicine and Health and Human Science, is the initiative to build a comprehensive, nationwide health promotion and disease prevention agenda for all the people in the United States. This agenda is to be carried out during the first decade of the 21st century. This document, well supported by scientific data, was developed through public consensus and is used as a measure of progress. The two primary goals of *Healthy People 2010* are to increase quality and years of healthy life and to eliminate health disparities.

Since the original document that was produced in 1979, *Healthy People: The Surgeon General's Report on Health Promotion and Disease Prevention,* the strong relationship between individuals' health and the community has become clear (Pelletier, 1991; Valuzzi, 2002). We can assume logically that occupational therapists and occupational therapy assistants can have a greater impact and a more diversified role in the community than in a hospital setting because the community is where the client lives and conducts his or her lifestyle. Home care offers an exciting opportunity to work with the client in his or her "natural habitat." By visiting the client in his or her home, the occupational therapy practitioner can evaluate risk management factors, architectural barriers, and variables that prevent the participation in activities of daily living. Home care also offers the possibility for engagement in avocational activities. In most cases, the home provides a familiar environment, a place where objects stimulate memories of an earlier lifestyle and help to maintain cognitive long-term memory. Using the *AOTA Occupational Therapy Framework* (AOTA, 2002) in the context of home care, the occupational therapy practitioner can evaluate performance skills (motor, communication, and process), performance patterns (habits, routines, and roles), activity demands (space, social, body function requirements, and other required actions), client factors (body functions and structure), and context (cultural, physical, social, personal, spiritual, temporal, and virtual).

As stated in *Healthy People 2010* (DHHS, 2001), the home and the community are where people engage in occupations that are meaningful to them. In part, the community determines health promotion and wellness. As stated in the document, "the health of the community and environment in which individuals *live, work and play*" is what determines health (p. 3).

## Demographics of Health

Demographics provide some interesting data that the occupational therapy manager might want to take into account for planning for the future. The following discusses how long we in the United State live, the prevalence of disability, and the growing need for services for the elderly population.

*Life Expectancy*

So far, the report card for the health and longevity of Americans is not very good. Data from the WHO, the United Nations, the Centers for Disease Control and Prevention (CDC), the National Center for Health Statistics, and other sources show that the United States continues to spend more per capita than any other developed country on health care yet ranks last in life expectancy. The data from 1999 suggest that men in the United States have a life expectancy of 72.5 years; women, 78.5 years. The country with the highest life expectancy is Japan: 76.4 years for men and 82.9 years for women. Many factors contribute to life expectancy. For example, people with higher household incomes live 3 to 7 years longer than do people with low incomes. Quality of life—that is, a general sense of happiness and satisfaction—and family support systems enhance life expectancy. Gender also seems to be another factor. In general, men have a life expectancy that is 6 years less than that for women. Men are more likely to die from unintentional injuries, whereas women are at a greater risk for Alzheimer's disease and are twice as likely to be affected by major depression (CDC, 1999a).

Race and ethnicity continue to be factors in the disparity of life expectancy. For instance, heart disease is more than 40% higher for African Americans than it is for White people. Latinos living in the United States are almost twice as likely to die of diabetes as are White people. Asians and Pacific Islanders are among the healthiest population groups in the United States (DHHS, 2001).

The *Healthy People 2010* (DHHS, 2001) document has provided "determinants of health." Briefly, the determinants are (a) biology, or an individual's genetic makeup; (b) behaviors such as poor health habits, cigarette smoking, and poor diet; (c) social environment, which involves interactions with family, friends, and other relationships; (d) physical environment, which includes elements that affect all of the senses or that pose risk for exposure to infectious agents, toxic substances, irritants, and other types of physical hazards; and (e) policies and interventions, which relate to public policy and campaigns to protect health, including efforts to prevent alcohol abuse and smoking and to require the use of safety belts in automobiles.

*Disability*

In the United States, approximately 21% of the population, more than 54 million people, have some degree of disability. People with disabilities report a higher incidence of sleep disorders, depression, pain, and anxiety. People with disabilities also report having fewer days of vitality than do people without activity limitations (CDC, 1999b).

*Emergence of the Elderly Population*

The baby boomers, who were born between 1946 and 1964, comprise approximately 76 million Americans. As these individuals grow older and retire, they are expected to place a big demand for services on the health care system (Haber, 1999). The aging population in the United States is increasing at a rapid rate. Between 1995 and 2030, the number of people who are ages 64 and older is anticipated to increase dramatically from

34 million to 70 million (Haber, 1999), whereas the population older than age 85 will triple during this time. Studies have shown that, of people from ages 65 to 69, 6% to 13% reported having difficulties performing activities of daily living. Of people age 85, 35% had difficulty performing activities of daily living (Guralnik, 1991).

According to Haber (1999), the leading chronic illnesses for elderly people are as follows:
- Arthritis, 50%
- Hypertension, 36%
- Heart disease, 32%
- Hearing impairment, 29%
- Cataracts, 17%
- Orthopedic, 15%
- Sinusitis, 15%
- Diabetes, 10%.

### Health Indicators

As occupational therapy managers carry out health promotion and wellness programs, they should be mindful of the *Healthy People 2010* (DHHS, 2001) report, which suggests that the following intervention strategies should address the leading health indicators (shown in parentheses):
- Physical activity (overweight conditions and obesity)
- Mental health (substance abuse)
- Responsible sexual behavior (environmental quality)
- Access to health care (risk-taking behaviors)
- Immunization
- Tobacco use.

### Causes of Death

The leading causes of death in the United States vary with age. For people aged 25 to 44 years, unintentional injuries top the list, followed by cancer and heart disease. In the 45–64 age group, cancer leads the list, and deaths from heart disease and unintentional injuries are far fewer. In the 65-and-older age group, heart disease is at the top of the list, cancer is second, and stroke is third (CDC, 1999a).

## Complementary/Alternative Medicine

In recent years, complementary/alternative medicine (CAM), which includes the use of relaxation training, herbal therapy, and various forms of body-work techniques, has been widely used in Europe, North America, and Australia (Wootton & Sparber, 2001). Exact figures are difficult to determine, but surveys show that approximately 1 in 10 Europeans use some form of CAM. In the United States, estimates suggest that 1 in 3 use some form of CAM.

Americans are spending out-of-pocket approximately $27 billion a year for complementary therapies. Estimates calculate that, in one year, Americans make approximately 33 million visits to primary care physicians and 435 million visits to seek out CAM practitioners. These estimates also indicate that approximately 83 million Americans (30% of the U.S. population) are using CAM (Astin, 1998; Eisenberg et al., 1998; Druss & Rosenheck, 1999). The National Cancer Institute and the National Institutes of Health conducted a study on adult patients who had participated in a clinical research protocol of a study (Wootton & Sparber, 2001). Out of a convenience sample of 100 participants, 63% of the patients reported that they used at least one CAM therapy; the average use was two CAM therapies per patient. The respondents who used CAM identified spiritual (94%) and imagery (86%) therapies as the most helpful.

Numerous surveys have revealed that patients are looking for a more humanistic approach to health care and are willing to explore CAM (Shapiro & Safer, 2002). In a meta-analysis of surveys concerning national health care trends, the literature suggested that CAM users were predominantly in higher-income groups, well educated, predominately more female than male, and in the mid-40s age group (Sparber, Bauer, Curt, & Eisenberg 2000; Wootton & Sparber, 2001). National surveys such as that done by Planta, Gunderson, and Petitt (2000) have shown that lower-income, middle-age patients are also using CAM to supplement Medicare services. In addition, studies (Kennedy, 2000; Vande Creek, Rogers, & Lester, 1999) have shown that patients with cancer will seek out CAM therapies because these treatments provide a better way of managing their symptoms and side effects than conventional biomedical interventions do.

The shift in interest toward using CAM as a complement to conventional medicine is the result of consumers becoming disgruntled with managed care and scientific medicine, which treat the patient as a passive recipient of external solutions (Cohen, 1998). Conventional medicine for chronic illnesses such as cancer and heart disease presents a higher risk of side effects. Many consumers have become fearful of the medical field's reliance on high technology and their loss of a personal relationship with the physician. They also fear iatrogenic illnesses, that is, the side effects that are caused by harsh treatments (Taylor & Saks, 1998). Consumers indicate that the therapeutic relationship with CAM practitioners is more satisfying.

Many consumers believe that they can influence their own health by making lifestyle changes and by achieving psychological balance. CAM is effective with endogenous conditions, which arise from within, including myofascial disorders, cumulative trauma, chronic pain syndromes, arthritis, respiratory conditions, skin disorders, and psychophysiologic disorders (Thomas, Carr, Weslake, & Williams, 1991; Wootton & Sparber, 2001). Consumers report that they feel better after they have visited a CAM practitioner because the practitioner takes more time to gather a full medical history and looks at all facets of the person's lifestyle, including beliefs, values, and relationships. The CAM practitioner understands the consumer or client as a person. CAM practitioners examine by touching and have less reliance on technology and mechanical devices. CAM practitioners discuss options and prognosis more fully, allowing the consumer to take a more active role. CAM practitioners are more willing to discuss emotional problems and spiritual perspectives. Consumers feel they are treated with respect and as peers (Astin, 1998).

Although engagement in purposeful activities and occupational roles are the cornerstones of occupational therapy, occupational therapists and occupational therapy assistants can use some of the complementary and alternative techniques as adjunctive methods under the occupational performance model (Pedretti & Early, 2001). For elderly people with chronic disabilities, once-valued occupations such as grooming, bathing, and dressing become less important to the person. Therefore, the motivation to engage in performance areas such as home management, educational activities, play, and leisure diminishes. Occupational roles such as returning to gainful employment can be a good diversion for the individual with physical and psychological trauma. However, in a managed care environment, the occupational therapist and occupational therapy assistant must address the immediate issues associated with adjusting to a catastrophic illness before engaging in individual purposeful occupations. These adjunctive methods become unique occupational therapy interventions because they are performed within the performance context of life cycle and health status. Many different health care practitioners can apply these techniques, but what makes occupational therapy's application unique is its theoretical frame of reference that focuses on the gradation of activities in an effort to reach higher levels of function and independence (Bottomly, Galentino, Umphred, Davis, & Maebori, 2001).

## Summary

As federal legislation has attempted to set limits on Medicare services, skilled nursing facilities have minimized the role of occupational therapy. Occupational therapists can perform home health care in community settings and receive direct payment for services as long as they work within the scope of occupational therapy practice. The philosophical underpinnings of occupational therapy are based on humanistic values and holism. Therapeutic occupations do not need to be action oriented or require activities that require manual manipulation of objects. The mind–body occupations such as deep-breathing exercises, visualization, and gentle forms of touch are appropriate adjunctive methods. The combination of these rather passive occupations promotes a shift in consciousness and a shift in the autonomic nervous system toward the parasympathetic end of the continuum. This therapeutic shift is authentic therapy because it enables the client to regain balance and a state of unity in the mind, body, and spirit.

## Systems Theory in Occupational Therapy

The rate of change that has occurred in society as a whole in the past 25 years is unprecedented in history. Individuals, groups, organizations, communities, and governments all have had to learn to adapt to change. As health professionals, occupational therapy practitioners will have to be prepared to help others cope with the changes that affect their lives.

In 1970, Alvin Toffler best described the change we face in his classic book *Future Shock:* "Change is the Process by which the Future invades our lives" (p. 1). He described the effects of the acceleration of societal changes as "future shock," or "the dizzying disorientation brought on by the premature arrival of the future," and he claimed that future shock may "be the most important disease of tomorrow" (p. 11). Although his words were written three decades ago, they are as pertinent today as they were then. To understand the changes that occur in our lives as well as those of our clients and to develop effective strategies to deal with the changes, we have to be cognizant of the environmental influences that bring about these changes.

Changes that have occurred in the health care industry include the managed care movement, which came about as a result of the spiraling costs of health care during the past 20 years. Considerable discussion ensued when government and the health care industry initially realized that health care expenses were escalating exponentially. Many theories and plans were developed to deal with what had become a crisis in health care in the United States. Organizations in both the public and private sectors of health care, all of which had been affected by these costs, attempted to develop new structures by reorganizing the system to address the changes.

However, health care in this country and in other highly industrialized countries does not exist in a vacuum. The growth and development of the health care industry is a result of many environmental influences on a variety of systems. Therefore, to understand health care today, with the fast pace of the many changes that have occurred in the past few decades, we must view the health care industry from a systems approach.

In general, a system may be defined as an organized complex of elements that are mutually interactive (Laszlo, 1972; Robbins, 1994; von Bertalanffy, 1968). The concept behind the systems approach, derived from both the biological and social sciences, is known as *systems theory.* Systems theory or a systems approach to health care helps the occupational therapy manager, entrepreneur, consultant, and practitioner understand the environmental factors that are affecting what is presently occurring in health care and what might be predicted for the future delivery of health services.

Environmental issues, both internal and external, affect individuals on a personal level and affect the practices of health care organizations on a societal level. All aspects of the social, political, and economic environment have affected the health care system today in ways that are more dynamic and complex than ever before. One can see the influence of systems theory by observing the effect that parts of social, political, or economic systems have on one another. The various forces in the environment affect one another, affect the health care system in general, and affect health professionals and clients (Jaffe, 1985a, 1985b; Kelly, 1970).

This section reviews systems theory from a historical background that takes into account the contributions of three perspectives: (a) the biological perspective; (b) the human occupation and psychological perspective; and (c) the organization and community perspective. These perspectives all have affected systems theory synergistically.

## Evolution of Systems Theory From a Biological Perspective

Systems theory originated from a biological perspective and, over the years, has evolved and been refined. The development of systems theory that has occurred largely from this biological perspective can be categorized as follows:

- General systems theory
- Open system theory
- Dynamic systems theory
- Ecological systems theory.

The following sections describe these developments in more detail.

### General Systems Theory

Systems theory was described originally by biologist Ludwig von Bertalanffy (von Bertalanffy, 1968). In the 1920s, during his early student years, von Bertalanffy studied life sciences and systems of biological organisms. He rejected the prevailing notion that organisms are simply aggregates of cells and questioned the assumption that the methods of physics are appropriate for all problems in science. His research attempts to understand biological phenomena led to his conclusion that linear causal trains of explanation were inadequate. Using the laws of biological systems, von Bertalanffy formulated some basic concepts to explain complex biological phenomena. He described any factor "not only in terms of its components or the sum of its properties, but also in regard to the entire set of relations between the components" (as cited in Jaffe & Epstein, 1992, p. 65; see also Laszlo, 1972).

He developed a systems approach that considered the interrelationship among all elements in living matter, an approach that might be used to consider either the biological study of a single cell or entire behavioral and sociological fields in society. He determined that living organisms maintain structure through continuous change. In 1947, von Bertalanffy proposed a model that would embrace all levels of science, providing general organizational principles that apply to a wide range of phenomena in nature. He referred to this model as "general systems theory" (von Bertalanffy, 1968).

*General systems theory* may be defined as follows: "Change in one part of the system causes inherent change in the total system" (von Bertalanffy, 1968, p. 115). Additionally, general systems theory describes an interrelationship among all elements in living matter that ranges from specific natural occurrences to general human behavior. "Each variable in any system interacts with the other variables, so that cause and effect cannot be separated" (Jaffe & Epstein, 1992, p. 65).

### Open System Theory

From the initial application of his theories within research in "organismic biology," von Bertalanffy began to look at social organizations and the influences in the environment that affected them. His studies led to his consideration of general systems theory for interdisciplinary applications, and it was embraced by the social scientists of the day (Katz & Kahn, 1978; Kuhn, 1970; Likert, 1967; Mann, 1957). During the 1960s, social and behavioral scientists, including social psychologists, sociologists, political scientists, and economists, were concerned with the social structure of society and the growing problems of social and political organizations (Kuhn, 1970). The concept of general systems theory was broadened to what Laszlo (1972), a disciple of von Bertalanffy, called "a new paradigm of contemporary thought" (p. 3). The scientists referred to general systems theory as the basis for a "systems approach" to address social problems. This interest in von Bertalanffy's concepts led to greater interdisciplinary research among the social and behavioral scientists.

von Bertalanffy refined and modified the biological aspects of general systems theory in the 1960s. He applied his concepts describing the inter-relatedness of components of living systems to the relationships between social phenomena and the environment. He referred to this modified concept as "open system theory." von Bertalanffy described the openness of all systems to environmental influences, and he postulated that this concept had applicability to all organizations. *Open system theory* expanded the initial concepts of general systems theory to a more global perspective; all of nature, including human behavior as well as most social structures and organizations, was considered interconnected by means of environmental influences.

An *open system* was defined as a system whose organization is characterized by exchanges of energy or matter with its environment (von Bertalanffy, 1968). For example, all living systems are considered open systems because they continually process energy or information from the environment, which is essential to their survival. Just as a baby develops from the energy and growth of internal parts and subsystems, he or she takes cues from the external environment, learning speech, social behaviors, and adaptation to environmental conditions.

However, not only living systems are considered open systems. Political and social entities also are in constant exchange with environmental influences. The social and behavioral scientists of the 1960s demonstrated considerable interest in the application of this theory to address the social–structural problems of the day. These scientists were part of a growing movement that referred to the concepts of open systems theory as the "systems approach" to social phenomena. Increased interdisciplinary research, called "systems research," resulted in the application of humanistic approaches to organizational structure.

By this time, systems theory was no longer the domain of scientists. Its practical application was introduced to corporations in the business world as well as to health care organizations and facilities. The need for increased management skills in health care industries had escalated as a result of the explosion of technology, biomedical science, social programs, and the health professions after World War II (Christiansen &

Baum, 1991; Crist, 1996; Jaffe & Epstein, 1992; Katz & Kahn, 1978; Laszlo, 1972; Likert, 1967; Lippitt, Watson, & Westley, 1958). As managers and administrators became more aware of the ways in which systems theory applied to organizational structure, they began to translate systems research into operational programs to address concrete societal, economic, and political problems.

The rapid societal changes, including social behavior that occurred during the last half of the 20th century, required organizations to be more aware of the effects of change on their systems. The need for adaptation led to changes in the organizations and to formations of new or different relationships to other systems. The open system approach flourished during this period. Management courses and workshops, which included some focus on systems theory, became the norm for new managers, recently hired middle managers, or those individuals promoted to higher managerial positions. The applicability of the open system approach in management was emphasized in many of these courses. Katz and Kahn (1978) described open system theory in relation to the cyclical events that occur in organizations—including budgeting, marketing, hiring, evaluation, and termination—and in relation to the organization's openness to environmental influences.

Capra (1982) postulated that the open system theory views the world "in terms of the inter-relatedness and interdependence of all phenomenon" (p. 43). Jaffe and Epstein (1992) stated that the "open system theory is a comprehensive approach to the study of every facet of organizational life and the interactions of the system with its environment" (p. 65).

von Bertalanffy (1968) also described the corollary to open systems, which he stated was a "closed system": a system with impermeable boundaries, which does not exchange matter or energy with its environment. In the biological sense, other organisms or living matter would not affect a closed system. In the sociological spheres, closed systems are neither affected by the external environment nor responsive to environmental issues, pressures, or needs. In these closed systems, activities, policies, and decisions may be made in a static, noninteractive state (Crist, 1996; Laszlo, 1972; von Bertalanffy, 1968). Closed systems may typify totalitarian states or organizations in which decisions are made for the expediency of government or internal business processes rather than as a result of studying the external environmental impacts.

The open system theory is used primarily in studies of human and organizational systems. It emphasizes the character of a system, including the dynamic events and predictable cycles that occur in organizations (Katz & Kahn, 1978). An important consideration of an open system approach is the identification of environmental influences, or input, on the activities of the system or organization. The subsequent processing and transformation of these influences, or throughput, and the final product or services, considered output, of the system is followed by the cycle of feedback to the system.

- *Input*—The process by which matter, energy, and information enter the system from the environment

- *Throughput*—The process of transformation of input into another form passing through the organism or system
- *Output*—The action of the system on the environment as a result of this throughput (transformation) of input (matter, energy, and information)
- *Feedback*—Information that results from the consequences of the system's output and that is subsequently returned to a system. (Negative feedback allows the system to correct problems or deviations from the planned course of action.)

Figure 4.1 illustrates the cycle involving these four components in a systems approach.

To illustrate the systems approach more specifically, consider this approach with respect to occupational therapy services in a school system. The key elements of an open system might be described in the following ways:

- *Internal Input*—The needs of the children to receive occupational therapy services, the other students in the class, the desires of parents, the constraints of the teachers, the facilities available, and the school policies and procedures
- *External Input*—School district policies, legislative mandates, economic constraints or resources, and community demands
- *Throughput*—Consideration of the internal and external input that are then transformed to develop an educational plan involving occupational therapy services
- *Output*—The result of the occupational therapy services in the school and the action of the school system on the school environment and community as a result of the throughput transformation
- *Feedback*—The reports from the parents, the teachers, and the school administration with respect to the results of occupational therapy intervention for the children who have received these services and, perhaps, the effect that occupational therapy may have had on the other children in the school—all of which allows the school system and the occupational therapy practitioner to correct problems, modify programs, or enhance and expand the services.

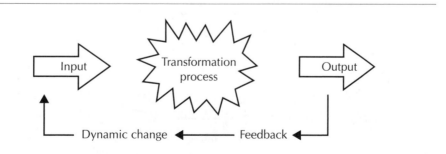

**Figure 4.1 Cycle of a Systems Approach.**

Therefore, a systems approach to management of an organization includes the study of all aspects of the environment: those aspects that are internal to the organization and the external environmental forces that can affect planning, policies, staffing, program development, services, financial issues, and future decisions. These aspects of an organization must be considered in all health care systems. Since the 1990s, health care has become a true business—with the focus being placed on controlling cost. However, consumer satisfaction and delivery of efficient services also must be factored into the overall organizational approach.

Figure 4.2 depicts a systems approach to the organization of a health care system. Crist's (1996) description of how the key components of the system interact with a health care setting will help readers understand this figure:

> Staff, facilities, capital, and equipment provide input to the health care system. The system *transforms* the *inputs* into *outputs,* such as interdisciplinary staff, coordinated services, product lines, and critical pathways. The success of this system depends on beneficial interaction with the environment, that is, with the groups and the institutions dependent on it: consumers, insurance providers, government agencies, and so forth. The system must provide continuing, cost-

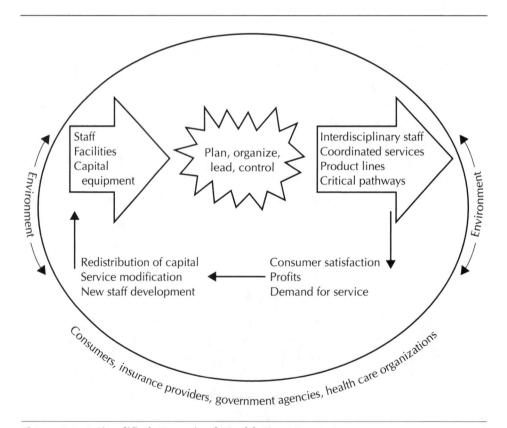

**Figure 4.2  A Simplified, Organized Health Care System.**

efficient, high-quality services to respond to environmental demands such as consumer satisfaction and profits, both of which either allow the system to continue or force it to dissolve. Consumer satisfaction and profits are forms of *feedback* that modify the organization of the system. (p. 173)

Using a systems approach enables organizational administrators (and the occupational therapy manager, entrepreneur, or consultant) to forecast environmental changes that may affect the organization. The systems approach allows the organization to be prepared for possible changes in reimbursement or staffing patterns, corporate culture, competitive markets, and legislative and economic trends (Jaffe, 2001; Pabst-Hunt, 2002).

### Dynamic Systems Theory

The basic concept of general systems theory and an open system approach was reformulated as *dynamic systems theory*. The dynamic nature of systems emphasizes the self-organizing processes of a system. This concept has been studied by several social scientists. In addition, Florence Clark, Ruth Zemke, and Diane Parham of the Occupational Therapy Department at the University of Southern California, as well as other investigators, have explored the relevance of dynamic systems theory to the science and study of the human as an occupational being (Zemke & Clark, 1996). Their work looks at the study of human occupation in attempting to bring about changes in the behavior patterns of people who are affected by illness or injury. Briefly, dynamic systems theory is described as the process in which patterns of stability and change emerge in human behavior and on which the focus is the dynamics of systems that change over time. Dynamic systems theory is based on the following framework (Kielhofner, 1997; Scaffa, 2001; Zemke & Clark, 1996):

- Systems evolve over time.
- Evolution or change is irreversible and, usually, inevitable.
- Organisms are complex, with varying degrees of freedom to interact.
- Systems exhibit self-organizing properties.
- Dynamic systems are heterarchical (influences on the system occur laterally) as opposed to hierarchical (influences occur vertically).
- Entities are not rigid structures but continually evolve and change spontaneously without causal mechanisms.

### Ecological Systems Theory

Another departure from general systems theory is the *ecological systems theory*, based on the concept that dynamic interactions occur among all components of a society. The theory is derived from basic concepts of ecology in nature that were developed into theories by the biological sciences and then adapted to the social sciences. Therefore, the ecological systems theory includes both biological and sociological theories of ecology. The biological aspects of the systems model focus on relations between organisms and their environment. Sociological aspects of human ecology consider the roles of people and institutions and their interdependency. Using ecological principles, which include the study and the assessment of the environment, human behavior and reactions can be analyzed. Institutional behavior patterns may be predicted from the characteristic responses of individuals or groups to certain environmental influences and settings. Additionally, the ecological systems approach forms the foundation for the model of occupational therapy consultation, described by Epstein and Jaffe in chapter 10 of this text.

The ecological systems theory may be used to determine the interrelationship of human systems to community services and may be studied in three ways:

- "The relationship between social or organizational systems and the impact of changes in one system on another" (Jaffe & Epstein, 1992, p. 694)
- The relationship between the physical environment and individual behavior (Kelly, 1970)
- "The relationship of the individual to his immediate social environment" (Jaffe & Epstein, 1992, p. 694; see also Kelly, 1970; Mann, 1957).

The ecological concept that forms the foundation of these three relationships is demonstrated by predictable individual behavior patterns that are characteristic of a social situation and individual behavior changes that occur in any newly defined social settings (Jaffe & Epstein, 1992; Kelly, 1970). Basic constructs of the ecological systems theory include enhanced interpretations of cultural and community mores and folkways. In using this approach, one's emphasis of intervention is on long-range changes in the social system. The literature is full of references to these theories (Brown & Weiner, 1984; Gardner, 1964; Hoffler, 1952; Jaffe, 1985a; Jaffe & Epstein, 1992; Kelly, 1970; Kielhofner & Burke 1980a; Lawrence & Lorsch, 1969; Mann, 1957). Although these concepts were originally described during the expansion of social theories in the late 1950s and 1960s, they are particularly timely and pertinent today for all health professionals who are working in this current era with its daily changes in present and proposed service delivery.

## Evolution of Systems Theory From a Human Occupation and Psychological Perspective

In addition to the biological perspective of system theory described earlier, scientists have described the relationship between changes in the environment and a person's physical and emotional health. Studies by many social scientists reveal that the health of an individual is intimately bound up with the adaptive demands placed on him or her by the environment and by the rate of life changes (Toffler, 1970). Hinkle (1964) termed this theory "human ecology" and wrote extensively about the importance of environmental factors in medicine.

Study of the environment, using a systems approach, has been described frequently in the occupational therapy literature. The human occupation perspective is documented in the work of Kielhofner, Burke, and others, based on general systems theory (Kielhofner & Burke, 1980a, 1980b). A conceptual model of human occupation considers human behavior as "occupation." A basic occupational therapy assumption suggests that occupation is a central aspect of the human experience. Using the framework of an open system approach, *man* represents the human system, and *human occupation* is considered the dynamic interaction of this system with the environment. Man's occupational behavior includes the mental, physical, and social aspects of occupation and is considered the output of the open system. Kielhofner and Burke (1980a) stated, "Within the model of human occupation, the environment is conceptualized as external objects, people, and events that influence the system's actions" and the "the physical, social, and cultural setting in which the system operates"(p. 573).

Human occupation evolves during the life span, driven by changes that occur in patterns of work and play throughout the developmental stages of life. The evolution in the human system occurs as man makes individual occupational choices (Kielhofner & Burke, 1980a, 1980b). Using the open system approach, the model of human occupation offers explanations for adaptive and maladaptive changes in behavior. In addition, Christiansen and Baum (1991) and Law et al. (1997) described occupational performance "as the transaction between the individual as an open system and the environment," forming the basis for the "Person–Environment–Performance Framework" (Christiansen & Baum, 1991, p. 18). This model identifies individual and environmental factors that have an impact on occupational performance. Application of these models is used in occupational therapy practice for assessment and intervention (Jaffe & Epstein, 1992; Kielhofner & Burke, 1980c, 1980d).

### Evolution of Systems Theory From an Organization and Community Perspective

Additionally, systems theory is described from the organization and community perspective as it relates to the various influences in social, economic, and political environments. The ability to understand and analyze the environment is an essential element of management, administration, entrepreneurship, and consultation. The use of a systems approach, including a review of the internal and external environmental factors that influence an organization, is particularly important with the change in the locus of occupational therapy practice. Emerging practice areas are concentrated more and more in the community. The expansion from traditional, medical-based, direct service practice to indirect service for community-based programs requires greater understanding of systems and environments. "As occupational therapy services in the community increase and as practitioners become more comfortable with indirect service provision and designing interventions for populations, the paradigm of community practice will evolve" (Scaffa, 2001, p. 33). According to Scaffa, "A systems perspective is extremely useful in conceptualizing community practice" (p. 31).

The emphasis in the community is on a broad, client-centered perspective. The term *client* may refer to an individual, group, or organization (AOTA, 2001, p. 4). The occupational therapy manager, administrator, entrepreneur, or consultant must assess the client system to ascertain the impacts on that system that affect all planning and program development. This analysis of environmental factors, including social, economic, demographic, and political trends or issues, is achieved with an environment and systems analysis (Epstein & Jaffe, 1996).

A systems analysis is the identification and determination of the state of the system. It includes a study and evaluation of all internal and external environmental factors influencing the system. A complex of internal and external factors on both macroenvironmental and microenvironmental levels influences individual or community behavior and organizational structure (Jaffe & Epstein, 2002). An environment and systems analysis should consider the environments that are defined in Table 4.1.

Readers will benefit from a more detailed understanding of the macro- and microenvironments that are listed in the table. The *macroenvironment* consists of forces in the external environment of the client system. These external factors or conditions include local or national legislative acts and regulatory policies; local or national economic concerns; the political climate; and the social and cultural mores, customs, attitudes, and values that shape occupational life. The *microenvironment* consists of forces close to the client system. These forces include administrative policies and procedures of the organization; internal resources of funds, personnel, and supplies; the corporate culture; and the mission and goals of the organization.

After identifying the macro- and microenvironments, the manager, administrator, entrepreneur, and consultant must consider the remaining specific environments that are described further in Table 4.2.

## Summary

The profound changes that occurred in the last century had a significant impact on all systems: human, natural, economic, political, and cultural. Social scientists, political scientists, and biological scientists recognized that all these forces shaped the environment and social structure. None of these forces can be studied or understood in isola-

**Table 4.1  Environment and Systems Analysis.**

| Environment | Systems Analysis |
| --- | --- |
| Human environment | Individuals who may influence the outcome |
| Macroenvironment | Forces in the larger environment |
| Microenvironment | Forces close to the issues |
| Natural environment | Particular setting or settings |
| Physical environment | External factors or conditions |

*Note.* From *Occupational Therapy Consultation: Theory, Principles, and Practice* (p. 65), edited by E. G. Jaffe and C. F. Epstein, 1992, St. Louis, MO: Mosby; A Consultative Approach to Occupational Therapy Practice by E. G. Jaffe and C. F. Epstein in *Willard & Spackman's Occupational Therapy* (10th ed.), edited by M. E. Neistadt, E. B. Crepeau, E. Cohn, and B. Schell, 2002, Philadelphia: Lippincott Williams & Wilkins. Adapted with permission.

**Table 4.2 Human, Natural, and Physical Environments.**

| Environment | Description |
| --- | --- |
| Human environment | Individuals who may influence the program or organization, including clients, administrators, staff members, families, teachers, health professionals, and others |
| Natural environment | The particular setting or settings in which the managerial, entrepreneurial, or consultation activities occur, including community agencies, schools, workplace settings, and health care facilities |
| Physical environment | External factors or conditions that influence the managerial, entrepreneurial, or consultation activities, including space, architecture, accessibility, and physical structure |

*Note.* From *Occupational Therapy Consultation: Theory, Principles, and Practice,* by E. G. Jaffe and C. F. Epstein, St. Louis, MO: Mosby; and "A Consultative Approach to Occupational Therapy Practice," by E. G. Jaffe and C. F. Epstein in *Willard & Spackman's Occupational Therapy* (10th ed.), edited by M. E. Neistadt, E. B. Crepeau, E. Cohn, and B. Schell, 2002, Philadelphia: Lippincott Williams & Wilkins. Adapted with permission.

tion, nor can they be considered as single causal factors but, rather, as part of many variables that influence the system. This concept formed the basis for von Bertalanffy's general system theory and for the further development of an open system approach that was followed by dynamic systems theory and, finally, by ecological systems theory (Jaffe & Epstein, 1992; von Bertalanffy, 1968). The rapid growth and development that were evidenced in all spheres of society during the last half of the 20th century do not show signs of slowing. If anything, the rapidity of social, biological, and technical change is escalating. Electronic equipment is a case in point. Purchases of electronic items are almost out of date before the ink dries on the purchase order. More than ever before, we must be aware of the environmental impacts on all systems, from three key perspectives:

- The biological perspective
- The human occupation and psychological perspective
- The organization and community perspective.

As occupational therapy practice transitions to more community-based environments, a systems approach to these changes is crucial. Without a systems approach to change, we will indeed face "future shock." The social, economic, political, technological, and human forces must be analyzed to provide an efficient framework for dealing with the myriad changes occurring almost daily in the health care system. Thus, managers, administrators, entrepreneurs, and consultants must be able to understand systems theory and use a systems approach to manage organizational structure, program planning, and interventions in current and future occupational therapy practice.

## Cultural Perspectives in Occupational Therapy

Our epistemology has long held that occupational therapy practitioners treat the "whole person." To understand the whole person, practitioners seek to learn how individuals operate in a variety of roles and how their development is shaped with others in their environment. Because our theory tells us that purposeful activity (i.e., physical, psychosocial, and spiritual activity) occurs within the unique cultural environment of the individual, occupational therapy practitioners need to acquire the knowledge and develop the necessary skills to serve an increasingly culturally diverse population.

Friedman (2000) wrote that our world has changed. There is an "inexorable integration of markets, nation-states, and technologies to a degree never witnessed before" (p. 8). The speed of communications, the mixing of belief systems, and a diminished clarity of social norms is causing value conflicts throughout the world. If we believe occupational therapy provides a means for optimal functioning, then we must accept the challenge to help our clients and coworkers "find a healthy balance between preserving a sense of identity, home, and community and doing what it takes to survive within the globalization system" (p. 41). The terrorist attacks of September 11, 2001, have made this management challenge even more urgent.

Predictions suggest that, inevitably, cultural diversity will increase in our organizations, both in the types of clients we serve and among coworkers within our profession's workforce. In the 1990 census, participants using write-in boxes identified almost 300 "races." These races included 600 Indian tribes, 70 Hispanic groups, and 75 combinations of multiracial ancestry. This past decade, the number of African Americans has increased by 13%, the Latino population has increased by 53%, the Native American population has increased by 37%, and the category "other race" has increased by 45% (Morganthau, 1995). California became the first large state to have a non-White majority, and projections point to one in four states having ethnic majorities by the next census in 2010 (Coile, 2001). As occupational therapists and occupational therapy assistants, we seek to communicate effectively with people who may look or act differently from ourselves and to plan appropriate treatment interventions. It becomes important to reflect on Meyer's (1922) observations that many "rhythms" shape the whole of a client's existence, including work, play, rest, and sleep. In a shrinking world where cultures meet, overlap, and at times clash, we must help our clients find what Meyer called the "pleasurable ease," an orderly set of natural rhythms.

As managers, how do we gain a set of skills that allow us to work effectively in the context of growing cultural differences? How do we develop competence in managing within multicultural organizations and communities? These questions highlight the challenge and opportunity for occupational therapy managers during the 21st century.

## Cultural Competence

What is culture? Helman (1990) defined *culture* as "a set of guidelines, which individuals inherit as members of a particular society, and which tells them how to view the world, how to experience it emotionally, and how to behave in it in relation to other people, to supernatural forces or gods, and to the natural environment" (p. 3).

American anthropologist Edward T. Hall (1966) further explained:

Most of culture lies hidden and is outside voluntary control, making up the warp and weft of human existence. Even when small fragments of culture are elevated to awareness, they are difficult to change, not only because they are so personally experienced but because people cannot act or interact at all in any meaningful way except through the medium of culture. (p. 188)

Basic interactions such as the selective use of touch, gentle or firm, or the physical closeness of a practitioner can be interpreted differently within a culturally diverse group of clients.

Guidelines that are "hidden," "outside voluntary control," and "difficult to change" suggest a real challenge for practitioners wanting to develop cultural competency. These descriptors also speak to the multifaceted dimensions of the concept and, as others have observed, to the need for a conceptual framework to organize these dimensions into a meaningful whole that provides direction for occupational therapists and occupational therapy assistants (Dumas, Rollock, Prinz, Hops, & Blechman, 1999; Sue, 2001). However, an agreed-on conceptual framework for achieving a cultural competence does not yet exist. Agreements on the definition of key terms in this emerging area of management are not complete and are still evolving. Skin color, race and ethnicity, social class, age, religion, gender, sexual orientation, and physical ability are social constructs of diversity that have changed over time.

Blue (2000) wrote that cultural competency in the context of providing health care involves a recognition that people of different cultures have different ways of communicating, behaving, interpreting, and problem solving. A client's cultural beliefs affect health beliefs; help-seeking activities; interactions with health care professionals; health care practices; and inevitably, health care outcomes, including adherence to prescribed regimens. He noted that, to provide optimal care for the client, health practitioners need to have an ability and willingness to adapt the way they work to fit the client's cultural and ethnic background.

Dillard et al. (1992) added that a culturally competent occupational therapy practitioner is one who will "reinforce the beauty of culture, incorporate it in therapy, and is open to different ways of engaging the patient" (p. 723). Different cultures have different sets of beliefs about correct behavior for preventing ill health, and sometimes, they have unique beliefs about healthy ways to eat, sleep, dress, work, play, and generally conduct one's life. Additionally, Helman (2000) reminded us that, in some societies, health is maintained by the use of charms, amulets, and religious medallions to ward off bad luck, including unexpected illness, and to attract good luck and good health.

Competent provider behavior reflects both cultural-specific knowledge and intercultural communication competence. To date, Anglo-American society has put a premium on cognitive competence and has minimized aspects of competence that involve linguistic skills, social–emotional sensitivities in the form of interpersonal skills, and practical problem solving (Dana, Behn, & Gonwa, 1992).

The problems associated with satisfactory communication between provider and client are of particular concern. We are learning that language barriers are a significant contributor to the racial and ethnic disparities that exist in interventions and outcomes. For example, a recent Robert Wood Johnson Foundation survey ("Foundation Program," 2001) revealed the desperate need to understand the language needs of certain communities. The survey found that, in the United States, 66% of Spanish-speaking Latino clients have concerns about using interpreters and that interpreter services are often makeshift and ineffective. Seventy-one percent of providers in the survey said that language barriers increase the risk of complications.

In addition to spoken language, miscommunication also can occur as a result of nonverbal communication such as body position, facial expressions, eye contact, choice of attire, physical closeness, and level of expressiveness shown by providers and staff members.

When a client cannot make a decision on the spot, providers can become very frustrated. Clients can be labeled as difficult or uncooperative. Providers can assume that they know what is best for the client and demand an answer to what they perceive is a simple decision. Individual clients are expected to understand their health conditions and consent to intervention without taking into consideration the support of extended family members—support that is often critical to the client.

The client's decision process may take longer, and the decision may not be made in the clinic but at the client's home, where the client is surrounded by cultural and spiritual support. We know that, in some cultures, the role of the extended family is emphasized. These cultures may not approve of making decisions, especially health care decisions, without consulting family members first. The extended family members are expected to identify and understand the level of the health risk. Sometimes, the risk information must be translated to the client and the family by one of the younger children who have learned English.

The use of children to provide interpretation services can cause many problems. Most children do not possess enough knowledge to understand medical terms, let alone the ability to interpret effectively their meaning to their relatives. By serving as an interpreter, the child can be placed in an adult role and become involved in adult conversation. Parents who are clients may feel powerless and resentful, and they may not divulge all of their symptoms out of embarrassment or out of fear that they will worry their children. In particular, gynecological issues for which sexual history is almost always needed can be extremely sensitive. Yet, using children as interpreters is a common practice.

Cultural competence also involves having a working knowledge of other systems of care that may be prevalent among the communities served. These domains and systems can include Ayurveda; traditional oriental medicine; Native American healing systems; herbalism; homeopathy; naturopathy; mind–body interventions such as prayer, meditation, and mental healing; biological based therapies such as megavitamin therapy, shark cartilage, and laetrile; manipulative and body-based methods; and energy therapies such as therapeutic touch, bioelectromagnetics, and spiritual healing.

These interventions may seem "alternative" to occupational therapy practitioners in the United States who have been trained in biomedicine's scientific paradigm, but to people throughout the world, these interventions may be "mainstream" in their cultures. People emigrating to the United States often bring their alternative remedies and their traditional healers along with them.

Today, legally sanctioned health care systems in the United States are largely based on Anglo-American cultural values, attitudes, and behaviors. Spiritual and religious beliefs of other cultures are not considered. The range of religious and spiritual beliefs related to pain, touch, and personal space can pose unique challenges to occupational therapists and occupational therapy assistants in a multicultural practice. A few examples may help to illustrate (Dumas, Rollock, Prinz, Hops, & Blechman, 1999).

- Many Koreans believe that hot water is safer as well as less shocking to the body and can speed recovery. To a Korean homemaker, preparing a warm cup of tea as part of occupational therapy may be preferable to mixing and then drinking a cold glass of lemonade.
- In China, the number 4 can be pronounced the same as the word for death. If an occupational therapy clinic is located on the fourth floor, Chinese clients may not return for their follow-up care.
- It is taboo for Native American children to be patted on the head, as their hair is spiritually important. Self-care activities should include the parent's approval.
- Asian Americans place high value on relationships that are established over time. Insurance methods and other payment schemes in the United States often force clients to move among a variety of health care providers, and clients may never establish a meaningful relationship.

Finally, a taken-for-granted clinic process like making an appointment can be unfamiliar in some cultures. Its relevance to receiving care can be a problem to clients who expect to be able to drop in and be treated immediately or to wait in line as they did in their former homeland. This problem will be exacerbated when the appointment system is not available in a language that is understood by the client.

A few comments about the use of interpreters may be helpful to occupational therapists and occupational therapy assistants. Currently in the United States, a patchwork of methods exist for communicating with clients who do not speak English. Lists of volunteer interpreters, flash cards with translations of key phrases, and wireless headsets connected to an interpreter who is located off-site are all examples of strategies to clarify communications in a health care organization that is serving diverse populations. McCormack (1987) advised practitioners to "use short sentences and concepts that would be understood by the patient if he spoke the same language"

(p. 31). He noted that "the therapist should talk to the patient, not the interpreter. Direct eye contact with the patient depends on his cultural background" (p. 31).

## National Systems of Care

The health care system found in the United States is remarkably pluralistic and complex. It is an expression of our values and our social structure. But occupational therapy practitioners working with people raised in other countries quickly learn that it is not the only way to organize health services. In fact, different countries produce varying systems and strategies in providing care to their populations.

When comparing industrialized nations, Frangos (2001) grouped nations into three basic categories: (a) tax-funded, national health services such as in Canada and Great Britain; (b) compulsory social insurance systems such as in Germany and Japan; and (c) primarily private systems such as in the United States. One society may see free (or relatively inexpensive) health care as a basic right of citizenship, whereas another society may see health care as a commodity to be bought only by those who can afford it.

For all nations, three competing priorities must be governed by public policy: cost, access, and quality of health care services. The three are interrelated, and a policy change in one affects the other two. National policy decisions lead to various health delivery patterns such as waiting lists for those needing care. Some countries have short waiting lists for procedures; others have long queues for procedures. In some systems, the use of specialists, expensive drugs, and interventions are restricted. In other countries, systems have fewer restrictions. Although large bureaucracies in some countries discourage entrepreneurs from creating new intervention alternatives, the governments in other countries encourage clinical experimentation and delivery options.

A report on world health in 2000 assessed and compared the health care delivery systems in 191 nations, ranking them according to how well they meet the needs of their people ("U.S. Health Care," 2000). Clearly, the United States was first in funding health care, spending a greater share of its gross domestic product on health care than any other nation. However, the United States ranked 37th out of 191 nations in terms of satisfactorily providing health care to its citizens ("U.S. Health Care," 2000). Satisfaction was defined as the overall heath of a nation's population, the inequalities within a population, how health care responses are distributed within a population, and the distribution of the health care costs among its population.

For those in the United States who have insurance, access to health care is impressive. On the one hand, the United States has the most advanced medical technology, the best-trained physicians, and unparalleled interventions for life-threatening diseases such as cancer and heart disease. On the other hand, those with less comprehensive coverage or no insurance experience much lower levels of care than either insured people in the United States or people in other developed countries. In a culturally diverse society like the United States, which has a significant immigrant population, we can expect that a client's assumptions about the health care system will vary greatly and might differ from our own expectations.

## Cultural Bias

Talking about prejudices is usually uncomfortable, but they are real and are manifested in the everyday behavior of health care professionals. Prejudice may be thought of as

> (1) a result of an individual's preconceptions or unfounded views against members of a group different from one's own or (2) a result of institutional assumptions, attitudes and practices that has an invisible-hand effect in systematically benefiting members of the more powerful groups and disadvantaging members of the less dominate groups. (Evans, 2001, p. 410)

Examples of institutional prejudice include culturally biased assessment and selection criteria, group norms that condone or permit racial or sexual harassment, and lower expectations for members of certain groups.

We often hear that actual practice in a health profession is based on both objective science and on a subjective art. Unfortunately, intervention decisions that are based on subjective judgment or opinions by occupational therapy practitioners can lead to unequal care. In the late 1960s, Katz, Cole, and Lowry (1969) examined the process of psychiatric diagnosis among British and American psychiatrists. Their study found marked disagreements in diagnosis between the two groups and differently perceived patterns of symptomology. Littlewood and Lipsedge (1989) suggested that prejudice plays an important role in how some African Caribbean patients in the United Kingdom are classified by psychiatrists as "mad," even when evidence points to the contrary. Van Os, Galdos, and Lewis (1993) studied the concepts of schizophrenia held by a sample of 92 British and 60 French psychiatrists and found major differences in how each group conceptualized the etiology, diagnosis, and management of the disorder.

Additionally, the evidence of unequal care to minorities is found in general medicine diagnoses. In repeated studies (Geiger, 1996) on American military veterans, Black patients with ischemic heart disease—even those enrolled in Medicare or free-care systems—were much less likely to undergo angiography, angioplasty, or coronary artery bypass grafting (CABG) than were White patients.

> Blacks were 33 percent less likely to undergo cardiac catheterization, 44 percent less likely to undergo angioplasty, and 54 percent less likely to undergo CABG than their white counterparts . . . With major confounding variables, increasingly controlled and adjusted for, investigators tend to invoke unspecified cultural differences, undocumented patient preferences, or a lack of information about the need for care as reasons for the differences. (p. 815)

Another study in the *New England Journal of Medicine* also argues that race, not financial factors, affects the type of intervention offered to minority clients.

> Since eligible veterans are not billed for admissions to VA hospitals, patients' fears about incurring large debts for the use of expensive procedures are also minimized.

Our analysis of a subgroup of veterans with more homogeneous incomes yielded results similar to those of the analysis of our entire study populations, further suggesting that differences in personal income do not underlie racial differences in the use of procedures. (Whittle, Conigliaro, Good, & Lofgren, 1993, p. 621)

It is understandable why some minority groups view the "medical establishment" as a whole with distrust. When a provider questions an individual's ability to pay because of a lack of health insurance or gives little attention to cultural variation, the client's lack of trust in the provider and the health care system is deepened further.

## Cultural Competence as a Strategic Objective

Health care organizations meet several societal goals. Often, they are the largest employer in a community, and some become complex commercial enterprises with various profit and nonprofit objectives. However, the primary role of our health care organizations in our communities must be to serve the health needs of individuals and families.

If demographic trends cited earlier are a harbinger of things to come, the increasing diversity of our communities makes cultural competence a strategic imperative for health care organizations. The benefits to human services agencies to become culturally competent organizations are many. In a guide to cultural competence in human services agencies, Nash (1999) described some of the many benefits of culturally competent organizations. First, culturally competent organizations are more effective because they understand and respond to the needs of the populations they serve. In addition, these organizations reflect the population served in their staffing and seek to make them more active in decisions that affect external customers. Finally, they "balance the needs of the organization, employees, and population served to achieve optimal results. They exhibit an appreciation of diversity and are perceived as a safe place for those seeking a supportive work environment" (p. 20).

## Role of an Occupational Therapy Manager

To manage diversity, the occupational therapy manager must acknowledge what he or she knows and what he or she does not know about the cultures of clients who are served by the department. Becoming culturally competent is difficult work, and managers need to seek out their own hidden biases. Humility is an important quality for an occupational therapy manager who is venturing into the realm of cultural competence.

Equally important is for the occupational therapy manager to inspire others in the department to search their minds and souls, to acknowledge and openly discuss differences, and to exchange ideas among one another. To achieve these goals, managers must first create a climate in which employees feel comfortable, accepted, and valued.

Because no clearly defined, straightforward map has been created to help us reach cultural competence, consciousness raising may begin at an informal roundtable discussion during which staff members share their experiences and strategies. Religious beliefs, cultural traditions and practices, clothing and food preferences, communication styles, socioeconomic differences, racial and ethnic issues, and generational differences are variables that may affect the therapeutic setting and are appropriate points at which to begin a dialogue.

The most vital message to convey is that cultural differences do matter in professional practice, and they deserve careful attention. All voices must be heard. One person at a staff meeting might be the lone voice that recognizes the struggle being felt by a client ethnic group, and that voice is important to hear. Alternatively, in some instances, the client may be saying "Don't stereotype me." According to Fernando (1995), an individual from a recognized ethnic group may have a complex relationship with the culture of that group. He or she may participate fully in the traditions and practices of the group, the client may identify more with the majority culture, or the client may be ambivalent with respect to group identity.

Dreachslin (1999) advised health care organizations to follow a five-part process toward cultural competence: discovery, assessment, exploration, transformation, and revitalization.

- *Discovery* refers to the emerging awareness that racial and ethnic diversity is a significant strategic issue. Occupational therapy managers can gather information that describes their service area's current and projected racial and ethnic demographics. The organization should emphasize the goal of ensuring equitable access for all the residents in the service area.

- *Assessment* refers to a systematic review of the organization's racial and ethnic climate. Occupational therapy managers can measure the satisfaction that diverse groups currently being served have with respect to services. Additionally, managers can measure employee satisfaction by surveying opinions within racial and ethnic groups. An action plan can then be developed to address those problems that surface, especially those that could have cultural implications.

- *Exploration* involves organizing and conducting systematic training initiatives to improve a department's ability to manage diversity effectively: The occupational therapy manager should ensure that important contributors have been invited to participate in the training, including administrators, key physicians, and other members of the multidisciplinary team. Nonclinical staff members should be welcome. Also, identified cultural healers may be invited. If important contributors are not invited to the training sessions, the reasons should be openly discussed. If the organization has no adequately skilled trainer on the staff, then the occupational therapy manager must assess the need and the budget options for using external consultants.

- *Transformation* refers to fundamental changes in organizational practices that result in a new departmental culture—one in which racial and ethnic diversity is valued and in which improving interaction with the population served is encouraged. Indicators can include mentoring programs for minority groups; rewards for delivery of culturally appropriate care; activities to celebrate diverse heritages; and strategies for recruiting diverse staff members, especially those from underrepresented groups. Additionally, the occupational therapy manager can make a difference by ensuring that the department is represented in community conferences where people of color are in the majority. The occupational therapy manager should look for opportunities to foster leadership throughout the organization, encourage staff members to become advocates and members of community advisory boards, and encourage staff members to speak to local civic groups about services and needs of the community. Finally, the occupational therapy manager should remember that change toward cultural competence is often gradual.

- *Revitalization* refers to the process of renewing and expanding racial and ethnic diversity initiatives to include additional identity groups and to reward change agents. The occupational therapy manager and staff members should focus on new diversity initiatives such as gender, sexual orientation, and disability issues. There is always room for improving cultural sensitivity. Cultural competence is seen as an ongoing process that is never quite completed.

## Role of the Internet

When developing business strategies, occupational therapy managers must consider future challenges and opportunities. Two things are clear to futurists: Institutions are becoming more global in character, and the use of the Internet will continue to increase. The health care marketplace is now the world, and forecasts predict that popular medical centers located in the United States will draw clients from a global pool (Giorgianni, 2000).

The Internet has been embraced faster than any technology in history. In the United States, a consumer-driven Internet is connecting everything and everyone, and it is changing the way health care is delivered. In particular, consumers are using the Internet to search for information that will empower them to take charge of their own health care. The Internet has inspired many potential applications and e-commerce opportunities for occupational therapy managers to consider, including the following:

- Provider advertising
- On-line shopping
- Referral assistance
- Advice Web sites
- Telerehabilitation
- Case conferences among specialists at distant locations
- Site visits within the client's home to monitor interventions.

The typical client in the 20th century often was confused and sought direction from a local health care professional. As the large cohort of post–World War II baby boomers retire, their demands on health care providers will increase, and their desire to control health care services will intensify. We may well be on the cusp of an entirely new concept of consumer-driven health care in which consumers even own and control their medical records. Cyberspace documents in which clients decide who will and will not be granted access are already being tested (van der Reis & Frey, 2001).

Predictions suggest that the typical client in the 21st century will be more of an "end user," that is, a client who seeks services from multiple organizations, perhaps through cyberspace. Health professionals who are practicing at times in cyberteams will simultaneously put in data and change data from different work stations at different geographical locations (Prins & Althof, 2000).

## World Federation of Occupational Therapists

No view of cross-cultural perspectives in occupational therapy would be complete without recognizing the work of the World Federation of Occupational Therapists (WFOT). Since 1952, WFOT has provided an international forum for occupational therapy practitioners, students, and related organizations to exchange ideas to improve the practice of occupational therapy worldwide. Often, participation in the federation's activities has fostered exchange opportunities for occupational therapy practitioners from the United States to visit with colleagues practicing in other countries. Also, occupational therapy practitioners from foreign countries continue to travel to the United States and share their knowledge and beliefs.

The first WFOT Congress was held in Edinburgh, United Kingdom. In addition to the United States and the United Kingdom, the founding members were Australia, Canada, Denmark, India, Israel, Sweden, New Zealand, and South Africa. Others attending that first congress included representatives from Ceylon, Egypt, Finland, France, Germany, Greece, the Netherlands, Norway, Poland, Rhodesia, and Switzerland. In addition to sharing clinical developments around the world, the international body has helped interpret the profession in worldwide political crises such as apartheid, reunification, and war. The federation has fostered the training of occupational therapy practitioners in developing nations, recognizing that different countries would have different priorities and needs.

In 1980, WFOT established the World Federation of Occupational Therapists Foundation to be used primarily for education and research. Awards are available for occupational therapy practitioners who are working in any area of occupational therapy and who are members of WFOT. Excellent histories of the federation were prepared by Alicia Mendez (2002) and Ruth Greenberg Harris (2002).

## Summary

Managing occupational therapy services in a multicultural society is the challenge of the 21st century. This challenge is magnified because occupational therapy managers have no clear road map to use in developing this new competence. Nevertheless, the demographic trends clearly show a need for occupational therapy practitioners to learn more about how our clients view their world and, in particular, how they view the health care delivery system.

## Conclusion

Organizational change is now a constant. Organizations can no longer operate in isolation, as they are influenced by both inside and outside forces. This change is occurring rapidly and is often derived from the effects of public policy and globalization.

Health care in the United States is changing. Expenditures have been increasing, but higher costs do not necessarily equate with better services. The federal government has sought to bring costs under control and in doing so has changed how medicine is practiced and how health care is accessed. Occupational therapy managers must stay informed of federal legislation issues to anticipate change and thus make relevant decisions.

Health care policy also is influenced by consumer needs. Complementary or alternative medicine is now commonly used in combination with conventional medicine. The definitions of health and wellness have evolved. Further, it has been suggested that home and community are where people really engage in occupations that are intrinsically important to them. Therefore, the provision of health care services—and occupational therapy services—are shifting out of large institutional organizations and into smaller, more community-based organizations.

The philosophical underpinnings of occupational therapy are based on humanistic values, holism, and treating the "whole person." Occupational therapy is a distinctive health profession using occupation to enable people to cope and adapt to disability and changes in their environment. Approximately 54 million Americans currently have some degree of disability, and as the population ages and life expectancy increases, the proportion of disability is likely to increase as well. Therefore, occupational therapy practitioners are well positioned to provide meaningful interventions in the community and deal with important life changes for a growing elderly population.

Systems theory is a useful model to understand how organizations maintain structure through continuous change. In this theory, all human behavior can be seen as occupation; therefore, occupation is central to human experience. Occupational therapy managers can use systems theory and the theory of human occupation to understand changes in the organizational environment and to explain adaptive and maladaptive behavior.

In the context of globalization, occupational therapy practitioners must face issues concerning race, ethnicity, culture, and other differences. Evidence has suggested that health care to ethnic minority people in not equal, and race seems to affect the type of intervention offered to patients. Cultural competence is a strategic imperative for occupational therapy mangers because evidence suggests that cultural diversity will continue to increase in health care organizations. Occupational therapy managers have a responsibility to create an intervention environment that values and respects people with diverse backgrounds.

Occupational therapy is a unique health profession because of its humanistic values and emphasis on holism and treating the whole person. As we seek to understand the whole person, we cannot overlook how public policy, the environment, and culture influence states of health.

Most occupational therapy practitioners will struggle with issues relating to race, ethnicity, culture, and cultural differences. Thus, occupational therapy managers have a particular responsibility to create an intervention environment in which diverse backgrounds of clients and staff members are respected and valued. Attention to cultural diversity is important both in reducing cultural bias and in promoting fair and effective care for all.

For the forward-thinking occupational therapy manager, competence in this new management expectation be will a strategic advantage in meeting the future demands of local and global markets.

# References

Aladana, S. G. (2001). Financial impact of health promotion programs: A comprehensive review of the literature. *American Journal of Health Promotion, 15,* 296–300.

American Occupational Therapy Association. (1995). Concept paper: Service delivery in occupational therapy. *American Journal of Occupational Therapy, 49,* 1029–1031.

American Occupational Therapy Association. (2001). *Occupational therapy practice framework: Draft XIII.* Bethesda, MD: Author.

American Occupational Therapy Association. (2002). *2000 AOTA member compensation survey.* Bethesda, MD: Author.

American Occupational Therapy Association. (2002). Occupational therapy practice framework: Domain and process. *American Journal of Occupational Therapy, 56,* 609–639.

Astin, J. A. (1998). Why patients use alternative medicine: Results of a national study. *Journal of the American Medical Association, 279,* 1548–1553.

Blue, A. (2000). *The provision of culturally competent health care.* Retrieved January 26, 2001, from http://www.musc.edu/deansclerkship/rccultur.html

Bottomly, J. M., Galentino, M. L., Umphred, D. A., Davis, C. M., & Maebori, D. (2001). Alternative and complementary therapies: Beyond traditional approaches to intervention in neurological diseases, syndromes, and disorders. In D. A. Umphred (Ed.), *Neurological rehabilitation* (4th ed., pp. 962–998). St. Louis, MO: Mosby.

Breslow, J. (1997). Social ecological strategies for promoting healthy lifestyles. *American Journal of Health Promotion, 10,* 253.

Brown, A., & Weiner, E. (1984). *Supermanaging: How to change for personal and organizational success.* New York: McGraw-Hill.

Capra, F. (1982). *The turning point.* New York: Bantam.

Centers for Disease Control and Prevention. (1999a). *Framework for program evaluation in public health* (MMWR 48, No. RR-11). Washington, DC: U.S. Department of Health and Human Services.

Centers for Disease Control and Prevention. (1999b). *Vital and health statistics.* Washington, DC: U.S. Department of Health and Human Services.

Christiansen, C., & Baum, C. (Eds.). (1991). *Occupational therapy: Overcoming human performance deficits.* Thorofare, NJ: Slack.

Christiansen, C., & Baum, C. (1997). *Occupational therapy: Enabling function and well-being.* Thorofare, NJ: Slack.

Clark, F., Azen, S. P., & Zemke, R. (1997). Occupational therapy for independent-living older adults: A randomized controlled trial. *Journal of the American Medical Association, 278,* 1321–1326.

Cohen, K. (1998). *Taoism: Study guide.* Boulder, CO: Sounds True.

Coile, R. (2001). Competing in a "consumer choice" market. *Journal of Healthcare Management, 46,* 297–300.

Crist, P. (1996). Organizational effectiveness. In M. Johnson (Ed.), *The occupational therapy manager* (pp. 173–174). Bethesda, MD: American Occupational Therapy Association.

Dana, R., Behn, J., & Gonwa, T. (1992). A checklist for the examination of cultural competence in social service agencies. *Research on Social Work Practice, 2,* 220–233.

Dillard, M., Andonian, L., Flores, O., Lai, L., MacRae, A., & Shakir, M. (1992). Culturally competent occupational therapy in a diversely populated mental health setting. *American Journal of Occupational Therapy, 46,* 721–725.

Dreachslin, J. (1999). Diversity leadership and organizational transformation: Performance indicators for health services organizations. *Journal of Healthcare Management, 44,* 427–439.

Druss, B. C., & Rosenheck, R. A. (1999). The association between use of unconventional therapies and conventional medical services. *Journal of the American Medical Association, 281,* 651–656.

Dubos, R. (1965). *Man adapting.* New Haven, CT: Yale University Press.

Dumas, J., Rollock, D., Prinz, R., Hops, H., & Blechman, E. (1999). Cultural sensitivity: Problems and solutions in applied and preventive intervention. *Applied and Preventive Psychology, 8,* 175–196.

Dunn, J. L. (1977). *High-level wellness.* Thorofare, NJ: Slack.

Edelman, C. L., & Mandle, C. L. (1998). *Health promotion throughout the lifespan* (4th ed.). St. Louis, MO: Mosby.

Eisenberg, D. M., Kessler, R., Foster, C., Norlock, F., Calkins, D., & Delbanco, T. (1998). Trends in alternative medicine use in the United States, 1990–1997: Results of a follow-up national survey. *Journal of the American Medical Association, 280,* 1569–1575.

Epstein, C. F., & Jaffe, E. G. (1996). Consultation: A collaborative approach to change. In M. Johnson (Ed.), *The occupational therapy manager* (pp. 533–574). Bethesda, MD: American Occupational Therapy Association.

Evans, R. (2001). Practitioner response to "Race, ethnicity, and careers in healthcare management." *Journal of Healthcare Management, 46,* 409–410.

Fernando, S. (1995). *Mental health in a multi-ethnic society: A multi-disciplinary handbook.* London: Routledge.

Finlay, L. (2000). Holism in occupational therapy: Elusive fiction and ambivalent struggle. *American Journal of Occupational Therapy, 55,* 268–269.

Fleming, M. H., & Mattingly, C. (1994). *Clinical reasoning: Forms of inquiry in a therapeutic practice.* Philadelphia: F. A. Davis.

Foundation program will address language barriers to health care. (2001, December 17). *AHA News*, p. 12.

Frangos, A. (2001, February 21). Model vs. model, a comparison of countries' health-care systems. *Wall Street Journal*, p. R4.

Friedman, T. (2000). *The Lexus and the olive tree*. New York: Farrar, Straus, & Giroux.

Furnham, A., & Vincent, C. (2001). Cultivating health through complementary medicine. In M. MacLachlan (Ed.), *Cultivating health: Cultural perspectives on promoting health* (pp. 113–131). New York: Wiley.

Gardner, J. (1964). *Self-renewal: The individual and the innovative society*. New York: Harper & Row.

Geiger, H. (1996). Race and health care—An American dilemma? *New England Journal of Medicine, 335*, 815–816.

Giorgianni, S. (Ed.). (2000). E-health care, the Internet information revolution. *Pfizer Journal, 4*(2), 4–36.

Golaszewski, T. (2001). Shining lights: Studies that have most influenced the understanding of health promotions financial impact. *American Journal of Health Promotion, 15*, 332–340.

Greenberg Harris, R. (2002). *A chronicle of the World Federation of Occupational Therapists*. Retrieved March 1, 2002, from http://www.wfot.org

Guralnik, J. (1991). Prospects for the compression of morbidity. *Journal of Aging and Health, 3*, 138–154.

Haber, D. (1999). *Health promotion and aging: Implications for the health professions*. New York: Slack.

Hall, E. (1966). *The hidden dimension*. Garden City, NY: International Universities Press.

Helman, C. (1990). *Culture, health, and illness* (2nd ed.). London: Wright.

Helman, C. (2000). *Culture, health, and illness* (4th ed.). Oxford, England: Butterworth, Heinemann.

Hinkle, L. E. (1964). The doctor, his patient, and the environment. *American Journal of Public Health, 54*, 11–17.

Hoffler, E. (1952). *The ordeal of change*. New York: Harper & Row.

Jaffe, E. G. (1985a). Transition in health care: Critical planning for the 1990s, part one. *American Journal of Occupational Therapy, 39*, 431–435.

Jaffe, E. G. (1985b). Transition in health care: Critical planning for the 1990s, part two. *American Journal of Occupational Therapy, 39*, 499–503.

Jaffe, E. G. (2001). *Systems theory lecture*, Samuel Merritt College, Oakland, CA.

Jaffe, E. G., & Epstein, C. F. (Eds.). (1992). *Occupational therapy consultation: Theory, principles, and practice*. St. Louis, MO: Mosby.

Jaffe, E. G., & Epstein, C. F. (2002). A consultative approach to occupational therapy practice. In M. E. Neistadt, E. B. Crepeau, E. Cohn, & B. Schell (Eds.), *Willard and Spackman's occupational therapy* (10th ed.). Philadelphia: Lippincott Williams & Wilkins.

Johnson, J. (1996). Wellness and occupational therapy. *American Journal of Occupational Therapy, 40*, 753–758.

Jona, S. (2000). *Talking about health and wellness with patients: Integrating health promotion and disease prevention into your practice*. New York: Springer.

Katz, D., & Kahn, R. L. (1978). *The social psychology of organizations* (2nd ed.). New York: Wiley.

Katz, M., Cole, J., & Lowry, H. (1969). Studies of the diagnosis process: The influence of symptom perception, past experience, and ethnic background on diagnostic decisions. *American Journal of Psychiatry, 125,* 109–119.

Kelly, J. G. (1970). Ecological constraints on mental health services. In P. E. Cook (Ed.), *Community psychology and community mental health* (pp. 54–62). San Francisco: Holden-Day.

Kennedy, P. S. (2000, November/December). An integrated alternative medicine program. *Oncology Issues,* pp. 14–16.

Kielhofner, G. (1997). *Conceptual foundations of occupational therapy* (2nd ed.). Philadelphia: F.A. Davis.

Kielhofner, G., & Burke, J. P. (1980a). A model of human occupation, part one. *American Journal of Occupational Therapy, 34,* 572–581.

Kielhofner, G., & Burke, J. P. (1980b). A model of human occupation, part two. *American Journal of Occupational Therapy, 34,* 657–663.

Kielhofner, G., & Burke, J. P. (1980c). A model of human occupation, part three. *American Journal of Occupational Therapy, 34,* 731–737.

Kielhofner, G., & Burke, J. P. (1980d). A model of human occupation, part four. *American Journal of Occupational Therapy, 34,* 777–788.

Kuhn, T. S. (1970). *The structure of scientific revolution* (2nd ed.). Chicago: University of Chicago Press.

Laszlo, E. (Ed.). (1972). *The relevance of general systems theory.* New York: Braziller.

Law, M., Cooper, B. A., Strong, S., Stewart, D., Rigby, P., & Letts, L. (1997). Theoretical contexts for the practice of occupational therapy. In C. Christiansen & C. Baum (Eds.), *Occupational therapy: Enabling function and well-being* (2nd ed., pp. 72–102). Thorofare, NJ: Slack.

Lawrence, P. R., & Lorsch, J. W. (1969). *Organization and environment.* Homewood, IL: Irwin.

Likert, K. (1967). *The human organization: Its management and value.* New York: McGraw-Hill.

Lippitt, R., Watson, J., & Westley, B. (1958). *The dynamics of planned change.* New York: Harcourt Brace & World.

Littlewood, R., & Lipsedge, M. (1989). *Aliens and alienists* (2nd ed.). London: Unwin Hyman.

MacLachlan, M. (2001). *Cultivating health: Cultural perspectives on promoting health. The American prospect.* New York: Wiley.

Mann, F. C. (1957). Studying and creating change: A means to understanding social organizations. *Research in Industry and Human Relations, 17,* 146–167.

Mattingly, C. (1991). What is clinical reasoning? *American Journal of Occupational Therapy, 45,* 979–986.

McCormack, G. (1987). *Culture and communication in the treatment planning for occupational therapy with minority patients: Social implications in treatment planning in occupational therapy.* Binghamton, NY: Haworth.

McCormack, G. (1994, September). Holism revisited: Toward a mind–body model for occupational therapy. *Physical Disabilities Special Interest Section Newsletter,* pp. 2–4.

Mendez, A. (2002). *A chronicle of the World Federation of Occupational Therapists, 1952–1982.* Retrieved March 1, 2002, from http://www.wfot.org

Meyer, A. (1922). The philosophy of occupational therapy. *Archives of Occupational Therapy, 1,* 1–10.

Morganthau, T. (1995, February 13). What color is Black? *Newsweek,* p. 64.

Moyers, P. A. (1999). *The guide to occupational therapy practice.* Bethesda, MD: American Occupational Therapy Association.

Nash, K. (1999). *Cultural competence: A guide for human service agencies.* Washington DC: Child Welfare League of America. (ERIC Document Reproduction Service No. ED 429 721)

Neistadt, M. E., & Crepeau, E. B. (Eds.) (1998). *Willard & Spackman's occupational therapy* (9th ed.). Philadelphia: Lippincott Williams & Wilkins.

O'Donnell, M. P. (1989). Definition of health promotion, Part III: Expanding the definition. *American Journal of Health Promotion, 3,* 5.

Pabst-Hunt, W. (2002). *Occupational therapy administration manual.* Albany, NY: Delmar.

Pedretti, L. W., & Early, M. B. (2001). *Occupational therapy: Practice skills for physical dysfunction* (5th ed.). St. Louis, MO: Mosby.

Pelletier, K. (1991). A review and analysis of the health and cost-effective outcomes studies of comprehensive health promotion and disease prevention programs. *American Journal of Health Promotion, 5,* 311–315.

Pelletier, R. R. (2002). A review and analysis of the clinical and cost-effectiveness studies of comprehensive health promotion at the worksite: 1995–2000 update. *American Journal of Health Promotion, 16,* 107–116.

Planta, M., Gunderson, B., & Petitt, J. C. (2000). Prevalence of the use of herbal products in a low-income population. *Family Medicine, 32,* 252–257.

Prins, C., & Althof, H. (2000, April). *The spotlight is on the client: Health information developments in the Netherlands.* The Hague: Dutch Association for Medical Records Administration.

Quiroga, V. A. M. (1995). *Occupational therapy: The first 30 years.* Bethesda, MD: American Occupational Therapy Association.

Robbins, S. P. (1994). *Management* (4th ed.). Englewood Cliffs, NJ: Prentice-Hall.

Scaffa, M. (Ed.). (2001). *Occupational therapy in community-based practice settings.* Philadelphia: F. A. Davis.

Shapiro, D. A., & Safer, M. (2002). Integrating complementary therapies in traditional oncology practice. *Oncology Issues, 18*(25), 35–40.

Smuts, J. C. (1926). *Holism and evolution.* New York: Macmillan.

Sparber, A., Bauer, L., Curt, G., & Eisenberg, D. (2000). Use of complementary medicine by adults participating in cancer clinical trials. *Oncology Nursing Forum, 27,* 2505–2514.

Sue, D. (2001, November). Multidimensional facets of cultural competence. *Counseling Psychologist,* pp. 790–821.

Swarbrich, P. (1997). Wellness model. *Mental Health Special Interest Section Quarterly, 20*(1), 1–4.

Taylor, D., & Saks, M. (1998). Medicine and complementary medicine: Challenges and change. In E. Scambler & P. Higgs (Eds.), *Modernity, medicine and health* (pp. 22–28). London: Routledge.

Thomas, C. L. (1989). *Taber's encyclopedic medical dictionary* (10th ed.). Philadelphia: F. A. Davis.

Thomas, K. J., Carr, J., Weslake, L., & Williams, B. T. (1991). Use of non-orthodox and conventional health care in Great Britain. *British Medical Journal, 302,* 210–297.

Toffler, A. (1970). *Future shock*. New York: Random House.

U.S. Department of Health and Human Services. (2001). *Healthy people 2010*. Washington, DC: U.S. Government Printing Office.

U.S. health care trails world. (2000, June 21). *The Contra Costa Times*, p. A14.

Valluzzi, J. L. (2002). Evaluating and monitoring community-based programs. *OT Practice, 7*(3), 10–13.

van der Reis, L., & Frey, W. (2001). *A bi-national study of the role of information technology in national healthcare systems: The Netherlands and the United States*. San Francisco: Quincy Foundation for Medical Research.

Van Os, J., Galdos, P., & Lewis, G. (1993). Schizophrenia sans frontiers: Concepts of schizophrenia among French and British psychiatrists. *British Medical Journal, 307*, 489–492.

Vande Creek, L., Rogers, E., & Lester, J. (1999). Use of alternative therapies among breast cancer out-patients compared with general population. *Alternative Therapy Health Medicine, 5*(1), 71–76.

von Bertalanffy, L. (1968). *General systems theory: Foundations, development, and application*. New York: Braziller.

Whittle, J., Conigliaro, C., Good, B., & Lofgren, R. (1993). Racial differences in the use of invasive cardiovascular procedures in the department of veterans affairs medical systems. *New England Journal of Medicine, 329*, 621–627.

Wootton, J. C., & Sparber, A. (2001). Surveys of complementary and alternative medicine: Part I. General trends and demographic groups. *Journal of Alternative and Complementary Medicine, 7*, 195–208.

World Health Organization. (1958). *The first ten years of the World Health Organization*. Geneva: Author.

World Health Organization, Canada, & Canadian Public Health Association, Ohawa Chapter for Health Promotion. (1992). *Health promotion*. Unpublished manuscript.

Yerxa, E. J. (1991). Seeking a relevant ethical and realistic way of knowing for occupational therapy. *American Journal of Occupational Therapy, 45*, 199–204.

Zemke, R., & Clark, F. (1996). *Occupational science: The evolving discipline*. Philadelphia: F. A. Davis.

# Planning

# Strategic Planning

Randy Strickland, EdD, OTR/L, FAOTA

*"Occupational therapy participation in strategic planning
helps to ensure a service delivery system that meets and
anticipates consumer needs."*

RANDY STRICKLAND

**Randy Strickland, EdD,
OTR/L, FAOTA,** has a
bachelor's of science
degree in occupational
therapy from East Carolina
University and a doctorate
in adult education from
North Carolina State
University. He is the chair
of the Auerbach School of
Occupational Therapy at
Spalding University in
Louisville, KY, and
president of the National
Board for Certification in
Occupational Therapy.
He is a former vice-presi-
dent of the American
Occupational Therapy
Association.

## Key Terms and Concepts

**Environmental analysis.** A snapshot of an organization's internal and external environments at any given time.

**Mission.** A common purpose that is understood, valued, and shared by members of an organization.

**Scenario planning (or scenario development).** Creative constructions of potential future realities for an organization.

**Stakeholders.** Groups or individuals with a vested interest in an organization's activities.

**Strategic management.** Process whereby an organization uses environmental analysis to establish and implement strategic initiatives.

**Strategic planning.** A "managerial process of developing and maintaining a strategic fit between [an] organization's goals [and] resources, and its changing market opportunities" (Kotler & Clarke, 1987, p. 90).

**Strategy.** A plan of action that enables an organization to achieve its goals.

**SWOT analysis.** An organization's internal analysis of strengths (S) and weaknesses (W) along with an assessment of both external opportunities (O) and threats (T).

**Vision.** Organizational or program aspirations for the future.

## Learning Objectives

After completing this chapter, you should be able to do the following:

- Describe the role of strategic planning in one's daily practice and organizational operations.
- Apply the concepts of environmental and SWOT analyses in strategic plan development.
- Identify the contributions and value of stakeholder groups in planning.
- Describe the process of strategic management, including strategic planning and strategy development.
- Use scenario planning concepts in the development of a strategic plan.
- Discuss the impact of strategic planning in occupational therapy management, advocacy, and leadership roles.

Strategic planning is a management concept that has received considerable attention from organizational leaders. The strategic planning process may appear vague and somewhat distant from the demands of daily practice that are experienced by the occupational therapist or occupational therapy assistant. In reality, strategic planning is a necessary and critical process for the ongoing success and even availability of occupational therapy services in varied settings. Occupational therapy practitioners may not be informed of or involved in the strategic planning initiatives in their work organizations. The occupational therapist's or occupational therapy assistant's participation in helping to plan, focus, and ultimately implement the strategic direction of the practice environment is an essential aspect of his or her professional role and contributions to the work setting's success in serving its clientele.

Strategic planning within an organization, whether it serves children, adults, older adults, or other populations, provides the direction for that organization over the next few years. Frequently, strategic planning efforts are incorporated into management operations, which may not be readily apparent or visible to the occupational therapy practitioner. The current efforts of the organization provide the data for assessing the present situation and status as well as for projecting its future viability and position in the community. Occupational therapists and occupational therapy assistants are knowledgeable and valued participants in promoting and delivering quality services; consequently, they should be included as contributors and participants in an organization's strategic planning efforts.

The occupational therapist or occupational therapy assistant is often assigned to a specific program or unit in an organization, for example, a public school setting, rehabilitation program, acute care hospital, senior citizen center, outpatient facility, or home health agency. In each setting, the practitioner has a vested interest in the organization's current and future plans for services. It is critical for the occupational therapy practitioner to participate in the strategic planning efforts and contribute toward defining the vision of the organization. From a strategic planning perspective, each organization should regularly examine its successes and challenges as well as reaffirm that its strategies not only are meeting current needs in the community but also are anticipating evolving needs and changes in the environment.

Proactive and community-focused organizations value their connection with the needs of society or the community. The participation of the occupational therapist or occupational therapist assistant in the strategic planning process links occupational therapy services with community needs. The organization's strategic planning must move beyond the board room or upper management and foster staff participation in charting the future. Including key players in strategic planning promotes the adaptation of service delivery environments that are geared toward present and future needs of individuals and populations.

## Key Concepts in Strategic Planning

The term *strategy* refers to a carefully crafted plan or approach that is key in operationally carrying out strategic planning. Kotler and Clarke (1987) defined *strategic planning* as the "managerial process of developing and maintaining a strategic fit between [an] organization's goals [and] resources, and its changing market opportunities" (p. 90). The organization's strategic plan identifies future goals and objectives as well as the strategies or methods that enable and support the attainment of those goals. An organization involved in strategic planning strives to critically review its internal operations and the external environment to ensure that its practices anticipate and respond to change. Organizations that are responsibly involved in strategic planning diligently pursue the ongoing development and refinement of plans that match its activities with established goals. Those who are defining and meeting an organization's goals must consider multiple points of view and the relationships of groups and individuals both within and outside of the organization. For example, a state-funded program that serves adults with developmental disabilities may be assessing the feasibility of closing an institution serving 100 residents and reallocating its resources for additional community programs. Regulatory, management, and financial perspectives may strongly support this action. Nevertheless, the opinions and input of the facility's residents and their family members must be considered when developing and selecting strategies.

Strategic planning decisions are best made by, first, thoughtfully examining the organization's foundation, including its mission and goals. The staff and leaders of an organization must understand its mission and core values. An organization without a clear understanding of its mission or core values is like a boat without a rudder. The effective mission statement creates a common guiding purpose that is understood, valued, and shared by all members of an organization. Pinchot (1998) described how the mission of the Sisters of Providence Hospitals organization allows its employees to meet traditional business measures such as patient census and cost containment requirements while remaining focused on meeting the needs of the community. This hospital system's mission, "to serve in whatever ways and means the people and the times require, consistent with the values of the Sisters of Providence" (p. 131), affirms the importance of a belief system as the basis for operations and planning efforts. An imbalance between the mission statement and the activities of the unit may minimize both the success and the appropriateness of the strategic plan until the disparity is addressed.

The identification of the organization's mission statement and core values are followed by the development of a vision statement. A vision statement projects where the program would like to be in the future. This projection is the statement of the ideal situation. Vision statements, although often expressed in the present tense, are intended as aspirations for the future. For example, the American Occupational Therapy Foundation (2000) included its vision statement along with its mission and organizational goals on its Web site:

> The American Occupational Therapy Foundation promotes a society in which individuals, regardless of age or ability, may participate in occupations of choice that give meaning to their lives and foster health and well being. Through its dedication to scientific inquiry, education and leadership development, the Foundation pays tribute to the significance of everyday activities in enabling those who face personal challenges to realize their full potential in society.

The coordination of an organization's mission statement, core values, and vision statement provides a starting point for future planning activities.

A key step in the strategic planning process is the completion of an environmental analysis. An environmental analysis is a snapshot of an organization's internal and external environments at any given time (see chapter 4, for additional information related to environmental analysis). This analysis provides the data for evaluating the organization's current operations and determining future areas of growth, development, and change. The environmental analysis focuses on stakeholders who are affected by or have a vested interest in the organization's activities. External stakeholders include a wide range of people such as patients and clients, other service providers, government agencies, payers, and community members or organizations. Internal stakeholders include employees, administrators and managers, staff members, and the organization's owners or board of directors. The combined internal and external environmental analyses, including the consideration of multiple stakeholder views and values, provide the core for strategic planning activities and connection with the community's perceived needs (Harrison & St. John, 2002).

A frequently used process in strategic planning is SWOT analysis. The SWOT analysis guides an organization's internal analysis of its strengths (S) and weaknesses (W) and an external assessment of opportunities (O) and threats (T), all of which could affect the viability of the organization (Mintzberg, Ahlstrand, & Lampel, 1998). The SWOT analysis is a progression of the environmental analysis. Frequently, opportunities for an organization may be embedded or represented in the identification of threats. Similarly, strengths and weakness may be synergistic and allow the organization to capitalize on what typically may be viewed as an internal disadvantage. Early and ongoing identification of strengths, weaknesses, opportunities, and threats propels the planning, creativity, and subsequent actions of the organization's members and promotes connections with the internal and external environments.

Scenario strategic planning is a critical process preceding the development of goals, objectives, and strategies. Scenario planning or development allows internal and, possibly, external stakeholders to construct possible future organizational realities. Often, these scenarios vary as to how realistic they might be and are not initially rated as desirable or undesirable options but simply as different sets of possibilities.

Through the scenario development process, one can envision various possibilities and select the most desired, most likely, or most beneficial choice or approach to which the organization could aspire. Schwartz (1996) clearly described the critical process of scenario construction and suggested for all planners (including occupational therapy practitioners) to consider the following:

> Not just our livelihoods, but our souls are endangered—unless we learn to distinguish the significant aspects of the future. The scenario method works in this respect. It is specifically based on our personal urgencies (or on a company's institutional urgencies). It uses our individual needs as a filter. . . . By imagining where we are going, we reduce this complexity, this unpredictability which . . . encroaches upon our lives. (p. 15)

The development of strategic scenarios challenges us to "think outside the box" and forces the organization to weigh alternatives critically in the development of its strategic direction. Strategic direction can include the establishment of long-term goals and objectives. This fundamental step is derived from the SWOT analysis and strategic scenario exercises. Strategic direction can support the organization's mission and vision aspirations. Additionally, strategies, including methods and measurement supports, are utilized to achieve the organization's goals. Harrison and St. John (2002) described *strategy* as "an organizational plan of action that is intended to move an organization toward the achievement of its shorter-term goals and, ultimately, toward the achievement of its fundamental purposes" (p. 6). Strategy formulation is enhanced by staff participation, including involvement of occupational therapists and occupational therapy assistants.

The establishment of strategies includes the assumption that various organizational units will cooperate to implement strategies and revise approaches as necessary. Gadiesh and Olivet (1997) stated that staff members in an organization must know the plan's purpose before they can implement and achieve new strategies and new goals. Simply informing staff members that change is required in a particular practice or procedure does not ensure that an organization will meet its stated objectives. Staff members must understand and appreciate how they work together in managing the strategic direction and plan. Teams are empowered by clearly established charges that clearly identify the organization's direction, objectives, goals, measures, limits, and focus. A common view of purpose and shared values allows the organization to attain and perhaps exceed its goals proactively (refer to chapter 13 for additional information).

## Strategic Planning Process

The strategic planning process includes six basic steps: (a) environmental analysis; (b) SWOT analysis; (c) strategic scenario development; (d) establishment of strategic goals, objectives, and strategies; (e) implementation; and (f) evaluation of results and ongoing review of the strategic plan (Fahey & Randall, 1994; Harrison & St. John, 2002; Kotler & Clarke, 1987).

Strategic planning is only one element of the comprehensive strategic management process. Harrison and St. John (2002) described *strategic management* as the process by which "organizations analyze and learn from their internal and external environments, establish strategic direction, create strategies that are intended to achieve established goals, and execute those strategies, all in an effort to satisfy key . . . stakeholders" (p. 4). Strategic planning is not a process that occurs once a year or that is stored in a file except for a cursory quarterly or annual review; rather, it is an integral part of strategic management, which is a dynamic, futuristic, ever-evolving, and entrepreneurial-oriented process.

## Environmental Analysis

The successful strategic management process, including strategic planning, strongly relies on a thorough assessment of an organization's internal and external environments. Various members of an organization may collect external data and provide this information for critical analysis. The occupational therapy practitioner can play an important role in both the internal and external analysis.

Wheatley (1999) supported group participation as a means to instill the employees' and community's ownership of the goals and strategies of the organization. She noted that "We live in a universe where relationships are primary. . . . Nothing exists independent of its relationships. . . . This is a world of process, the process of connecting, where 'things' come into temporary existence because of relationship" (p. 69). Relationships with the internal and external communities are critical to achieve success in strategic management and in the actual development of a strategic plan and future direction of an organization. Consideration of varied stakeholders' views with respect to an organization's current and potential strategic initiatives promotes buy-in and, more importantly, helps to ensure that the plans of the organization are congruent with the community. Analysis of external and internal stakeholders' views provides the opportunity to identify areas of possible conflict and collaboration.

External environmental analysis considers both the global environment and specific stakeholders. Harrison and St. John (2002) cited the broad environment, including sociocultural, economic, technological, and political forces, as significantly influencing an organization's capacity to plan for its enhancement, renewal, creation, or survival (see chapter 4, for additional information on environmental analysis). The broad environment model provides a framework with which to identify external stakeholders such as patients, clients, and family members; payers; federal, state, and local governments; vendors; activist groups; professional associations; and competitors. For example, the concept of continuing competence and professional development depicts the impact of the broad environment including external stakeholders on the daily practice demands in occupational therapy settings. Occupational therapy clients expect to receive intervention that is culturally sensitive and cost-effective and that reflects a therapist's knowledge and skills in a changing service delivery environment (Law & Baum, 1998). Third-party payer expectations require that occupational therapy services provide tangible outcomes. Watson (2000) analyzed occupational therapy payer expectations and stated:

> We are moving away from an era where service delivery systems could offer an unlimited array of health services to a climate that focuses on the equitable allocation of cost-effective services. The identification of cost-effective services requires that all service providers have an understanding of the cost and outcomes of the services that they render. (p. 7)

Meanwhile, other organizations such as state regulatory jurisdictions, the National Board for Certification in Occupational Therapy (2002), and the American Occupational Therapy Association (AOTA, 2002) are developing requirements, standards, or programs for continuing competence. The occupational therapist's and occupational therapy assistant's practice is affected by these and other influences as they strive to deliver professional and ethical occupational therapy services that are client-centered and cost-effective. Many current work settings require ongoing self-assessment in light of continual role changes and performance demands.

Additionally, the environmental analysis considers the internal stakeholders such as employees, administrators and managers, board of directors, and owners. Harrison and St. John (2002) recommended that an assessment of the views and skills of the organization and its internal stakeholders include "all of the organization's resources and capabilities to determine strengths, weaknesses, and opportunities for competitive advantage, and to identify organizational vulnerabilities that should be corrected" (p. 5).

## SWOT Analysis

Completion of the environmental analysis creates a basis and logical transition for developing a SWOT analysis. Where the environmental analysis provides an assessment of both the internal and external environment with specific emphasis on the perspectives and influences of stakeholder groups, the SWOT analysis is essential to delineate an organization's strengths, weaknesses, opportunities, and threats. The results of the internal environmental analysis may be used to compile a listing of the organization's strengths and weaknesses; similarly, data from the external environmental analysis assist in determining opportunities and threats (Fahey & Randall, 1994). The input of various constituent groups and individuals supports the development of a strategic plan and initiatives that are attuned to both organization and community needs.

The completion of the SWOT analysis requires the informed judgments of the organization's management and staff. The occupational therapist's or occupational therapy assistant's skills in the specific practice setting may add needed validation with respect to the value or weight that should be placed on a particular internal or external issue. The information that is discerned by doing a SWOT analysis does not constitute a decision as to a strategic direction for an organization, program, or department. The SWOT analysis serves as an initial step in the prioritization of internal and external issues deemed as influential in strategic plan development.

## Strategic Scenario Development

The creation of a strategic plan is an ongoing process that ideally involves participants from throughout the system. One step in this process that is significantly enriched by staff involvement is scenario development. Staff members may have varying degrees of participation in the process; however, all staff members must be aware of the process and its relationship to their current roles and, even more important, their future ones. Although one approach would be simply to take the completed environmental and SWOT analyses and develop long-range goals and short-term objective and strategies, the more prudent approach is to capitalize on the organization's most powerful and useful resource—its employees.

Using scenario development as a component of the strategic planning process fosters the creative juices that are inherent but often untapped in staff members. Mintzberg et al. (1998) expanded on scenario planning and stated that "if you cannot predict the future, then by speculating on a variety of them, you might open up your mind and even, perhaps, hit upon the right one" (p. 58). To further the science and art of developing strategic scenarios that can provide a springboard for both futuristic proactive planning and, ultimately, organizational success in achieving its mission or vision, Schwartz (1996) suggested eliciting staff members' and stakeholders' participation in strategic dialogues about possible options, including the engagement of staff members and other stakeholders in a permanent strategic conversation.

Both the environmental and SWOT analyses included consideration of the views and perspectives of stakeholders. Scenario development adds two important features: the evaluation of multiple options and the inclusion of stakeholders in the dialogue. These features may be illustrated by considering a recurring challenge in many occupational therapy practices—scheduling clients for services, which could be categorized under the broad strategic goal "Ensure customer satisfaction." Varied scheduling systems and software may be used to resolve the problem, but identification of the true problem requires a review of multiple factors such as referral patterns and, most certainly, patient preferences. Using various "what-ifs" in the scheduling scenarios along with participation from a wide range of stakeholders may yield a more effective solution. In addition, this technique may be used for a customer- and staff-focused strategy addressing customer satisfaction in general.

## Establishment of Goals, Objectives, and Strategies

Scenario analysis by internal and external stakeholders is pivotal for establishing the plan's actual strategic intent. Jacobs (1994) suggested that

> this process of thinking together leads to more individual perspectives being shared, a more holistic view of the organization's collective reality and ultimately, a more informed change effort overall. . . . Business as usual is not an acceptable outcome from strategic change process. (p. 23)

At this juncture—after the analyses and the scenario development—the organization performs a reality check of possible strategic goals and assesses their fit with the mission and vision; that is, it begins to develop a strategic plan. Identification of new or revised goals for the organization requires that the responsible decision makers (administrators, managers, board of directors, and possibly staff members) determine whether the goals reflect integrity and fiduciary responsibility. Selection of goals as well as subsequent objectives and strategies implies ownership by the organization. Perry (2002) described the role of an organization and its decision makers as being "willing to stand up, be open and accountable to stakeholders by exposing the reasoning for the decision. This requires a willingness to be tested, questioned, and judged by others. . . . Durable decisions usually follow thorough dialog, consultation, and collaboration" (p. 28).

Within a strategic plan, goals are typically broad intentions that may number as few as two or three. For instance, a goal for a hospital system's programs for individuals with acquired brain injury may be stated as the following: "A comprehensive, seamless service delivery model for individuals with acquired brain injury will be implemented." After goals are identified, specific and measurable objectives, which quantify the expectations and benchmarks (outcomes), are then listed under the goals. The number of objectives for each goal will vary by setting and by the scope of the goal. A companion objective for the hospital system goal might be stated as the following: "Each individual with an acquired brain injury will be referred for an outpatient transitional program evaluation prior to discharge from the acute rehabilitation unit in the hospital system." The stated strategies for this goal and objective might include the following:

> "(1) The outpatient program representative (rotating among occupational therapist, speech–language pathologist, and psychologist) will attend weekly rounds for the brain injury team; (2) the brain injury case manager will monitor discharges daily, recommend outpatient referrals, and inform the outpatient administrative assistant of any planned or unplanned discharges from the unit; and (3) the outpatient transitional program evaluator (occupational therapist) will initiate the evaluation process within 24 hours of receipt of the referral."

## Implementation

The establishment of goals, objectives, and strategies is very similar to the occupational therapy evaluation and intervention process. The objectives and strategies embedded in a strategic plan will have designated measures, timelines, and responsible staff members. The expectation of occupational therapists and occupational therapy assistants that they will be accountable and responsible for their program's meeting objectives and strategies is very likely.

Implementation of the strategic plan is an ongoing activity for managers and staff in an organization. For example, in the previously cited program objective, "the outpatient transitional program evaluator will initiate the evaluation," assigned staff are responsible for focusing on the implementation of the strategies needed for the goal and objective achievement. Strategy implementation requires the prioritization and allocation of the organization's human resources and budget for task completion. Management emphasis on staff commitment to the process and time for strategy implementation is critical. Additionally, staff and management have a joint accountability for ensuring that staff have the knowledge and skills to use and evaluate identified implementation strategies.

## Evaluation of Results and Review of Strategic Plan

The development of an organization's strategic plan is based on environmental and SWOT analyses; possible scenarios for the future; and a set of goals, objectives, and specific strategies that are developed from those analyses and scenarios. The plan's basic foundation is the organization's mission and its vision or aspirations. Within the organization, an individual or group will be responsible for monitoring and evaluating the plan's status and currentness on a regular basis.

In the past, plans may have been reviewed on a yearly basis and may have undergone a major overhaul every 3 to 5 years. Today's environments are demanding, and more careful scrutiny of an organization's strategic plan and strategies is common. The formation of new goals, objectives, and strategies or the revision of existing ones occurs frequently, with some plans being monitored as frequently as once weekly. Generally, the monitoring process may be less frequent than a weekly review, but commonly, successful organizations find that the shelf life of a plan is relatively short and needs to be reviewed often. The occupational therapy practitioner and other staff members may be expected to assess the plan's progress in assigned areas. Additionally, because a successful organization is planning on a formative basis, most staff members will contribute regularly to plan review in some capacity.

## Strategic Planning Precautions and Precepts

Mintzberg et al. (1998) listed three common fallacies of strategic planning:
- The strategic plan can predict all things.
- The strategic plan allows management to become detached from the daily life of the organization.
- The strategic planning system inevitably becomes overly bureaucratic and prescriptive.

In fact, reliance on the organization's strategic plan to accurately forecast the future and ensure success can create a false sense of security. Certainly, management needs to be attuned to the daily life of the organization to better adjust or completely redesign the strategic plan. And history shows us repeatedly that the successful organization is adaptive and does not act as if it were restricted by a rigid document.

Strategic planning must be an inclusive and participatory process rather than a rigid adherence to a linear and hierarchical management approach. Strategic planning identifies and achieves organizational priorities through strategy selection and implementation. The success of the process is directly influenced by the synthesis of information that is obtained from the organization's internal and external stakeholders. Obtaining information and assistance in the total strategic planning process requires stakeholder ownership. At a minimum, the process must be transparent and ensure accountability for the organization's actions. If planning occurs in a vacuum, disregards the organization's mission, or discounts the stakeholders' perspectives, then it may jeopardize the likelihood that the programs or services will reflect the community's needs. Finally, the strategic planning process and the resulting plan and strategies must be tangible, uncomplicated, easily understood, and actually used as a part of the staff's daily assignments.

The ultimate measure of a plan's usefulness is its relevance and performance in assisting the organization to meet ongoing and emerging challenges as well as mission or vision expectations in its ever-changing work environment. Ongoing planning ensures an organization's capacity to make future role changes while promoting achievement of its mission and goals.

## Occupational Therapy Leadership and Strategic Planning Connections

Initially, the connection between the occupational therapy practitioner and strategic planning may seem ambiguous or, at least, minimal. Yet the future viability of occupational therapy is directly influenced by the planning efforts of varied organizations. If occupational therapists and occupational therapy assistants are not active participants (internal stakeholders) in the planning activities within their workplaces, the results may prove to be detrimental for the individuals and groups who require occupational therapy services. The perspectives provided from occupational therapists and occupational therapy assistants can support the goals of the organization. Occupational therapy staff members cannot abdicate their responsibility to engage actively in their employer's planning initiatives; at the very minimum, practitioners must remain informed as to the organization's direction and engage in the strategic dialogue at all possible levels. Involvement in these activities is both an opportunity and an expectation for all staff members and is not restricted only to designated managers or supervisors. Practitioners must understand that the business of planning and management may affect their ability to provide needed services within an environment that fosters both quality and productivity. Being strategic in one's thinking and actions is an attribute of a highly skilled, effective, and reflective practitioner.

Occupational therapists and occupational therapy assistants who are cognizant of the organization's strategic thinking and plans can enrich daily practice and better assess intervention effectiveness. The occupational therapy profession, like many other health professions, is responsible for providing services that produce outcomes that are cost-efficient, cost-effective, and client focused. The mantra of evidence-based practice is not an academic ideal but a reality in service delivery environments, where needs often exceed available resources, particularly staff and funding. The profession's members can participate in varied strategic planning exercises and contribute to highly innovative strategic scenarios that can value occupational therapy intervention. However, all of these efforts, no matter how valiant, are for naught if the evidence of occupational therapy intervention is not readily apparent and strategically embedded in the organization's analysis of pertinent data. Holm (2000), in her Eleanor Clarke Slagle Lecture, rightfully and strongly advocated that practitioners develop two new habits for the new millennium:

> We have an obligation to become competent in, and make a habit of, searching for the evidence, appraising its value, and presenting it to those we serve in an understandable manner. . . . We also have an obligation to improve our research competencies, to develop the habit of using those competencies, to develop the habit of using those competencies in everyday practice, and to advance the evidence base of occupational therapy in the new millennium. (p. 584)

Strategic planning has tremendous application possibilities for the practitioner who is developing a new practice or program. Limiting the application of strategic management, strategic planning, and scenario development concepts to established practice settings omits the very situations in which a strategic and innovative focus is most needed. The practice of occupational therapy is evolving to meet emerging community needs. Continued growth in education and community-based practice along with expansion in medical settings affords numerous options for the practitioner to further define and, in some instances, reclaim the vital contributions of occupational therapy for varied populations and settings. By using business savvy skills and the creative use of evidence-based practice in daily practice, today's practitioners can exert considerable influence and have a tremendous impact on the lives of service recipients.

This chapter has emphasized how an occupational therapist or occupational therapy assistant can have an impact as an internal stakeholder on the strategic planning process in the work setting. Perhaps the greater challenge and opportunity occurs as practitioners direct their attention toward other stakeholders who may actually control, sanction, or persuade the development of policy, regulation, funding, or even recognition of occupational therapy's scope of practice. Thinking strategically and collaboratively with payers, government agencies, consumers, and many others is a forward-thinking approach. Although no one individual can be totally engaged in all arenas at local, state, and national levels, occupational therapists and occupational therapy assistants must consistently monitor the external environment for issues that influence their daily practice and the profession. Involvement in professional associations such as AOTA and state occupational therapy associations as well as in the regulatory and certification activities provides excellent stages for providing input into the strategic thinking and plans of the profession. The larger challenge is to enter the dialogue with others who are not within this profession. Creating linkages and alliances with other groups and individuals strengthens the profession and the individual practitioner as well as provides for delivery and creation of more appropriate programs and services for diverse needs.

The challenge to connect strategic thinking, occupational therapy leadership, and management extends to each occupational therapist and occupational therapy assistant; to ignore this challenge is to shirk one's professional duties. Occupational therapy leaders in this decade have an excellent and perhaps time-sensitive opportunity to strategically advance and promote this profession.

## Case Example

The following case example describes an occupational therapy program in a public school district; however, occupational therapy practitioners in an extensive range of practice settings can assume active roles in charting the organization's direction. Application of the strategic planning process can be best understood by becoming involved in the process.

### Background

A local school district has a long history of using contractual occupational therapy services for all of its programs. The district has used several companies and numerous therapists over the years. In fact, the entire process has been rather uncoordinated and, often, at the discretion of each individual school principal. Feedback from teachers and parents has indicated a general satisfaction with services in a select number of schools. Recent district funding concerns and possible management changes have indicated that one cost-saving plan may be for the district to employ occupational therapists. The district currently contracts for the equivalent of 4.5 full-time equivalents (FTEs) for occupational therapy services. The director of district special education has engaged a respected local occupational therapist, who has previously contracted with the district, to develop a plan for employing occupational therapists as staff members. The director also hopes to recruit this consultant as the district coordinator of occupational therapy services.

### School District Strategic Plan

An occupational therapist and the district director of district special education have collaborated to develop a strategic plan for implementing district occupational therapy services. (Readers will note that this strategic plan provides a highlight of key areas; a complete plan may require several pages.) The actual application of this example plan would evolve as the occupational therapists and occupational therapy assistants became members of the district staff.

#### *Environmental Analysis*

Internal stakeholders (parents, school principals, and selected teachers) were interviewed to obtain their input with respect to possible concerns about current services and areas for development. District records, including a sample of individual education plans and other related services documentation, were analyzed for state and federal compliance. A similar review process for external stakeholders included a review of federal and state regulations as well as consultation with three school districts. The board of directors of the Council for Individuals with Developmental Disabilities participated in a focus group. In addition, contractual staff members and the local occupational therapy association leaders were surveyed.

### SWOT Analysis

Strengths (S) include the district's willingness to initiate a new service delivery model, sufficient funding for up to six FTEs, a competitive benefits package for employees, and the superintendent's personal support for needed changes. Weaknesses (W) include a desire by the principals to maintain all authority for hiring staff members, a lack of any standard operating procedures for using occupational therapy services, and the identification of handwriting and sensory integration as the only accepted interventions with no transitional services for older students. Other concerns include a projected caseload of at least 500 students and teachers' perception that the therapists are costly and, perhaps, not a value-added service when compared to the option of hiring more aides. Opportunities (O) include greater availability of occupational therapists, reduced occupational therapy salary expectations as compared to when the district last considered employing its own occupational therapy staff, and a possible district contractual arrangement to provide services for the local council. Threats (T) include possible litigation over insufficient services, community practitioners who are uncertain of the district's support, and a possible shortage of occupational therapists and occupational therapy assistants with school experience.

### Strategic Scenarios

Options examined by a representative group of teachers, principals, district physical therapists, speech and language pathologists, and psychologists included the following: (a) continue with the current system with potential litigation and unsatisfactory experiences for students; (b) do not recruit and retain therapists, and therefore, the district will be forced to contract at even higher rates, with less predictable staffing; and (c) develop a model program with a stable staff and excellent support of students' educational needs and experiences. The district decided to develop its own model program to meet the educational needs of its students.

### Strategic Goals

The district planning group outlined the following goals:
- Develop a district-wide model for staffing occupational therapy services programs.
- Implement a plan that ensures that all state and federal laws and regulations for related services are met or exceeded.

### Strategic Objectives

The district planning group developed the following objectives:
- Develop position descriptions and hire an occupational therapy coordinator (1 FTE), occupational therapists (4 FTEs), and occupational therapy assistants (1 FTE).

- Implement standard procedures for occupational therapy delivery.
- Develop a plan for professional development and continuing competency for newly hired staff members.

### Strategy Development, Implementation, and Evaluation

The occupational therapy consultant will assist the special education director in implementing a recruitment plan and developing job descriptions. This process will be initiated in February prior to the new school year beginning in August. An initial review of assessment procedures and programs will be completed by August. The newly hired coordinator (employed by July) will conduct a two-day planning session for all new staff members in early August; this session will include orientation and the development of plans to begin educational efforts with teachers and school administration in the joint development of revised or new programs, including assessment protocols. From early July until the beginning of the school year, the special education director and district occupational therapy coordinator will have joint responsibility for the plan's objectives. Later, education and occupational therapy staff members will assist in the identification and selection of other objectives and strategies. The district's annual program evaluation system will be used in conjunction with the strategic plan to assess progress toward the two goals established prior to the beginning of the academic year. During the first year, all occupational therapy staff members will regularly review the program's status in collaboration with internal and external stakeholders.

## Conclusion

The strategic planning process is a dynamic interaction involving internal stakeholders (such as staff members and managers) and external stakeholders. Ideally, this process is based on the organization's mission and vision. Consideration of both the internal and external stakeholders' perspective provides the basis for a complete environmental and SWOT analysis. The SWOT analysis builds on the organization's internal strengths and weaknesses and balances this information with external opportunities and threats. The development and review of varied strategic scenarios assists the organization in formulating a strategic plan that includes goals, objectives, and strategies. This plan is then implemented and evaluated on a regular basis so adjustments can be made that respond to an ever-changing environment.

Strategic planning is an important process influencing the daily practice environment for the occupational therapist and occupation therapy assistant. Recognition of one's responsibility to become an active part of developing the future for occupational therapy services in an agency is an important management practice. Delivering strategic occupational therapy services is optimized when occupational therapists and occupational therapy assistants are involved in planning the course for the occupational therapy service unit or program. Delivery of these services is strengthened further by including the occupational therapy perspective in strategic planning and management tasks throughout the organization.

# References

American Occupational Therapy Association. (2002). *AOTA strategic plan*. Bethesda, MD: Author. Retrieved May 29, 2002, from http://www.aota.org/members/area6/links/LINK06.asp

American Occupational Therapy Foundation. (2000). *The mission of the American Occupational Therapy Foundation*. Bethesda, MD: Author. Retrieved May 21, 2002, from http://www.aotf.org/html/mission.html

Fahey, L., & Randall, R. M. (1994). *The portable MBA in strategy*. New York: Wiley.

Gadiesh, O., & Olivet, S. (1997). Designing for implementability. In F. Hesselbein, M. Goldsmith, & R. Beckhard (Eds.), *The organization of the future* (pp. 53–65). San Francisco: Jossey-Bass.

Harrison, J. S., & St. John, C. H. (2002). *Foundations in strategic management* (2nd ed.). Cincinnati, OH: South-Western Thomson Learning.

Holm, M. (2000). Our mandate for the new millennium: Evidence-based practice. *American Journal of Occupational Therapy, 54*, 576–585.

Jacobs, R. W. (1994). *Real-time strategic change*. San Francisco: Berrett-Koehler.

Law, M., & Baum, C. (1998). Evidence-based occupational therapy. *Canadian Journal of Occupational Therapy, 65*, 131–135.

Kotler, P., & Clarke, R. N. (1987). *Marketing for health care organizations*. Englewood Cliffs, NJ: Prentice-Hall.

Mintzberg, H., Ahlstrand, B., & Lampel, J. (1998). *Strategy safari*. New York: Free Press.

National Board for Certification in Occupational Therapy. (2002). *Certification renewal handbook* [Brochure]. Gaithersburg, MD: Author.

Perry, F. (2002). *The tracks we leave*. Chicago: Health Administration Press.

Pinchot, G. (1998). Building community in the workplace. In F. Hesselbein, M. Goldsmith, R. Beckhard, & R. F. Schubert (Eds.), *The community of the future* (pp. 125–138). San Francisco: Jossey-Bass.

Schwartz, P. (1996). *The art of the long view* (2nd ed.). New York: Doubleday.

Watson, D. E. (2000). *Evaluating costs and outcomes: Demonstrating the value of rehabilitation services*. Bethesda, MD: American Occupational Therapy Association.

Wheatley, M. J. (1999). *Leadership and the new science* (2nd ed.). San Francisco: Berrett-Koehler.

# Financial Planning and Management

Janet Jabri, MBA, OTR, FAOTA

*"Understanding, implementing, and effectively managing a budget empowers you to manage the service quality of your department or business."*

JANET JABRI

**Janet Jabri, MBA, OTR, FAOTA,** is the executive director for Gentiva Rehab Without Walls, in San Jose, CA. She has over 20 years of operations experience that includes increasing responsibility and accountability for the financial management of various departments and businesses. This includes the development, interpretation, and daily management of budgets ranging up to $15 million a year.

## Key Terms and Concepts

**Budget.** A budget is the detailed and coordinated revenue and expense plan for a business (Moore, Jaedicke, & Anderson, 1989).

**Financial management.** Financial management is the process of developing and executing an effective financial plan for a business unit. The process includes developing the objectives, establishing the budget, and managing the financial results. Standards are set for managing financial activities and systems, and tools are developed to monitor and affect results and business practices.

**Financial planning.** Financial planning is the overall process of developing a financial course of action for a business entity. In conjunction with the strategic planning process, planners develop financial analyses to determine viability of identified business goals and objectives.

**Strategic planning.** Strategic planning is the process to determine the viability of the business activities or services. Through an analysis of internal and external environments, planners establish a business plan with specific goals and objectives. The plan includes the overall company vision, values, and mission as well as operational and financial objectives.

## Learning Objectives

After completing this chapter, you should be able to do the following:

- Understand the annual financial planning and management cycle.
- Understand the basic components needed in analyzing the internal and external factors affecting successful financial planning.
- Develop a basic department or small business budget to include setting specific revenue and expense projects.
- Read and understand financial results presented on statements of income.
- Learn to interpret results and implement basic corrective action plans.

This chapter presents a basic financial management framework for occupational therapy managers. The framework explains the financial management cycle, which includes completing the initial strategic and financial plan, developing the department budget, implementing the budget plan, and managing the financial results.

The text discusses how a strategic planning process is used to establish a sound financial plan, reviewing the internal and external factors affecting the health care environment and, specifically, occupational therapy practice. In addition, the text reviews guidelines to establish a viable line-item budget. Finally, specific concepts and strategies are presented to provide the manager with the tools to effectively implement, interpret, monitor, and adjust the budget plan through the business cycle.

The information in this chapter is directed toward occupational therapy departments that are part of a larger business entity such as an acute hospital, large outpatient clinic, or psychiatric facility. However, this information also provides basic elements for those occupational therapists who are managing a private practice as a sole proprietorship or partnership.

## Financial Management and Occupational Therapy

Financial management is the process of developing and executing an effective financial plan for a business unit. Through the strategic planning process, a business entity will establish a set of operational goals and objectives along with a financial plan (see chapter 5, Strategic Planning). Successful strategic and financial planning involves researching the internal and external factors that will affect the business unit. The goal is to determine the strategies to optimize strengths and opportunities while minimizing weaknesses and threats.

Examples of a business entity or unit include a large corporation with many subsidiary businesses, a single hospital setting, an outpatient clinic, or a small occupational therapy private practice. Unless the occupational therapy service is a private practice operating as either a sole proprietorship or small partnership, the service will generally be identified as a department within a larger business unit. Each department of the company is identified as its own responsibility center and will have its own revenue and expense line-item budget. Ultimately, the budgets for each responsibility center will be consolidated into one overall financial plan for the entire company.

The occupational therapy department's overall program goals and objectives will determine the parameters of the department's financial plan. These objectives will always be developed in conjunction with the company's objectives. If the occupational therapy department provides a service for a fee, then it will be identified as a *revenue center*. The financial plan will include projected revenues along with related costs connected to the delivery of the defined services.

Some therapy departments provide a service but do not generate direct revenue from the service. These departments may help the company meet overall business objectives. The income from the occupational therapy services might be either bundled into a per diem fee that includes all therapy services or received through some other kind of allocation system. For example, in a psychiatric day treatment or school-based therapy program, the occupational therapy department will be included in overall objectives that are generated from the larger business entity, and the occupational therapy budget will be focused only on the costs for the department. Departments such as these are referred to as *cost centers*.

Whether the occupational therapy department is a revenue or cost center, the financial plan and detailed budget ensure that the department will be a viable operation. The financial plan is the overall roadmap, and the budget provides the detailed directions. With ongoing and regular monitoring of financial results, managers can adjust and correct for unforeseen changes in the plan.

## The Strategic and the Financial Planning Process

Financial objectives need to be considered early in the strategic planning process. Part of the strategic plan will include an analysis of the external and internal factors that will affect the financial viability of the company. An external analysis focuses on the opportunities and the threats existing in the community marketplace. An external analysis in the health care environment may include assessments of the potential community population that could be served, receptiveness of referral sources within the community, payer reimbursement potential, availability of staff members to provide the service, and market share currently held by competitors.

An internal analysis will focus on the company's strengths and weaknesses. In the health care environment, this analysis may include the evaluation of organizational efficiencies, the availability of qualified staff members, access to needed resources such as equipment and space, and the ability to demonstrate successful service outcomes.

The financial considerations of the data gathered for this internal and external analysis must be aligned with each opportunity, threat, strength, or weakness that is identified. For example, if a payer is going to pay only 50% of the expected billing rate, then the financial impact of that information must be calculated. If the department is unable to recruit qualified staff members within the current salary scale, then the financial impact of raising salaries or of not filling positions must be determined.

When an occupational therapy department is part of a larger business entity, such as a hospital, it will be important to understand the company's overall strategic plan objectives. The financial parameters established by the overall hospital plan are important to incorporate into the department plan and budget. The specific kind of information that is needed from the larger business unit is discussed below.

A private practice is the entire business entity. The internal and external analyses are very important. Internally, the private practice must focus on the strengths and weaknesses of its available resources whether they are funding, available capital equipment, or sufficient but affordable personnel support. For example, having sufficient cash flow may be a critical internal issue when considering the necessary funding needed for paying personnel, making lease payments, or paying monthly utility bills. If this is not available, the business may be in great jeopardy. Externally, the private practice must evaluate the community for potential competition and gaining market share or for available funding and reimbursement sources. This strategic planning process is critical when establishing presence and reputation within that community.

## The External Analysis

The external analysis is a key strategic planning process. In health care, many factors may present opportunities or threats to the viability of occupational therapy services. One primary factor is reimbursement for services rendered (See chapter 17, Reimbursement). It is important that the occupational therapy manager understand the evolution of third-party reimbursement systems and the factors that drive decisions for systems such as Medicare, Medicaid, and various private insurance companies.

Understanding the relationship of the provider, patient, and payer of the service will help in understanding the complexities of the system (see chapter 17). In health care, this relationship is different from a typical relationship between a business and a customer. In typical business transactions, the receiver of the service is also the one who pays for the service. As a result, the transaction is negotiated between only two parties, and once agreement is reached, the service is provided and the payment for the service is made. Similar to the business relationship, the patient is the receiver of the health care service, and the therapist is provider of the service. However, in most health care situations, a third party is the reimbursement agent or the payer for the service.

Adding this third party significantly complicates the business transaction. Now, the transaction requires full agreement by three separate participants. Often, these parties have difficulty reaching a mutual agreement with respect to what services the patient needs and wants, what the provider wants to bill for those services, and what the reimbursement agent is willing to authorize and pay. Sometimes the insurance company may not reimburse the full amount that the provider charges. Instead, the company may pay a defined "usual and customary" charge for an occupational therapy evaluation. This amount may be only 80% of the actual provider charge. At this point, the service provider has to decide whether it can afford to provide the service at a lower rate. This concept is common in the health care industry and becomes a critical factor when conducting financial planning for the department or private practice. Predicting an accurate occupational therapy financial plan depends on having a full understanding about what will be paid for and the amount that will be paid.

Over the past 20 years, dramatic changes have occurred in reimbursement systems within the government and in the private sector. Table 6.1 shows the actual and projected increasing costs of these expenditures between 1990 and 2010. These costs

**Table 6.1  Actual and Projected U.S. Health Care Expenses.**

| Year | Dollars (in billions) |
|------|----------------------|
| Actual | |
| 1990 | 696.0 |
| 1995 | 990.3 |
| 1998 | 1,149.8 |
| 1999 | 1,215.6 |
| 2000 | 1,299.5 |
| Projected | |
| 2001 | 1,423.8 |
| 2002 | 1,545.9 |
| 2003 | 1,653.4 |
| 2004 | 1,773.4 |
| 2005 | 1,902.2 |
| 2006 | 2,036.2 |
| 2007 | 2,174.9 |
| 2008 | 2,320.0 |
| 2009 | 2,476.1 |
| 2010 | 2,639.2 |

*Note.* From National Health Care Expenditures Projections—Table 1 by the Centers for Medicare and Medicaid Services, Office of the Actuary, Washington, DC, March 2002. Retrieved September 2002 from http://www.cms.gov.

will nearly quadruple over this 20-year period of time because of trends anticipated in an increasing elderly population (Centers for Medicare and Medicaid Services, 2001a).

Table 6.2 depicts the distribution of health care spending among the market share of the various payer sources in 1999 (Centers for Medicare and Medicaid Services, 2001b). Noting the percentage of payer dollars by source will affect the kind of service that can be provided and will guide health care business decisions such as where and how services will be provided.

Government-funded programs such as Medicare have implemented dramatic changes in reimbursement for all levels of care. Hospital admissions and the patient's

**Table 6.2  U.S. Health Care Spending by Payer Source, 2000.**
**Total Expenditures = $1,299.4 (in billions)**

| Payer Source | Dollars (in billions) | % |
|--------------|----------------------|---|
| Private insurance | 443.9 | 34.2 |
| Federal funds | 411.5 | 31.6 |
| Out-of-pocket payments | 194.5 | 15 |
| State and local funds | 175.7 | 13.5 |
| Other private funds | 73.8 | 5.7 |

*Note.* From National Health Care Expenditures Source of Funds and Type of Expenditures 1995–2000 by the Centers for Medicare and Medicaid Services, Office of the Actuary, Washington, DC, July 2002. Retrieved September 2002 from http://www.cms.gov.

length of stay have significantly decreased through the diagnosis-related group (DRG) system (Centers for Disease Control and Prevention, 1999). Skilled nursing, home health, and acute rehabilitation reimbursement has shifted to complicated prospective payment systems (PPS). Reimbursement agencies have established many more screening procedures to ensure that patients meet certain clinical levels to secure payment for services. Outpatient service providers must match services to specific *Current Procedural Terminology* (CPT) codes to ensure that services will be covered. Reimbursement fees are attached to each CPT code.

All of these reimbursement changes have shifted payment for Medicare services from a less controlled retrospective payment system to a highly controlled prospective and predictable payment system. The DRG system defines planned care for specific diagnoses and sets a defined dollar amount for the expected clinical care needed (Jacobs & Logigian, 1999). The PPS system uses key clinical factors to determine needed services such as therapy treatment and sets reimbursement based on specific cost analysis of providing that therapy service. For example, Medicare determines the cost to provide 720 minutes of therapy in a skilled nursing facility (Baker, 1998). As mentioned above, Medicare defines each service that may be used in outpatient therapy and attaches a CPT code with a reimbursement rate to that defined service. Costs are controlled because reimbursement for each CPT code is preset. These codes are adjusted for regional differences but are set at a specific reimbursement rate regardless of whether costs are greater or less for that particular program or facility. All of these changes have made Medicare costs more predictable and controllable for Medicare. In other words, Medicare has shifted the responsibility for managing the actual cost of care for each patient by setting these fixed reimbursement rates.

In the private sector, the evolution from indemnity plans to health maintenance organizations (HMOs) and preferred provider organizations has been dramatic, and tremendous shifts have occurred in the kinds of payer sources available. The growth in HMO enrollment is demonstrated in the following statistics (see Table 6.3). In 1992, 14.7% of the population was enrolled in an HMO, and in 2000, 28.1% of the population was enrolled. The actual number of enrollees increased from 37.6 million in 1992 to 81.1 million in 1999, and in the past 2 years, enrollment has slightly decreased by 2.4% down to 79.5 million (U.S. Census Bureau, 2001).

All of these reimbursement changes have created a tremendous shift in the type of setting in which patients are treated. The shift from hospital inpatient stays to outpatient services has resulted in the closing of 279 community hospitals in the United States. The average hospital length of stay has decreased from 8 days to 5 days. And the number of health care outpatient visits almost doubled in 10 years, from 301,329 visits in 1990 to 592,673 visits in 2000 (American Hospital Association, 2001).

Understanding the specific changes in Medicare regulations will assist an occupational therapy manager in identifying threats that affect current services and in optimizing opportunities to create new treatment options. After analysis, the manager may

**Table 6.3  HMO Growth Rates.**

| Year | Number of Enrollees (in millions) | % U.S. Population Enrolled in HMOs | % Annual Growth Rate |
|------|------|------|------|
| 1992 | 37.6 | 14.7 | 7.1 |
| 1993 | 41.0 | 15.9 | 9.0 |
| 1994 | 45.2 | 17.3 | 10.2 |
| 1995 | 50.1 | 20.3 | 10.8 |
| 1996 | 58.2 | 24.0 | 16.2 |
| 1997 | 66.9 | 27.0 | 14.9 |
| 1998 | 76.2 | 29.0 | 13.9 |
| 1999 | 81.1 | 30.0 | 6.4 |
| 2000 | 80.4 | 28.1 | −0.9 |
| 2001 | 79.5 | Not Available | −1.1 |

*Note.* From HMO Growth Rates, by the U.S. Census Bureau, 2001. Retrieved June 2002 from http://www.census.gov.

discover that it is more financially feasible to shift a particular service from an inpatient setting to the outpatient clinic. In addition, understanding rules for the private insurance sector will allow the manager to more effectively align service definitions with HMO policies to secure authorization and payment.

The same external analysis is needed to ensure success for occupational therapy programs that are funded in other ways, such as through grant funding, state or federal mandated laws, government allocations, or donations from charitable organizations. The benefit inherent in applying for grant funding is that the requesting agency must propose a program that fits into the grant's defined parameters. However, a business must be careful not to compromise its own long-term mission and objectives to meet a grant's specified objectives. Dramatically changing an established strategic plan can result in weakening the internal workings of the business, and it will impact the business's overall success. When applying to receive grant funds, the applicant is obligated to develop a plan and attach the costs related to implementing the plan. Viability of continued grant funding will depend on the applicant's ability to demonstrate past and continuing financial success. Therefore, good financial planning and management are critical to success.

Understanding how the government allocates dollars for children with special needs in the schools may be more difficult. Learning what services are included and, more important, knowing what dollars are allocated and what services must be provided are critical to the development of a viable occupational therapy service. An excellent way to learn and understand these government processes is to seek information through key government agencies, for example, the Centers for Medicare and Medicaid Services, the Office of Special Education and Rehabilitation Services, and local or state government groups. Using the Internet, one can easily find current information on regulatory changes, reimbursement levels, and upcoming legislation.

## The Internal Analysis

Most occupational therapy departments fit into a larger business entity, whether it is a hospital, an outpatient clinic, or a large corporation that owns many business lines. As a unit of a larger entity, the occupational therapy department will be affected by systems and mandates that may or may not directly apply to the department but that are necessary for the operation of an entire company. In addition, understanding the vision, mission, values, mandated policies, financial objectives, and rationale for business decisions made by the company is critical to ensuring that department goals and objectives are aligned with the organization's interests.

A wide range of information must be gathered when completing an internal analysis. The information will range from details of organizational structure to the specific guidelines the company gives managers to determine the department's objectives and financial plan. General questions that are usually researched about the business entity are listed below. Answers to these questions can help the occupational therapy manager establish a full understanding of the organization and work environment. The information will allow the manager to capitalize on the strengths and adjust for the weaknesses when developing the department's strategic plan and final financial plan.

*What is the organizational structure of the business entity?* Besides the occupational therapy department, what other departments are included within the business entity? Which departments directly affect occupational therapy services and vice versa? Does the company comprise many business lines (e.g., the company may own 10 hospitals, 30 skilled nursing facilities, and 5 outpatient clinics).

*If the entity is a public school system, how does the state structure its schools?* Are the schools grouped into districts? Does the local government have any part in the management of the systems? Does each district run differently?

*What are the business entity's vision and mission statements?* Are the occupational therapy department's vision and mission statements aligned with those of the larger organization?

*What are the overall goals of the business entity?* Is the company focused on financial goals? Are the goals focused on community service? Do the company goals reflect the mandates of government or other regulatory agencies?

*How is the business entity operated?* Is it a for-profit business? Is it publicly traded on the stock market? Is it a nonprofit organization? Who owns and operates the company? Does the entity have a board of directors that oversees all business activities? Is the business operated by a government agency?

*Who are the stakeholders served by the business entity?* Are there stockholders? Who are the patients served? Are the third-party payers viewed as customers? Has the company identified the employee as a customer? What community agencies are involved in the business? (This information can offer a perspective of the company's attitudes and related business goals. If the stockholder is considered the primary customer, then the focus of the company may be strongly directed toward financial outcomes. A company that views the patients and the community as the primary customers may focus on quality outcomes and high customer satisfaction ratings.)

*How is the business entity organized?* What is the organizational structure? Who leads the business? Who oversees the occupational therapy manager? Who oversees that person? Which departments are the revenue producing departments and which departments are not?

*How is the organization funded?* Who are the third-party payers? Are government funds allocated to the facility? Is occupational therapy a funded service? Is occupational therapy a mandated service but one that is not directly funded through a fee-for-service billing system?

## Business Practices and Budgetary Expectations

The occupational therapy manager will be required to understand the company's specific operating practices and budgetary parameters before he or she can complete the strategic plan. This information will help to ensure that program and financial expectations are met and are presented in a manner that matches the rest of the business entity. These business practices and expectations include understanding various parameters such as the designation of the fiscal year and the guidelines for developing and adjusting budget expectations.

### The Fiscal Year

The budget cycle runs for 1 calendar year or another period of 52 weeks, and it is referred to as the *fiscal year*. Generally, the date that starts a fiscal year falls at the beginning of one of the four commonly identified quarters, which are January, April, July, and October (Fess & Warren, 1985).

A quarter is further divided into periods, which can be months or specific, equal weeks. Sometimes, companies define exact start days of their quarters so that the length of the periods is equal. There are significant advantages in analyzing equal periods. Months vary in length from 28 to 31 days, so comparisons among uneven months can be skewed. Equal periods can be compared much more accurately.

Dividing the budget year into smaller units allows the company to present actual financial results regularly, which gives the company the opportunity to analyze and affect these results through the year. Quarterly results are also used as report cards for businesses to show investors and interested parties the progress that has been made toward financial objectives. This information could make a difference in stock prices for publicly traded companies or in the ability to obtain investment money from future investors (Moore, Jaedicke, & Anderson, 1984).

### Budget Expectations and Adjustments

Some business decisions will be made on the basis of the external and internal analysis completed by the larger entity, which will affect the work of the entire facility. Business decisions that directly affect the occupational therapy department must be incorporated into the department's overall plan. These decisions could include the facility canceling two key insurance contracts, decreasing inpatient census by 10%, adding a new pediatric outpatient clinic, setting expectations that each revenue producing department will increase revenues by 10%, or expecting a 5% increase in work productivity for revenue or nonrevenue producing departments.

The occupational therapy manager may see opportunities arise from some of these business decisions and may be able to develop some effective goals, for example, "the Occupational Therapy Department will increase its total service volume by 5% and maintain a 10% department profit margin for the fiscal year" or "the Occupational Therapy Department will establish a new pediatric outpatient program and will increase overall revenues by 10%." With these goals, occupational therapy managers can then develop specific objectives and include identified detailed needs and requirements. For example, specific objectives might be stated as "an increase of 500 occupational therapy visits will be provided during the fiscal year" or "with the addition of the hospital pediatric clinic, 25 pediatric outpatients will be seen by the Occupational Therapy Department during the 3rd and 4th quarters of the fiscal year." It becomes easier to apply a financial analysis to these specific objectives. Acceptance of the objective will often be determined by ensuring a positive financial outcome.

Ideally, the financial plan should be based on sound operational objectives, which make it easier to adjust budget projections up or down and to align those changes directly with operational consequences or opportunities. For example, if the department was requested to cut its workforce by one staff person, then the occupational therapy manager with a solid business plan would be able to minimize the consequences of that cut. The manager might be able to determine, for instance, that the way to achieve the least impact from that sort of cut would be to delete one aspect of service, such as pediatric outpatient services, rather than to compromise treatment in all areas. Alternatively, the manager might be able to review objectives and determine how to avoid the cut by finding a way to increase the work volume without adding any new staff members, thereby saving the potential layoff of a staff member.

## Financial Resources

The strategic plan will have global goals and specific objectives, and the financial plan will support the successful execution of the objectives. The final step of the budget process is to establish a detailed annual budget, which involves developing a line-item budget and projecting all specific revenues and expenses. The larger organization will consolidate all department budgets to create one larger budget. If other business units, such as multiple hospitals, are involved, then this consolidation process will continue until the larger organization establishes one overall budget for the entire corporation.

It is unlikely that the occupational therapy manager will be solely responsible for the full development and management of all the department's financial aspects. The company more likely will provide a budget template, which may include some valuable historical data. The template may include projections based on the current year's activities. For example, if the budgeting process starts in August for the upcoming fiscal year beginning in January, then current year-to-date revenues and expenses can be annualized. In this case, the numbers from January through July would be used. The year-to-date figures would be divided by 7 months to get a monthly average. This monthly average would then be multiplied by 12 months to get annualized estimates. Annualizing actual financial results creates an initial draft budget and gives the manager a starting place from which to work. Adjustments can be made up or down depending on identified objectives in the strategic plan.

As seen in Table 6.4, the current budget and actual numbers through June of the year are given. Annualized actual numbers are then determined by dividing June's actual numbers by 6 months (January through June) to give an average monthly dollar amount. For example, Medicare revenues were $4,000 from January through June which, when divided by 6, yields a monthly average of $666.66. This monthly average is multiplied by 12 months (a full fiscal year) to determine a projected annualized budget of $8,000 (rounded to the whole dollar). However, the proposed budget for Medicare revenues is $10,000. Clearly, the proposed budget will not likely be met, and actual figures are going to total $2,000 less than anticipated, or 20% less than what was budgeted. The manager can then use this information along with information obtained from the internal and external analysis to decide that Medicare revenues will return to this year's expected budget level and, thus, propose a budget of $10,000 again. The same analysis needs to be completed for each payer classification designated (e.g., Medicaid, private insurance).

This process is also completed for each revenue and expense category. The annualized numbers help managers to understand current trends, consider them with

**Table 6.4  Budget Projection Using Annualized Financial Information.**

| Gross Revenue | Account Medicare | Private Insurance | Total |
|---|---|---|---|
| Current budget | $10,000 | $25,000 | $35,000 |
| Year-to-date actual (through June) | $4,000 | $15,000 | $19,000 |
| Annualized actual | $8,000 | $30,000 | $38,000 |
| Variance (current budget vs. annualized actual) | −$2,000 | $5,000 | $3,000 |
| Variance (current budget vs. annualized actual) | −20% | 17% | 9% |
| Proposed budget | $10,000 | $35,750 | $45,750 |
| Variance (annualized vs. proposed) | $2,000 | $5,750 | $7,750 |
| Variance | 20% | 16% | 17% |

respect to anticipated future trends, and derive a projected budget based on both sets of data.

It is also important for the manager to be aware of other resources available to assist with the financial management process. Most companies will have a chief financial officer (CFO) who oversees all financial aspects of the business, including the development of budgets, the management of financial operations, and ongoing reporting of the financial results. Several departments under the direction of the CFO assist in the budgeting and ongoing financial activities of an organization: the billing department, where all bills for services are generated; accounts payable, where invoices for purchased goods and services are paid; payroll, where compensation for all staff members is processed; accounts receivable, where all dollars owed to the company are collected; and accounting, where expense and revenue transactions are recorded.

## The Budget Process in General

The budget template is divided into revenues and expenses. *Revenues* are the charges that are billed after the delivery of a service. *Expenses* are generally divided into direct and indirect costs. Table 6.5 shows a sample breakdown of these categories for a department and how they relate to one another.

*Direct costs* are those expenses that are directly related to providing the service. These expenses fluctuate depending on the workload. When volume goes up, costs will generally go up and vice versa. Therefore, these costs can also be referred to as *variable costs*. In occupational therapy, staffing costs are generally the largest portion of the direct expense. In a product-driven company, variable expenses will include not only the staff but also the materials needed to make the item.

*Operating costs* or *indirect costs* are those expenses that sustain the overall operation of the business. These expenses are not directly related to the delivery of services

**Table 6.5 Sample Occupational Therapy Department Budget.**

| Budget Category | Budget ($) | % Profit Margin |
|---|---|---|
| Revenues | | |
|   Gross revenues | 500,000 | |
|   Contractual allowances | 10,000 | |
|   Net revenues | 490,000 | |
| Expenses | | |
|   Direct expense | 200,000 | |
|   Gross profit | 290,000 | 58 |
|   Operating expense | 150,000 | |
| Department contribution | 140,000 | 28 |
| Total corporate allocations | 29,400 | |
| Total bad debt and recoveries | 500 | |
| Profit | 110,000 | 22 |

but, rather, to the support of the overall department operation. The majority of expenses in this category (such as salaries) do not vary from month to month, so most of these expenses can also be referred to as *fixed costs*. In other words, the costs are incurred regardless of the total volume of work produced. The department manager's salary, the department's phone bill, or the department's office supplies are all examples of operating costs.

Adding together the a department's direct expenses and operating expenses will determine the total department expenses. Once a department's revenues and expenses are identified, the department contribution can be determined easily by subtracting total net revenues from total expenses. Finally, corporate overhead allocations will be entered along with any bad debt resulting from noncollection from payers. Corporate overhead includes costs that are generally spread over all departments such as the expenses incurred by nonrevenue producing departments (e.g., admitting, personnel, or administration). There are different methods a corporation may use to allocate these costs. Some businesses set a defined percentage of revenue earned. For example, if the occupational therapy department uses 1,000 square feet, and this equals 5% of the total space in the facility, the department may be responsible for 5% of the total facility costs for these areas. A profit or loss can be calculated by subtracting overhead allocations and bad debts from the department contribution. More detail on each of these major budget categories is provided below.

## The Budget Process in Detail

The description provided above is a simplistic overview of the budget template. Many other components must be considered when developing a budget. For example, the revenues that are billed may not be the revenues that are finally collected. In addition, companies may choose to subdivide revenues into different programs, such as inpatient, outpatient, and day treatment, or subdivide them by payer source, such as Medicare, Medicaid, and private insurance. To manage the variety of expenses incurred, a company will set up a chart of accounts so it can effectively capture like expenses in defined categories. These assigned accounts ensure appropriate allocation of revenues and expenses and they establish an accounting framework within which to calculate business taxes, project future revenues, or manage overall costs.

### Projecting Revenues
When establishing a budget, it will be important to accurately project revenues.

#### Gross Revenues
*Gross revenues* are the expected work volume multiplied by the billed charges. The first step in calculating gross revenues is to estimate that volume. Data gathered in the business plan and from other historical data can be used to estimate potential work volume. Note that external and internal market changes will have significant impact

on this estimate. Factors such as the hospital's closing of a particular program, changes in referral patterns from outside sources, changes in reimbursement systems, or changes in grant funding can affect the projections.

Two approaches can be used to estimate work volume. The first method is to consider the department's total work opportunities. This would include meeting all service needs possible, including new and expanded programs. The manager determines how many staff members would be needed to provide the service based on the projected potential workload. The second method could be used when the department has fixed resources such as limited staff or space and, as a result, can perform only a limited amount of work. For example, if the clinic space can accommodate only five patients per hour, then projections would need to be based on the confined space and the hours the space is available.

Work volume should be expressed in work increments or service units that can easily be translated into a dollar amount. Some examples of work increments may include a 15-minute unit of service, a visit, a per-day treatment, or a procedural unit that is based on the specific service provided (e.g., an occupational therapy evaluation or an activities of daily living [ADL] treatment).

The second component of estimating gross revenues is to establish the charge, or fee, for each service unit. A fee for each service unit—whether it is a 15-minute unit (e.g., $25 per 15 minutes) or a visit rate (e.g., $75 per 45-minute treatment visit)—must be assigned.

Now that the work volume has been converted into work increments and the fee for each work increment is set, the gross revenues can easily be calculated by multiplying the two numbers together. If the department provides services in varying work increments and at varying charges, gross revenues will be determined by calculating the gross revenues for each service and then adding all the products together. For example, a work volume consisting of 100 45-minute treatment visits at $75 each ($7,500) and 500 15-minute specialized treatments at $30 each ($15,000) will produce gross revenues of $22,500.

As mentioned above, some health care systems may want to divide revenues into different payer categories such as Medicare, Medicaid, insurance, or private pay. If this system applies, then the gross revenues will need to be allocated to each category. Once again, historical data (annualized revenues) may be helpful in determining the expected workload for each of the categories. Reimbursement changes that are identified in the external analysis will also provide valuable information for preparing accurate projections.

### Contractual Allowances

Once the fees for the occupational therapy services are set, they are identified as the published charge for the service. However, as mentioned above, the facility may negotiate a lower fee with a payer, or a payer such as Medicare may reimburse at a regulated set rate. As a result, the published fee will be what is billed, but the lower fee is what the facility will be paid. The discount given is entered into the budget as a *contractual allowance*. For example, if the facility has negotiated and established a contract with Blue Cross for a 20% discount on billed services, then a contractual allowance would be calculated for all Blue Cross patients seen by the department. In other words, if the treatment fee is $100 an hour, then Blue Cross will pay $20 less, and the $20 would be applied as a contractual allowance.

Not all contractual allowances are determined by a straight percentage discount from the published charge. For example, Medicare Part B Occupational Therapy services are reimbursed using an established fee schedule based on CPT codes. Thus, the published department charge may be $25.00 for 15 minutes, but the CPT code rate for an ADL service may be only $15.00, and a mobility training CPT code may be $18.00. As a result, the contractual allowance for these services will be different: $10 for the ADL service and $7.00 for the mobility training. It is critical that these lower rates never exceed the published therapy rate. If the discounted rate exceeds the published rate, then the contractual allowance will be a negative number, and in the case of Medicare, the lower of the two rates will be paid. For example, if the published rate is $25.00 for 15 minutes and the CPT code reimbursement is $28.00, then Medicare will pay only $25.00 and the department will lose $3.00 per treatment.

### Net Revenues

If a department's budget contains contractual allowances, then the department will need to create another revenue category called *net revenues*. Net revenues accurately reflect the real dollars that will be collected. This number is used to determine the true profitability of the department. The net revenue is calculated by subtracting the contractual allowance from the gross revenue. For example, if $25 (gross revenue) is billed for a 15-minute treatment session, but Medicare reimbursed only $20, then $5 (contractual allowance) is subtracted from the gross revenue, and the actual amount collected (net revenue) will be $20.

## Projecting Expenses

Whether a department is a revenue center or cost center, expenses will always be attached to the unit. The two primary categories of expenses are direct costs and operating expenses. If the department is a revenue center, then expenses will be projected based on the anticipated workload and the resources necessary to effectively complete the workload. If the department is a cost center, then expenses will still be based on an expected workload projection. The company will likely provide the occupational therapy manager with these projections. The projections could be in the form of total patients treated during the year, total bed days (the days each bed in the facility will be filled), anticipated day treatment patients, or projected number of students to receive services during the school year.

### Direct Expenses

Direct expenses are those costs that are directly related to the delivery of the service. In other words, if the treatment takes place, then costs occur related to that treatment or work increment. If the treatment is not provided, then the cost was not incurred. Total direct costs are determined by adding together all costs directly related to providing and processing a billable service. These costs may fluctuate from day to day or month to month, depending on changes in the volume of treatments that are provided. Direct costs are the primary areas that managers can control when the patient census increases or decreases. Understanding the relationship between staffing and caseload is critical in analyzing the department activity. Having the means to take action when costs are too high is critical to managing a successful budget.

*Determining direct costs: Method 1.* One approach for projecting direct expenses is to project the exact and full cost to provide one unit of treatment. Thus, a 60-minute treatment segment requires 60 minutes of staff time for treatment and 15 additional minutes to cover the setup and documentation of services provided, so the total time is actually 75 minutes even though the therapist may bill for only 60 minutes. In addition, there is an estimated $5.00 cost for materials used during the treatment. It is important that all relevant staff salaries, costs of fringe benefits, and materials charges be included in the calculation.

*Determining direct costs: Method 2.* Another method takes into account the fact that, most often, staff costs represent the primary expense of a treatment segment. This method for projecting expenses determines how many staff people are required to meet the total workload standard. This projection would require that a productivity standard be established for the staff. For example, if the billable productivity standard is 75%, then each full-time employee would need to bill 6 out of 8 hours worked each day or, if using 15-minute units, 24 units a day. The remaining 2 hours reflects the nonbillable time to complete all billable work. These figures can be calculated to determine a weekly, monthly, or annual expectation of work volume. One can determine the needed staff by dividing the expected staff units into the total expected work volume already projected. Knowing the total staff needs, costs can then be applied for each of the appropriate accounts. For example, if 25 hours of treatment are projected for each day of work, we can determine how many therapists are needed for each day by dividing how many daily units a therapist can provide into the total units for that day. If a therapist's productivity was expected to be 6 hours per day, then 4.16 therapists would be needed to complete the work each day. Other analyses can also be completed using this method. These include evaluating the impact of using more efficient treatment strategies such as groups or staggered treatment sessions. These alternative treatment regimes would increase the number of treatments a therapist may provide in a day, and the end result would be a decrease in the total staff needed.

One must remember that costs used in this second method must include salary plus benefits such as health insurance, worker's compensation insurance, unemployment taxes, and malpractice insurance. Most facilities will have formulas based on state and federal standards and company insurance policies that they will use to determine the cost of these categories. In addition, in this second method, direct costs related to any materials that are needed to provide the treatment (e.g., cooking supplies for the home-making session) may be estimated by historical data figures or by projections of the quantities of materials that are expected to be used.

### Operating Expenses

The final budget estimates needed are the operating expenses or indirect costs. Because these expenses must be paid regardless of the work volume, indirect costs are more difficult to adjust on a day-to-day basis. The first category of operating expenses is for the administrative staff. This staff can include the department manager, a department secretary, or other staff members who do not provide direct treatment services. In determining costs for these staff members, allocation of benefits is calculated as it is for the treating staff.

Other operating expense categories will vary depending on the needs of the specific department. These expense categories include costs for lease or space, office supplies, telephone service, utilities, business meetings, staff education seminars, advertising for recruitment, marketing services, postage, equipment leases, and equipment maintenance. The company will provide a standard list of accounts that are used along with guidelines to determine the kinds of expenses that go under each of those accounts. These guidelines ensure consistency for the entire company and uniform understanding for accountability.

Depreciation and amortization also are included under operating expenses. In this category, the cost of capital equipment (usually equipment that cost more than $500 or $1,000) is divided up and distributed over a period of 3–5 years or over the projected life of the piece of equipment. This procedure more accurately reflects the actual cost of doing business over time.

As mentioned above, overall operating expenses are not easy to adjust when quick changes occur in the department's activities (e.g., outpatient visits dropping for 1 month). However, when the service volume goes up again and no additional operating expenses are added, the costs will balance out. When volume increases, the fixed expenses become a smaller percentage of the overall costs, and savings that were made during periods of low volume are noted. When budgeting a department's operating expenses, a manager should consider the minimum amount of service volume that is needed to support all the projected operating expenses. If this figure is calculated, then the manager can more easily determine the efficiency of the department and the resulting impact on the budget when the minimum standard is not met.

## Other Operating Allocations

Once the department budget is determined, there may be other allocations that will affect the ultimate profitability of a department. Often, these allocations and expenses are not within the control of the occupational therapy manager, and the manager will not be held accountable for the expenses. These expenses can include services from the hospital administration, accounting department, human resources department, housekeeping, dietary staff, or maintenance department. Generally, the expense is entered in the department budget as one set dollar amount that covers the department's share of the general overhead for the business entity. These allocations cover the costs of nonrevenue producing services that are necessary for the effective operation of the business unit.

One method companies use to determine the allocation is to calculate a percentage of revenue dollars generated by the department. For example, if $100,000 is billed, then $600 or 6% of the revenue might be allocated as overhead expense.

## Bad Debt and Recoveries

Bad debt write-offs are another set of expenses that are added to the budget. These expenses are dollars that cannot be collected from the payers. If the insurance company has denied the charges and there is no further recourse, then the facility will decide to write off this amount as a loss. This loss is subtracted from the total profit of the department. If these write-offs are large, then a profitable department may actually reflect a total loss. Occasionally, some of these bad-debt dollars that have been written off may be recovered, and at that time, the dollars will be added back into the department.

## Profit–Loss Calculations

Revenue producing departments will conduct a profit or loss calculation. Business performance and success are ultimately measured by the profit of the department or the company as a whole. Subtracting expenses from net revenues determines the profit or loss for a business entity. Companies usually set a specific goal for how much profit is expected in a specified period of time. This number is stated in terms of dollars expected in the first quarter. However, to better measure the effectiveness of the company, a profit margin will also be set. This number is a percentage and is calculated by dividing actual profit dollars by total revenues (e.g., a $50,000 profit is divided by the $500,000 net revenues, showing a 10% profit margin). By calculating the percentage, the manager can determine whether the ratio of revenues to expenses was maintained, especially during periods when revenues may have fluctuated as a result of increases and decreases in census. Even if net revenues are below expectations, the manager will want to strive to maintain the profit margin, which means managing costs in relationship to the actual workload.

A profit and profit margin may be calculated in various places within the budget plan. The various calculations provide different information and can be helpful in analyzing why budget shortfalls occur. These calculations include determination of gross profit, department contribution, branch profit, and pretax and after-tax profit.

### Gross Profit

*Gross profit* measures the relationship of direct costs and net revenues. This margin is key in determining the effectiveness of managing variable costs and related workload. If the margin is lower than expected, then it suggests that more dollars were spent to produce the revenue and efficiency was compromised. If the margin is higher, then it indicates that efficiencies were optimized and resulted in a better financial outcome.

### Department Contribution

The *department contribution* is calculated by subtracting all direct and operating costs from net revenues. This figure is not the ultimate branch profit number but, rather, a calculation of the portion of the budget over which the manager has the most control. The manager has direct control over the majority of expenditures for the department and, as a result, this profit number becomes a key indicator for measuring the manager's overall effective performance.

### Branch Profit

The *branch profit* is calculated after the corporate overhead costs are allocated to the department. This number also reflects adjustments for bad debts or recovery of uncollected dollars. These losses or recoveries are an important variable for reflecting the true revenues for a department or company. As mentioned above, large write-offs for bad debt are critical to the solvency of any business entity.

### Pretax and After-Tax Profit

The final two profit calculations are the *pretax profit* and *after-tax profit*. All business income is taxable. Tax laws mandate how taxes are calculated. All income statements and other financial records are structured and aligned to meet these rules so that management of the tax process is clear and can easily demonstrate the business activity. The pretax profit calculation indicates the tax liability for each department. The after-tax profit calculation indicates the true profitability of the company.

## Finalizing the Annual Budget

Once the annual budget is established, the budget numbers for each account must be divided so revenues and expenses are defined for each quarter or period. There are several ways to divide the budget:

- It can be set up as a straight line budget in which the annual budget is divided into 12 equal segments.
- If the expectation is that the program will gradually grow throughout the year, then the budget may be set up so that revenues and respective expenses increase throughout the year.
- If work is seasonal, then the budget may be allocated according to anticipated fluctuations. Choosing the option that best reflects the expected performance

is critical to ensure that performance is more accurately measured and that predicted shortfalls do not affect overall ongoing period and quarterly financial results.

## Capital Budgeting

Another component of the annual budget process includes budgeting for capital equipment, property, or plant changes. These assets are classified as capital and are based on a minimum cost for the equipment or asset and on its useful life. The company sets the minimum cost of the asset (e.g., $1,000), and the item is assigned an expected useful life (e.g., 3 or 5 years).

If the occupational therapy department needs a new piece of equipment, such as a treatment table, the manager will need to prepare a capital budget request. This request involves determining the costs, including taxes, shipping, installation, and then writing a justification for the equipment to support the expenditure. The justification will include the reason for the equipment; the direct cost benefit if the equipment will help to generate revenue; and a description of either the impact on the program (e.g., not meeting regulatory requirements) if the equipment is not purchased or the positive effect the purchase will have on the overall quality of services. The request will also include an estimate of the useful life of the equipment. Once the equipment is approved and purchased, the expenses will be depreciated over the period indicated as the useful life of the equipment. For example, if the useful life were 5 years, then the department would have an allocation of $10,000 a year for a $50,000 piece of equipment.

Remodeling projects, certain moving expenses, or purchase of a building are other examples of plant and property assets that will also be depreciated over time or amortized if the project is funded through a loan.

## Cash Flow

To successfully operate a business, one must have some kind of revenue stream that will cover expenses incurred, and this revenue stream involves the movement of cash. Cash comes in for services rendered, and cash goes out to pay bills incurred. In most health care companies, the cash transactions do not occur in real time. Services are provided and billed, and then payment follows 30 to 60 days later. Expenditures for the services are generally processed before payment is received. Salaries are paid, and supplies are purchased and stocked in advance. Because of the varied timing of these transactions, a company must monitor its cash flow. The stability and value of a company is often rated on its available cash. When a company cannot collect money that is due and must extend payment schedules for products and services that have been provided, the solvency of the company is at risk.

In any business, accounts receivable and accounts payable must be managed in tandem. The company must closely monitor and address receivables that are not collected in a timely manner. Until money is collected, an account receivable is only a revenue figure entered onto an accounting report. When money is collected, the account receivable becomes real income. When receivables exceed income, the company is at risk because it does not have the cash in hand to operate its business. As a result, the company will have to borrow the money, creating more debt, or delay payments of outstanding bills incurred.

The occupational therapy manager may not be asked to actively participate in the collection of billed services, but the manager does have a role in ensuring that all services are authorized correctly and provided as authorized. This responsibility includes accurately documenting the services provided so retroactive denials do not occur. In addition, managers may be asked to manage expenditures more closely during times when cash is not readily available so accounts payable issues can be managed more effectively.

As mentioned earlier in this chapter, cash flow is a daily consideration for small private practice businesses. It is critical that income for services is received quickly. Some payers hold payments for 90 days or more before paying. This delay can have a serious impact in paying ongoing payroll and other monthly expenses. The private practice must be able to predict delays and be aggressive about collecting receivables to remain an ongoing viable business.

## Interpreting and Managing the Financial Results

Once a budget is completed, the primary focus will be to manage the ongoing financial results. Every business unit will have its own unique formats and processes to accomplish the budgeting task. Different computer programs and financial systems may be used depending on the complexity of the business and the reporting structure that is needed to meet the business needs. For larger businesses, the computer system may be designed specifically to meet the unique needs of the company. To further complicate the process, health care companies need to integrate with existing Medicare and Medicaid systems that require automated transmission of bills. The volume of a business's activity may also create more system complexities. In general, it is important for the occupational therapy manager to have a basic understanding of the system and its capabilities to effectively participate in the financial process.

A small private practice will generally use one of the standard over-the-counter accounting systems that collects financial information in a way that meets standard accounting practices for tax reporting purposes. Some of these programs can also generate a bill, create productivity reports, and manage receivables as well as payables. In addition, some of these systems are set up to include managing payroll and the related tax and social security payment issues.

The company will generate different reports to assist in the monitoring and interpreting of financial results. The reports will answer certain questions for particular performance issues and may create questions about the impact the results had on other performance areas. The manager will be required to respond to and justify objectives that were not met, and at the same time, the manager will have the opportunity to evaluate successes and work toward maintaining positive trends.

## Financial Statements

Each company will choose the financial tools and reports that best meet the information needed for the operation of the business. Some of these reports will be used for internal analysis only, and other reports will be used for outside public purposes such as presenting information to the stockholders, filing with the Internal Revenue Service, or seeking money from investors. Types of commonly used internal analysis reports include statement of income, rolling income statement, detailed transaction report, payroll report, and productivity report.

### Statement of Income

The primary document that is provided each month or period is the *statement of income*. This report states the actual financial results by revenue and expense categories. It generally will match the same sequence used for the budget process. Table 6.6 shows a sample.

Formats for the report will vary but will often include the actual performance for the current period as well as year-to-date performance. The actual numbers are also compared to the budget, and a variance is calculated to show whether the item was over or under the budgeted dollar amount. The variance can be translated into a percentage so the manager can easily determine relatively how much the budget was over or under projected amounts. Variances can also be calculated to compare the total expense cost to the percentage of the total revenue. For example, the department may spend $20,000 for staff salaries to bill $50,000 in revenue. This translates to salaries being 40% of revenues earned. This variance becomes a helpful benchmark in assessing whether the department is maintaining a set correlation of staffing expense to expected revenue despite revenues rising or falling. If revenues are up, actual salary costs will go up, but the benchmark of a 40% variance ensures that the costs are relative to the revenues earned. The statement of income provides the majority of the information that the manager will need to analyze the success of the department. Evaluating each of the category numbers and comparing them to expected budgeted figures will help to explain why profit margins were met or not met. The report is used to investigate where financial problems may lie or where positive results may have been attained.

### Rolling Income Statement

The *rolling income statement* provides much of the same information as in the regular statement of income. The primary difference is that, in the rolling income statement, results from each of the previous 6 months are reflected. In addition, the same month from the previous year is also reflected. Year-to-date figures are also compared with

**Table 6.6  Monthly Income Statement, Occupational Therapy Department, Period 4—April.**

| | | Current Period | | | | |
|---|---|---|---|---|---|---|
| Account Description | Actual | % of Revenues | Budget Plan | % of Revenues | Variance | % Variance |
| Gross revenues | 125,435 | 100.0 | 115,000 | 100.0 | 10,435 | 9.1 |
| Contractual allowances | 8,000 | 6.4 | 10,000 | 8.7 | (2,000) | −20.0 |
| Net revenues | 117,435 | 93.6 | 105,000 | 91.3 | 12,435 | 11.8 |
| Direct expense | | | | | | |
| Salaries | 42,460 | 33.9 | 40,250 | 35.0 | 2,210 | 5.5 |
| Benefits | 8,405 | 6.7 | 8,000 | 7.0 | 405 | 5.1 |
| Supplies | 275 | 0.2 | 500 | 0.4 | (225) | −45.0 |
| Total direct expense | 51,140 | 40.8 | 48,750 | 42.4 | 2,390 | 4.9 |
| Gross profit | 66,295 | 52.9 | 56,250 | 48.9 | 10,045 | 17.9 |
| Operating expenses | | | | | | |
| Admin salaries | 22,500 | 17.9 | 23,000 | 20.0 | (500) | −2.2 |
| Benefits | 4,500 | 3.6 | 4,600 | 4.0 | (100) | −2.2 |
| Temporary help | 1,200 | 1.0 | 750 | 0.7 | 450 | 60.0 |
| Office supplies | 275 | 0.2 | 250 | 0.2 | 25 | 10.0 |
| Phone | 195 | 0.2 | 150 | 0.1 | 45 | 30.0 |
| Postage | 55 | 0.0 | 75 | 0.1 | (20) | −26.7 |
| Recruitment/ advertising | — | 0.0 | 250 | 0.2 | (250) | −100.0 |
| Travel | — | 0.0 | 300 | 0.3 | (300) | −100.0 |
| Dues/education | — | 0.0 | 500 | 0.4 | (500) | −100.0 |
| Depreciation | 500 | 0.4 | 500 | 0.4 | — | 0.0 |
| Equipment repairs | — | 0.0 | 125 | 0.1 | (125) | −100.0 |
| Lease | 2,000 | 1.6 | 2,000 | 1.7 | — | 0.0 |
| Miscellaneous | 125 | 0.1 | 125 | 0.1 | — | 0.0 |
| Total operating expenses | 31,350 | 25.0 | 32,625 | 28.4 | (1,275) | −3.9 |
| Department contribution | 34,945 | 27.9 | 94,500 | 20.5 | 12,708 | 13.4 |
| Corporate allocations | 7,526 | 6.0 | 6,900 | 6.0 | 626 | 9.1 |
| Bad debt and recoveries | 565 | 0.5 | 1,150 | 1.0 | (585) | −50.9 |
| Department profit before taxes | 26,854 | 21.4 | 62,300 | 13.5 | 14,758 | 23.7 |

(*continued*)

the prior year-to-date numbers. This statement is an excellent tool to evaluate trends. The manager can see whether growth is actually occurring as planned and whether the department is doing better or worse than last year at the same time. It can also reflect whether workload consistently fluctuates in certain months.

**Table 6.6** *(Continued)*

| | | Year-to-Date | | | | |
|---|---|---|---|---|---|---|
| **Account Description** | **Actual** | **% of Revenues** | **Budget Plan** | **% of Revenues** | **Variance** | **% Variance** |
| Gross revenues | 452,500 | 100.0 | 460,000 | 100.0 | (7,500) | −1.6 |
| Contractual allowances | 32,600 | 7.2 | 40,000 | 8.7 | (7,400) | −18.5 |
| Net revenues | 419,900 | 92.8 | 420,000 | 91.3 | (100) | 0.0 |
| Direct expense | | | | | | |
| Salaries | 153,850 | 34.0 | 161,000 | 35.0 | (7,150) | −4.4 |
| Benefits | 30,462 | 6.7 | 32,000 | 7.0 | (1,538) | −4.8 |
| Supplies | 1,800 | 0.4 | 2,000 | 0.4 | (200) | −10.0 |
| Total direct expense | 186,112 | 41.1 | 195,000 | 42.4 | (8,888) | −4.6 |
| Gross profit | 233,788 | 51.7 | 225,000 | 48.9 | 8,788 | 3.9 |
| Operating expenses | | | | | | |
| Admin salaries | 90,500 | 20.0 | 92,000 | 20.0 | (1,500) | −1.6 |
| Benefits | 18,100 | 4.0 | 18,400 | 4.0 | (300) | −1.6 |
| Temporary help | 4,730 | 1.0 | 3,000 | 0.7 | 1,730 | 57.7 |
| Office supplies | 876 | 0.2 | 1,000 | 0.2 | (124) | −12.4 |
| Phone | 695 | 0.2 | 600 | 0.1 | 95 | 15.8 |
| Postage | 179 | 0.0 | 300 | 0.1 | (121) | −40.3 |
| Recruitment/ advertising | 300 | 0.1 | 1,000 | 0.2 | (700) | −70.0 |
| Travel | 100 | 0.0 | 1,200 | 0.3 | (1,100) | −91.7 |
| Dues/education | 600 | 0.1 | 2,000 | 0.4 | (1,400) | −70.0 |
| Depreciation | 2,000 | 0.4 | 2,000 | 0.4 | — | 0.0 |
| Equipment repairs | 375 | 0.1 | 500 | 0.1 | (125) | −25.0 |
| Lease | 8,000 | 1.8 | 8,000 | 1.7 | — | 0.0 |
| Miscellaneous | 125 | 0.0 | 500 | 0.1 | (375) | −75.0 |
| Total operating expenses | 126,580 | 28.0 | 130,500 | 28.4 | (3,920) | −3.0 |
| Department contribution | 107,208 | 23.7 | 94,500 | 20.5 | 12,708 | 13.4 |
| Corporate allocations | 27,150 | 6.0 | 27,600 | 6.0 | (450) | −1.6 |
| Bad debt and recoveries | 3,000 | 0.7 | 4,600 | 1.0 | (1,600) | −34.8 |
| Department profit before taxes | 77,058 | 17.0 | 62,300 | 13.5 | 14,758 | 23.7 |

*Note.* Fiscal Year = January to December.

### Detailed Transaction Reports

When questions arise on certain revenue and expense accounts, further detail can be attained through a *detailed transaction report*. This report will provide information on each invoice that was paid. For example, in Table 6.6, the income statement may show an actual figure of $275 for office supplies and a budgeted figure of $250. The transaction report will list each invoice paid in this budget category so the manager can ensure these were invoices that should have been charged to the department. This kind of investigation is necessary when income statement numbers appear to be too high or too low. The detailed report can identify whether invoices are missing, have not been paid, or have been incorrectly applied to the wrong department.

### Payroll Reports

*Payroll reports* detail staff salary expenditures. They generally will reflect what the staff person was paid and will also include all deductions made for the employee. These reports may be especially important to review if staff members are shared among cost centers or if payroll mistakes are made.

### Productivity Reports

*Staff productivity,* which a manager can monitor through staff productivity tracking forms, is a key indicator of efficiency and is especially helpful when census dramatically fluctuates. Managers may use a productivity report to react immediately to these fluctuations by determining staffing needs on a daily or weekly basis. Staff schedules can be adjusted to meet the need, and unnecessary expenses will be avoided.

## Analysis of Specific Financial Problems

The following problems describe typical situations that an occupational therapy manager might face when managing a budget. The analysis provides guidance about how to resolve these problems.

### Problem 1

The income statement reflects that revenues are below budgeted projections and that direct costs are higher than the expected budgeted numbers.

In reviewing this scenario, one might first assume that there were too many staff people working and not enough work was available to ensure that department productivity standards were met. The manager will want to research further to attempt to determine why this imbalance happened and how this problem can be avoided in future months.

Evaluating productivity reports may help to pinpoint where the problem lies. Was one particular program having a problem? For example, did the new pediatric outpatient clinic have fewer patients than expected? Was there an unusual number of patient cancellations? Did the staff have any additional in-service time or meeting time that would have cut into treatment time? All these questions can be answered with some additional investigation, and if it is determined that the issue is an ongoing problem, then action plans can be implemented to correct the problem. If the problem was only incidental, then the manager will be able to explain the reason, and the supervisor will know that this imbalance is not an ongoing problem.

## Problem 2

On first review of the income statements, the manager realizes that the temporary staffing agency bill for $4,000 has not been paid and applied to the current monthly financial figures.

Monitoring the payment and accounting of large expenses incurred by a department is critical to accurately reflect revenues and expenses. Ideally, all the costs incurred for a month of service should be reflected in the month they occurred, especially in the case of the $4,000 temporary staffing agency cost, where additional outside help was needed to meet increased volume needs. Without the reflection of this $4,000 expense, direct costs will be too low, and the gross profit margin will be too high. These numbers will give a false reflection of the actual service efficiency, which will skew overall results.

When this kind of problem is discovered, it is important for the manager to note the discrepancy and potentially refigure the numbers using the correct total direct costs. The manager will then be able to inform the supervisor of the discrepancy and provide the supervisor with the true financial picture. In addition, the manager should notify the larger business entity so figures for the entire operation can be adjusted.

If this information were not noted, two problems could happen. The supervisor would assume that the efficiencies were real and would make decisions on staffing needs using the wrong information. In this particular case, the decision could be to increase expectations of staff members and not allow for needed additional support when the census rises even higher. Second, the temporary staffing agency bill will be processed and likely will be reflected in the next period's income statement. At that time, the ratio of revenue to direct cost will look worse because an additional $4,000 was added to the staffing costs. Thus, it will appear that more staff people provided less service.

Although these numbers will even out when looking at year-to-date numbers, they will provide inaccurate information for rolling income reports and could distort analyses made by comparing previous year's reports for the same month. The manager will always want to review the year-to-date numbers in a case like this one to ensure that the unpaid invoice was the only problem in attaining the projected gross profit.

To avoid these kinds of problems for future periods, the manager may want to monitor expected large invoices. If the invoice is going to be processed late, then the manager may have an opportunity to inform accounting of the situation and ask the accounting department to accrue for this unpaid invoice. Accruals are an option to book dollars into the financial record even though they have not yet been processed and paid. By doing this procedure, the income statement results will reflect the real cost of doing the business provided during that period.

## Problem 3

Recruitment has been a major issue, and the occupational therapy manager decides that advertising in the newspaper will help in finding additional staff people. The advertising expense was not budgeted. The supervisor approves the $1,500 expenditure, and now, this expense is reflected on the income statement.

There will always be some unforeseen expenses, and it will be difficult to plan and predict for all contingencies. This expense will skew operating expenses and ultimate profits, but the consequences of not advertising may be more negative. When presenting the problem to the supervisor, the manager will want to understand the full impact to the budget. The short-term impact will be the cost of the advertisement, but if the recruitment of staff members is not done, the long-term impact will be a staff that is insufficient to meet the workload. In a revenue producing department, the value of hiring a full-time employee can be measured in lost opportunity to bill for services. This kind of financial analysis can assist the manager in developing a justification for the $1,500 expenditure.

## Summary

This chapter has presented the components for effective financial management for an occupational therapy department:

- Planning the budget—Considering the company's overall business plan and practices, developing department goals and objectives, aligning a financial plan with those objectives, and creating a line-item annual budget from the framework of the financial plan
- Monitoring and analyzing financial results—Using various reports and tools to manage and enhance department performance and to handle specific budget problems.

## References

American Hospital Association. (2001). *Hospital statistics: Hospital admission and outpatient visits for the past 10 years.* Chicago: Author.

Baker, J. (*1998*). *Prospective payment for long-term care.* Dallas, TX: Resource Group.

Centers for Disease Control and Prevention. (1999). *1999 National Hospital Discharge Survey.* Hyattsville, MD: Author.

Centers for Medicare and Medicaid Services. (2001a). *National healthcare expenditures.* Baltimore, MD: Author.

Centers for Medicare and Medicaid Services. (2001b). *U.S. healthcare spending by payer source for 1999.* Baltimore, MD: Author.

Fess, P., & Warren, C. (1985). *Financial accounting* (2nd ed.). Cincinnati, OH: South-Western.

Jacobs, K., & Logigian, M. (1999). *Functions of a manager in occupational therapy* (3rd ed.). Thorofare, NJ: Slack.

Moore, M. C., Jaedicke, R. K., & Anderson, L. K. (1984). *Managerial accounting* (6th ed.). Cincinnati, OH: South-Western.

U.S. Census Bureau. (2001). *HMO growth rates.* Washington, DC: Author.

## Additional Resources

Baker, J. (1998). *Prospective payment for long-term care.* Dallas, TX: Resource Group.

Brigham, E. (1986). *Fundamentals of financial management* (4th ed.). New York: CBS College.

Gilkenson, G. E. (1997). *Occupational therapy leadership.* Philadelphia: F. A. Davis.

# Marketing

Tammy Richmond, MS, OTR

*"Efforts and courage are not enough without purpose and direction."*

JOHN F. KENNEDY

**Tammy Richmond, MS, OTR,** is currently chief operating officer of Ultimate Rehab, LLC, and www.ultimaterehab.com, a consulting company in rehabilitation practice and management with on-line presence, based in Los Angeles, CA. She also continues to work in her own private practice, Hands 4 Health, in Los Angeles. She lectures frequently on various private practice issues, has written articles on similar topics, and is actively involved in national and state occupational therapy associations.

# Key Terms and Concepts

**Environmental assessment.** "Evaluation of all forces and changes affecting the organization's ability to conduct business effectively within the market" (Kotler, Armstrong, & Cunningham, 2000, p. 100).

**Market.** "All actual or potential buyers of a product, service, or idea" (Jacobs, 1987, p. 316).

**Market analysis.** The use of information to "define the market and determine if the organization's perception of the wants and the needs of the market are valid" (Shoemaker & Wheeler, 1996, p. 110).

**Marketing management.** "The analysis, implementation, and control of programs designed to create, build, and maintain beneficial exchanges with target buyers, so as to achieve organizational objectives" (Kotler & Armstrong, 1991, p. 10).

**Organizational assessment.** An organization's reevaluation of its effectiveness relative to the patient population, the community, and the health care system itself (Shoemaker & Wheeler, 1996, p.108).

**Place (or distribution).** Where and how the organization will make the products or services accessible and available to the target market (Kotler, 1975, p. 190).

**Position.** "The place that a product holds among similar products in the marketplace" (Shoemaker & Wheeler, 1996, p. 106).

**Target market.** The segment of the market with similar characteristics and needs that are measurable and desirable for an organization to influence.

# Learning Objectives

After completing this chapter, you should be able to do the following:

- Define marketing and the objectives of marketing.
- Define and compare the concepts of market and target market.
- Describe the four steps of market management.
- Distinguish between the two types of market analysis.
- Name the components of a marketing plan.
- Describe the 4 *P*s of marketing strategy.
- Name the three action elements of marketing implementation.
- Describe market measurements.

Marketing is often used synonymously with *selling* or *advertising*. However, marketing is much more than that. In the business world, it can be the difference between success and failure. Many thousands of dollars are spent attempting ultimately to make a profit by appealing and stimulating consumers to purchase a product that is particular to a consumer's wants and needs. Similarly, in health care, marketing is an essential function of the overall organization's strategic plan (or business plan) to grow and succeed by increasing consumer awareness of services, which eventually leads to financial profits and consumer value.

In the past, the health care environment was generally described as moving from being a provider-driven industry to a payer-driven industry on its way to a consumer-driven industry. Today, we are at the forefront of a consumer-driven environment in which the consumer's needs and wants determine the design and delivery systems of products and services. Moreover, consumers have multiple choices as to whom and where they should go for health care products and services and how much they should spend. Therefore, occupational therapists and occupational therapy managers must become knowledgeable and skilled in marketing and marketing management to be competitive and financially successful.

## Marketing Fundamentals

*Marketing*, a basic business function, is defined as "a social and managerial process by which individuals and groups obtain what they need and want through creating and exchanging products and values with others" (Kotler & Armstrong, 1991, p. 5). Marketing facilitates the identification and development of a unique product that will meet the personal expectations and values of a particular group of consumers. In marketing, the unique product must become visible and accessible to the consumer by means of various communication strategies so the exchange can take place. In occupational therapy, the product is generally thought of as a service or program. However, keep in mind that tangible health care products such as educational materials or equipment are marketable items that occupational therapy practitioners also should consider including in the service or program.

Marketing objectives can be both humanistic and managerial. The humanistic objectives of marketing include the following:

- To identify and meet consumer needs and wants
- To create awareness of the product or service and increase accessibility to the consumer
- To persuade the consumer to purchase the product
- To build consumer loyalty.

The managerial objectives of marketing are as follows:

- To encourage strategic planning
- To meet the social, managerial, operational, and financial business goals

- To develop standards and policies that integrate with business objectives
- To increase profits.

Determining the organization's marketing objectives gives guidance and direction to the marketing process. Once objectives are identified, the organization must understand its market and how to manage marketing approaches to effectively reach its goals.

## Market

*Consumers*, as previously noted, are individuals who buy products and services. Health care providers usually think of consumers as patients or clients. However, the evolution of the health care industry dictates that the traditional patient–practitioner relationship is now better thought of as a business–consumer relationship. Within the realm of business operations, consumers are considered to be the market.

The *market* consists of all actual or potential buyers of a product, service, or idea (Jacobs, 1987). To health care providers, the market is anyone (buyer) who will buy or pay for products or services. Within the health care market are several types of buyers and, often, multiple buyers, such as with an ergonomic program in which the buyer can be both the consumer and employer. These buyers are generally lumped into three categories:

- Consumers and potential consumers
- Physicians
- Third-party payers.

However, buyers of occupational therapy products or services can also include these additional categories:

- Public or private businesses
- Nonprofit organizations and charities
- Provider networks
- Other allied health care providers or alternative and complementary practitioners
- E-health care or Internet information systems
- Legislative groups.

Instead of attempting to appeal to a market base that is too large and too varied, successful organizations customize the marketing of products or services to selective target markets. *Target markets* are segments of a market with similar characteristics and needs that are measurable and desirable for an organization to influence. Target markets have four common characteristics: particular needs, money to buy the product, decision-making power, and easy access to the product or service (Wood, 1999). For example, the optometrist identifies the need to hire an occupational therapy practitioner who will provide services in his or her clinic for the existing client population with low-vision difficulties. The present client base has a need, has accessibility, makes decisions about what additional services on which to spend money, and potentially would use the occupational therapy services related to their need.

In occupational therapy, examples of typical target markets include the following:
- School administrators
- Assisted living centers
- Optometrists.

Other appropriate target markets could also include the following:
- Medical spas
- People with disabilities in developing nations
- Low-income mothers with premature babies
- Cancer survivors
- Private insurance contract managers
- Health clubs with pools
- American Diabetes Association
- Novarits Foundation for Gerontology.

An organization identifies target markets by recognizing either an emerging trend or the need for a new service or program and by conducting operational assessments. The organization must thoroughly understand the target market and the organization's relationship to it to develop marketing strategies that will result in new or increased profits. For example, the occupational therapist or occupational therapy manager recognizes the fact that many of the facility's present client population are diagnosed with a form of arthritis. The therapist or manager contacts the nearby community center that contains a therapeutic pool to establish a new aquatic program for the client base.

## Market Management

*Market management* "is the analysis, implementation, and control of programs designed to create, build, and maintain beneficial exchanges with target buyers, so as to achieve organizational objectives (Kotler & Armstrong, 1991, p. 10). Market management is the systematic approach used to identify, persuade, and secure a target market for value and profit.

In today's consumer-driven market, analysis of the environment must be performed first before any goals or planning can take place. This approach differs from the traditional health planning model adapted from Berkowitz and Flexner (1978) in which analysis of the situation or consumer was not considered until the goals and strategies were developed (see Figure 7.1).

Marketing management involves four steps:
- Analysis
- Planning
- Implementation
- Measurements.

These steps are described further in the sections that follow.

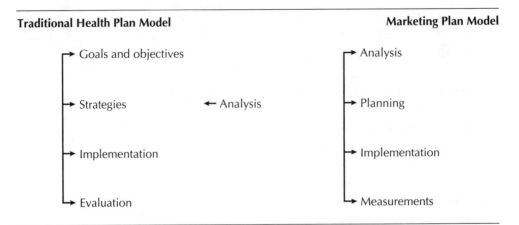

**Figure 7.1 Traditional Health Care Model vs. Today's Marketing Plan Model.**
*Note.* Adapted from "The Marketing Audit," by E. N. Berkowitz and W. A. Flexner, *Health Care Management Review*, Vol. 3, No. 4, 1978, pp. 51–57. Used with permission.

## Analysis

*Market analysis* is the use of information to "define the market and determine if the organization's perception of the wants and the needs of the market are valid" (Shoemaker & Wheeler, 1996). Market analysis can be consolidated into two main assessment methods: the organizational assessment and the environmental assessment. Market research is the most critical step to market management and is the most time-consuming. Gathering, organizing, and assessing the information during this discovery phase will establish the key elements of the marketing plan.

The goals of a market analysis are as follows:
- To identify current trends, opportunities, and threats
- To access consumer needs and demands
- To determine target markets
- To identify and compare competition and position in the market
- To develop and enhance products and services.

An organization can gather marketing information in various ways. MacStravic (1981) divided the marketing process into two methods: (a) market audit and (b) market analysis, consisting of various smaller components such as consumer analysis. Kotler and Armstrong (1991) examined the environmental forces affecting the organization as micro and macro environmental forces (information). Epstein (1992) adapted the micro and macro environmental forces (information) as interactions among business, markets, competitors, and publics. Jacobs and Logigian (1999) suggested that the analysis process consists of a self-audit, consumer analysis, an analysis of other providers with similar services, and an environmental assessment. Shoemaker and Wheeler (1996) identified the components of information gathering as organizational assessment, environmental assessment, market analysis, and communications. Obviously, several approaches to the market analysis have been developed. The commonality among these assessment methods is the need to address both the internal and external factors affecting the organization and the organization's relationship with the consumer and business market.

### Organizational Assessment

The *organizational assessment* is an organization's evaluation of its effectiveness relative to the patient population, the community, and the health care system itself (Shoemaker & Wheeler, 1996). This evaluation can be accomplished by identifying the strengths, weaknesses, opportunities, and threats—a SWOT analysis (Aldag & Stearns, 1987; Fahey & Randall, 1994)—of various internal and external operational factors of an organization. The SWOT analysis is also presented in chapter 5 as the tool used to complete the first step in strategic planning. The internal issues that should be addressed include the daily operations of the occupational therapy organization such as customer service, staffing, and program development. The external issues that should be addressed include current patient populations, competition, and other factors that directly influence advantages and disadvantages of the present organizational operations.

To complete a SWOT analysis of an occupational therapy program or organization, gather information from various sources:
- Operational documentation
- Outcome measurements
- Staff members
- Risk management programs
- Medical records
- Products and services
- Regulatory bodies
- Internet.

Defining the strengths, weaknesses, opportunities, and threats of internal and external operational factors allows the organization to achieve a clear representation of its own internal emerging trends and changes (see Table 7.1).

### Environmental Assessment

*Environmental assessment* is the evaluation of all forces and changes affecting the organization's ability to conduct business effectively with the market (Kotler et al., 2000). Similar in theory to the organizational assessment, the environmental assessment seeks to identify emerging trends and changes as they affect the organization's relationship to the market. In addition, the environmental assessment helps to define and explain the purchasing behaviors of the target market. (See chapter 4 for more information on environmental analysis as well as internal and external factors.)

**Table 7.1 SWOT Analysis.**

| Internal Factors (Strengths and Weaknesses) | External Factors (Opportunities and Threats) |
| --- | --- |
| Staffing | Patient populations |
| Customer service | Competition |
| Programs | Regulations |
| Quality assurance | Technology |
| Risk management | Health care trends |

*Note.* Adapted from *The Portable MBA in Strategy,* by L. Fahey and R. M. Randall, 1994, New York: Wiley. Copyright 1994 by Wiley. Used with permission.

Five important factors affect the environmental assessment:

- Cultural trends
- Demographics
- Economics
- Political and regulatory issues
- New technologies.

The following sections describe these factors more fully.

*Cultural trends.* "Trends in the cultural environment include the persistence of cultural values, shifts in secondary cultural values, and changes in people's views of themselves, of others, of organizations, of society, of nature, and of the universe" (Kotler et al., 2000, p. 93). Cultural and cross-cultural populations have already affected the global economy and, in some cases, have determined the next trend in products and services. Occupational therapy practitioners need to evaluate their immediate environmental surroundings according to cultural makeup and purchasing habits. For example, an occupational therapy practice that services an area with a large Latino pediatric population with juvenile diabetes may consider creating diabetes educational software for multilingual children.

*Demographics.* Information such as population, age, housing, sex, ethnicity, educational levels, income, growth, and labor force projections can be easily found on the Internet or in libraries. Seeking current statistical information about the demographics of the organization's current consumer and potential consumer bases assists in determining target markets and the services and products that the target markets will either engage in or purchase. Understanding the target market and its living habits provides vital analytical support to the marketing plan. For example, the success or failure of a new senior citizens' fitness program depends on whether enough individuals older than age 65 live within a 5-mile radius of the program's location and whether their socioeconomic status could support paid participation.

*Economics.* Economics is the science that deals with the management of the income, resources, organization, and expenditures of a government, business, community, or household. Changes in the condition of a financial system such as governmental spending or financial markets will influence consumer confidence and purchasing patterns. Understanding economic issues that are relevant to a particular market can guide product or service development. For example, more than 55% of all children ages 6 and younger who are living in the United States are living in a female-headed household that is under 100% of the poverty standard (U.S. Bureau of the Census, 2000). An occupational therapy nonprofit life skills program targeting low-income mothers may be an appropriate program to address this issue.

*Political and regulatory issues.* Occupational therapy practice is heavily affected by state and federal legislative rules and guidelines. Products and services developed for target markets must comply with standards of practice, the code of ethics, reimbursement procedures, and regulation within the field of occupational therapy as well as with local, state, and federal laws and regulations related to business and taxes. The state and national organizational bodies such as the Occupational Therapy Association of California (or other professional state organizations) and the American Occupational Therapy Association are valuable resources of information. Additionally, reimbursement strategies may fall under regulatory limitations. Understanding the political and regulatory parameters of products, pricing, and promotional strategies is essential to marketing implementation. For example, the development of a new home health practice to evaluate would be subject to regulatory laws.

*New technologies.* The explosion of information technology systems such as personal computers, hand-held devices, and assistive technologies has already affected health care significantly. As consumers demand real-time communication and treatment strategies to manage their health at home, those strategies that capture the World Wide Web or the Internet are becoming vital tools to marketing promotions. Telemedicine and home modification programs are examples of existing integrated service technologies.

Occupational therapy practitioners need the information gathered from both organizational and environmental assessments to make effective marketing decisions (see Figure 7.2, which shows the market analysis process using the organizational and environmental assessments). Most important, the assessments should answer these questions:

- What are the emerging trends?
- Who is my target market?
- What is my unique product or service?
- Who is my competition?

## Planning

The next step in marketing management is the development of the marketing plan. The marketing plan, like a strategic plan or business plan, is a tool (a) to coordinate and use information about the organization, its product or services, and its objectives and

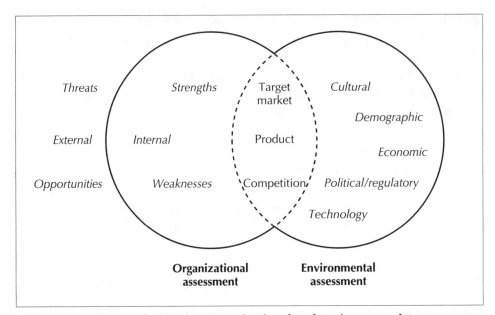

**Figure 7.2 Market Analysis Using Organizational and Environmental Assessments.**

strategies and (b) to stimulate the outcome of marketing activities. The marketing plan should contain these components:

- Company description
- Mission statement
- Target market
- Product or service
- Identification of competition
- Marketing objectives
- Marketing strategies
- Action plan
- Measurements.

Company description, mission statement, target market, product or service, and identification of competition are all derived from the information gathered and evaluated from the market analysis. Marketing objectives are the humanistic and managerial goals that direct the plan. Marketing strategies are further explained in the following sections. The action plan and measurements are carried out in the implementation and measurement steps of market management and are explained in later sections.

## Marketing Strategies

*Market strategies* are the essential schematic processes used to achieve marketing objectives. A comprehensive marketing plan typically uses multiple marketing strategies to be effective. Traditionally, these processes are called the 4 *P*s: product, place, price, and promotion. Marketing experts also add a fifth *P* to the basic concepts: position.

*Product.* A *product* is "anything that can be offered to a market for attention, acquisition, use or consumption and that might satisfy a need or want" (Kotler & Armstrong, 1991, p. 7). In occupational therapy practice, the product typically refers to services and programs. To develop promotional materials, it is important for the organization to describe the product in terms of its features and value. Before the consumer will purchase the product, it has to do several things: fill a need, appeal to the target market, have value and purpose, and provide advantages over another similar product. For example, an occupational therapist develops a women's health program that includes treatment for incontinence and osteoporosis. Biofeedback devices, fitness and nutritional services, and educational materials for the various related health care issues are included in the program. The promotional materials will need to highlight the product's (the program's) benefits and advantages and explain what needs are being satisfied.

*Price.* The *price* is the amount of money charged for a product or service or the sum of the values that consumers exchange for the benefits of having and using the product or service (Kotler et al., 2000). Basically, it is the monetary exchange between the buyer and the seller. In today's market, the seller is the occupational therapist or occupational therapy manager, and the buyer (or target market) could comprise several groups such as the consumer and third-party payers. In some cases, the price or pricing components fall under regulatory bodies and are already established. For example, the cost of a class to an aquatic program should be competitively priced to area programs or established by averaged local third-party payers' reimbursement. In other situations, the occupational therapist or manager will have to establish a price. To estimate the price of the product or service, the practitioner must determine the following:

- Costs to develop and produce the product or service
- Fair market value
- Fee options (flexibility)
- Sales and taxes
- Third-party payer rates
- Competitor's pricing
- Revenue needed to maintain customer service
- Other overhead costs such as permits and licenses
- Consumer's perception of value relative to costs.

The goal of pricing is to make a profit. Pricing should never be thought of as static. Constant changes in the marketplace warrant regularly revisiting the price of the products or services.

*Place.* *Place* is where and how the organization will make the product or services accessible and available to the target market (Kotler, 1975). Place may commonly be described as *distribution*. The obvious access is the actual physical location where occupational therapy is provided. However, place should be viewed more completely as how, when, where, and through what types of communication strategies the product or service is provided. For example, the consideration of place is particularly important when marketing an after-school program for adolescents and parents called "Violence and Drug Prevention," which is provided on the campus of a middle school that has a history of school violence. Clearly, the participation in and success of the program are connected to where it is offered.

*Promotion.*  Marketing is typically thought of as *promotion,* which is defined as the method of communicating information to the consumers about the product's benefits, place, and price. Visibility and costs are determining factors in selecting types of promotional strategies. The ultimate goals of marketing promotions are to create awareness of the product and to persuade consumer purchasing. Successful promotional campaigns integrate several types of marketing strategies over a designated period of time. The occupational therapist and manager must constantly monitor the target market to respond quickly to any new trends and changes.

Several guidelines are important to keep in mind when deciding which promotional strategies to integrate. Target markets want to be informed about convenience, costs, product comparison, the organization's ability to provide services, and accessibility. The image created by the marketing strategies should be clear and simple, and it should demonstrate added value. Market "branding" by the use of slogans, tag lines, logos, colors, and other persuasive techniques also provides valuable promotional advantage. For example, the yellow arches of McDonald's automatically create an image and awareness of what the product is without having to be told. In occupational therapy, the slogan "OT makes it possible" is an example of creating product awareness or branding.

Promotional strategies can be grouped into four categories:

- Advertising
- Sales promotion
- Public relations
- Personal selling.

Advertising is generally accomplished as paid media. Business cards, brochures, and ad placements in magazines or on an Internet Web site are examples of advertising. Advertising may be regulated by several federal and state laws, including the Occupational Therapy Code of Ethics and state occupational therapy licensing (Hertfelder & Crispen, 1990). Occupational therapy practitioners should become familiar with the specific rules and regulations in their state before generating advertisements.

Sales promotion is the use of a wide variety of short-term incentives to encourage purchase of the product (Jacobs & Logigian, 1999). Often the incentives have value to the consumer, for example, coupons, free assessments, or free samples. Similarly, scheduling a free follow-up screening 6 weeks after discharge not only allows the occupational therapist or manager to gather additional outcome measurements but also promotes good customer service and return business.

"Public relations is doing good things and telling people about them" (Hertfelder & Crispen, 1990, pp. 2–18). News releases, articles, and donations to charities are all examples of strategies by which the practitioner can create an image or opinion of the organization. Publicity efforts are most viable when they are visible to the target market that an organization wishes to influence.

Personal selling is the most effective and can be the least expensive type of promotion. It can include face-to-face communications or word-of-mouth referrals. It also can include electronic mailings through the Internet or World Wide Web. (Although marketing and promotional plans do not usually deal with individuals' protected health information, the occupational therapy manager should follow appropriate Health Insurance Portability and Accountability Act privacy regulations for electronic mailings, which are discussed more in chapter 9.) Consumers place value on the opinions of others, especially if the opinion is coming from someone they trust such as a physician or occupational therapy practitioner. However, health care providers are generally uncomfortable personally promoting themselves or their services to consumers. Therefore, networking and focus groups are two excellent personal selling strategies. Professional contacts are a way to share information and offer support. Similar relationships are affiliated partnerships or strategic alliances. Customer service is very important to the success of personal selling. As a general rule, a pleased consumer tells three other people who, in turn, continue to promote the benefits of a new product or service.

*Position.* *Position* is the place that a product holds among similar products in the marketplace (Shoemaker & Wheeler, 1996). The occupational therapist or manager needs to evaluate closely the competition and compare product advantages and disadvantages. Attempting to market an elbow brace against numerous other elbow braces that already have a history in the marketplace is an example in which position may have a negative influence on the success of the product. Ultimately, the success or failure of a new product can be determined by market position.

## Implementation

*Implementation* is the organized process of carrying out the marketing plan. It is the action function of the marketing plan and has the purpose of increasing business growth and financial success. Implementation involves three action elements:

- *Identify the marketing budget*—Marketing budgets depend on the organization's ability to raise or set aside business capital, but they do not have to be expensive; creative thinking and organizational input can produce more for less.
- *Identify the promotional strategies*—Determining which promotional strategies to implement depends on finances, time, and personnel power (hosting a seminar is a great way to self-promote without spending money).

- *Create a time line*—The general rule with respect to time lines is one marketing strategy type per 3 months or nine types per 18 months.

## Measurements

Outcomes measurements are very familiar to occupational therapy practitioners, and the same basic operational guidelines apply in measuring marketing results as in measuring occupational therapy practice outcomes. Determine what elements to measure, how to calculate change, and when to reassess the measurements.

Monitoring and assessing the marketing strategies allows the organization to redirect the marketing effort if necessary. Customer surveys are one way to gain knowledge of the current and potential consumer's expectations and responses about the effectiveness of the market strategy.

## Conclusion

Marketing is a basic organizational business function that promotes an exchange of products and values with others by a social and managerial process (Kotler & Armstrong, 1991). The health care market comprises buyers and sellers of health care products, services, or programs. The occupational therapy practitioner and manager play the role of seller, and numerous individuals or agencies act as buyers, including patients, third-party payers, and private businesses. Target markets are segments of a market with similar characteristics and needs that are measurable and desirable for an organization to influence. Marketing management involves identifying the target market in which the organization wants to exert influence.

Marketing management involves four steps: analysis, planning, implementation, and measurements. Market analysis can be consolidated into two main assessments, the organizational assessment and the environmental assessment. The organizational assessment is the reevaluation of the organization's effectiveness relative to the patient population, the community, and the health care system itself (Shoemaker & Wheeler, 1996). The SWOT analysis is a good organizational tool to use for assessing the internal and external factors affecting the business operations of an occupational therapy organization. The environmental assessment examines the forces and changes affecting the organization's ability to conduct business effectively within the market (Kotler et al., 2000). The functional outcomes of the assessments are the identification of emerging trends, target markets, unique products or services, and competition. The marketing plan is the tool to coordinate and use the information gathered during the market analysis.

Marketing strategies can be thought of in terms of the 4 Ps (product, place, price, and promotion) plus a fifth P (position). Product is "anything that can be offered to a market for attention, acquisition, use, or consumption and that might satisfy a need or want" (Kotler & Armstrong, 1991, p. 7). Place is where or how the organization will make the products or services accessible and available to the target market (Kotler, 1975). Price is the amount of money charged for a product or service or the sum of the values that consumers exchange for the benefits of having and using the product or service (Kotler et al., 2000). Promotion is the method of communicating information to the consumers about the product's benefits, place, and price. Position is the place that a product holds among similar products in the marketplace.

Implementation involves three action elements: identifying the market budget, identifying promotional strategies, and creating a time line. Market measurements, the last step in market management, require establishing a systemic approach to measuring data that are collected after implementing marketing strategies that are directed at the target market in a given time frame. The results provide useful information for future selection of marketing strategies in response to target market trends and changes. To be successful in today's consumer-driven environment, occupational therapists and managers must understand as well as become comfortable with and skilled in marketing and marketing management.

## References

Aldag, R. J., & Stearns, T. M. (1987). *Management*. Cincinnati, OH: South-Western.

Berkowitz, E. N., & Flexner, W. A. (1978). The marketing audit: A tool for health service organizations. *Health Care Management Review, 3*(4), 51–57.

Epstein, C. F. (1992). Marketing: A continuous process. In E. G. Jaffe & C. F. Epstein (Eds.), *Occupational therapy consultation: Theory, principles, and practice* (pp. 655–659). Chicago: Mosby YearBook.

Fahey, L., & Randall, R. M. (Eds.). (1994). *The portable MBA in strategy*. New York: Wiley.

Hertfelder, S., & Crispen, C. (1990). *Private practice: Strategies for success*. Bethesda, MD: American Occupational Therapy Association.

Jacobs, K. (1987). Marketing occupational therapy. *American Journal of Occupational Therapy, 41*(5), 316.

Jacobs, K., & Logigian, M. (1999). *Functions of a manager in occupational therapy* (rev. ed.). Thorofare, NJ: Slack.

Kotler, P. (1975). *Marketing for nonprofit organizations*. Englewood Cliffs, NJ: Prentice-Hall.

Kotler, P., & Armstrong, G. (1991). *Principles of marketing* (5th ed.). Englewood Cliffs, NJ: Prentice-Hall.

Kotler, P., Armstrong, G., & Cunningham, P. (2000). *Principles of marketing* (5th Canadian ed.). Upper Saddle River, NJ: Prentice-Hall.

MacStravic, R. E. S. (1981). Market research in ambulatory care. *Journal of Ambulatory Care Management, 4*(2), 33–40.

Shoemaker, T., & Wheeler, C. (1996). *The occupational therapy manager* (rev. ed.). Bethesda, MD: American Occupational Therapy Association.

U.S. Bureau of the Census. (2000). *Current population reports: March current population survey, consumer income.* (Series P-60). Retrieved June 10, 2002, from http://www. childstats. gov/ac2000/econ1a.asp

Wood, J. (1999). *Marketing research: Basics 101.* Retrieved from http://www.online. wbc.gov

**Additional Resources**

Centers for Disease Control and Prevention—www.cdc.gov
Centers for Medicare and Medicaid Services—www.cms.hhs.gov
SBA Online Women's Business Center—www.onlinewbc.gov
U.S. Department of Health and Human Services—www.dhhs.gov

# CHAPTER 8

# Starting Up a New Program, Business, or Practice

Gordon Muir Giles, PhD, OTR, FAOTA

*"I'm a great believer in luck, and I find the harder I work the more I have of it."*

THOMAS JEFFERSON

**Gordon Muir Giles, PhD, OTR, FAOTA,** is associate professor at Samuel Merritt College, Oakland, CA, and director of neuro-behavioral services at Crestwood Behavioral Health, Inc., Stockton. In 1993, Dr. Giles was responsible for opening the first county-funded neurobehavioral program for people with acquired neurological impairments. He currently is responsible for a 60-bed neuro-behavioral program in Fremont and a 40-bed Med/Psych program in Sunnyvale.

## Key Terms and Concepts

**Break-even point.** This is the point at which revenues from services provided equal the cost of providing services. Revenues above the break-even point result in profit.

**Executive summary.** A short, clear, and compelling statement of the place of the proposed business in the market and of how the proposed business or program can be successful.

**Market analysis.** Examines the number of potential consumers, discusses the potential growth rate of the market for the service, describes the program or service (including strengths and weaknesses) in comparison with the competition, and details marketing strategies.

**Nonproductive time.** In a fee-for-service model, the time during which a staff person is not engaged in revenue-generating activity.

**Program proposal.** This is the first description of the program's goals and how the program can be successful. It should include the resources required, including facilities, management, and staffing, as well as an estimate of expenses and revenues. It is circulated to key decision-makers. Approval of the program proposal results in the development of a business plan.

**Referral patterns.** Detail the source, frequency, and variability of referrals to the program or service.

**Staffing patterns.** Describe the number of staff needed in particular job categories in relation to the type of service provided, number of clients, clients' medical acuity, and need for service.

## Learning Objectives

After completing this chapter, you should be able to do the following:

- ■   Justify the need for a program and describe how the program can be successful.
- ■   Write a program proposal.
- ■   Write a business plan for program development.
- ■   List the key elements of a staffing pattern.
- ■   Describe how the program's location and physical structure can affect the program's success.

hange in the health care environment has led many occupational therapists to engage in program development. Closure of many hospital-based programs has increased the number of practitioners working in the community. The decline in traditional, institution-based occupational therapy mental health services has led to an expansion of community mental health programs (Bailey, 1998). Continuing changes in the health care industry will lead occupational therapists to develop new ways to serve existing service sectors and to develop new services (see chapter 9). Occupational therapists are involved in developing occupational therapy services and interdisciplinary services. Despite the wide variety of clients, program types, reimbursement sources, and environmental contexts, important commonalities can be found in the requirements of program development.

The evolving nature of health care delivery requires that practitioners adapt services to the changing needs and expectations of the client base. For many therapists, program development and program transition will affect the way that they work within the same company or within the same job position. Successful programs are likely to be those that respond to changes in client population, referral patterns, and reimbursement. Meeting the challenge of the changes in patterns of care and service delivery models is imperative if practitioners are to remain innovative providers of essential health care services.

Introductory sections of this chapter describe how an initial program idea may be developed. The typical contents of a one- or two-page program proposal are described. Further development of the idea is described under headings appropriate in a business plan. Vignettes describing the planning and development processes of five programs are included in Appendix 8.A and are referred to throughout the chapter. Emphasis is placed on staff selection, development, and training.

## Development of a Program Idea

The idea for a program may come from many sources. Observation of referral patterns at a setting may indicate a sufficient number of individuals in an underserved population to justify the development of a specialty area. A public or private agency (e.g., federal, state, local agency, or a private charity) may put out a call for a proposal. Alternatively, a group of individuals, an institution, or an agency might wish to develop a program and may investigate the need for a service in the community. Individuals may want a career change, more independence, or the opportunity to use or develop a skill and may develop a program or service that enables them to fulfill these goals.

Going from an initial program idea to a functioning program is often a long and arduous task. A single individual rarely has all the requisite knowledge and resources; thus, program development is usually a team undertaking. Even individuals who are developing a private practice will need to call on multiple sets of resources and do a considerable amount of research before start-up. Involving key stakeholders early in the process increases the chances for the program idea to receive wide support; additionally, interested outside agencies (i.e., foundations) should be involved at an early stage. For example, in developing a hospital-based outpatient traumatic brain injury (TBI) program, the rehabilitation manager may wish to involve staff therapists from each discipline, referring physicians, the facilities manager, and representatives of consumer advocacy and service agencies.

An initial written proposal is required in most circumstances. First-time proposal writers should avoid "reinventing the wheel" and should plan to consult early and often with someone who is knowledgeable about the process of writing proposals. Proposals that have been successful within the same corporation or funded by the same agency may be used as a starting point. Although the initial proposal serves a multitude of functions, it should be brief, no more than one or two pages. The goals of the initial proposal are to justify the need for the program and to describe how the program can be successful. If the proposed program is to be part of an existing institution or business, the initial proposal needs to demonstrate that the program is consistent with the goals and culture of the existing entity or that it would complement previously existing services. For example, when developing a proposal for a long-term psychiatric services company to provide a medical and psychiatric program based in a skilled nursing facility (SNF), the proposal writers needed to show how a medical service could maintain clients within the system and provide a service that was important to key referral agencies (see program vignette 2, Appendix 8.A).

The initial proposal should describe the population to be served, the program's goals and objectives, and the proposed services. A needs assessment should be conducted and should include an estimate of the number of clients who would make use of the service and for what length of time. The proposal should describe target outcomes as well as benefits to the population served and to the organization. It should also include what resources are required, including facilities, management, and staffing as well as an estimate of expenses and revenues. However, proposal writers should resist the temptation to go into too much detail. At this point, it is only necessary to obtain the approval of key decisionmakers for further investigation and for approval of the resources necessary to develop a business plan. The proposal should be circulated to potential stakeholders for input. Favorable reception to the initial proposal permits the development of a more detailed document, referred to as a *business plan* (Abrams, 2000). The business plan includes an executive summary (a two- to three-page summary of the business plan) that is similar to the initial proposal but provides more detail.

## Development of a Business Plan

An outline structure for a business plan is provided in Appendix 8.B. The detailed structure and content of the business plan vary, depending on the type of program, the program's needs, and the type of information required by stakeholders. Individuals who are contemplating opening a private practice should develop a business plan before embarking on a program with a significant financial risk (Edwards, Edwards, & Economy, 2000). The remainder of this chapter examines in more detail the content of a business plan to develop a new program and includes case study descriptions of different types of programs developed by occupational therapists. The content of some sections of a business plan are described in greater detail in other chapters of this book and are not discussed in depth here.

## Nature of the Service Sector

The first section of the business plan provides a description of the population and the service environment. This section should include the population of potential clients, the nature of the problem to be addressed, and current service delivery models. Many sources can be used to develop background information, including epidemiological databases and population projections, literature reviews, analysis of business trends, previous referral patterns, information about competitors, and requests from referral agencies.

## Problem Statement

The problem statement describes the nature of the problem or resource deficit to be addressed by the proposed program. It may be a very brief section that simply states the unmet need in the community.

## Market Factors and Future Trends

The description of market factors and future trends examines possible directions in the market sector and describes how trends are likely to affect the proposed business. It is important to note whether the population to be treated in the proposed program is expanding (e.g., people older than age 65, people with autism) or contracting (e.g., people with postpolio syndrome). Changes in the health care market often result from the evolution of service delivery models and changes in reimbursement. Giles and Clark-Wilson (1999) described the expansion and contraction of transitional living services for people with TBI as a result of changes in the willingness of third-party payers to fund services. Most Alzheimer's programs have moved from SNFs to residential care facilities (RCFs) as a result of changes in funding and the development of new service delivery models. The introduction of caps on rehabilitation reimbursement in SNF-based, subacute rehabilitation funded by the Medicare program provides an example of how market factors affect service delivery.

## Services

### Description

The business plan describes the population to be served, the type of problems to be addressed, and the nature of the service to be delivered. It should provide a clear definition of the service user and a description of the treatment criteria, including whether the service is going to be inpatient or outpatient, what disciplines are delivering services, and how many hours per day and how many times per week services are provided. The target population should be defined as specifically as possible with inclusionary criteria (i.e., the defining characteristics such as age, diagnosis, type of problem, severity of the problem that make clients eligible for the program) and exclusionary criteria (i.e., the characteristics such as age limitations, problem complexity, dual diagnoses, medical stability, and behavioral problems that make clients ineligible for the program). See program vignette 5, Appendix 8.A, for an example.

### Unique Program or Features

The program proposal or business plan should describe the unique characteristics of the program under development that make it superior to other available services. For example, the program may offer a unique service delivery model or represent evidence-based practice. A computer search and a review of the literature using an appropriate database (e.g., Index Medicus, Cinahl) normally finds reports of model programs and practice or treatment guidelines. Textbooks provide a place to start in thinking about model program approaches, and their reference lists provide a place to begin finding literature (Neistadt & Crepeau, 1998). Commercial search engines provide many useful Web sites, and the American Occupational Therapy Association (AOTA) materials and listserv resource can be helpful.

Programs with a similar focus that are already in operation provide an invaluable resource for the practitioner who is intent on developing a program. Observing other programs can highlight both advantages and disadvantages of various approaches to the requirements (e.g., physical plant, staffing, organizational structure) of the particular program under development or expansion. Building on the strong points of existing programs and evidence-based practice allows the clinician to develop an appropriate service model. For example, the author, working as a consultant, conducted a computer search and literature review to establish guidelines for an RCF-based Alzheimer's disease program. Incorporation of the treatment approaches derived from the literature review led to improved client and family satisfaction, increased staff morale, and increased referrals.

## Market Analysis
### Target Market and Characteristics

The market analysis is conducted to estimate the population of potential service users in the market area. The market analysis addresses the question of whether the area has a sufficient number of individuals who can get to the point of service, who need the service, and who can pay enough to support the service. When many people need the service in a given community, customers are easier to attract because they do not have to travel far to the point of service.

Fettig and Riegel (1998) described a market analysis performed for a proposed adult day care center. The authors used U.S. Census data to describe the population of the county in which the day care center would operate and to quantify the number of individuals living in the county who were ages 60 years or older and who would meet the age criteria. Median income of the population was included because day care services were out-of-pocket expenses. The analysis included the fact that the center was located in a rural area (without local competition).

The nature of the service dictates the number of new admissions needed to support the program. For example, program vignette 2 in Appendix 8.A shows that a long-term, 30-bed, combined medicine and psychiatric program involving an average length of stay of 6–12 months needs an average of 50 admissions a year to stay viable. Similarly, program vignette 5 in Appendix 8.A shows that a pediatric outpatient program with an average overall treatment duration of 1–2 years and a maximum capacity of 13 clients needs fewer than 13 new clients per year. A practitioner in an orthopedic program with an average number of 2–3 visits and 75% productivity requires 10 new clients per week.

### Strengths and Weaknesses of Competitors

Knowing the number of potential clients provides only part of the information needed in estimating the potential use of the service; one must also estimate potential market share. Most programs have competitors of one form or another (even if the "competitor" is no treatment). Reviewing the strengths, weaknesses, opportunities, and threats (a SWOT analysis) may prove helpful in evaluating the market potential of a new program (Abrams, 2000).

Practitioners should determine the "selling points" of their service. What advantages does the new service offer over the programs to which clients are currently referred? Cost is often an important determinant in choosing a program, but it may not be the decisive factor: Many individuals will pay more for perceived quality or may not consider cost at all if the payment will be covered by insurance. For example, staff members of a subacute rehabilitation program emphasized the availability of therapies 7 days per week, intravenous therapy, and total parenteral nutrition as factors that set their program apart from their competitors' programs.

## Marketing

### Advertising

AOTA promotes the profession of occupational therapy to the community at large to increase the awareness of occupational therapy among the U.S. public and core user groups. For most programs, however, advertising should be highly focused toward a group that will be likely to use the service. Occupational therapists may use free or low-cost advertising methods such as disseminating press releases and newsletters as well as making presentations to special interest community groups (Opila-Lehman,

2002). Practitioners should consider the audience they are attempting to reach. For example, rehabilitative services may be marketed in retirement communities, clubs, and organizations in which individuals may either need services themselves or know others who need services. Specialized services and services for which clients are not self or family referred are unlikely to benefit from general advertising.

### Marketing Strategy

The marketing strategy is influenced by knowledge of pre-established relationships and by service and referral patterns in the community. Individuals who refer clients for services (i.e., hospital or insurance case managers) need a reason to alter their established referral patterns. Thus, practitioners need to introduce the new service to potential referrers. Inviting potential referrers to see the program and to meet the staff helps to increase the referrers' knowledge of the services offered. An open house provides an opportunity to showcase the program. (Marketing is described in detail in chapter 7.)

Diverse factors may influence referral patterns and program reputation. Practitioners are usually focused on the quality of the services and pay less attention to other factors that may influence program acceptance, including whether the facility is clean and well decorated and whether staff members are courteous and appear professional.

Once a program has begun to receive referrals, these sources of clients should be treated as a valuable resource. Referrers want to know that the people they are sending to the program are obtaining appropriate care. Wherever possible, outcome information should be provided to the referral agency.

### Management and Ownership

A company's investors and managers want to know that qualified personnel are available to open the program. The individuals who are listed as key personnel should be committed to the program, have the necessary knowledge and skills, and have the time to ensure that the program is successful. Résumés that detail requisite training and experience of staff members should be included in an appendix to the business plan (see Appendix 8.B). Gaps in expertise can be filled by the use of consultants. Some programs are practical only with certain key posts filled, and a plan should be established to ensure that appropriate individuals are recruited.

## Staffing

### Staffing Patterns

Staffing patterns should be developed before opening the program. The need for particular staffing levels and staff qualifications varies with client acuity and type of services (i.e., direct individual intervention, group intervention, consultation). The number of occupational therapists, occupational therapy assistants, and aides as well as the "mix" of these staff people are affected by client acuity and program model. Programs that involve direct intervention are different from those programs in which the occupational therapist assesses the clients and then develops a plan to be carried out by nontherapy personnel (i.e., care providers in a board and care home).

The program model and the responsibilities of staff members are important in assessing the number of staff people required. *Nonproductive time* is the term used to describe the time during which the staff person is not engaged in direct intervention (i.e., generating revenue in a fee-for-service model). Some models include nonproductive time for staff meetings, family meetings, documentation, scheduling, student supervision, and other non-direct-care activities. Some models of service are communication intensive (usually programs that have a high need for coordination of services) and, therefore, have more nonproductive time. Knowing how many hours of direct intervention are needed is important in developing a staffing pattern. For example, in an Alzheimer's disease day program, maintaining the program's routine of activities (e.g., lunch, snack breaks) and managing behaviors is as important as providing direct intervention. Thus, it is necessary to know who will help with meals, when staff members will take breaks, and when meetings will occur. In an SNF, more intervention may occur in the morning so that self-care retraining can be provided to the maximum number of individuals. Outlining the staffing structure for a typical day and a typical week can assist in determining staffing needs.

Table 8.1 presents a spreadsheet showing a simplified rehabilitation staffing pattern that also estimates hours of direct intervention and labor costs for a subacute rehabilitation unit. The staffing projections can be used to demonstrate when staff hours need to be added or subtracted in a program as the census changes. Similar methods can be applied to labor and cost projection in other types of programs.

In the table, a module is a 15-minute period of direct therapy. The number of modules (mods) per day is derived from the number of beds multiplied by use assumptions. To derive the number of hours required for client treatment, divide the number of mods by 4 and multiply the quotient by 3 (75% productivity estimate). The staffing pattern is derived by estimating appropriate staff mix based on client acuity and totaling the necessary number of hours. Hours per patient day (HPPD) are derived from dividing total hours by census. As a check on accuracy, HPPD must total the number of mods per client plus nonproductive time (actual staff hours per patient day).

Projections differ depending on acuity and diagnosis of clients. (For example, people with cerebrovascular accident may require extensive intervention from three therapy disciplines, whereas clients with knee replacement will require more physical therapy but little occupational therapy and no speech therapy.) Assumptions about the amount of direct intervention per client are based on a mix of client acuities (hours of direct intervention needed will change depending on the client's use of individual disciplines).

Note that practitioner hours increase predictably as the client census increases. For example, a minimum requirement for full occupancy in a 12-bed unit might be one full-time practitioner in each discipline. However, if census falls to seven clients

## Table 8.1  Rehabilitation Staffing Patterns.

| Assumptions | Modules | | | | | |
|---|---|---|---|---|---|---|
| PT = 4.0 Mods/Rehab Patient | 4.0 | | | | | |
| OT = 3.0 Mods/Rehab Patient | 3.0 | | | | | |
| ST = 2.0 Mods/Rehab Patient | 2.0 | | | | | |
| Productivity—75% | 75% | | | | | |

| Rehab Census | # of Mods | # of Hours | PT Hours | PTA Hours | PT Aide | Total | HPPD |
|---|---|---|---|---|---|---|---|
| 20 | 80 | 26.67 | 8 | 8 | 11 | 27 | 1.35 |
| 19 | 76 | 25.33 | 8 | 8 | 9 | 25 | 1.32 |
| 18 | 72 | 24.00 | 8 | 8 | 8 | 24 | 1.33 |
| 17 | 68 | 22.67 | 8 | 8 | 7 | 23 | 1.35 |
| 16 | 64 | 21.33 | 8 | 8 | 5 | 21 | 1.31 |
| 15 | 60 | 20.00 | 8 | 8 | 4 | 20 | 1.33 |
| 14 | 56 | 18.67 | 8 | 5 | 6 | 19 | 1.36 |
| 13 | 52 | 17.33 | 8 | 5 | 4 | 17 | 1.31 |
| 12 | 48 | 16.00 | 8 | 0 | 8 | 16 | 1.33 |
| 11 | 44 | 14.67 | 8 | 0 | 7 | 15 | 1.36 |
| 10 | 40 | 13.33 | 8 | 0 | 5 | 13 | 1.30 |
| 9 | 36 | 12.00 | 7 | 0 | 5 | 12 | 1.33 |
| 8 | 32 | 10.67 | 5 | 0 | 5 | 10 | 1.25 |
| 7 | 28 | 9.33 | 5 | 0 | 4 | 9 | 1.29 |

| Rehab Census | # of Mods | # of Hours | OT Hours | COTA | OT Aide | Total | HPPD |
|---|---|---|---|---|---|---|---|
| 20 | 60 | 20.00 | 8 | 8 | 4 | 20 | 1.00 |
| 19 | 57 | 19.00 | 8 | 7 | 4 | 19 | 1.00 |
| 18 | 54 | 18.00 | 8 | 7 | 3 | 18 | 1.00 |
| 17 | 51 | 17.00 | 8 | 6 | 3 | 17 | 1.00 |
| 16 | 48 | 16.00 | 8 | 5 | 3 | 16 | 1.00 |
| 15 | 45 | 15.00 | 8 | 7 | 0 | 15 | 1.00 |
| 14 | 42 | 14.00 | 8 | 6 | 0 | 14 | 1.00 |
| 13 | 39 | 13.00 | 8 | 5 | 0 | 13 | 1.00 |
| 12 | 36 | 12.00 | 8 | 4 | 0 | 12 | 1.00 |
| 11 | 33 | 11.00 | 8 | 3 | 0 | 11 | 1.00 |
| 10 | 30 | 10.00 | 8 | 2 | 0 | 10 | 1.00 |
| 9 | 27 | 9.00 | 8 | 1 | 0 | 9 | 1.00 |
| 8 | 24 | 8.00 | 8 | 0 | 0 | 8 | 1.00 |
| 7 | 21 | 7.00 | 7 | 0 | 0 | 7 | 1.00 |

| Rehab Census | # of Mods | # of Hours | ST Hours | | ST Aide | Total | HPPD |
|---|---|---|---|---|---|---|---|
| 20 | 40 | 13.33 | 8 | | 5 | 13 | 0.65 |
| 19 | 38 | 12.67 | 8 | | 4 | 12 | 0.63 |
| 18 | 36 | 12.00 | 8 | | 3 | 11 | 0.61 |
| 17 | 34 | 11.33 | 8 | | 3 | 11 | 0.65 |

(continued)

**Table 8.1**  *(Continued)*

**Rehab**

| Census | # of Mods | # of Hours | ST Hours | ST Aide | Total | HPPD |
|---|---|---|---|---|---|---|
| 16 | 32 | 10.67 | 8 | 2 | 10 | 0.63 |
| 15 | 30 | 10.00 | 8 | 0 | 8 | 0.53 |
| 14 | 28 | 9.33 | 8 | 0 | 8 | 0.57 |
| 13 | 26 | 8.67 | 8 | 0 | 8 | 0.62 |
| 12 | 24 | 8.00 | 8 | 0 | 8 | 0.67 |
| 11 | 22 | 7.33 | 7 | 0 | 7 | 0.64 |
| 10 | 20 | 6.67 | 7 | 0 | 7 | 0.70 |
| 9 | 18 | 6.00 | 6 | 0 | 6 | 0.67 |
| 8 | 16 | 5.33 | 5 | 0 | 5 | 0.63 |
| 7 | 14 | 4.67 | 5 | 0 | 5 | 0.71 |

*Note.* HPPD = hours per patient day. Contributed by Araceli D. Antonio, RN, MSN, Nursing Consultant, Antonio and Associates, Dale City, CA. Reprinted with permission.

or fewer, less than a full-time therapist may be required in each discipline. The use of therapy aides and assistants can reduce cost but should be determined according to client complexity.

Once salaries are averaged across hours for each staff qualification level (occupational therapist, occupational therapy assistant, occupational therapy aide), an average salary expense can be calculated. After the average salary cost per discipline has been established, the cost of the staff per client day can be estimated according to census. This method allows therapy labor costs for the program to be estimated. Similar staffing patterns can be developed for nursing, clerical, and ancillary labor. The estimation of these costs can assist in determining how much the program will need to charge for the service (see the "Finances" section in this chapter).

### Qualifications and Numbers of Personnel

In some circumstances, existing staff members in an organization can begin a program. However, many programs require the recruitment of new staff people (Shermerhorn, Hunt, & Osborn, 1994). Careful consideration should be given to the professional qualifications and the personality characteristics of individuals recruited for a start-up program. Are they self-starters? Are they flexible in approaching problems, and do they tolerate ambiguous situations and task demands well? New programs often go through periods during which personnel must work in less-than-ideal conditions. Frequent review of the entire program model and changes in staff members' responsibilities may continue every 3–6 months for 2 to 3 years in a new program or may need to occur for even longer as the program changes and develops and new organizational needs emerge (see program vignette 3 in Appendix 8.A). Individuals who enjoy the excitement of a start-up program may not enjoy the more routine aspects of service delivery and vice versa.

Managers should keep in mind that 200% staff turnover is not unusual in the first 2 years of a new program. Managers need to decide what qualifications and experience staff members should have and whether new graduates or individuals with limited experience in the service sector are appropriate. Note, however, that personnel with limited experience can offer advantages; they may have less to unlearn and may make fewer assumptions that are unhelpful in a novel service model. The roles and responsibilities of staff members should be defined as clearly as possible in written job descriptions.

### Recruitment and Salaries

The recruitment and retention of staff members are important considerations in program development. Availability of potential staff members may vary depending on program location, number of occupational therapy training programs in the area, and the number of new graduates entering the profession. The program's ability to attract staff may depend on the reputation of the company in which the program is being developed and the desirability of the service sector (e.g., acute rehabilitation and pediatrics may be regarded as desirable practice areas).

Staff recruitment can be costly and time-consuming. Various methods can be used to recruit staff, including advertising through newspapers and professional publications, Internet job listings, and listings maintained by state and local organizations. Staff recruitment may also occur through word of mouth, attendance at job fairs, contact with occupational therapy training programs, or the use of professional recruiters. As in other types of marketing, consideration should be given to the selling points of the position (i.e., factors likely to attract appropriately experienced and qualified therapists). For example, a new program may appear to lack stability, but the company may be well established, and participation in a start-up venture may offer many opportunities for personal and professional development.

Average regional salary levels may be obtained from professional groups and discipline-specific publications. Salary levels are affected by many factors such as specialized training, experience, and expertise. Salary structures also may be predetermined in an already existing organization.

### Training

How much training staff requires depends on the staff qualifications and experience as well as the degree of specialization of the service. Over much of the past 20 years, occupational therapists have been taught to expect to practice in a fee-for-service, direct intervention model (e.g., program vignettes 1 and 5 in Appendix 8.A), and older practice arenas such as mental health have been de-emphasized in many occupational therapy training programs. With rapid change in the health care environment, practitioners are working in more varied service structures, including industry, wellness, and community case management services. For individuals who have not worked in these new arenas, the practices and expectations may be different from those they were taught in school and may necessitate continuing education to remain current.

Training requirements may include the content of the intervention service, the program goals, and the program philosophy. Written policies and procedures should be available to the staff. Early in the development process, individuals need to be trained in basic practices. Once these practices are established, new staff members can learn by on-the-job training with experienced staff members. Ongoing training can occur regularly during the week at times when other staff can meet client needs.

## Finances

Realistic financial performance expectations need to be established for the program. For example, it is important to establish whether a program is expected to be viable immediately or within 1 to 2 years.

A private practitioner should establish how the start-up period of limited income and significant expenditure is to be managed. If money is to be borrowed, then time-lines and repayment procedures must be determined. In most instances, financial projections are necessary. Financial projections are based on assumptions about the market, the client base, payer sources, and the competition.

One-time start-up costs for building alterations, renovations, and equipment should be estimated. These line-by-line costs are listed on an expense sheet. A staffing structure with salary and cost of benefits (usually 20%–30% of salary) should be included in the financial projection. These costs are considered direct expenses. Indirect expenses (particularly for a program housed within a larger facility) include the allocated amounts of rent, heating, lighting, housekeeping, telephone services, and maintenance costs. Factors such as estimates of use and customary charges in the community as well as fixed and variable costs may contribute to how charges for services are set. With this information, it is possible to determine the cost of opening and operating the program (see chapter 9).

Many institutions will be looking at 2- and 5-year financial projections for the program. Important milestones are the "break-even" point and the point at which the start-up costs are recouped. If a program can never be cost-effective, then sources of additional funding need to be investigated.

Many basic financial concepts are described in detail in texts on how to write a business plan or start a business (Abrams, 2000; O'Donnell, 1991). For illustration, the process for deriving the break-even point for a program that bills for direct intervention by modules is described here. The break-even point is reached when fixed costs and variable costs equal revenue. First, monthly fixed costs are established. Fixed costs such as facility rent, telephone, and copier rental are expenses that do not vary from month to month (Perinchief, 1998). If the fixed cost for operation of the new program is determined to be $10,000 per month, then this amount needs to be covered whether

or not clients are admitted. Second, overall profit margin should be established by determining the cost of labor per hour of direct intervention plus the cost of supplies. If
the actual cost of direct intervention is $70 per hour (including nonproductive time)
and if the program bills $140 ($35 per 15-minute module) for an hour of direct intervention, then the overall profit margin is 50% (half of the $140 revenue is variable
cost, so half is profit). Dividing the monthly fixed costs of $10,000 by the overall profit
margin of 50% gives a result of $20,000. So the program has to bill out $20,000 in
services to break even (i.e., to cover fixed and variable costs). Revenues of more than
$20,000 are 50% cost and 50% profit.

## Facilities

The facilities in which services are provided are often a key factor that influences
whether or not a program is successful. The extent to which the location and the nature of the facilities affect service delivery depends on the type of service, client variables, and problems treated.

### Location

A person's willingness to travel to a health care provider is influenced by many factors. If individuals are to attend frequent appointments, then getting to the point of
service must be practical for them. Some programs provide transportation to increase
the access for potential users of the service. Other programs locate in an area close to
the population to be serviced. For example, Citywide Case Management (see program
vignette 3 in Appendix 8.A) is located in a run-down area of town that has a high concentration of individuals who need the service it provides (providing this access has
the disadvantage of placing the program in an area that has high drug and crime levels, but the low-cost housing used by the clients is located here). A community reentry
program should be close to community-based amenities such as shops, restaurants,
recreational facilities, and potential work settings. An acute hospital might be located
on the outskirts of town because clients will not need community services while hospitalized and will be transported by relatives or by ambulance. An outpatient clinic for
people with TBI needs to be accessible to public transportation because clients will
need to attend the clinic many times and may be unable to drive.

### Licensing

Numerous federal and state laws regulate the service that may be provided in any given
facility. However, expert consultation should be obtained with respect to regulatory issues because the service provider is responsible to ensure that the service meets regulatory requirements. Typically, the state department of health or department of social
services licenses services that are provided by occupational therapists. Federal, state, or
local requirements for access and egress, living space, bathroom access, fire safety, and
occupational safety also must be met. Reimbursement agencies such as the Centers for

Medicare and Medicaid Services may have very specific rules for the physical layout of the facilities whose reimbursed services are provided.

### Building and Space Requirements

Facilities need to meet the minimum physical requirements of clients (e.g., enough space for the number of clients using wheelchairs), but facilities should also support the delivery of services. Structure should follow function; however, actual facilities are often far from ideal. Programs often operate in facilities that make service delivery difficult. Appropriate facilities can be important in maintaining the health and welfare of staff members and clients. For example, Citywide Case Management (program vignette 3 in Appendix 8.A) screens clients daily before allowing them into the program to ensure that they are not under the influence of illicit drugs or alcohol and do not have a behavior disorder. The facility has a system by which clients are allowed onto the unit only after they have signed in and have been observed by the "officer of the day" through a security window. Alzheimer's disease care units are often structured in ways that provide clients with the ability to walk around in a safe and secure area (e.g., no access to stairs) and that disguise exits so clients who are confused and repetitively seek exits are not continually trying to leave. The facility design also can influence the number of staff members required for supervision and management of clients, thereby affecting overall costs of providing care.

### Equipment and Supplies

In planning a program, equipment requirements can be divided into "needs and wants." Different programs need different types of equipment. Certain types of equipment are required to provide services for all or almost all clients, and other types of equipment are required for only a small proportion of clients served. The latter type of equipment may be appropriate for purchase later in the growth of the program. Capital equipment usually costs more than $500 and includes items such as computers, refrigerators, office furniture, wheelchairs, therapy tables, mats, equipment for modalities, and expensive testing equipment. This type of equipment is itemized and is listed in an appendix of the business plan. Less costly equipment, such as tools, pots and pans, dishes, and heat guns are not itemized, and only an overall sum for the purchase of these items is included in the business plan. Supplies (or expendable supplies) are items that that are consumed in their use, including splinting materials, coloring books, and crayons. Some insurance systems allow some expendable supplies to be billed to the members' insurance plans; however, some insurance systems do not reimburse for these costs of providing services. A system needs to be in place to track supplies so billable items can be billed out and so needed items are available.

## Program Evaluation

In defining a program, it is also vital to define expected outcomes (Valluzzi, 2002), how the program is to be evaluated, and the indicators to be used. One set of indicators includes revenues and whether the program is on budget and meeting financial projections. Other potentially important indicators are the number of clients treated, client improvement as measured by standardized functional measures (e.g., Functional Independence Measure scores), rapidity of discharge to a lower level of care, and reduced recidivism (see program vignette 3 in Appendix 8.A). Follow-up evaluations may include objective measures of outcome appropriate for the client population. Client satisfaction surveys provide another set of important indicators (Forer, 1996).

The health care sector typically serves two (or more) types of customers: the end user, or client, and the third-party payer, or funding agency. Goals and quality indicators are likely to be different for each of these customers. The client is most likely to be concerned with the quality and convenience of the service. The third-party payer may be interested in cost containment and in avoiding the use of more expensive acute services. For example, in program vignette 2 (Appendix 8.A), program goals are for the clients to be discharged to a lower level of care and for clients to need minimal use of further acute medical or psychiatric services.

### Risks

A business plan should include a consideration of the risks involved in entering the service area. Discussion of risks can include inevitable risks, potential risks, and worst-case risks (Abrams, 2000). Inevitable risks include the financial loss associated with start-up. Potential risks include not meeting client projections. Worst-case risks include failure to obtain clients or catastrophic outcomes for clients.

## Private Practice and Small Business Ventures

Many individuals dream of going into private practice or of opening a small business (e.g., adult day health, board and care home). Private practice has advantages for some individuals: schedule flexibility, the absence of a supervisor, and potentially increased income. However, considerable planning needs to put into entering private practice or consultant work. Many of the issues that pertain to program development for a corporation also apply to private practice. Questions to consider include whether the person has the expertise and experience necessary to treat the target population; whether the person has established networks that will provide him or her with clients and, if not, whether he or she has another source of clients; how the person will determine pricing; and whether the person can provide competitive services. In addition, a person entering private practice should look into an office, equipment, appropriate insurance and permits, a source of money to pay the bills and expenditures associated with the business before it generates enough revenue to pay a salary, and a plan to handle cash flow if insurance is to be billed. Many resources are available to help the new entrepreneur; some popular books are included in the reference list at the end of this chapter.

## Conclusion

Program development is exciting because it requires personal and professional self-examination, adaptability, and the ability to tolerate risk. Recent unevenness in the employment market may have contributed to a renewed spirit of entrepreneurship as members of the profession have explored new markets and new service delivery models for occupational therapy. As a result of the success of many of these ventures, occupational therapists have a renewed sense of enthusiasm about the opportunities and contributions to be made by members of the profession.

## References

Abrams, R. (2000). *The successful business plan: Secrets and strategies* (3rd ed.). Palo Alto, CA: Running 'R' Media.

Bailey, D. M. (1998). Legislative and reimbursement influences on occupational therapy: Changing opportunities. In M. E. Neistadt & E. B. Crepeau (Eds.), *Willard & Spackman's occupational therapy* (9th ed., pp. 763–771). Philadelphia: Lippincott-Raven.

Edwards, P., Edwards, S., & Economy, P. (2000). *Home-based business for dummies.* New York: Hungry Minds.

Fettig, E. R., & Riegel, D. R. (1998). Adult daycare: An entrepreneurial opportunity for nursing. *Nursing Economics, 16,* 189–195.

Forer, S. (1996). *Outcome management and program evaluation made easy: A toolkit for occupational therapy practitioners.* Bethesda, MD: American Occupational Therapy Association.

Giles, G. M., & Clark-Wilson, J. (Eds.). (1999). *Rehabilitation of the severely brain-injured adult: A practical approach* (2nd ed.). Chichester, UK: Stanley Thornes.

Mastboom, J. (1992). Forty clubhouses: Models and practices. *Psychosocial Rehabilitation Journal, 16,* 9–23.

Neistadt, M. E., & Crepeau, E. B. (Eds.). (1998). *Willard & Spackman's occupational therapy* (9th ed.). Philadelphia: Lippincott-Raven.

O'Donnell, M. (1991). *Writing business plans that get results: A step-by-step guide.* Lincolnwood, IL: Contemporary Books.

Opila-Lehman, J. (2002). Marketing 101. *OT Practice, 7*(1), 18–21.

Perinchief, J. M. (1998). Management of occupational therapy services. In M. E. Neistadt & E. B. Crepeau (Eds.), *Willard & Spackman's occupational therapy* (9th ed., pp. 772–790). Philadelphia: Lippincott-Raven.

Schermerhorn, J. R., Jr., Hunt, J. G., & Osborn, R. N. (1994). *Managing organization behavior* (5th ed.). New York: Wiley.

Valluzzi, J. L. (2002). Evaluating and monitoring community based programs. *OT Practice, 7*(3), 10–13.

## Appendix 8.A    Five Program Vignettes.

### Program Vignette 1: A Pediatric Hand Therapy Clinic in a Children's Hospital

*Concept.* The program is intended to provide a designated area for a pediatric hand therapy clinic in a children's hospital.

*Program goals and objectives.* Inpatients and outpatients with conditions of differing severity were treated together in the general pediatric rehabilitation department. Younger children were not developmentally able to dissociate their own condition and experience from that of more severely injured inpatients (i.e., the younger children were traumatized by seeing older, more seriously injured children in distress). A major goal, therefore, was to separate the outpatient hand therapy clients from the more involved inpatients. Additional goals were related to the size and physical organization of the department. The distribution of supplies was inefficient, and it was difficult to establish a treatment area. In addition, the department did not have a hygienic area for hand washing. The program's goals were consistent with the goals and values of the institution.

*Program benefits (how the proposed program benefits clients, the organization, the community, and other key players).* The program is intended to reduce stress on clients who are receiving hand therapy. A designated clinic is intended to increase efficiency and improve compliance with accreditation standards by having a hand-washing sink. Locating the clinic in the same suite as the primary referrer is intended to increase ease of referral and communication. Development of a specialized clinic is expected to increase the visibility of the pediatric hand therapy service, thereby increasing both in-house and community referrals.

*Services.* Clients include children with hand trauma, cumulative trauma, fractures, soft tissue injuries, burns, congenital hand anomalies, and postsurgical corrective procedures for congenital anomalies. Type and range of services include outpatient treatments, inpatient consultation, attendance at team hand therapy clinics, splinting, prosthetic training, and measurement for customized garments. Frequency and intensity of service is two to three times per week (a 1-hour assessment and 45-minute treatment sessions). Length of stay varies from a single visit to three visits per week for 4–6 months. Some children use the service repeatedly throughout their developmental period.

*Facilities, equipment, and supplies.* The pediatric hand therapy clinic is located in a children's hospital in the outpatient center and is licensed as an outpatient clinic. Facilities include one small room that houses a sink, hydroculator, paraffin unit, supply cabinet (with wound care supplies and splinting supplies), a locked closet for hazardous materials, a small pediatric table, and a larger table for older children. An electrical stimulation unit and an ultrasound machine have been requested for the capital budget (this equipment currently needs to be borrowed). Supply needs include splinting materials, wound care supplies, therapeutic media (paint, crayons, toys, theraputty), and scar management supplies.

*Staffing qualifications and numbers.*  The principal clinician was mentored by an experienced clinician and visited other hand clinics to observe how to set up a clinic for efficiency as well as to examine client education materials and clinic procedures. The clinician is a certified hand therapist and has obtained extensive continuing education in hand therapy.

*Implementation and timelines.*  An original two-page proposal was submitted 3 years before the opening of the clinic.

*Risks and problems.*  The clinic is efficient for the purposes of treatment but is administratively inefficient. Difficulties arise because the clinic is physically removed from the department and from administrative support (support requirements include client registration, taking phone calls, and assembling new client charts).

*Source: Contributed by Ginny Gibson, MS, OTR, CHT, Oakland, CA.*

## Program Vignette 2: A Medical–Psychiatric Unit in a Locked Skilled Nursing Facility

*Concept.*  The program is intended to provide service to individuals who have a combination of medical and psychiatric illness. Treatment goals vary by client: Some clients are rehabilitation candidates and are able to move to a lower level of care; other clients need long-term medical and psychiatric support and management.

*Program benefits (how the proposed program benefits clients, the organization, the community, and other key players).*  Clients who have both medical and psychiatric needs are often difficult to manage in standard treatment programs and, as a result, occupy acute hospital beds long after their need for acute services has ended. The program is based on a modified clubhouse model (Mastboom, 1992) that provides psychiatric services as well as the opportunity to engage in practical activities of each client's choice at the rate and intensity that each client can tolerate. The program developed within the context of a corporation providing a range of psychiatric services, including long-term care, psychiatric rehabilitation, and board and care services. Clients often fail at these programs because concurrent medical conditions result in frequent acute hospitalizations and negative client outcomes. The addition of this service allows the corporation to provide greater range and continuity of services to county mental health departments. Community members had identified this service sector as an unmet need.

*Define service user.*  Clients admitted for treatment have both medical and psychiatric disorders (e.g., schizophrenia and chronic obstructive pulmonary disease, insulin-dependent diabetes, and bipolar disorder) that cannot be managed in a nonspecialized program and that require specialized services. Clients can be adults of any age but are typically older than 40 years, with the majority in their 50s–70s.

*Marketing.*  The clinical director and administrator met with County Mental Health directors and senior county placement personnel. The management team met with County Mental Health and Aging and Adult Service managers to introduce the new service. Key players with referral agencies were invited for facility tours. Soon after the program opened, some very difficult clients were accepted into the program, and their outcome was managed aggressively.

*Facilities.* The service is housed in a distinct unit in a 180-bed locked SNF. The distinct unit itself contained only 42 beds. The program took over one nursing station as well as one dining room for dining and group activities and decreased the bed capacity from 42 to 36 to create more group and treatment space.

*Staffing qualifications and numbers.* Licensed and certified nursing staff levels were established at a level typically found in a subacute program (i.e., the program was "staff-plentiful"). In addition, four occupational therapists and four occupational therapy aides were recruited to provide services for 36 clients. The clinical director and external consultants provided training.

*Startup funding needs.* The corporation accepted significant financial losses to support the program in the first 18 months of start-up.

*Implementation and timelines.* The clinical director was hired 4 months before the program opening to oversee program development and physical plant changes. Three significant program and staffing reorganizations occurred in the first 18 months, with a 50% turnover of therapy staff members. A census of 35 was achieved following 18 months of operation, and plans were made to open an additional unit because of the program's success. The corporation views the program as significantly expanding its range of services, and the program is highly regarded by referrers and clients. No clients have required more than short-term psychiatric rehospitalization despite the sometimes very severe nature of their psychiatric disorders.

*Source: Contributed by Gordon Muir Giles, PhD, ORT, FAOTA, Director of Neurobehavioral Services, Crestwood Behavioral Health, Inc., Stockton, CA.*

## Program Vignette 3: Forensic Treatment Services for Mental Health Clients

*Concept.* The program is intended to provide mentally ill offenders with an integrated service agency focusing on stabilized housing, substance abuse management, and management of mental health symptomatology to reduce jail recidivism.

*How new service augments or differs from other available services.* The new service (Citywide Case Management Forensics Project) specifically targets individuals with mental health and substance abuse problems who are cycling through the criminal justice system and who are not receiving mental health services. The program is part of an experimental project to evaluate how to best serve this population and reduce the incarceration of mental health service recipients.

*Program benefits (how the proposed program will benefit clients, the organization, the community, and other key players).* Outcome goals are to achieve a 35% reduction in days in jail; fewer arrests; fewer parole revocations; reduced criminal justice costs; reduction in the rate of violent crimes, depressive symptoms, and self-reported use of drugs; and increased ratings on quality of life and health status measures. The program is conducted in the same space as Citywide Case Management and allows the organization to service another section of its core client population.

*Services.* Clients have *DSM-IV* Axis I mental health diagnosis, may have a co-existing substance abuse diagnosis in addition to a personality disorder diagnosis, and have had two previous bookings in addition to an incarceration since 1993. Some individuals are mandated to receive treatment rather than to remain in jail. Offered services include the following: linkage from jail or prison (clients are first enrolled when still in jail), court advocacy, intensive case management, individual psychotherapy, a wide range of groups (e.g., symptom management, support groups, substance abuse groups, money management, leisure groups, and medication monitoring), outreach, after-hours crisis intervention, prevocational and vocational services, and linkages to housing or residential programs. An occupational therapist was recruited to develop the group program, lead groups, and develop prevocational and vocational programs.

*Frequency and intensity.* The program provides services to 25–60 clients a day, with a total of 150 clients enrolled. Clients may come daily Monday to Saturday and attend up to four groups a day. Individuals may receive services for an indefinite period. The program has seen a 10% loss of clients since opening, and many of these clients have been unavailable for contact or follow-up.

*Facilities and operations.* The program is located on the fourth floor of a downtown office building in an area of low-income housing and residential hotels, and it is secured. Clinical staff members function as gatekeepers to ensure that individuals entering the program are evidencing appropriate behavioral control. Facilities include a café, an art area, a food bank, a food preparation area, two group rooms, seven interview rooms, and staff offices.

*Funding types and sources.* The program is funded by the California Board of Corrections "Mentally Ill Offender Grant." Forty counties applied for the grant, and 17 were funded. Programs are funded for 5 years and will seek alternative funding after the grant period.

*Ongoing development issues.* Initially, the program used a psychoeducational model focusing on abstinence. Attendance declined, and clients appeared to disengage from the staff and from one another. Staff members began to be reluctant to lead groups because the interactions and relationships were not positive. After a year of operation, the program model was changed to a harm reduction process group model (i.e., a model to minimize harm related to substance use), which produced an improvement in client and staff morale.

Staff members describe the positive aspects of working in a start-up as having one's own vision actualized, working as part of a team, and having the ability to modify things that are not effective. Negative aspects include the awareness that more always needs to be done, the need to continue to do things that do not work until the program can be changed, staff turnover, and the sense of loss that goes with this staff change. Other negative aspects include wanting to be able to carry out more individual assessments and one-to-one interventions. Outcome data are being collected as part of an ongoing analysis but are not yet available.

*Source: Contributed by Gregory Jarasitis, MOT, OTR, Occupational Therapist II, Citywide Case Management, San Francisco, CA.*

### Program Vignette 4: A Student Clinic in a Graduate Program

*Concept.* The program is intended to provide a free occupational therapy clinic run by faculty and staffed by students as part of the students' coursework.

*Program goals and objectives.* The goals of the program are to augment the training of students in a master's of occupational therapy (MOT) program and to provide real-life skills in client evaluation and treatment. Additionally, the clinic offers a service to the community in an inner-city environment.

*Program benefits (how the proposed program benefits clients, the organization, the community, and other key players).* On a "student climate" survey, students had indicated a desire for more clinical exposure. Participation in the clinic allows students to use interview skills, apply evaluation tools and methods, apply documentation skills, apply theoretical approaches to treatment, learn practical ethics, and experience writing home-programs for clients. The student clinic increases the visibility of the MOT program and the college in the community by way of service announcements, newspaper pieces, and press releases. Initially, the college administrators needed to be convinced about the benefits of a student clinic. Administrators were concerned with liability issues, start-up costs, and the availability of faculty to supervise clinic operations.

*Services.* Individuals accepted for the program are clients who need and desire occupational therapy to treat physical disabilities, are medically stable, are not currently receiving occupational therapy services elsewhere, and have the ability to get to the clinic (free parking is provided). Services are offered for 1 hour once per week over a 14-week period. Individuals may return to the clinic in subsequent years as space permits.

*Market.* The clinic is the only free occupational therapy student clinic in northern California, and clients' lack of financial resources is not a barrier to treatment. Therapists may refer clients when funded services have run out and when it is believed that the client may continue to benefit from treatment. Referrals come from physicians, through the college's Web site, through press releases, and by word of mouth in the local community.

*Facilities and operations.* The clinic is located in a wheelchair-accessible clinical classroom suite that includes private treatment areas, a pediatric room with a two-way mirror, and an adjacent lounge for the parents to wait while the child is being treated. Faculty members oversee all treatments.

*Funding types and sources.* The college provides faculty salaries for supervising clinic operations, parking reimbursement for clients, and the facilities. All materials and supplies required for the clinic were previously used to teach students in the class-room and therefore do not represent an additional cost.

*Implementation and timelines.* A faculty member was funded for one semester unit to write the proposal. The proposal was reviewed by the department chair, the academic vice president, the college president, and by the board of regents. The clinic was approved and began the next semester. Initially, the clinic provided services to adults but later was divided into an adult clinic one semester and a pediatric clinic the next. More than 30 clients are treated per year, with many repeat users and an overall high level of client and student satisfaction.

*Source: Contributed by Kate Hayner, EdD, OTR, Samuel Merritt College, Oakland, CA.*

## Program Vignette 5: Pediatric Sensory Integration Home Clinic

*Concept.* The program is intended to provide sensory integration pediatric services in a home-based clinic.

*Program goals and objectives.* The program provides direct intervention to chil-dren with sensory integrative dysfunction and sensory defensiveness to improve their function at home and at school. The program educates families with respect to the phys-ical, behavioral, emotional, and social implications of sensory integrative dysfunction and educates parents about how to manage their child's difficulties at school and at home.

*Service.* The age range of clients accepted for treatment is from 2 to 12 years. The typical presenting problems of the children are lack of coordination, poor fine and gross motor skills, decreased organizational skills, difficulty with writing and draw-ing, and poor school performance. Parents may describe their children as clumsy, awk-ward, or poorly coordinated; socially isolated; getting along better with adults and younger children than with peers; easily frustrated and anxious; and having poor self-esteem. Children who are severely involved are not accepted for treatment (e.g., no children with orthopedic involvement). Children who have severe emotional or be-havioral disorders cannot be accommodated in the location. Hours of service are Saturday mornings and after school for 2 hours, 4 days per week. Length of treatment varies from 6 weeks to 2–3 years or longer. Average treatment duration is once per week for 12–18 months. The program can accommodate a maximum of 13 children a week. An intensive summer plan is offered for families interested in treatment 5 days a week for 6 weeks.

*Market.* The practice is situated in a relatively affluent suburban area. No mar-ket research or market development activities were performed. The practitioner was in contact with a local therapist who had more referrals than could be accepted. Be-fore opening the practice, the local therapist said that she would refer her "overflow" clients. The practitioner started seeing clients on Saturday mornings; after-school hours were added after 1 year. After 2 years, most clients are being referred by word of mouth. Current referrals come from behavioral pediatricians, neuropsychologists,

psychologists, or other occupational therapists who want to refer to a specialist in sensory integration.

*Facilities and operations.* Children are treated in the garage space of the practitioner's home. The practitioner states that, although she provided a safe environment for treatment, she initially was concerned about the appearance of the treatment setting, but parents' responses were uniformly positive. After 1 year, alterations were made to the garage space to improve professional appearance and storage capacity. The business is a sole proprietorship and requires a city business license and permission to have an educational practice in a residence.

*Expenses.* Start-up expenses included professional and general liability insurance, an average of $2,500 for equipment each year for the first 3 years, and approximately $500 each year for supplies. Major equipment purchases included a computer and printer, video camera, mats, ceiling hooks and chains, and suspended equipment. Equipment and supplies continue to be purchased for specific clients' needs and as new materials become available. Continuing education and professional books are an ongoing expense. Changes to the treatment space described earlier also represented a capital investment.

*Revenues.* Insurance companies typically do not pay for the types of problems seen, so the majority of clients are private pay. The practitioner charges at the lower end of the local market rate because of low overhead. Running the business out of the home allows for a home-office tax write-off.

*Background and experience.* The practitioner's first formal instruction in sensory integration occurred at occupational therapy school. A research project carried out at the MOT program was developed into a publication on sensory integration for use by occupational therapists, teachers, and parents. The practitioner is certified to administer the sensory integration and praxis test.

*Future directions.* The program venture generates enough work for a full-time private practice; however, the practitioner prefers the regular income, benefits, and security of being a school employee. Thus, the practitioner collaborates with other professionals who provide consultation or direct services to her clients. The practitioner envisions providing a multidisciplinary service to clients who could benefit from co-treatments and a team approach. The practitioner expects that earnings will go up by one third over the next year because of increased hours of operation and then remain stable after reaching the maximum hours available to work.

*Source: Contributed by Nan Arkwright, MOT, OTR, instructor at Samuel Merritt College, Oakland, CA; private practitioner for a pediatric practice specializing in sensory integration; and occupational therapist for the Walnut Creek and Orinda School Districts.*

## Appendix 8.B   Outline Business Plan.

Executive Summary

1. Background and trends of the service sector
   a. Nature of the service sector
   b. Problem statement
   c. Market factors and future trends

2. Services
   a. Description
   b. Unique program or features

3. Market analysis
   a. Target market and characteristics
   b. Comparing strengths and weaknesses of competitors

4. Marketing
   a. Advertising
   b. Marketing strategy

5. Management and ownership
   a. Key players' qualifications and experience
   b. Administrative personnel
   c. Professional support
   d. Ownership
   e. Directors, advisors, community representation

6. Staffing
   a. Staffing patterns
   b. Qualifications and numbers of personnel
   c. Recruitment and salaries
   d. Training

7. Finances
   a. Funding requests and investments
   b. Financial statements
   c. Expenses
   d. Revenues
   e. Financial projections
   f. Assumptions

8. Facilities
   a. Location
   b. Licensing
   c. Building and space requirements
   d. Equipment and supplies

9. Program evaluation

10. Risks
    a. Problems
    b. Inevitable risks
    c. Potential risks
    d. Worst-case risks

# Entrepreneurial Ventures

Sara Pazell, MBA, OTR, CSCS
Evelyn G. Jaffe, MPH, OTR, FAOTA

*"A banker is a person who is willing to make a loan if you present sufficient evidence to show you don't need it."*

—HERBERT HOOVER

**Sara Pazell, MBA, OTR, CSCS,** is the new international business development manager with the Division of Health Sciences at the University of South Australia. She is a graduate of the University of South Australia with BS in occupational therapy. She completed her MBA at the University of LaVerne, San Luis Obispo, CA.

**Evelyn G. Jaffe, MPH, OTR, FAOTA,** is an assistant professor at Samuel Merritt College, Oakland, CA. She has been a consultant in occupational therapy for over 35 years, specializing in community mental health, high-risk infants, school-age parents, and primary prevention in the workplace. She earned her master's degree from the School of Public Health at the University of Michigan.

## Key Terms and Concepts

**Business plan.** The statement that describes and analyzes the business concept; provides projections about the future; projects financial and other resources needed; and describes target markets, competition, strategic plans, and marketing ideas.

**Entrepreneur.** One who conceptualizes, originates, materializes, organizes, manages, and assumes the risk of a business or enterprise.

**Intrapreneur.** One who harnesses the resources within an organization to develop, improve, promote, extend, or enhance a new or existing program.

**Market test.** The business assessment of the viability of an idea and market conditions, effectiveness of proposed marketing and operations plans, adequacy of financial support, and accuracy of projections.

**Proposal.** The initial written request submitted to a funding source that identifies the purpose, major goals, intended plans, and desired outcomes for a venture.

**Window of opportunity.** A period within a business cycle during which available skills and resources match the needs of consumers and market conditions.

## Learning Objectives

After competing this chapter, you should be able to do the following:

- Define the term *entrepreneur*.
- Identify entrepreneurial traits and characteristics.
- Define the term *intrapreneur*.
- Identify sources that lead to the genesis of a new idea.
- Identify the American Occupational Therapy Association's 10 emerging practice areas.
- Define the term *window of opportunity*.
- Describe key principles and components of proposal writing.
- Identify components of a business plan.
- Assess the viability of a business opportunity.
- Identify basic strategies to develop a business for occupational therapy services, a business to sell or produce occupational therapy products, or both.

O ccupational therapy practitioners who are innovators should be celebrated. Those who generate new programs, expand and diversify service delivery, and collaborate with other agencies have intrapreneurial tendencies. Their actions support their employers and their communities. Entrepreneurial occupational therapists open their own businesses, risk their finances, and create new avenues to access occupational therapy services. This chapter is dedicated to exploring entrepreneurial and intrapreneurial characteristics, activities, skills, tools, and methodologies.

## Entrepreneurial Ventures: An Overview

Entrepreneurial ventures serve as the cornerstone of our modern economy. The entrepreneur may be credited as the most influential factor contributing to economic growth in the United States, rising above the economic influence of Fortune 500 companies, the president of the United States, and Congress (Ernst & Young, 1998). Entrepreneurialism represents power, virility, resourcefulness, creativity, optimism, hard work, personal achievement, and risk taking. In addition, it represents visionary leadership, management, sales ability, intellect, goal setting, planning, personal assertion, pioneering activity, competitiveness, individuality, a hunger for success, and an internal locus of control (Ernst & Young, 1998; Hamilton, 2000; Mazzarol, Volery, Doss, & Theirn, 1999; Miner, 2000; Morrison, 2000; Ryan, 2000; Thompson, 1999; Van Auken, 1999). Estimates suggest that, at any given time in the United States, almost 4% of working-age adults are either evaluating or jump-starting a new business venture (Reynolds, 1994). This figure may be markedly higher, given the proliferation of Internet technology and e-commerce business start-ups.

Undoubtedly, an entrepreneur is a do-er. An *entrepreneur* may be defined broadly as one who conceptualizes, originates, materializes, organizes, manages, and assumes the risk of a business or enterprise to gain profit, freedom, or independence.

### Culture, Characteristics, and Traits of Entrepreneurs

The culture within the United States, which is considered to be capitalistic and fiercely competitive, fosters an entrepreneurial spirit (Cullen, 1999). Hofstede's (1991) cultural dimensions of entrepreneurial activity lend an understanding to the nature of an entrepreneur; these five cultural factors stimulate entrepreneurial activity:

- *Low power distance* exists when the hierarchical power differences among supervisors and the line staff are not significant (e.g., staff members may be rewarded when they demonstrate innovation). Other examples of low power distance are the following: The staff is empowered with decision-making; the dress code for the line staff and the supervisors is the same; all staff members are enabled to work as a team to provide customer support rather than to serve upper management; inequality with superiors is diffused; and people are encouraged to believe that they, too, may act as leaders.

- *Low uncertainty avoidance* exists when norms, values, and beliefs tolerate conflict (e.g., people are rewarded for ideas that are unique, unusual, or different; a break from consensus is valued rather than shunned), and it enables the entrepreneur to accept and be excited by uncertainty rather than to avoid it.
- *High individualism* exists when people are encouraged to value themselves and others for personal achievements, status, and unique characteristics.
- *High cultural masculinity* is associated with a tendency to seek advancement, success, money, competition, decisiveness, risk taking, and machismo (in a culture that supports their independence, women also may act in a manner that reflects cultural masculinity).
- *High long-term orientation* reflects a willingness to plan and invest for the future as well as the belief that persistence and hard work are necessary to achieve goals.

At a macro level, the American culture is considered to rate on the high end as one that encourages and fosters entrepreneurial activity (Cullen, 1999).

At a micro level, the traits and characteristics of individual entrepreneurs become important to consider. A review of current literature (Ernst & Young, 1998; Hamilton, 2000; Mazzarol et. al., 1999; Miner, 2000; Morrison, 2000; Pazell, 2000; Ryan, 2000; Thompson, 1999; Van Auken, 1999) reveals the following common traits among entrepreneurs:

- Is able to identify windows of opportunity
- Is a risk taker, a pioneer
- Functions as a visionary leader
- Functions as a leader of change
- Has incessant curiosity
- Has a strong intellect
- Is competitive
- Is highly creative and resourceful
- Functions as an individual and an independent
- Maintains an internal locus of control (has self-efficacy and a belief that one's own actions can affect the world)
- Is optimistic
- Is hungry for success
- Holds a customer service orientation
- Is not adverse to hard work, is persistent
- Is attracted to power and feelings of virility
- Has the ability to recognize skill sets in others and to motivate others
- Is instinctive
- Is impulsive
- Communicates and networks effectively
- Negotiates effectively
- Is ethical and trustworthy

- Maintains a willingness to find and learn from mentors
- Is a big thinker
- Shows interest in others and in the opinion of others
- Exhibits a sense of humor, is able to laugh at self
- Has emotional intelligence
- Is assertive
- Is innovative
- Is market driven and quality driven.

Occupational therapists and occupational therapy assistants have the opportunity to embrace an entrepreneurial spirit and ride the wave of influential business practice. To do this, they must identify their own inherent entrepreneurial traits and develop business skills to recognize and capitalize on windows of opportunity. In-depth interviews with a sample of occupational therapy entrepreneurs ($n = 6$) revealed that, consistently, these entrepreneurs were able not only to recognize their entrepreneurial traits but also to recognize the qualities and skill sets that were needed in others to help them move forward in business (Pazell, 2000).

According to the Occupational Therapy Association of California, less than 9% ($n = 226$) of its membership designates their work as private practice. The number of these respondents who owned their own practices and those who were simply affiliated with a private practice is unknown (C. Strauch, personal communication, August 6, 2000). The ratio determined by the California group is consistent with the national statistics of the American Occupational Therapy Association (AOTA, H. Hostetler, personal communication, August 11, 2000). Industry leaders admit that occupational therapy practitioners who are functioning as entrepreneurs are a poorly researched and ill-represented group. In-depth interviews of a sample of occupational therapy entrepreneurs in California ($n = 6$) revealed that the majority entered their business by accident; they created an opportunity out of necessity (Pazell, 2000). Occupational therapy practitioners can and should embrace their entrepreneurial traits, harness the support of and forge partnerships with others, seek mentors to guide the path, and develop the business acumen and skills necessary to start a business when the opportunity is ripe. Wood (1998) reminds us that "when we honor the genius within our field . . . we simultaneously honor the genius within every human being" (p. 324).

## Intrapreneurial Ventures: An Overview

Intrapreneurial activity reflects the qualities of good management and leadership that help to build a team, diversify programs, and provide for stellar customer services. Intrapreneurs are also innovators, but they are distinguished from entrepreneurs because their ideas are fostered, nurtured, and developed within an existing organization. The ultimate financial risk of their energetic activity is borne by a third party. An *intrapreneur* is one who harnesses the resources within an organization to develop, improve, promote, extend, or enhance a new or existing program.

Intrapreneurs are typically highly effective managers and leaders. Their skills are extremely useful during company reorganization, staff development, and program development. They are often discovered working within programs that advance social development. Intrapreneurs are often leaders of change, and their skills, attitude, and aptitude motivate others to reach a new level of performance. Consequently, intrapreneurs do not work completely without risk; intrapreneurial innovations may carry the risk of affecting professional reputation or may lead to job loss. Failure of a new program can consume limited resources and affect the freedoms of the organization to diversify and continue taking risks. Intrapreneurs, however, are typically lauded for their ability to help a company achieve positive growth and are found in both the private and public sector. They are innovators, skilled with the ability to predict change and capitalize on growth trends and, thus, must have the skills to justify their ideas to a management team or payer source.

Many occupational therapy practitioners who are in positions of organizational leadership may find that they are intrapreneurial by nature. Intrapreneurs, like entrepreneurs, are likely to possess skills that help them identify new opportunities. Whether a new idea is to be launched within a current organization or a new business is to be developed by an entrepreneur, similar steps must be followed:

- Harness a new idea.
- Identify the window of opportunity.
- Develop a proposal and a business plan.
- Secure financing and resources.
- Test market the idea.
- Receive and review feedback.
- Launch the new business, service, or program, which includes assessing growth, cost effectiveness, cost–benefit, value, customer satisfaction, resource management, quality controls, competition, and outcomes.

## Genesis of an Idea

The business idea is paramount; it is the starting point for further investigation. An idea implies intelligence. Although ideas may seem to come more naturally to some people than to others, many sources of information can help the occupational therapy practitioner become an "idea person." He or she can develop skills to filter favorable ideas from unfavorable ones as well as assign priority and weight to those ideas having the greatest potential. One approach to generating ideas is to ask questions of those in the immediate environment. Another approach is to consider ways to extend and diversify the environment, especially by gaining exposure to new ways of doing things.

Ideas may arise from anyone, from anywhere, and at any time (see Exhibit 9.1). The entrepreneur and the intrapreneur must be receptive to a wide variety of ideas. The following sections further describe the sources for new ideas listed in Exhibit 9.1.

**Exhibit 9.1  Sources of New Ideas.**

| | |
|---|---|
| Customers | Vendors and sales representatives |
| Employees and employers | Outside industry contacts |
| Professional contacts | Regulatory and reimbursement trends |
| Trade shows and conferences | Literature review and current affairs |
| Professional associations | Environmental scan |
| Research publications | Existing business or franchise |
| Educational institutions | |

*Customers.* Listen to clients, medical professionals who make referrals, family, and caregivers because they can offer an abundance of information. Often, they can identify what works well and what could be improved in the profession. Clients may offer solutions for their own needs. For example, if clients report that they could benefit from wheelchairs that allowed them to pedal with their legs rather than use their upper-body strength, then others also may benefit from the suggestion. In addition, market research and sampling among a wider population helps quantify market demand.

*Employees and employers.* Interview past and present employees, employers, supervisors, and representatives of the competition because they typically offer a wealth of information. Frequently, employees have stimulating ideas about what could be designed to make their jobs easier. Ask, and a new niche for consulting services may arise. For example, an occupational therapy practice may find that billing and documentation software are not adequate to meet the needs of the practice organization. The entrepreneur may work as a consultant to bridge the gap between software manufacturers and practitioners.

*Professional contacts.* Inform professional colleagues of your intent to try something on your own. This approach can be a simple way to gather and generate ideas. In the course of the conversation, you might say, "I would like to eventually work for myself. Have you heard of any ideas that you think are worth developing?" Surprisingly, most people like to share what they know.

*Trade shows and conferences.* Attend trade shows to see the newest, latest, and greatest among the trends, services, and products on display. Observing new trends with a critical but enthusiastic eye can spark new ideas.

*Professional associations, certification boards, and licensing bodies.* Read professional publications, volunteer to chair a committee, and stay abreast of the trends by affiliating with trade associations. These strategies are an efficient way to receive information about new professional developments as well as expand and diversify your circle of professional contacts. AOTA (2003) has identified 10 emerging practice areas (see next section of this chapter). These areas may serve as the framework for stimulating new ideas.

*Research publications.* Review professional journals and reports from research institutions or corporations, which can be highly informative. These periodicals and organizations have thoroughly researched the available resources, have identified flaws in systems of service, or have recognized the need for new products. This information can foster the genesis of a business idea.

*Educational institutions and providers.* Contact continuing education providers and educational institutions, which are alert to the heartbeat of innovation. Educational providers have access to a wide variety of practitioners from whom they quickly learn of developing trends and unmet needs.

*Vendors, suppliers, and sales representatives.* Become familiar with vendors and sales representatives. Sales representatives are the first point of contact between industry and practitioners. Larger companies will have research and development departments to help them predict industry change and drive sales. Invite reputable sales representatives to lunch. Ask them to describe what they see as industry trends, how their companies are preparing for change, and what they believe is needed in the future.

*Outside industry contacts.* Look beyond the occupational therapy industry to obtain new ideas. By attending chamber of commerce events, for example, you may hear from other industry representatives about innovations that might be carried over into the field of occupational therapy. In most communities, councils that are focused on workforce development, economic vitality, and private industry provide information about some of the most creative and successful businesses in the area. Call business representatives and ask to visit their operations. Similarly, overseas travel and observation of other cultures can reveal new ideas. Make a list of fabulous ideas and use them to improve or enhance your business. This approach can be as simple as more attentively observing a business that you typically frequent. For example, your hairdresser's invitation for water or coffee and a 2-minute forehead massage on arrival may be a strategy that can be used in occupational therapy practice. Complimentary drinks and purposeful human touch may be just the distinguishing factor to help establish a new practice.

*Regulatory review and reimbursement trends.* Observe regulatory change by reviewing the *Federal Register* on-line, reading Web site announcements of professional associations, scanning new state assembly bills, and reading professional newsletters. For example, if state licensure requirements dictate the need to increase continuing education, then the entrepreneur may discover a method to provide accessible, high-quality, on-line education for practitioners.

*Literature review and current affairs.* Choose a period of time—the past month, the past 3 months, or the past year—for a literature review. Make a record of the types of stories that have been published by identifying the main subjects of the stories and attempting to categorize them. You may be able to identify new needs by discerning recurring themes. For example, the recent surge of interest in alternative health, wellness, yoga, and the Pilates method may mean that you could provide niche services in a new way to clientele by becoming certified as an instructor.

*Environmental scan.* Observe current or potential competitors. A new service or product that is offered by competitors through an aggressive entry strategy, such as heavy advertising, may create an opportunity for a competitive reaction, allowing you to replicate, improve, or promote a similar idea. If the service or product is in the early stages of development and a trend is growing, a strong reaction that provides additional consumer options adds to the competitive mix.

*Existing businesses or franchises.* Approach owners of an interesting business with a proposal for purchase. Many business owners are more adept at running their businesses than they are at selling them. They may have been thinking of retirement but did not know what to do with the business. Alternatively, an owner may be prepared to help the entrepreneur by franchising his or her operation, lending a creative hand, offering good advice, or selling intellectual property and products.

## Entrepreneurial Ventures in Emerging Practice Areas

AOTA (2003) describes 10 emerging practice areas that offer numerous opportunities:
- Services to address the psychological needs of children and youth
- Design and accessibility consulting and home modification
- Driving rehabilitation and training
- Ergonomics consulting
- Health and wellness consulting
- Low-vision services
- Private practice community health services
- Development and consulting services related to technology and assistive devices
- Ticket-to-work services
- Welfare-to-work services.

Each emerging practice area provides the practitioner with the opportunity to develop niche expertise, new programs, or new business. Additional training or certifications may be necessary, but given the right market conditions, the payoff may involve more than enough business. Whether the occupational therapist branches out to start a new business or helps to build, expand, and diversify the business of an existing organization, these emerging practice areas may enable him or her to meet growing needs of the community. The following sections further describe these emerging practice areas.

*Services to address psychological needs of children and youth.* These services require that the practitioner have skills-based training to help children effectively deal with their social environment. Johansson (2003b) reports that community needs for occupational therapists to help reduce violence in the school setting are growing. Intervention for youth may include consulting about vocational skills, coping strategies, and life planning. Within the context of current events, the practitioner may assess and mitigate the impact that the war on terrorism has had on the psychological balance of children and youth. The occupational therapist may work with these children to foster lifesaving responses to possible dangerous situations.

*Design and accessibility consulting and home modification.* Universal design ensures access to environments by a wide range of people, including those with disabilities and those who are aging. Occupational therapy practitioners can provide prime consultation services to commercial and residential builders with respect to accessibility. Recommendations made during these consultations should include removing barriers early in the design of a building, a topic that has received growing media attention in local communities, especially as affordable housing and drive-through businesses stay in the news. A practitioner may choose to partner with a behavioral architect who creates designs that accommodate the differences in gender, age, or specific environments to support certain behaviors. For example, the architect and occupational therapist might create healing environments in hospitals or calming environments for mental health settings or correctional facilities. In addition, they could ensure safety and ergonomic design for children's playgrounds and public outdoor spaces as well as creative design for compatible house-sharing arrangements.

*Driver rehabilitation and training.* "The recent landmark decision by the American Medical Association to assign physicians the ethical responsibility to address driver safety issues with patients will boost the demand for driver rehabilitation services" (Johansson, 2003a). Occupational therapists might provide consultation to physicians who will be required to make this important decision on behalf of their patients. In addition, occupational therapy practitioners might play an important role in developing alternative transportation systems for clients who no longer drive safely (Johansson, 2003a).

*Ergonomics consulting.* Ergonomics (or human factors) evaluation and training is a field that continues to grow and diversify. At a national level, increasing legislative attention has focused on workplace safety. Mounting research continues to show evidence that the health and safety of employees can be improved by putting into effect rigorous ergonomic safety standards. Ergonomic services may include the following:

- Evaluations of office or industrial workers in their work environments
- Train-the-trainer education
- On-site health care intervention, including traditional hands-on rehabilitation for orthopedic or musculoskeletal injuries
- Delivery of wellness programs such as therapeutic exercise with yoga and the Pilates method
- Orientation and safety training for newly hired employees
- Consultation during occupational health and safety meetings
- Consultation for the development and management of programs focused on illness, injury, and prevention
- Consultation for the ordering and administration of assistive technology
- Review and editing of job descriptions, specifically those involving lifting requirements or compliance with the Americans with Disabilities Act
- Delivery of work hardening programs, especially in industrial settings.

*Health and wellness consulting.* Health and wellness consultation is a growing element in occupational therapy practice. Occupational therapists have reported developing allergy clinic programs in which they provide consultation to those suffering from allergies. Services include helping people to identify allergens, modify the home environment to deter the buildup of allergens, and modify their activity (Pazell, 1999). *Feng shui*, the Chinese art and science of arranging one's environment to enable free flowing *chi* ("good energy") has become a popular focus among mainstream interior designers and architects. *Feng shui* consultation has been incorporated into occupational therapy consultation services to help clients remove clutter from their homes and organize space for efficiency, relaxation, and auspicious life events. In addition, health insurance providers, county health services, women's health and outreach programs, and educational institutions are hiring health and wellness coordinators.

*Low-vision services.* With the advent of growing collaboration among optometrists and outpatient occupational therapists, low-vision services are becoming a new area for practice. Ophthalmology retinal specialists may welcome the idea of employing an occupational therapist to provide services to their low-vision clients. Nationally, departments of rehabilitation have continued to allocate resources that will help support elderly people with low vision. The occupational therapy practitioner might consult with these government agencies and provide relevant services. In addition, the occupational therapy practitioner might develop expertise in helping people with ocular vision loss or neurological vision loss (Pazell, 1998). Services may include providing low-tech solutions to the challenges involved with training people to operate high-tech devices such as electronic reading appliances, speech output systems, electronic screen magnifiers, and closed-circuit televisions.

*Private practice community health services.* A wide variety of opportunities exist for occupational therapy practitioners who operate private practices to provide community health services. For example, private practitioners might start their own businesses or work with a physician or similar health care provider to expand services in the community. Fitness centers may want to develop comprehensive services, which could include occupational therapy lifestyle management consulting or traditional rehabilitation services. Residential care facilities and adult day health care centers frequently need occupational therapy consulting services. Private practitioners may contract directly as vendors with state vocational rehabilitation centers for return-to-work consultation, including psychosocial intervention or ergonomic and assistive technology services. Goodwill Industries nationwide offers many training services to support hard-to-place vocational applicants, and these programs could provide an opportunity for occupational therapists to help clients augment their vocational training. Innovative private practice may include software consulting to build in accessibility features or consulting to bridge the gaps among billing, client record keeping, and administrative database software. In addition, few occupational therapy consultants are currently available to help occupational therapists open their own businesses. Therefore, providing organizational development consultation to other occupational therapy practitioners may be a lucrative service for practitioners with business experience.

*Development and consulting services related to technology and assistive devices.* Assistive technology specialty services may include consultation with respect to augmentative communication systems; electronic aids to daily living; accessibility technology for home, school, or work; low-vision technology; indirect or direct computer access systems; and seating system design. Direct services may be provided through contracts with vocational training vendors, regional centers, hospitals, and school districts. In addition, occupational therapy practitioners with an aptitude for sales might consider becoming representatives for reputable manufacturers. In this area of technical specialty, sales representatives are typically required to provide in-depth training to clients and their families.

*Ticket-to-work services.* Practitioners can develop contracts with the state departments of rehabilitation services, independent living centers, vocational training centers, and educational institutions to advocate for people with disabilities. These services may include helping people with disabilities to find and retain employment as well as developing work-related program strategies.

*Welfare-to-work services.* Occupational therapy practitioners who are interested in economic vitality projects might consider providing consultation services for welfare-to-work clients and employers. The practitioner can partner with local private industry councils, workforce development agencies, chambers of commerce, economic development departments, vocational training centers, departments of social services, and employment development departments. This practitioner might help a client with lifestyle management; provide case coordination to locate child care options; develop problem-solving, time management, budgeting, transportation, worksite behavior, and performance strategies; or help a client with job procurement and retention—in effect, act as a job coach. As a complement to this service, practitioners might help employers to understand the benefits they might gain when hiring welfare-to-work applicants. The development of retention and training programs is very important to ensure long-term, beneficial employment outcomes for the employee and employer.

## Identifying Windows of Opportunity

A *window of opportunity* exists when the time is ripe to capitalize on a new idea or growth period. Just as a window in our home consists of glass, a frame, and sound structural support and provides a view and visions beyond the horizon, a window of opportunity in the business world also has many interdependent elements. These elements include the conception and development of an idea, favorable market conditions, suitable timing, growing consumer demand, adequate current or potential resources, and the business acumen of the person or people driving the idea. A window of opportunity is not stagnant; it is a dynamic phenomenon occurring in a world of constant change (Timmons, 1999). It is defined as a period in a business cycle when available skills and resources match the growing needs of consumers during supreme market conditions.

If a window of opportunity exists, then the launch of an appropriate new idea should lead to success. The generator of the idea, of course, defines success. In an existing organization, it may be determined by improved customer satisfaction, timely clinical intervention, increased generation of revenue, improved collections and reimbursement, improved staff morale, and increased productivity. For the entrepreneur, success might simply mean financial self-sufficiency. The practitioner will best prepare to assess whether a window of opportunity exists by researching and testing the market conditions, drafting a proposal to submit to potential funding sources, and developing a business plan. The following three sections describe these activities in more detail.

## Assessing the Viability of a Business Idea

The entrepreneur or intrapreneur should clearly understand the viability of his or her business idea. Personal interest and passion aside, the idea must make business sense. To pursue a business opportunity, particularly if seeking outside funding, the entrepreneur should be prepared to demonstrate convincing, positive results of a market test.

A *market test* is defined as the business litmus test to assess the viability of an idea. A market test helps determine favorable market conditions, the effectiveness of proposed marketing and operations plans, the adequacy of financial support, and the accuracy of projections. The entrepreneur can use the checklist shown in Exhibit 9.2 to assess the viability of a business idea. The following sections provide more explanation about the various elements of this checklist.

### Favorable Market Conditions

An objective evaluation of market conditions will help the entrepreneur understand whether an idea has merit and can be considered as an opportunity. The deeply rooted concept of creating potential value for a wide array of clients while ensuring favorable

**Exhibit 9.2  Business Viability: A Checklist of Considerations.**

| | |
|---|---|
| Favorable market conditions | Plans to address uncontrollable factors |
| Potential for value creation | Effective marketing plan (the 5 *P*s) |
| Fragmented or emerging market structure | Realistic operations plan |
| Ideal market size | Sustainable competitive advantages |
| Trends that demonstrate market growth | Superior management team |
| High estimated market share potential | Adequate start-up capital and cash flow |
| Thorough competitive analysis | Business potential (adequate profit and |
| Targeted customer base |    return on investment) |

returns to the provider is one to be considered and comprises the areas described in the following sections.

*Value creation.* Does the idea serve a market niche and add new benefits to life in a radical manner? Will the idea change the way people live or behave? Brand loyalty among consumers is lowest when a new service or product markedly changes the way things have been done in the past. If the idea does not change life in a radical fashion, then does it represent significant value-added benefits to current products or services? Does the idea hold potential for long-term revenue generation? Will consumers continue to require services or products on a recurring basis, and will the market expand with the sale of product extenders? For example, a wellness studio may grow as a result of the general population's increasing awareness of and curiosity about services such as yoga and meditation. Aromatherapy products, yoga mats, soothing music, video education, relaxed clothing, as well as training events and retreats represent product extenders that help to promote this industry. Product extenders are products or services that complement a core service or product, increase value to the customer, and increase sales revenue potential for the entrepreneur.

*Market structure.* A fragmented, imperfect market or an emerging industry often will reveal opportunities (Timmons, 1999). This fragmentation may be evidenced by inadequate supply to meet consumer demand. Additionally, inadequate distribution channels, poor access to services, low price sensitivity among consumers, or significant barriers to entry are further conditions of a fragmented market. In the example of the wellness industry, a structural shift in the health care market has led to an increase in the number of third-party payers that include wellness intervention as a covered service.

*Market size.* Venture capitalists typically refrain from investments in markets that represent less than $20 million of national sales per annum. A more attractive market size is represented by sales potential of $100 million to $1 billion per annum (Timmons, 1999). For example, the emergence of consulting services for universal design and accessibility that support new engineering and architectural projects vastly broadens a market previously limited to consulting for people with disabilities. This increase in market size may stimulate potential funding sources.

*Market growth and trends.* The entrepreneur will want to consider the following questions with respect to market growth and trends. Is the market growing? According to demographic statistics, providing services to people over the age of 50 could be a growing market around the nation. Can a growth rate of 30% to 50% or more be achieved? Is market demand far in excess of supply? Can the entrepreneur establish a niche before current providers expand service outlets and saturate the market? Does a competitive analysis—an analysis of a business's strengths, weaknesses, opportunities, and threats—reveal greater strengths and opportunities than threats and weaknesses? Will the political and reimbursement climate encourage long-term growth (over a 7-year period) for the industry? Are there few barriers to entry? For example, if one is opening a new facility for aged care, is a certificate of need required by the state, or is the process relatively unencumbered?

*Estimated market share.* Business plans should reflect expectations of market share growth within each successive year after start-up. Is it possible to capture at least 20% of the potential market share in a given region? An objective analysis also would include consideration of competitors and substitutes. Substitutes refer to those products or services that do not replicate existing commodities but that consume the same expendable dollar. For example, among occupational therapists, alternative health care providers may represent a substitute for traditional occupational therapy services.

*Business potential and exit strategies.* Does the business demonstrate the potential to produce high returns for a relatively low initial investment? The potential to add value by using new technology or strategies is important. From the inception of the business idea, the entrepreneur should formulate plans to demonstrate book value (actual value) and perceived value (potential value) to attract prospective buyers of the business, which is considered a favorable exit strategy. By following this approach, the entrepreneur's business will be in a better position for strategic change, mergers, or expansion, regardless of whether the entrepreneur plans to keep or sell the business.

## Recruiting and Retaining Customers

The entrepreneur must develop strategies to retain customers and recruit new customers. Two important rules should be considered:

- *The 80/20 rule:* Invest 80% of the customer service effort toward retaining current customers, and invest 20% of the effort toward recruiting new customers. Satisfied customers will act as sales agents to promote goods or services.
- *Not all customers think and act alike:* In terms of buying behavior, not all customers do not respond at the same speed. The most influential customers are those who purchase products after their introduction to the market has demonstrated the products' early success. These customers are the opinion leaders, and their satisfaction greatly affects future sales (Dalrymple & Parsons, 2000).

*Recruitment.* Have the customers adequately been targeted? Are the customers well defined, and does this definition include their demographics and spending patterns? What are the customers' levels of expendable income, purchasing habits, brand loyalty, and expectations for service and access?

*Retention.* Dalrymple and Parsons (2000) describe a five-step model of buying behavior. First, customers identify an unmet need. Second, they recall methods to purchase what they believe they need. This step is strongly influenced by exposure to advertising and the beliefs and purchase patterns of friends, colleagues, or other influential characters. Third, the customer evaluates options for purchase. Subjective valuation is most influential at this stage. What will others think? Does the packaging of the product represent their personality and lifestyle? Cost considerations also influence this stage. Is the product or service worth paying for? What is sacrificed to make this purchase (i.e., what is the opportunity cost)? Fourth, a transaction may occur. The goods and services must be easily accessed for purchase. Fifth, the marketer must determine the level of post-purchase satisfaction, a vital element to ensure repeat business. Customer retention plans may include making follow-up phone calls, providing ongoing product support, or guaranteeing product durability with long-lasting beneficial outcomes (Dalrymple & Parsons, 2000).

## Effective Marketing Strategies

Chapter 7 describes the five *P*s of marketing: product, price, place, promotion, and position. The entrepreneur should prepare effective marketing strategies that reflect consideration of these factors. Do the products or services create value for the customer? Can tangible and intangible qualities of the product be merged? For example, a client receiving an ergonomic evaluation receives intangible intellectual property and education as a service as well as concise and pertinent ergonomic reports as a tangible product, but could more tangibility be introduced? An effective marketer might consider also providing photographs that illustrate before-and-after intervention conditions, a thank-you bonus of ergonomic software that illustrates dynamic stretch breaks to improve office routine, or an illustrated coffee mug that shows a cartoon about work causing pains in the neck.

Where does the product stand in relation to competitors? On a perceptual map, will the product be perceived to be of superior quality, elite and prestigious; affordable and practical; conservative and safe; flamboyant and fun; or a hybrid of these qualities? How will the product be distinguished and assigned value? Are community opinion leaders willing to promote the product? Is the market price elastic or inelastic? Does an increase in price affect demand? Is the product accessible and easy to find?

## Effective Operational Planning

Operational considerations include the expectations of seasonal growth and staffing, the beginning and end of the fiscal year, site location of the business, and access to customers and suppliers. Other considerations include business facilities; maintenance and planned improvements; insurance needs; legal and accounting support; operational structure as a sole proprietor, limited liability company (LLC), partnership, or corporation; and licensing and accreditation requirements. The next two sections provide more specific questions that one should consider with respect to operational planning.

*Developing the management team and staff.* Does the management team demonstrate the leadership and visionary qualities necessary to effect positive growth? Are staff members invested in the outcome of the business? Can the business afford adequate employee compensation, benefits, and stock options to ensure competitive staff recruitment and retention? Are qualified staff members readily available? How is the organizational chart structured? Does the business allow for other investors? Are investors silent, or do they markedly influence the direction of the business?

*Sustainable competitive advantages.* Do the services offer competitive advantages? Are these advantages sustainable? Are they difficult for others to replicate? What company advantages can be demonstrated that help make the business seem attractive to investors? For example, will operations occur in a family-owned building, thus containing occupancy costs and improving profit margins? Will employees be allowed profit-sharing arrangements as an incentive to ensure their commitment to the company, thus reducing recruitment and training costs? Is the product trade-marked, licensed, or otherwise legally protected?

## Preparation for Uncontrollable Factors

The five primary sources of uncontrollable effects on business are regulatory events, technological events, societal events, economic events, and competitive events. Although these events are difficult to predict, it is prudent to explore these elements, consider potential threats, and create defensive strategies for business survival. For example, regulatory change may influence insurance reimbursement for services. A defense strategy is to diversify funding and include options for clients to pay out-of-pocket. Occupational therapy practices also charge clients up front for service delivery. The client is then responsible for obtaining reimbursement from his or her insurance carrier. If demand for services is high and is expected to remain high, then this strategy may prove profitable for a provider. In general, when profit margins can be sustained at a high level, it is easier to insulate the business against eventual slumps in revenue.

*Acts of God* are natural disasters that can devastate operations, for example, fire, earthquake, floods, tornado, or similar disasters. When writing a business plan, consider including insurance for these events.

## Justifying the Financial Merits of a New Business

Starting a new business, expanding an existing business, or developing a program within an institution requires some consideration of finances. Bottom-line figures matter to the investor, to the entrepreneurial team, and to institutional management. Chapter 6 provides details about managerial accounting and financial analysis in the health care setting. The following sections describe financial variables that can guide an assessment to determine whether a business or business expansion is viable.

*Start-up capital requirements.* A venture that requires low up-front capital investments is most desirable. Capital may be required for marketing and advertising activities, legal and accounting fees, outside contracted consultant activities, office supplies, new equipment, down payments for the lease of physical space, or similar expenditures.

*Profit margin analysis.* Gross margins represent the selling price of the unit (a good, service, or product) minus all direct and variable costs (e.g., clinical staff and supplies). Gross margins representing an increase of 40%–50% or more typically represent financial "wiggle room" in the event of an error, wastage, staff turnover, or similar circumstances. High gross margins, in turn, typically reveal high profits after taxes. Ideally, one's after-tax profits should represent an increase of 10%–20% or more. Anything representing an increase that is at or less than 5%–9% represents an opportunity that is fragile at best. Even with the most thorough planning, however, unexpected events can be unexpectedly costly.

*Cash flow, break-even, and profit-and-loss analyses.* The statement of cash flow can prove to be one of the most vital elements to business success. It indicates how much money is in the checking account to pay the monthly bills. An analysis of cash flow can help determine whether to purchase or lease equipment, negotiate fair rental agreements for physical space, and determine opportunities for staffing growth. This measure of predictive analysis can influence decisions about profit-sharing plans, the amount solicited for start-up capital, and the amount solicited for credit lines. Break-even analysis indicates the point at which sales revenue and costs are equal. At the break-even point, the business realizes no net income or loss. Beyond this point, the company should realize a profit. The following equations and definitions describe financial terms that the entrepreneur should know.

- *Fixed costs:* Costs that are constant (e.g., administrative salaries, insurance, building occupancy costs, property taxes, facility maintenance costs, and depreciation)
- *Variable costs:* Costs that vary directly with the change in volume of sales (e.g., direct clinical staff costs or supplies used on a per-client basis)
- *Basic profit equation:* Net income = revenue − total variable costs − fixed costs
- *Contribution margin equation:* Contribution margin = revenue − total variable costs
- *Contribution margin ratio:* The contribution margin per unit; contribution margin ratio = contribution margin by unit/selling price per unit
- *Break-even (BE) units:* The number of units that must be sold to reach the break-even point; BE units = fixed costs/contribution margin per unit
- *Return on investment (ROI):* Income expressed as a percentage of assets; ROI = income/investment.

Work with a qualified accounting professional to develop pro forma income statements, balance sheets, cash flow analysis, and break-even analysis.

*ROI and internal rate of return (IRR) potential.* ROI is attractive at 25% or more per annum. IRR is subjective, but for appealing returns, the business should deliver five to ten times the original investment in a period of 5 to 10 years.

*Cost control measures.* Cost drivers represent those items that cause variable costs to rise. For example, costs for therapy supplies can add to the cost of providing service. Control measures should be addressed in a business plan. These measures might include strategies such as joining a group purchasing organization to achieve the lowest possible supply costs or recruiting a mix of practitioners that includes occupational therapists and occupational therapy assistants to keep service costs affordable.

## Writing a Proposal or Grant

The occupational therapy practitioner may be responsible for drafting a proposal to justify a program, purchase capital equipment, or procure funding to support the development and growth of a new service (see chapter 8). Typically, the intrapreneur frequently will write proposals. The proposal has many similarities to the business plan, and it is usually the precursor to a detailed business plan.

If the intention is to apply for a grant, then one also needs to identify possible granting agencies, including private foundations and government agencies. The intrapreneur might request support from a local, state, or federal government agency; from private individuals; from private foundations; or from other businesses. To start, the intrapreneur should research potential funders by identifying those sources most likely to support the proposal. This research should identify the monetary amount of budgets typically funded and the average annual contributions to similar programs as well as the mission and specific priorities of the funder, including the types of projects funded, any exclusions to funding, and turnaround schedules (Zlotnick, 2001). Regardless of the funding source, a written proposal stating exactly what is being requested and why is essential.

Determining which of the many different kinds of proposal formats to use depends on the nature of the request. Some funding agencies, especially private family foundations, may request a brief, informal description of what is planned. Others, including governmental agencies, require extensive, comprehensive, formal grant proposals that may be many pages long. The informal type of proposal may be somewhere between a brief letter of intent and a complete grant proposal.

When writing a proposal or grant, a good maxim to follow is "Never overestimate your audience's knowledge, and never underestimate its intelligence." Regardless of the format, certain key questions (Jaffe, 2000) should be answered before beginning to write the proposal:

- What do you want to change, improve, enhance, or augment?
- What target population will you serve?
- What resources do you have?
- What do you anticipate needing?
- What do you want to accomplish during the first year?
- What are your specific goals (stated in measurable terms)?
- What do you want to accomplish during the second year?
- What opportunities are available to you?
- What risks do you perceive in meeting your initial goals?

The proposal should be clear and accurate, providing information that is currently available, well written, and "packs some punch." It should clearly express the major objectives and purpose of the venture to any reviewer who may not be versed in the particular product or service being proposed. In other words, write for the layperson. Do not load the writing with professional jargon in an attempt to sound erudite. Just explain clearly why starting this new program, venture, or corporation would be productive or important.

## Key Principles of Proposal or Grant Writing

Before writing anything, review the granting agency's guidelines for funding applications. These may require that applicants submit a query letter or letter of interest before beginning the actual application process. The following principles offer universal guidance for writing grants and proposals.

- Know the priorities or interests of the foundation or agency to which you are submitting the proposal. (Usually, the granting agency makes its funding decisions not according to need but, rather, in accordance with the agency's interests.)
- Be clear about the request, know what the grantor wants, and determine whether the request and the requirements match.
- Tailor the proposal to the grantor's priorities.
- Identify what initial funding or support is needed—usually start-up funds or seed money. (Possibilities for permanent or ongoing support also should be mentioned.)
- Demonstrate what support the project has generated from the community, other professionals, or other businesses.
- Develop an outline for the proposal or grant. Writing the proposal is easier with a draft outline, which helps determine the contents of a section or subsection.
- Establish the "theme of the proposal": What is the nature of the venture or business, and why?
- Identify the "message," or key point, of the proposal: What is the unique or special product or service that is involved?
- Submit the draft to a reviewer, such as a friend or family member who is not necessarily familiar with the project, and request his or her opinion (which will reflect the reaction of a typical layperson).
- Submit the proposal on time, or if possible, earlier.
- Be patient. Some granting agencies reveal when the applicant will receive confirmation of receipt as well as acceptance or rejection of the proposal. Others may not give a time line.

## Proposal Writing

A proposal typically incorporates key elements that organize the request: the letter of intent, the introduction, the goals, the objectives, the methods and operational strategies, the time frame and milestones, the management and organizational structure, the evaluation plan, the request for funding, and an indication of collaboration. The following sections describe in more detail what should be included in each of these typical elements.

### Letter of Intent

The letter of intent, or query letter, should be brief, usually no more than two to five pages, and should convince the granting agency to look at the proposal. This letter should include

- A statement about the venture or organization
- A brief statement describing the needs of the project
- A description of the methods or interventions planned
- A projection of the outcome or results desired and
- The budget requested as well as the time period for use of the funds.

The letter should be succinct and direct, without jargon or excess verbiage, and should be clearly understandable to laypeople. Demonstrate that the mission of the venture is consistent with the mission of the funding agency. Illustrate that funding this project will help the funding agency achieve its mission and goals. Direct the letter of intent to the appropriate project officer or administrator in the granting agency if possible. Acceptance of the letter of intent is usually followed by an invitation to submit an application or proposal, which demonstrates some interest in the project by the funding agency (Zlotnick, 2001).

Granting agencies usually have guidelines and a specific format for proposals. Review each section heading, and follow the guidelines, including page limits, if any. Exhibit 9.3 shows the components of most proposals.

### Proposal Introduction

The proposal should have an overall introduction. The proposal is the initial request for support for the ideas that will develop the business or corporation. Therefore, the introduction is extremely important. It makes the first impression on the funding or supporting agency. However, writing an effective, attention-grabbing introduction is difficult to do until the what, the why, and some of the hows within the body of the proposal are answered. Therefore, before writing this component, first develop the ideas, formulate an outline, and prepare the draft. Then, write the introduction last, when the information that has already been organized can be explained briefly, yet cogently, as to why this venture is important. The introduction should be no more than one page.

**Exhibit 9.3  Components of a Proposal.**

| | |
|---|---|
| Introduction | Management/organizational structure |
| Goals/business concept | Evaluation |
| Objectives | Funding request |
| Methods/operational strategies | |

*Note.* From *Writing a Good Proposal* [Lecture], by E. G. Jaffe, 2000, Oakland, CA: Samuel Merritt College.

The introduction describes the current issues and concerns that have led to the ideas of the venture and that are related to the effects of the environment on the system. The introduction presents the project organization as well as the capabilities and qualifications of a professionally competent group. It may demonstrate that this venture is the first to introduce this product in this way or the first to provide certain unique services to the community. It is the opening statement and must grab the reader's attention. Therefore, it must be well written, concise, and yet contain enough information to entice the reader (i.e., the reviewer) to read on.

The vision statement may be included in the introduction. Additionally, the introduction provides the needs or problem statement, which substantiates the need for this venture and justifies the basis for the request to develop the organization or program by verifying the need with basic statistical information, if available, or with social indicators that provide the market for the organization. If possible, include information from surveys, censuses, and organizations that are providing similar services or products, yet demonstrate how this venture is different or more cost-effective (see also chapter 8). In addition, include changes in market share or shifts, community descriptors, and demonstration of community support, which is obtained from the initial analysis of the surrounding environment (as described in chapter 4). Statistics should be relevant to the corporation's end product or service. Remember, just one powerful statistic that relates to the specific product is worth ten statistics that, even if interesting, are merely tangential and can actually be distracting.

Finally, the introduction describes the nature of the business, including its locus, form of business, personnel (staff employees, contracted employees), and type of end product or community service. A description of the setting (e.g., major city, suburban town, rural community) in which the venture will operate is important because the setting will affect the general philosophy and structure of the organization. A preliminary environmental and systems analysis will help determine the appropriate setting and overall nature of the business or venture (refer to chapter 4).

### Proposed Goals

Goals are the broad statement of overall purpose. They identify the general direction and the concept on which the venture or business is based. Describe the problem or issue, the product or service, the target market, and where or how the specific location of the organization affects implementation. The mission statement should be included in this section. As an example, the goal or mission of the venture may be to improve worker health and productivity in community-based workplaces by providing comprehensive health promotion and wellness programs.

### Proposed Objectives

Objectives demonstrate how the organization is going to achieve the goal or purpose. Objectives have three characteristics: They must be specific, time-oriented, and measurable. Additionally, objectives can be classified into three types:

- *Process objectives* are based on the process or methods rather than the end result (e.g., the organization will provide stress management counseling sessions to employees once a month).
- *Product objectives* involve the development of a tangible product (e.g., by the end of the year, the organization will have an employee wellness and living skills program).
- *Outcome objectives* reflect the desired results or outcome, effect, or change (e.g., the stress management and wellness program will produce a 75% reduction in employee stress-related absenteeism).

Note that baseline data must be provided when using a percentage for a comparison. In the example used in the list above, data can be added to demonstrate the current absenteeism rate. However, exact information about statistical outcomes may not be possible to provide when the proposal is being written. This detailed information may require further research (e.g., a literature search, data gathering, etc.). Nevertheless, the outcome objectives can state a ballpark figure for the desired results.

### Proposed Methods and Operational Strategies

The methods are the action steps that describe how the objectives are to be operationalized. The methods are the blueprint for how objectives are to be accomplished at this stage in the development of the organization. (The final business plan will be more detailed and will include the strategic plan). Depending on the depth of information requested in the initial proposal, this section should describe to some extent the preliminary steps that will be taken to plan and develop the organization, the meetings that will be required, and the information or data that will be gathered. Describe the action steps or operational strategies in measurable terms (e.g., 1. Visit and observe three corporations in the community that have high incidences of employee absenteeism; 2. Interview four employees in each corporation who have experienced stress-related absenteeism during the past year; 3. Review and compare the corporate structure, health benefits, corporate culture, and employee policies and procedures of each corporation).

### Proposed Time Frame and Milestones

Regardless of whether the organization is service oriented or product based, consider the initial activities and timetable for the organization and for the development of each division needed to implement the services or produce the product. Again, the amount of detail in this section depends on whether the proposal is a full grant request or an initial proposal to assess interest in the organization or program. Describe the preliminary processes required, when each component of the activities may be accomplished, and the logistics of when and how long each component occurs. Include overall planning meetings, division meetings, development of assessments or evaluation tools, data to be recorded, and information to be tracked and monitored.

A process to pilot new techniques or programs may be essential to determine final activities. State what must be done to determine the final activities, and provide projected completion dates of steps to develop the organization and move the venture forward. Outline the phases and time frames for the organization's activities, and project when each component will be at a fully operational level. This information will be detailed in the business plan.

### Proposed Management and Organizational Structure

Provide an overview of the proposed organizational structure. Describe the administrative configuration of the organization and the expertise and experience of the people involved in this venture, especially the administrative team. Briefly emphasize previous accomplishments of these people, summarizing their experience in this field. Include an organizational chart that describes the staffing patterns needed, including management and support staff, and on what level executive decisions are determined. In addition, this section should describe any advisory groups (e.g., community support through local advisory boards) and organizations providing matching funds, which may be required in some grants.

Even if matching funds are not required, the organization should demonstrate that project personnel and other supporters are committed to the product or service and that the people involved are dedicated to its success. A valuable addition would include a brief description of any "contribution" by the organization to the outcome (e.g., employees of the organization will devote volunteer time to a community agency that supports the general concept of the venture, with the organization providing all administrative costs).

### Evaluation Plan

A proposal must include an evaluation plan that describes how a vigorous and effective evaluation of the intervention or activities will be conducted. The evaluation plan should flow from the previous sections. If the objectives are clear and measurable, the methods specific and relevant, then the evaluation section should follow easily. The evaluation section should answer two questions:

- How will progress be assessed?
- Who will analyze the information?

When objectives and methods are clear, the evaluation plan may need only monitoring and tracking information such as how data will be recorded and the reporting schedule. The evaluation section also should include the manner in which reports or information are to be disseminated. Some funding agencies or boards of directors require bimonthly reports; others, quarterly reports. Briefly outline the reporting mechanism that is being proposed (subject to change as strategies are refined), which will be based on what is relevant for the organizational activities. That report also serves as a management tool for tracking activities, identifying problems or issues, and resolving problems.

An individual or a division in the organization should be responsible for evaluation of the organization's activities. Regardless of who provides funding, related agencies and even clients and their families will want to know how the activities will be monitored and evaluated. The inclusion of a statement with respect to evaluation procedures may well be the determinant for future funding.

### Funding Request

The funding request is the budget description of the projected initial estimate of funds that are needed to set up the organization—the initial start-up funds. Two key components of a sound budget are consistency and realistic figures. Include realistic estimates of funds to cover the following costs: administration (overhead, janitorial, computer and copying maintenance, administration of the grant); phone; postage; expendable supplies and capital equipment; personnel and benefits; transportation; and capital expenses, including office or clinic rental.

The initial request for funds must be realistic and consistent with the type of organization, objectives, and methods being proposed. Requested funding for all items must be justified. For example, a grant proposal that requests funds for expensive video equipment when the project description, objectives, or methods make no mention of videotaping would most likely be rejected.

Specify any matching funds that are available, as mentioned above, either as direct cash contributions or as in-kind contributions (e.g., administrative services, space, clerical support, supplies, personnel, etc.). If the venture expects to receive matching or in-kind contributions, they can be outlined in the grant proposal by having two columns: requested funds and donations.

Many granting agencies, particularly government agencies, want to see an indication that this project can be replicated in other areas. Therefore, include a request for funds to disseminate outcome information (e.g., in-service training workshops, community or professional seminars, and presentations at conferences).

If possible, include some projection of potential earnings and ROI, with a payback period specified. If accepted, most proposals are given only seed money. Therefore, describe a permanent funding plan to demonstrate how the project will be perpetuated in the future. This plan may change as the organization develops, but funding agencies look more favorably on proposals that demonstrate an attempt at securing future funding and do not suggest dependency on the agency for continual money.

### Collaboration

Funding agencies frequently are interested in other organizations that will collaborate with the venture or business. Especially if the funding agency is community-based, the directors will want to know whether the community accepts the venture and whether collaborative relationships are planned. Include a description of the particular community system (such as the schools) and the collaborative activities that are proposed.

"Collaborations may broaden the scope of the activities, increase the number of clients served, and strengthen your infrastructure" (Zlotnick, 2001).

## Mistakes to Avoid

Developing a proposal or grant request can be time consuming and challenging; however, one commits the necessary time and energy to developing a quality request with the expectation that funding will follow. In addition, competition for funding is often intense, which increases the need to create a first-rate proposal. Unfortunately, despite these efforts, not all proposals receive funding. The following list describes the most common reasons that proposals are rejected. Make every effort possible to avoid them.

- The proposal as a whole is not focused; it is too wordy, attempts to be all inclusive, and is not to the point.
- The issues are not clearly expressed and do not convey the purpose of this venture.
- The proposed activities do not demonstrate an essential, special, or unique product or service.
- The identified problem or need does not fit the objectives.
- The objectives are not measurable.
- The identified problem or need does not match the methods, or the proposal does not clearly show how management will accomplish the objectives.
- The projected budget or the costs and resources that are requested do not fit the project (e.g., they are unrealistic, are either too big or too small, or are not justified).
- The proposal does not present enough information to demonstrate that the organization can do what is proposed.

## Summary

The proposal presents a basic statement of the overall issues, the qualifications of the principals of the venture, and their interest and commitment. It describes the venture, including the major goal and desired outcomes, and the phases and time frame for the organization's activities. It provides enough information so the reviewer in the funding agency has a clear picture of what this organization is all about, what outcomes are expected, how they will be achieved, and how much money it will take to get the venture going.

The proposal is really a sales pitch and should be relevant, professional, to the point, and directed to the decision-making authority of the potential funders or supporting organization. Ideally, it describes the purpose in proposing this venture and relates to the environmental impacts on the given community or system, to the direction of the heath care delivery system in general, or to the future of occupational therapy practice in particular. A well-written proposal provides the foundation for the development of the detailed business plan.

# Developing a Business Plan

The entrepreneur can use the process of business planning to help guide his or her assessment of a new business venture. The answers to questions typically asked by lending institutions may help to determine the worthiness of a business idea. A *business plan* is defined as the business blueprint in the form of a written statement that describes the business concept, explains the window of opportunity, defines the strategy, explains the resources and people behind the idea, provides projections about the expected outcomes, analyzes the market conditions, and entices investors to provide support.

As in a proposal, the language in the business plan should be clear, concise, and simple so the layperson can understand the concepts that are presented. A business plan provides a road map for the entrepreneur but, more important, the business plan should speak to the investor. With the fast pace of business events, the document may be out of date the day after it is printed. Nevertheless, the business plan sells the idea. An investor wants to see a realistic picture presented. If the idea were truly one that cannot miss, an investor would not want to say no to the opportunity presented in the entrepreneur's business plan.

A sample of occupational therapists–entrepreneurs studied in California ($n = 6$) revealed that the majority self-funded their ventures (Pazell, 2000). However, a business that has extra capital and free cash flow can better accommodate growth, fluctuations in business seasons and cycles, competitive pressures, and staffing fluctuations. To gain strength and viability in business, the occupational therapist–entrepreneur should embrace the opportunity to plan his or her business, argue its viability, and procure funding from appropriate lending institutions.

The business plan should include a vision and mission statement, strategic plans, target markets, customer analysis, competitive analysis, and market analysis (see chapter 5, Strategic Planning). The plan should also include the organizational structure, the entrepreneurial team, the marketing plan, the operations plan, revenue forecasts, financing strategies, available and needed resources, physical plant and geographic location, as well as critical risks and assumptions (Evanson, 1998; McKeever, 1999; O'Donnell, 1991).

Exhibit 9.4 presents a sample business plan. In addition, for a detailed description of business planning, see chapter 8. Simply put, the business plan describes the what, why, how, who, where, and when of the venture:

- *What* the business hopes to achieve—its major goals and objectives
- *Why* the business is important to the community and the health care industry, including occupational therapy practice
- *How* the business will be conducted; the vision, mission, strategic planning, operational plan, marketing strategies that are involved as well as the resources that are required to start the business entity

**Exhibit 9.4   Business Plan Outline.**

## I. Executive Summary
a. Description of the business, the idea, the opportunity, the vision, the mission, the goals and objectives, the strategy
b. Description of the target market and an overview of sales projections
c. Distinguishing factors of the business; competitive advantages
d. General estimates of profitability and long-term potential
e. Description of the leadership

## II. Industry Entrance
a. Information about the industry; the company and the concept as related to the industry; specialized products or services
b. Barriers to entry and strategies to mitigate these barriers
c. Entry and growth strategies

## III. Market Research and Analysis
a. Definition and description of the customer
b. Definition and description of market size, growth potential, and trends
c. Competitive analysis, or SWOT (strengths, weaknesses, opportunities, threats) analysis
d. Estimated market share and sales

## IV. Marketing Plan
a. Description of marketing strategies that reflect the five Ps: product, positioning, pricing, promotion, place
b. Description of strategies in the event of the five uncontrollable factors: regulatory, technological, societal, economic, competitive
c. Description of supply chains
d. Strategic planning, distinguishing factors of the company, sustainable competitive advantages

## V. Operations Plan
a. Operating cycle
b. Geographical location; access to customers and suppliers
c. Facilities, including maintenance and improvements
d. Regulatory and legal considerations

## VI. Management Team and Staffing
a. Organizational chart
b. Leadership team and staffing strategies
c. Other investors
d. Compensation plans, benefits, stock options, profit sharing, similar methods of employee reimbursement
e. Recruitment and retention strategies

## VII. Business Economics and Financial Plans
a. Proposed capitalization: Use of capital funds and investor's returns
b. Pro forma income statements, balance sheets, cash flow analysis
c. Fixed and variable costs
d. Break-even and positive cash flow expectations
e. Return on investment and internal rate of return
f. Cost control measures and other considerations

## VIII. Critical Risks, Problems, and Assumptions

## IX. Exit Strategies and Strategies for Divestiture

## X. Any Other Special Considerations

- *Who* will form the entrepreneurial team—the skill set, history of success, and commitment of each director and officer of the organization and who will form the customer base
- *Where* the business will occur—the locus of the business
- *When* the business can proceed—an estimate based on obtaining start-up funds and when the company will meet its short- and long-term objectives.

## Understanding Business Financing

For an entrepreneurial idea to be attractive, it must make good business sense. Bottom-line figures do matter. The majority of small businesses fail within their first 3 years of operation, often because of inadequate financing (Glancey, 1998; Mazzarol et al., 1999). Lending institutions will want to see rigorous and realistic financial plans. For many lenders, the financial pages are the first places to examine in a business plan. Lenders will look to see that personal financial commitment exists and that the lender is not being asked to become the sole source of funding. Financing options include personal financing, recruitment of investors, leveraging of other business capital to invest in a new business, outside funding from a traditional lending source for capital financing and jumbo loans, and lines of credit to assist with operational cash flow shortages.

After the entrepreneur writes a business plan, which will translate ideas of the venture into realistic goals, he or she must be able to identify the funding source for the start-up business. Evanson (1998) refers to this process as finding the appropriate "angels" and describes five basic types:

- *Corporate angels* may be retired corporate executives looking for another management position who, typically, will make one major investment.
- *Entrepreneurial angels* usually own and operate their own successful businesses and are looking to create synergy.
- *Enthusiast angels* usually are independently wealthy individuals who like to be involved in "deals."
- *Micromanagement angels* are serious investors who may demand a seat on the board.
- *Professional angels* come from a particular field to invest in products or services with which they have interest and some experience.

In addition, McKeever (1999) describes the seven most common financial resources in order of their frequency:

- The entrepreneur's own savings
- Funds provided by friends and family
- Equity investments by an investor who shares profits and losses up to the amount of initial investment
- Funds gained by borrowing or selling equity from other assets or properties
- Financial backing by external (or community) supporters of the venture

- Bank loans, such as start-up capital, lines of credit, or equity loans
- Venture capital
- Grants (in particular, grants from private or government granting agencies for the expansion or start of new programs in occupational therapy services).

Several types of funding are available for small businesses and new programs. Among these are *contracts*, "legal instruments that reflect a relationship between two entities where the purpose is to acquire goods or services"and *grants*, "financial mechanisms whereby money is provided to carry out approved activities" (Zlotnick, 2001). The contract is a legal document that demonstrates expectations and certain outcomes. A contract usually allows more give and take than a grant, which is very specific to the granting agency.

## Starting a Business

After a business idea has been tested against market conditions and an opportunity has been found to exist, then the next step is to take the idea from concept to reality. The following sections describe this process, which involves deciding on a business structure and initiating the start-up process.

### Deciding on a Business Structure

In the early stages, the entrepreneur should consider options for a business structure. The entrepreneur should consult an attorney and a tax accountant to help determine the best organizational structure to suit the needs and long-term plans for the business. A significant decision is the legal form under which to operate a business. Most businesses fall into one of four legal forms: sole proprietorship, partnership, LLC, and corporation. The following sections describe these forms as well as their advantages and disadvantages (Pazell, 1998).

*Sole proprietorship.* The simplest, most common from of a small business organization is a sole proprietorship. The owner of a sole proprietorship is personally responsible for all business debts and liabilities. All business profits are considered personal income and taxed accordingly. Establishing a sole proprietorship is typically the least expensive and least complicated organizational form. When conducting business under a trade name, a business name certificate should be filed with a county register or local paper and a local business license obtained.

The advantages of a sole proprietorship include:

- Control over determining business standards and making decisions
- Flexible working hours
- Control over the volume of business accepted
- Choice of office site and arrangements

- Control over fees for services (unless accepting assignment by third-party payers).

The disadvantages of a sole proprietorship include

- Risk of feeling overwhelmed and isolated
- Limited coverage for vacation, illness, and other absences
- Illness, injury, or death that threatens the viability of the business
- No unemployment benefits if the business fails
- Risk of financial insecurity as the sole owner
- Liability that extends beyond the business; personal property is unprotected.

*Partnership.* A partnership is the association of two or more people who have agreed to accept responsibility and share resources to operate and manage a business. The partners must agree on the following:

- The amount, type, and valuation of property that each partner will contribute
- The method of disbursement of profits and liabilities
- A plan for sharing gains, losses, deductions, and credits
- A provision for changing the conditions of the partnership, including accommodating the loss or death of one of the partners.

The advantages of a partnership include

- Shared financial, legal, and emotional risk
- Opportunities to harness a variety of entrepreneurial skills within the leadership team
- Availability of coverage for decision-making events in case of illness, vacation, and so forth
- Additional credibility when associated with a group practice
- Opportunities from many sources to increase start-up capital funds and operating cash.

The disadvantages of a partnership include

- Challenges in establishing mutual agreement on professional ethics, standards, and business objectives
- Shared profits
- Difficulties involved in dissolving the partnership without causing harm to operations
- Shared liability even when risky behavior is associated with only one partner
- Liability that extends beyond the business; personal property is unprotected.

*Limited liability company.* An LLC is a separate legal entity, and personal liability is, for the most part, protected. Some states prohibit the formation of an LLC by physicians, attorneys, or other state-licensed persons. Some states restrict ownership to two or more people, although most states allow one person to form an LLC. LLCs offer advantages and disadvantages similar to corporations,' although the two entities do have differences. Most striking, pass-through taxation is available to LLCs, whereas corporations risk double taxation. Another difference is that LLCs have less restrictive requirements for documentation of corporate functions.

*Corporation.* A corporation is formed by law as a separate legal entity, distinct from the people who own, manage, control, and operate it. A corporation allows other investors to contribute funding but remain silent or own less weight in the decisions that affect operational management. Start-up funds are generated by shareholders in exchange for stock. A corporation may be private or public. A board of directors makes decisions for management and directors, and officers legally may obligate the business. Articles of incorporation must be filed to notify the state franchise board of board members, directors, and officers. The firm's banking institution typically requires a copy of these articles on file.

The advantages of a corporation include

- Limited personal liability; liability generally limited to the amount of venture capital invested
- Business life span that is independent of its owners
- Ownership transferred by the sale of stock
- Additional operating capital obtainable through the sale of stock
- Separate credit rating.

The disadvantages of a corporation include

- Expensive start-up costs, including legal fees and state franchise taxes
- Strict compliance required with corporate functions, including filing articles of incorporation; appointing a registered agent, a board of directors, officers, and shareholders; and conducting regular, documented meetings
- Taxation reporting and annual state filing requirements
- Required maintenance of separate banking transactions; personal funds of shareholders not to mix with corporate funds
- Additional, hidden expenses in the form of higher bank fees or extra liability insurance, including coverage for officers, board members, and executive management.

## Starting Up

Once the organizational structure is determined, various actions are required to start the business. These can include some or all of the following:

- Confirm the business structure by filing applications with the appropriate organization. Typically, the secretary of state's office will have forms available online for applications to incorporate or form an LLC. Produce articles of organization, a name availability inquiry letter, and a statement of information to disclose details of ownership. An attorney can help prepare these documents. Many of these documents also are available in generic form at large office supply stores or on-line.

- Name the business. A company name that describes exactly what the business does will help potential consumers remember it (e.g., "WorkRite: An Ergonomic Training Center" is easier to understand than "The Body Factory"). Check with city and county records to make certain the business name is not already being used, and conduct a Web search to determine whether the business name is not already registered on-line.
- File a business name statement with a county clerk recorder or a local paper.
- Apply for a business license if required for occupancy by the local government.
- Create a chart of accounts. This chart can be prepared by an accounting professional to help plan for the allocation of expenses.
- Create pro forma financial tools (such as invoices) and procedures (such as determining when new staff may be added or predicting sales revenues and expenses). Those documents and procedures will be needed if loans are to be solicited.
- Recruit qualified personnel, remaining constantly vigilant for potential staff members who are committed to customer service. Plan for an office manager, and prepare to delegate.
- Investigate billing software, particularly if traditional insurance payers will be billed.
- Become an official employer. If employees will be hired, apply for a federal employer identification number, IRS Form SS-4, which can be downloaded from http://www.irs.gov/businesses/small/article/0,,id=97860,00.html.
- Open a separate bank account. Share business plans with the banker, who should know how to help leverage funding sources or be able to help with business loans. In addition, banks have information about obtaining loans through the Small Business Administration (SBA). Other sources of assistance include local private industry councils, SBA centers and economic development departments.
- Obtain insurance for professional liability that reflects the organizational structure of the practice. Insurance also should be obtained for the business if it is a separate legal entity. A qualified insurance agent should be able to advise what insurance is appropriate for the specific needs of the business.
- Put the business plan into action.

## Purchasing an Existing Business

Existing businesses have great merit to an entrepreneur who is creative and can incorporate into the business new technology, new operational strategies, or both. Many strategies and calculations can be used to help determine the value of the business. One simple but effective strategy can assess a business according to the fundamentals of tangible and intangible assets. In this process, the purchaser can inquire about the physical and nonphysical assets by asking the following questions:

- What are the physical assets of the company? External consultation can help evaluate the fair market value of therapy equipment, devices, and buildings (if included as an item for sale).
- What is the worth of the company's intangible assets, including intellectual property and community goodwill? Has the company developed a market niche with specialized services that are not easily replicated by a competitor? Is the practice in a growth phase, or has there been an attenuation of new clients?

Consistent with industry standards, a gross calculation of the goodwill value for a rehabilitation practice is 35%–40% of average annual gross receipts for the most recent 3-year period of operation. This calculation assumes that the business is unencumbered and that it has not experienced a dramatic attenuation of business transactions or client interactions.

Of course, a business is worth only what someone will pay. Premium practices command higher awards; practices that are sold in declining markets are worth less. A declining business may be seen as an opportunity, depending on the entrepreneur's vision of possible change. However, a business should be purchased according to historical performance rather than potential. This approach enables the buyer to negotiate a competitive purchase price. In turn, the challenge to market the business according to historical performance should provide incentives for business owners to consider shaping a possible sale by demonstrating that their revenues consistently sustain growth.

## Case Study

The following case study considers the intangible and tangible assets of a business as one would evaluate them for possible purchase.

Mary Jane has worked for the last 12 years in business and industry as an occupational therapy ergonomics consultant. She has worked out of a home office facility. The majority of her assets are soft assets: the relationships she has developed; her name and reputation; access to her services, including a Web site and the business's phone number and e-mail address; and the contracts she has negotiated. Her soft assets also include her intellectual property—her knowledge, the forms she has developed for report writing, her contacts with vendors, her awareness of industry trends, and similar expertise. The rates that Mary Jane has negotiated for her services represent an investment of her time and business savvy. In addition, her hard assets include a computer system, software, and peripherals; evaluation and assessment equipment, such as a goniometer, an ErgoMeter muscle-action biofeedback device, some adaptive keyboards, mice and trackballs, footrests, ergonomic chairs, and similar assistive technology.

The resale value of her hard assets may be very low, but the entire package of a thriving, growing business has greater value. That "goodwill" value is determined by the seller and buyer and should reflect the reality of the business, including an ever-increasing number of referrals, cash-flow history of the business, new contracts for service delivery, or recent media exposure and press releases. If Mary Jane introduces a prospective buyer to her contacts, then together, they may be more likely to develop positive relationships and make referrals. Relationships and reputation have value in business. If Mary Jane were to wait until her business had dwindled and referrals had slowed before she considered selling it, then the majority of her business's soft assets would be harder to sell.

Anecdotal evidence from a sample of occupational therapists has revealed that these therapists have not thought about how to sell their enterprises, especially those with single-person, sole-proprietor establishments. Instead, those therapists believed that their businesses would no longer exist once they decided to retire from their consulting services (Pazell, 2000). Obviously, for the profession of occupational therapy to have greater merit in the community at large, the economic strength of its constituents matters, and occupational therapy businesses must be validated by economic worth. Occupational therapy practitioners should be encouraged to engage in long-term, strategic planning for business. They should, and can, value their skills and learn to prepare a business for realistic valuation and sale. The enterprising practitioner can use the selling of his or her business as an opportunity to mentor others.

In turn, practitioners who wish to start their own business should consider the prospects of proposing the purchase of an existing business, an approach that can save a great deal of time and expense over the long term. However, as indicated by the anecdotal evidence referred to earlier, prospective buyers should be prepared to propose the idea of buying an existing business because, although the owner of an occupational therapy venture may be considering closing the business, he or she may not be making a considered effort to sell it.

## Conclusion

The skills required of intrapreneurs and entrepreneurs have many similarities. These skills and tools include generating new ideas, seeking windows of opportunity, enlisting financial analysis, conducting competitive analysis, strategizing marketing and operations plans, writing business plans or proposals, and market testing. Intrapreneurs and entrepreneurs are innovators. Each shares risk when putting forth a new idea. However, the intrapreneur's ideas are fostered, nurtured, and developed within an existing organization. The ultimate financial risk of their energetic activity is borne by a third party. The entrepreneur has personal financial risk at stake.

Intrapreneurs, especially occupational therapists who demonstrate innovation within organizations, should be celebrated for their ingenuity and their inventive nature. Entrepreneurs in the field of occupational therapy should be applauded for adding strength and visibility to the profession. Generally, the entrepreneur is considered a formidable and highly influential element in the nation's economy.

The occupational therapist's business idea is the first step in a long ladder of business formation. A business idea implies intelligence, and intelligence gathering is a skill that can be acquired. An idea has merit when it makes good business sense—when it is financially prudent; when market conditions are favorable; and when customers believe they need the product, good, or service that will be brought to market. Occupational therapists have brought to market some stellar and diverse business ideas, including allergy clinic management, corporate wellness programs, ergonomic training programs, and sales in assistive technology.

Only a relatively small percentage of professional association members have identified their employment as private practice. The time is ripe for occupational therapists to develop their business acumen and venture into businesses of their own. An entrepreneurial presence in the community will strengthen the image and political command of the profession.

# References

American Occupational Therapy Association. (2003). *Emerging practice areas*. Retrieved March 3, 2003 from http://www. aota.org/members/area7/index.asp

Cullen, J. B. (1999). *Multinational management: A strategic approach*. Cincinnati, OH: International Thomson.

Dalrymple, D. J., & Parsons, L. J. (2000). *Marketing management: Text and cases* (7th ed.). New York: Wiley.

Ernst & Young. (1998). *Ernst & Young survey conducted by Roper Starch: Leading Americans assess entrepreneurship*. New York: Roper Starch Worldwide.

Evanson, D. R. (1998). *Where to go when the bank says no: Alternatives for financing your business*. Princeton, NJ: Bloomberg.

Glancey, K. (1998). Determinants of growth and profitability in small entrepreneurial firms. *International Journal of Entrepreneurial Behaviour and Research, 4*(1), 18–27.

Hamilton, B. H. (2000). Does entrepreneurship pay? An empirical analysis of the returns to self-employment. *Journal of Political Economy, 108*, 604–631.

Hofstede, G. (1991). *Cultures and organizations: Software of the mind*. London: McGraw-Hill.

Jaffe, E. G. (2000, October). *Writing a good proposal*. Lecture given for Administration/Management course, Samuel Merritt College, Oakland, CA.

Johannson, C. (2003a). *AMA guideline will boost demand for drive assessment*. Retrieved March 30, 2003 from http://www.aota.org/nonmembers/area1/links/link55.asp

Johannson, C. (2003b). *Let's take a stand on school violence*. Retrieved February 17, 2003 from http://www.aota.org/ nonmembers/area1/links/link55.asp

Mazzarol, T., Volery, T., Doss, N., & Theirn, V. (1999). Factors influencing small business start-ups: A comparison with previous research. *International Journal of Entrepreneurial Behavior & Research, 5*(2), 48–63.

McKeever, M. (1999). *How to write a business plan*. Berkeley, CA: Nolo.com.

Miner, J. B. (2000). Testing a psychological typology of entrepreneurship using business founders. *Journal of Applied Behavioural Science, 36*(1), 43–69.

Morrison, A. (2000). Entrepreneurship: What triggers it? *International Journal of Entrepreneurial Behaviour & Research, 6*(2), 59–71.

O'Donnell, M. (1991). *Writing business plans that get results.* Chicago: Contemporary Books.

Pazell, S. (1998). Implementing a visual rehabilitation program. *Caring Magazine.*

Pazell, S. (Ed.). (1999). *Branching out: Private practice and beyond.* Sacramento: Occupational Therapy Association of California.

Pazell, S. (2000). *Entrepreneurial spirit: The experience of therapists.* Unpublished master's thesis, University of LaVerne, San Luis Obispo, CA.

Reynolds, P. (1994, August). *Reducing barriers to understanding new firm gestation: Prevalence and success of nascent entrepreneurs.* Paper presented at the Academy of Management Meeting, Dallas, TX.

Ryan, V. (2000). Anatomy of an entrepreneur. *Telephony, 238*(15), 36–44.

Thompson, J. L. (1999). A strategic perspective of entrepreneurship. *International Journal of Entrepreneurial Behaviour & Research, 5*(6), 1355–1554.

Timmons, J. A. (1999). *New venture creation: Entrepreneurship for the 21st century* (5th ed.). Boston: Irwin/McGraw-Hill.

Van Auken, H. E. (1999). Obstacles to business launch. *Journal of Developmental Entrepreneurship, 4*(2), 175–187.

Wood, W. (1998). The genius within. *American Journal of Occupational Therapy, 52,* 320–325.

Zlotnick, C. (2001, February). *Grant writing.* Lecture given for Professional Development course, Samuel Merritt College, Oakland, CA.

## Resources

The Foundation Center (a collection of information on private foundations that provide funding): http://www.fdncenter.org

U.S. Department of Health and Human Services: http://www.dhhs.gov

PART

# Consultation

# Consultation: Collaborative Interventions for Change

Cynthia F. Epstein, MA, OTR, FAOTA
Evelyn G. Jaffe, MPH, OTR, FAOTA

*"My greatest strength as a consultant is to be ignorant and ask a few questions."*

PETER DRUCKER

**Cynthia F. Epstein, MA, OTR, FAOTA,** is the president and executive director of Occupational Therapy Consultants, Inc., in Somerset, NJ. She has over 30 years of experience as a consultant, practicing in such diverse areas as vocational rehabilitation research and program development, adult day treatment, wheelchair management, school-based programming, and long-term care. She earned her master's degree in vocational rehabilitation at New York University.

**Evelyn G. Jaffe, MPH, OTR, FAOTA,** is an assistant professor at Samuel Merritt College, Oakland, CA. She has been a consultant in occupational therapy for over 35 years, specializing in community mental health, high-risk infants, school-age parents, and primary prevention in the workplace. She earned her master's degree from the School of Public Health at the University of Michigan.

# Key Ideas and Concepts

**Client.** The person or the system seeking and receiving help.

**Consultant roles.** Multiple sets of behaviors that may be performed by a consultant in the course of a consultation, including those of adviser, helper, facilitator, outsider, change agent, evaluator–diagnostician, clarifier, trainer, planner, and extender.

**Consultation.** The interactive process of helping others solve existing or potential problems by identifying and analyzing issues, developing strategies to address problems, and preventing future problems from occurring.

**Consultation process.** A process through which a client receives help from a consultant by means of an interactive, egalitarian relationship based on mutual respect.

**Environment.** A complex of internal and external conditions or factors that surround an individual or a community and that influence behavior or organizational structure.

**External consultant.** An independent agent from outside the organization with whom the client contracts to provide consultation services.

**Internal consultant.** An employee of the client system who is asked to provide consultation services within the organization.

**Levels of consultation.** A conceptualization of consultation as occurring on three possible levels: case centered (focused on a specific person), educational (focused on a specific client group), and program or administrative (focused on a specific system).

**Preventive outcomes.** Results (outcomes) that are achieved through consultation activities and are described in terms of the level of their potential for preventive programming in social, organizational, and health contexts.

**Theoretical models of consultation.** A conceptualization of consultation drawn from specific theoretical frames of reference and having nine possible foci, each calling for different consultant strategies: clinical model, collegial model, behavioral model, educational model, organizational development model, process management model, program development model, social action model, and systems model.

# Learning Objectives

After completing this chapter, you should be able to do the following:

- Define the basic concept of consultation.
- Describe the nine theoretical models of consultation that determine the various consultative approaches.
- Describe the levels of consultation that form the foundation of consultative activities, including the focus and goal of each level.
- Define preventive outcomes and determine their relationship with the levels of consultation.
- Describe evolving practitioner roles and the multiple dimensions of the consultant's roles.
- Define the difference between an internal and external consultant.
- Describe the consultation process, including the stages and basic steps of consultation.
- Compare the process of clinical intervention with the process of consultation.
- Describe important consultant marketing strategies.
- Identify emerging consultative practice arenas for occupational therapy practitioners relative to changes in occupational therapy practice.

Consultation is an important component of the occupational therapy intervention process (American Occupational Therapy Association [AOTA], 2002). Today's practice environments require the use of a collaborative approach to resolving client problems, which is the essence of consultation. The changing nature of health and human services delivery has created challenges for the occupational therapy practitioner and has increased opportunities for a consultative approach. Stringent criteria for approval of services coupled with time-limited appropriations, fixed payments, and increasing competition for funds from other disciplines call for practitioners who are knowledgeable, skilled, and responsive. Practitioners must diagnose an individual's functional problems effectively while considering problems in the system's organization and processes that may affect intervention outcomes. Consultants are trained to analyze systems and develop problem-solving strategies within a client-centered, collaborative relationship. Successful practitioners, therefore, must understand and use principles of consultation in all areas and at all levels of occupational therapy practice to expand the potential for successful client outcomes.

Every practitioner may be called on to provide consultation within the context of his or her job. Those possessing particular expertise may provide consultation as their primary role (AOTA, 1993b). Whether consultation is a secondary or primary role, one must understand how to use principles of consultation to meet client needs.

Consultation is the interactive process of helping others solve existing or potential problems by identifying and analyzing issues, developing strategies to address problems, and preventing future problems from occurring. Key elements in consultation, in addition to occupational therapy expertise, are an understanding of (a) systems (see chapter 4), (b) organizational development, (c) behavior, and (d) principles of prevention. The consultant must have not only the ability to listen and communicate effectively but also a capacity to diagnose and facilitate resolution of existing or potential problems (Yerxa, 1978).

Occupational therapy consultants provide services in varied settings. These include not only traditional environments such as hospitals, long-term care facilities, and schools but also the growing arenas of industry, community programs, regulatory agencies, professional organizations, and international health programs. Consultant services may be requested by individuals, departments, or entire systems, and they may involve a brief intervention or an extended relationship. Services are delivered using a client-centered approach that emphasizes an interactive relationship between consultant and client (AOTA, 1995, 2002).

A consultant may be from a private practice or from another type of organization outside the system that is requesting help. Alternatively, a consultant may be an employee of the organization that is seeking consultation. Any occupational therapy practitioner might, then, receive a request to provide consultation to a department or staff in his or her organization. The client (the individual, group, or system seeking help) uses consultation to improve planning; participation; and interaction with colleagues, consumers, or employees. The consultant helps the client to mobilize internal and external resources that will foster change and lead to problem resolution (Lippitt & Lippitt, 1986; Ulschak & SnowAntle, 1990).

In the course of consultation, the client is offered suggestions for new or revised elements, information, concepts, perspectives, values, attitudes, and skills. During this time, the consultant must view problems from a broad, client-centered perspective and must consider systems, theoretical models, and environmental contexts as an integral part of the decision-making process (AOTA 1993a, 1995, 2002; Dunn, Brown, & McGuigan, 1994; Jaffe & Epstein, 1992a).

Inherent in occupational therapy practice is the enabling of the client through occupation. Engagement in occupation supports client participation in the many contexts in which daily life activities occur. Client and practitioner work collaboratively to design and carry out required interventions (AOTA, 2002). Similarly, occupational therapy consultation requires collaboration between client and consultant. The goal of consultation also is to enable the client. The consultant's task is to identify or collaboratively develop enhanced environments in which positive change can take place, thereby leading to improved client performance.

Jaffe and Epstein (1992c) have proposed a theoretical model of consultation that "integrates occupational therapy and consultation concepts within an ecological framework" (p. 709). The model relates the principles, philosophical assumptions, and theoretical premises of occupational therapy to those of consultation. It recognizes ecological contexts as a critical factor in goal achievement for both occupational therapy and consultation. AOTA's (2002) *Occupational Therapy Practice Framework* supports this perspective. Jaffe and Epstein's (1992c) model incorporates and acknowledges "the synergetic relationship between occupational therapy, human ecology, and consultation" (p. 677).

The model is based on

- The milieu or environment in which the consultative activities occur;
- The application of the human ecological perspective of the client;
- Collaboration between consultant and client;
- The adaptation or change brought about by this collaborative approach; and ultimately,
- Enablement of the client to achieve improved function and to maximize his or her human potential.

Concepts of prevention are basic to this model because the ultimate goal of consultation is to help the client develop skills to prevent future problems. Consultation, therefore, enables the client to assume a proactive stance and, thus, anticipate and forestall situations that could lead to further problems or dysfunction.

Occupational therapy practice environments require that practitioners provide efficient and cost-effective responses to the varied needs of their clients. Knowledge and understanding of occupational therapy consultation principles and processes will enhance the practitioner's ability to make these responses. This chapter provides an overview of consultation concepts and the process of consultation as well as the important skills and concepts needed to perform the role of consultant. Additionally, the chapter addresses marketing and business as they relate to establishing a consultation practice.

## An Expanding Marketplace

Changing legislative priorities, economic and social issues, continued advances in technology, and an expanding system of managed care in the delivery of health services (see chapters 3 and 17) have had a profound influence on the growing demand for consultation services. Federal mandates, including the Americans with Disabilities Act (ADA) of 1990, the Individuals with Disabilities Education Act Final Regulations of 1999, the Ticket to Work and Work Incentives Improvement Act of 1999, and the New Freedom Initiative Executive Order of 2001 (Croser, 2002), have increased consumer awareness of the need for skilled occupational therapy consultants.

These mandates target disability and community concerns across the developmental spectrum. Additionally, the global information highway and growing assistive technology options have created new and exciting options for people with disabilities. This fast-paced and continuously evolving environment requires consultants with expertise, including occupational therapists, to help health and community planners, managers, and consumers move successfully through the process of change.

Health care now operates under a system of managed care and many similar plans that emphasize cost containment. In controlling cost and access, systems influence how occupational therapy services are provided. Traditional one-on-one intervention may be limited. Indirect services, including consultation and case management, may become the primary choice for many health care providers. Consultation skills to help consumers, families, employers, and communities assess needs, identify strengths, and develop and coordinate resources are essential for today's practitioner (Jaffe, 1996).

The consultant is usually found at the leading edge of practice, initiating occupational therapy services in new markets, especially in the community. For example, the Ticket to Work legislation provides opportunities for individuals with disabilities to seek and select services necessary to obtain and retain employment. As an evaluator, analyst, and trainer, the occupational therapy consultant may help identify and select work-training programs for these individuals. In addition, the training of program staff members frequently requires consulting services to assist with configuring jobs to address client needs.

Best, Noblitt, Synold, and Hughes (2001) explored emerging areas of occupational therapy practice. Their research indicated opportunities in case management, driver rehabilitation, ergonomics, wellness, forensics, and low-vision rehabilitation—all of which have a consultation component. For example, Lori Basey, an occupational therapist in Oklahoma City, was involved with the City Rescue Mission, where initially, clients with psychiatric histories were unable to participate in a community reentry program. Basey and university fieldwork students collaborated with mission staff members to develop a program teaching self-sufficiency skills. This program became the preliminary step clients needed to become eligible for the mission's employment training program (Diffendal, 2001).

Schools and early intervention programs constitute the largest practice setting for occupational therapists and the second largest for occupational therapy assistants (AOTA, 2001). Consultants with expertise in pediatrics and knowledge of educational systems are in demand to develop educationally related programs for children in these settings (Dunn, 2000).

Educators use occupational therapy services for children with special needs. However, mandates for cost containment and educational relevance require a change in how these services are provided. The traditional "pull-out," direct intervention one-on-one model, has given way to in-class support and inclusion services. This current model requires understanding and use of a consultative approach. The practitioner–consultant applies consultation principles and expertise within classroom settings (Dunn, 2000; Rainville, Cermak, & Murray, 1996; Swinth & Mailloux, 2002). Using a collegial model of consultation (see Exhibit 10.1), the consultant establishes a supportive milieu for collaborative problem solving. The expertise of both teacher and consultant is recognized for the benefit of the students with special needs and the classroom as a whole (Dettner, Dyck, & Thurston, 1999).

Needs for consultation also are increasing at the opposite end of the human developmental spectrum. The preferred option for long-term care is maintenance of older people in their homes. The need for community-based occupational therapy services, therefore, will continue to grow. Consultants help develop programs, provide case consultation, and train staff members (AOTA, 1996; Epstein, 1992c; Maddox, 2001).

Other growing markets include those related to technology and accessibility. Assistive technology enables many people with disabilities to achieve greater independence and productivity. This intervention includes providing technological assistance in seating, positioning, and mobility for clients who are developmentally disabled; consulting on the use of environmental control units for people who are physically challenged; and fostering consumers' use of effective communication technology (Bender & Davidson, 2002; Mann, 2001).

Accessibility issues resulting from the ADA have created countless opportunities for occupational therapy consultation to industries, private and public businesses, and corporations. City planners, developers, architects, and others involved in designing living space need consultation services, as do employers and lawyers concerned with employment of people with disabilities. The occupational therapy consultant is uniquely qualified to help develop reasonable accommodations for job performance and to conduct work capacity evaluations for employees with disabilities (Hoelscher & Taylor, 2000).

## Exhibit 10.1 Theoretical Models of Consultation.

### Clinical or Intervention Model
Patient- or client-focused model based on diagnosis and recommendations for intervention, frequently in a specific case; often considered case consultation

### Collegial or Professional Model
Peer-centered model based on egalitarian, problem-solving relationships with professional colleagues; considered collaborative consultation

### Behavioral Model
Behavior-focused model based on control, adaptation, modification, or change of learned behavior

### Educational Model
Information-centered model with consultant acting as educator and trainer to enhance the staff's knowledge and skills that can support desired consultation outcomes

### Organizational Development Model
Management-focused model based on examination of organizational structure, leadership styles, and interpersonal communication and relationships

### Process Management Model
Group-based model focused on process dynamics of client, with consultant acting as a catalyst for staff development and the building of group skills to manage organizational process more effectively

### Program Development Model
Service-centered model focused on development of new programs or modification of existing programs to improve services; involves assessment, design, implementation, and evaluation

### Social Action Model
Social reform model focused on social values and policies, with consultant acting as advocate to foster social change

### Systems Model
Overall system-centered model based on specific values and culture of client (e.g., school, corporation, health facility, community agency); focused on understanding the system's mission and goals to effect change in system

*Note.* From "Theoretical Concepts of Consultation," by E. G. Jaffe, in *Occupational Therapy Consultation: Theory, Principles, and Practice* (pp. 44–46, Table 2.1), edited by E. G. Jaffe and C. F. Epstein, 1992, St. Louis, MO: Mosby/YearBook. Copyright 1992 by Mosby/YearBook. Adapted with permission.

Changes in health care delivery models and recent technological advances will continue to expand consultation opportunities. For example, as increasing numbers of older and younger individuals survive due to life-sustaining technologies, the need for technology consultation services will grow (Technology-Related Assistance for Individuals with Disabilities Act of 1988). Building a core of consultants begins with expanding the knowledge base of prospective consultants. The information presented in this chapter is intended to widen the perspective of occupational therapy students and practitioners by providing an overview of the basic concepts, process, and practice of consultation.

## Concepts of Consultation

Consultation is a multidimensional, highly complex, dynamic activity. Successful consultation is not happenstance but the result of knowledge, skill, and grounding in the theoretical foundations of the activity. It requires careful study and understanding of (a) a client's environment, (b) the various models or approaches that a consultant might use, (c) the different roles and styles appropriate to a specific system, and (d) the process of consultation. Before undertaking consultation, a prospective consultant should have a thorough knowledge of the concepts that provide a theoretical framework for consultation.

Models of consultation are drawn from many fields of study, including sociology, psychology, education, medicine, and business. Jaffe (1992c) identified nine theoretical models, shown in Exhibit 10.1, and three levels of consultation activity, shown in Exhibit 10.2.

Consultation may involve only one theoretical model and one level, as is frequently the case when a consultant is called in as an expert to help resolve a clinical problem. This kind of situation usually requires evaluation of a specific individual and the development of recommendations to be carried out by people on-site. For example, an older adult, who uses a wheelchair and has a diagnosis of rheumatoid arthritis, is a participant in a community day program center. Her current wheelchair is impeding independent mobility. Staff members ask an occupational therapy consultant to provide a wheelchair assessment. They want to improve the woman's functional independence at the center and at her home.

The consultant, Betty, shares her findings and recommendations with staff members and the client. She identifies a list of medical equipment dealers who are knowledgeable with respect to the type of wheelchair suitable for the client. Using this information, a medical equipment dealer is chosen. Before leaving the center, the consultant indicates that she is available, if needed, for a follow-up visit. The vendor brings several chairs to the center so the client can make a final choice, possibly with help of the consultant (Epstein 1992a). In this example, the consultant uses the Clinical or Intervention Model, at Level I, Case-Centered Consultation (see Exhibits 10.1 and 10.2).

## Exhibit 10.2  Levels of Consultation.

### Level I: Case-Centered Consultation

Focused on a specific person, with the goal of achieving appropriate behavioral or physical change; derived from traditional Clinical or Intervention Model; usually involves specialized assessments to diagnose problem

### Level II: Educational or Collegial Consultation

Focused on a specific client group (e.g., staff members, clinicians, teachers, administrators), with the goal of improving function, efficiency, and ability; derived from Educational Model; involves in-service training or staff development

### Level III: Program or Administrative Consultation

Focused on specific system (e.g., school, agency, corporation, health facility), with the goal of promoting institutional change; derived from Systems, Program Development, and Organizational Development models; involves program planning, administrative and management skill development, and strategic planning

*Note.* From "Theoretical Concepts of Consultation," by E. G. Jaffe, in *Occupational Therapy Consultation: Theory, Principles, and Practice* (pp. 44–46, Table 2.1), edited by E. G. Jaffe and C. F. Epstein, 1992, St. Louis, MO: Mosby/YearBook. Copyright 1992 by Mosby/YearBook. Adapted with permission.

In most situations, consultants are asked to address more complex issues. This process requires use of multiple theoretical models and levels of consultation. For example, Jane is assigned to provide consultative occupational therapy services in a local school system. She recently evaluated 8-year-old Bobby, a pupil in a regular classroom who was referred because he could not pay attention. Jane recommended use of the program "How Does Your Engine Run" (Williams & Shellenberger, 2001), which she suggests is most appropriate for Bobby. She adds that this program is designed to help all students attend more successfully. Although Jane started her consultation at Level I, she is now quickly moving to Level II, Educational or Collegial Consultation.

Training of the school's staff, especially the teacher and aide in Bobby's classroom, was the first step. Jane used Educational and Collegial or Professional models to bring needed information to the group and to collaborate with the teacher and aide on carrying out the program in Bobby's classroom. As she progressed with the training phase, Jane realized that some staff behaviors were impeding rather than advancing the progress of the program. She then applied strategies related to the Behavioral Model to help staff members change their approach.

During the training phase, the classroom aide went to the principal and asked for a raise. The aide based her request on the new training, stating that this new approach required a higher level of skill. Jane was now propelled into Level III, Program or Administrative Consultation. Using approaches from Organizational Development and Program Development models and from the Systems Model, Jane developed a report for the principal, illustrating the benefits that all classroom staff members and students were realizing through the new program. The principal (administrator) used Jane's consultative skills and report information to help address the aide's request. The goal was to help all staff members, including the aide, understand that the program provided another way to support the delivery of the classroom curriculum. As everyone became more involved in the program, they realized its significant benefit to the school as a whole. During this turn of events, the aide became one of the program's strongest supporters.

Figure 10.1 illustrates the fluid nature of consultation when different levels and models are applied during the consultation process. These levels and models provide an organizing framework for analyzing, planning, and implementing any given consultative experience.

## Environment and Systems Analysis

Successful consultation outcomes begin with careful analysis and planning. An environment and systems analysis is an important preliminary step (see chapter 4). The systems in which occupational therapy consultation may take place include health care facilities, schools, social agencies, the community, industry, regulatory agencies, and

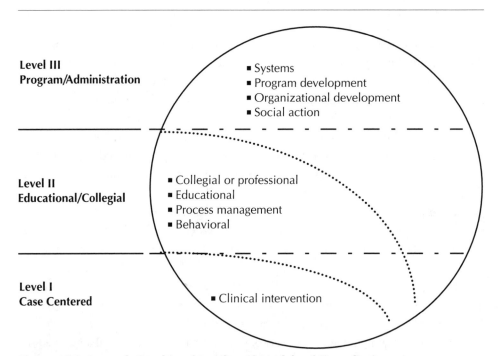

**Figure 10.1 Interrelationship of Levels and Models of Consultation.**

*Note.* From "Theoretical Concepts of Consultation," by E. G. Jaffe, in *Occupational Therapy Consultation: Theory, Principles, and Practice* (p. 51, Figure 2.1), edited by E. G. Jaffe and C. F. Epstein, 1992, St. Louis, MO: Mosby/YearBook. Copyright 1992 by Mosby/YearBook. Adapted with permission.

political arenas. The analysis should ascertain the state of the system. A thorough study and evaluation of all influential internal and external environmental factors will help determine consultation goals and strategies.

The environment is a complex of internal and external conditions or factors that surround an individual or a community. These factors influence behavior or organizational structure. The external environment includes political, economic, social, demographic, cultural, and physical factors. The internal environment includes personal and organizational goals, resources available, power and control, organizational structure, the physical environment, and more. Analysis of these factors helps determine the consultation frame (or frames) of reference.

## Consultant Roles and Relationships

The actual role of the consultant involves many dimensions. Natural role shifts occur at various stages of consultation as relationships develop, new information becomes available, and the consultant fosters change. The consultant may be an internal consultant, employed within the system, or an external consultant, brought in from outside the system. He or she may assume a singular role or, more usually, take on multiple roles as the consultation progresses, providing a variety of services depending on the needs and the setting of the client.

### Internal and External Consultants

The way in which the consultant perceives a client and is perceived by the client depends to a large extent on whether the consultant is inside or outside the system. An internal consultant is an employee of the client system who is asked to provide consultation services within the organization. An external consultant is an independent agent, outside the organization, with whom the client contracts to provide consultation services.

Role expectations for client and consultant are directly related to the consultant's relationship with the system. The consultant's behavior, identified frames of reference, and role choice influence the development of the consultation. The internal consultant, an employee, is an integral part of the system and has knowledge of the corporate culture as well as the strengths and weaknesses of the organization. This connection may or may not be considered an advantage, depending on the organization's needs. The external consultant, as an outsider, may have a fresh, objective perspective. Each type of consultant has advantages and disadvantages. The client is wise to consider specific system problems and needs before choosing an internal or an external consultant (Jaffe & Epstein, 1992c).

### Evolving Roles: Practitioner to Consultant

The occupational therapy practitioner uses meaningful occupation-based intervention strategies. Time constraints and mandates for cost effectiveness may require that the practitioner assume a consultative role as the intervention proceeds. Consultation approaches become embedded in the practitioner role as intervention shifts from a direct to an indirect perspective. Occupational therapy practitioners recognize that, to maintain functional outcomes, the human and nonhuman environments that support the client must be considered. This concept is described in chapter 4.

As practitioner–consultant roles gradually evolve, direct client intervention still occurs. However, indirect intervention, directed to client support systems, becomes increasingly visible. The practitioner–consultant now assumes roles such as trainer, collegial collaborator, problem-solver, information specialist, and clarifier (Lippitt & Lippitt, 1986).

Use of this embedded, indirect perspective will encourage the client, the client system in which intervention occurs, or both to change the understanding of the consultant's role. As an adviser, helper, or facilitator with occupational therapy expertise, the consultant focuses on a collaborative intervention process. To maintain and solidify functional achievements, the role of consultant gains importance. The consultant helps the client to function within systems that are an identified part of the client's lifestyle. In this role, the consultant uses knowledge of systems and an understanding of the client's goals and objectives to effect and support positive change.

Figure 10.2 illustrates the evolution from the practitioner's direct intervention role to the indirect consultant role. It identifies activities that are expected at each role

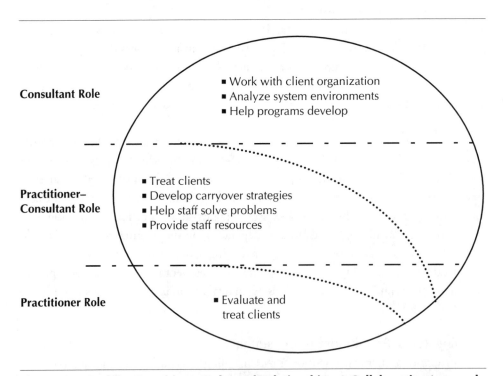

**Consultant Role**
- Work with client organization
- Analyze system environments
- Help programs develop

**Practitioner–
Consultant Role**
- Treat clients
- Develop carryover strategies
- Help staff solve problems
- Provide staff resources

**Practitioner Role**
- Evaluate and treat clients

**Figure 10.2  Evolving Practitioner Roles and Relationships: A Collaborative Approach.**

level and recognizes that, as is true in Figure 10.1, the roles and activities of consultant and practitioner maintain a fluid relationship during a given client intervention process.

## The Consultation Process

Occupational therapy consultation is a process through which a client receives help through an interactive, egalitarian relationship based on mutual respect. Problem solving is a key component, involving identification and analysis of issues as well as resolution of problems. Consultants use a systems perspective to develop an environmental analysis, identify available internal and external resources, and foster interactive communication.

Consultation occurs in four stages: (a) initiation and clarification, (b) assessment and communication, (c) interactive problem resolution, and (d) evaluation and termination. Within these stages are eight basic steps, which are shown in Exhibit 10.3. These steps can be used for consultation that (a) is a short-term, problem-specific intervention; (b) is provided at predetermined intervals; or (c) occurs on a continuing basis as needed. Continuing consultation needs are usually community based and include school systems, community mental health centers, assisted living centers, adult day programs and workshops, and other community facilities.

Regardless of the setting, the four stages and the eight basic steps provide the foundation for all consultation. These stages and steps can be used in the consultation process to clarify the roles and the functions of the consultant as well as the expectations of the client and to assist the consultant in providing successful consultation activities and strategies.

### Initiation and Clarification

In some scenarios, the initial identification of a need or a problem may precipitate a request for consultation services. In other scenarios, the consultant may see a need

**Exhibit 10.3  Basic Steps of Consultation.**

---

- Entry into system
- Negotiation of contract
- Diagnostic analysis leading to problem identification
- Goal setting and planning through establishment of trust
- Maintenance phase of intervention and feedback
- Evaluation
- Termination
- Possible renegotiation

---

*Note.* From "The Process of Consultation," by E. G. Jaffe, in *Occupational Therapy Consultation: Theory, Principles, and Practice* (p. 136), edited by E. G. Jaffe and C. F. Epstein, 1992, St. Louis, MO: Mosby/YearBook. Copyright 1992 by Mosby/YearBook. Adapted with permission.

within a particular system and present a proposal. In early meetings with the client, the consultant delineates his or her knowledge and experience. The client presents an overview of the system and enumerates the desired outcomes of the consultation. During these interactions, the parties have an opportunity to clarify roles, expectations, and goals that can lead to a formal contract.

### Entry Into the System

Entry into the system or the organization is the first step in the consultation process. The entry is based on exploration of the potential for consultation in the system (Jaffe & Epstein, 1992b) and may develop in one or more of four ways:
- *Planned entry*—Individual develops a strategy and presents a proposal
- *Opportunistic entry*—Situation arises spontaneously, and individual seizes the moment
- *Uninvited entry*—Individual perceives a need and attempts to enter the system
- *Invited entry*—Individual is invited because of specific skills.

Planned, opportunistic, and uninvited entry provide methods to obtain a foothold for the formalized consultation. This type of entry allows the consultant to help the client appreciate the benefits that can be derived through the consultation process. However, unless the consultant is finally invited to enter the system, the actual consultation may not be successful. During the entry step, the consultant considers certain factors. These include the potential for a mutual relationship, an initial assessment of needs, the client's readiness for change, and possible consultation activities.

### Negotiation of a Contract

Clear communication and understanding are essential in establishing a collaborative relationship. This stage culminates in the contract, which both parties sign. This formal document defines the purpose of the consultation; describes the qualifications of the consultant; identifies the obligations and the expectations of both parties; and delineates procedures, time constraints, and the method and amount of compensation.

## Assessment and Communication

Once the consultant has formalized a contract and effective communication is established, assessment of the problem begins. The consultant draws on professional knowledge, experience, and resources in conjunction with an in-depth study of the client's competence and knowledge. Special terminology and procedures used in the setting are identified and noted to ensure effective communication and accurate identification of the client's problems or needs (or both). External sources of power such as regulatory agencies, funding sources, and community consumer groups are considered. These may have a direct influence on the system and the issues for which consultation has been requested.

### *Diagnostic Analysis Leading to Problem Identification*

Preliminary diagnostic work in the entry phase prepares the consultant to perform a more intensive diagnosis of the system. This work is essential to consultation success. Study must include an environmental and systems analysis that reveals the organizational structure; the internal and external trends and resources that affect the system; and the corporate culture, mission, and goals (see chapter 4). During data collection, the consultant should identify not only forces that impede movement but also forces that facilitate progress (Lewin, 1951).

### *Goal Setting and Planning Through Establishment of Trust*

In addition to helping the consultant identify the needs and the problems of the system, the diagnostic process provides the framework for the next step in consultation—collaborative goal setting and planning. This step aids the consultant in establishing the mutual respect necessary for a successful consultation. The consultant must develop a good working relationship with the client to identify the desired outcomes of the consultation. Knowledge of formal and informal lines of communication, system politics, key power figures, and the ways in which decision making occurs in the system will enhance the planning phase.

## Interactive Problem Resolution

After thoroughly studying the situation and carefully analyzing gathered data, the consultant begins the process of interactive problem resolution. First, the consultant shares data with the client. Decisions remain the province of the client. To help effect change in the system, the consultant must collaborate with the client. Interactive problem resolution demonstrates the consultant's commitment to helping the client effect change through collaborative strategy development. This collaborative strategy development has a basis in the consultant's role as a trainer, a facilitator, an educator, a communicator, and a resource person. Through participative decision making, the consultant helps the client to identify multiple strategies for consideration. Additionally, the consultant must demonstrate a commitment to confidentiality and an adherence to professional ethics (see chapter 21). The consultant and the client build a relationship of mutual trust and respect, establishing an open environment in which the client can consider change strategies by using the perspective and the suggestions offered by the consultant.

## Maintenance

Putting into effect the plans that emerge from the consultation leads to the maintenance phase. During this phase, an internal and external communication network or feedback system is developed that supports a review of observations, perceptions, and progress. Through communication and sharing of knowledge, the client and other members of the system develop greater understanding and appreciation of the consultant's occupational performance perspective. During data gathering, the consultant interviews and meets with a variety of people who are concerned with the issues, including key power individuals in the system (e.g., administrators, managers, directors) and the general staff. These occasions provide further opportunities to observe the system in action and to consider possible solutions. The consultant must be aware of the needs of the people working in the system and of the difficulties that they face when the system is considering change.

During this stage, the consultant should identify sources for feedback and reflection. If the consultant is an outsider, he or she may not always perceive and interpret actions and information as they are viewed by the system. The consultant must verify the information and data using a variety of analysis techniques, including interviews, surveys, group discussions, and documentation.

## Evaluation and Termination

The final stage of the consultation process is evaluation and termination. An exit or summary conference usually occurs between consultant and client to provide an opportunity for clarification, feedback, evaluation, and discussion of any remaining areas of concern. The consultant prepares a final report containing the following information: dates of service, individuals and departments involved, and a plan of action for both the consultant and client. The report also contains data-gathering methodology; findings; assessment; collaborative strategy development; and recommendations, including possible follow-up to allow an avenue for further communication as needed.

### Evaluation

The feedback network provides information for evaluation of the consultation. Throughout the consultation activities, the consultant monitors and evaluates the outcomes of the intervention. "The evaluation process is an integral part of planning and implementation," providing the data necessary "to clarify goals, refine or revise intervention strategies, and develop future plans" (Jaffe & Epstein, 1992b, pp. 147–148). Similar to the data gathering that is performed during the diagnostic phase, evaluation includes both formal and informal methods of assessment. Informal evaluation occurs during the consultant's periodic observations of and feedback from the client, either independently or in collaboration with the client. "Formal evaluation consists of data collection and analysis based on the specific outcome objectives desired from the consultation" (Jaffe & Epstein, 1992b, p. 149).

### Termination

The consultant and the client should prepare for termination during development of the initial contract, when preliminary goals and time frames are established. Termination may occur at any time during the consultation, either when the consultant or client mutually agree that goals have been achieved or when further intervention is no longer appropriate.

*Possible Renegotiation*

Contracts may include the possibility of renegotiation at any time in the consultation process to allow for changes in or expansion of the goals of the consultation. After termination of the original contract, the parties may decide to renegotiate if the client requests additional help.

# Principles of Prevention

The ultimate goal of consultation is to help clients assume a proactive stance, enabling them to anticipate or forestall problems that otherwise could lead to dysfunction. Concepts of prevention are, therefore, inherent in all consultation. They are also inherent in occupational therapy practice, and many authors have discussed them (Epstein, 1979; Grossman, 1977; Jaffe, 1980, 1986, 1992c; West, 1969; Wiemer, 1972). The basic principles of prevention follow:

- *Primary prevention*—Activities undertaken before the onset of a problem to avoid occurrence of malfunction or disability in a population potentially at risk
- *Secondary prevention*—Early diagnosis, identification, and detection of at-risk populations to prevent chronic dysfunction or permanent disability
- *Tertiary prevention*—Rehabilitation and remediation of a problem or illness to prevent further problems, loss, or disability.

The basic principles of prevention listed above are applied to the three levels of consultation (see Exhibit 10.2) to achieve preventive outcomes. As the consultant addresses the specific issues, consultation strategies are based on the levels at which the activities occur. Included in the strategy plan is the consideration of the preventive outcome that can be expected at that level. Enablement of the client is another inherent goal for occupational therapy practitioners. Merging the concepts of prevention with occupational therapy consultation practice at various levels ensures appropriate outcome expectations and fosters proactive approaches by clients and consultants that acknowledge the important relationships among client, consultant, and the environment. Three levels of preventive outcomes are directly related to the three levels of consultation.

## Tertiary Preventive Outcome

At Level I, Case-Centered Consultation, the preventive outcome expected is tertiary prevention. Modification of the specific client behavior occurs as a result of remediation or maintenance activities. In the Level I consultation scenario of 8-year-old Bobby, the suggestion of a specific program to aid his attention deficit is an example of modification of client behavior with a tertiary preventive outcome.

## Secondary Preventive Outcome

As that Level I consultation progressed to Level II, Educational Consultation, which entailed training the school's staff and Bobby's teacher to carry out the program in the classroom for all of Bobby's classmates, the preventive outcome expected is secondary prevention. The entire class was at risk of distraction because of Bobby's behavior.

## Primary Preventive Outcome

In the school scenario, the occupational therapy consultant, Jane, progressed to Level III, Program or Administrative Consultation, as she demonstrated the benefits of the program to the school principal. She suggested instituting the program in the entire school, for all students, before similar disruptive behaviors could occur. Thus, the preventive outcome at Level III is primary prevention. Before the onset of a problem, strategies were suggested for that school system as a whole.

## Consultation Skills and Knowledge

The occupational therapy philosophy of helping others do for themselves carries over naturally into consultation. Knowledge and professional competence in occupational therapy practice as well as an understanding of professional ethics and behavior (see chapter 22) can provide a sound foundation for developing consultation skills. Numerous authors have identified areas of knowledge that are critical in consultation. These include systems theory and behavioral sciences; developmental theory as it applies to individuals, groups, organizations, and communities; education and training methodologies, including problem solving and role playing; human occupation and personality, attitude formation, adaptation, and change; and self-knowledge (Dunn et al., 1994; Gallessich, 1982; Gilfoyle, 1992; Grady, 1995; Jaffe, 1992b; Jaffe & Epstein, 1992b; Lippitt & Lippitt, 1986).

"A mutually supportive and synergistic relationship can exist between direct treatment roles and indirect consultation approaches" (Jaffe & Epstein, 1992c, p. 683). In both cases, recognition and appreciation of the environment are critical factors. Principles of human ecology also apply (see chapter 4). "Understanding and effectively utilizing these approaches help reinforce the important role for the environment for both therapist/consultant and patient/client. Thus, the occupational therapy treatment/consultation interaction bonds these processes together" (p. 683). Figure 10.3 illustrates the similarity between these two processes while acknowledging the uniqueness of each.

Key skills that the consultant must possess are communicating, educating, diagnosing, and linking. To use these skills successfully, the consultant must be able to establish effective interpersonal relationships. Attitudes and attributes such as flexibility, creativity, maturity, and self-confidence help the consultant function successfully in varied environments.

## Communicating

Communicating is a primary consultation skill. It encompasses more than verbal and written abilities. It also includes one's use of body language, role modeling, and analogies as well as one's ability to reflect and confront. In addition, listening skills

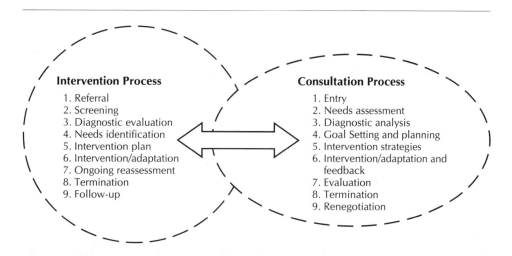

**Figure 10.3 Comparison of Intervention and Consultation.**

*Note.* From "Toward a Theoretical Model of Occupational Therapy Consultation," by E. G. Jaffe and C. F. Epstein, in *Occupational Therapy Consultation: Theory, Principles, and Practice* (p. 51, Figure 2.1), edited by E. G. Jaffe and C. F. Epstein, 1992, St. Louis, MO: Mosby/YearBook. Copyright 1992 by Mosby/YearBook. Adapted with permission.

play a role of the utmost importance (see chapters 11 and 13). What is or is not said and how a message is presented provide valuable insight. The consultation environment plays an important function in communication. A working space where walls are covered by lists of rules, regulations, and procedures expresses a very different message from a space where walls and shelves contain interesting artwork and growing plants.

Written and oral communication must express differences in language usage as it applies in any given consultation setting. In school settings, industry, and day care centers, for example, catchphrases or special terms may be used as part of the communication process. Outsiders, unfamiliar with this language, may feel cut off from meaningful dialogue. As consultants, we must define our terms in the client's perspective, often using the client's language.

## Educating

Training and educating are basic components of consultation. A variety of methods may be used to help broaden client skills and further develop abilities to effect independent change. Designing and leading workshops is one of these methods ( Jaffe, 1992a). This approach allows the consultant to present new material as the client participates actively through experiential learning. Specialized materials and instructional programs may be used, allowing the client to proceed at a comfortable pace that includes built-in opportunities for feedback and discussion. The materials must be presented clearly and must be relevant for the client.

## Diagnosing

Occupational therapists and occupational therapy assistants are most familiar with assessment technology as it pertains to diagnosis and direct intervention for people who have mental or physical dysfunction. Consultation calls for a more global perspective. Moving into a dysfunctional system, the consultant must gather data from a variety of sources in collaboration with the client. As the consultant reviews and assesses data, feedback is obtained to help verify and clarify issues before a final diagnosis or conclusion is reached. The consultant must have the ability to diagnose problems; to locate sources of help, power, and influence; to understand the client's values and culture; and to determine readiness for change (Jaffe & Epstein, 1992a; Lippitt & Lippitt, 1986).

## Linking

Linking is a skill that comes naturally to occupational therapists and occupational therapy assistants. As proponents of adaptation, they constantly identify resources and alternative methods to help achieve a particular goal. The consultant links the client to appropriate resources both within and outside the consultation environment. A consultant, for example, may learn about new and competitive sources for equipment and supplies when consulting with one organization. He or she may link these resources to another client, when appropriate.

## Establishing Effective Relationships

An understanding of the client's value system and attitudes as well as the external and internal pressures on the system are essential to establish effective interpersonal relationships. These factors all have a bearing on the capacity to change. For example, pressured by time and environment, an aide finds it quicker, easier, and less frustrating to feed a child even though that child has the ability to eat independently with adaptive equipment. The consultant's task is to help the aide and other team members understand the importance of this daily living task so independence becomes a first priority. Additionally, the consultant works with the aide's supervisors to modify time and environmental constraints, thereby fostering change in the aide's behavior. To develop this kind of collaborative relationship, the consultant must have a sincere interest in the client and must gain the confidence and respect of the team and the client (LaGrossa & Saxe, 1998).

## Incorporating Key Attitudes and Attributes

Consultation requires a high degree of self-direction, comfort with taking risks, and ease in working without a formalized support system. Satisfaction for a job well done comes through success achieved by the client. To be fulfilled by this indirect type of gratification, the consultant must have a strong sense of security and self-confidence. In addition, maturity, flexibility, a sense of humor, and a sense of timing are important. At times, a crisis may cause the original consultation problem to be put aside.

The consultant may come prepared to deal with one problem and find the system's priority to be quite different. At a moment like this, staff members are not amenable to considering other issues, and the consultant must help resolve the more pressing problem. The consultant must make a realistic appraisal of his or her limitations and abilities. Everyone cannot be an expert at everything. When additional skills are required, the consultant should have the confidence to acknowledge this fact and to suggest other resources, one of which may be the client.

## On Becoming a Consultant

When forging into new and less secure settings, consultants should follow the Scout motto, "Be prepared." They should consider current and future consultation environments. They also should create business and marketing plans based on careful study of economic factors (see chapters 7 and 9). Further, they should develop and use resources appropriately. The "business of being in business" can then become a reality.

### Considering Current and Future Consultation Environments

Occupational therapy consultants can be found in private practices, school systems, industry, hospital departments, rehabilitation centers, and community agencies as well as in schools of occupational therapy whose faculty members provide community- and campus-based consultation. A few serve as administrative consultants for governments, national health organizations, insurance companies, accrediting agencies, and other concerned health groups. Some provide services in unusual settings, including prisons, Native American reservations, programs dealing with abuse of children and elderly people, homeless shelters, and women's crisis centers. In addition, consultants advise architects and designers, analyze the occupational performance of employees, and design appropriate and efficient work environments.

Current health planning finally has moved toward firm support of health promotion models of care. The emphasis on primary prevention can be seen in the growing use of alternative health practitioners and health plans that include routine health screenings and other preventive measures (Allison, 1999). The outcome of these primary prevention activities will involve systemwide programming.

As more and more consumers have recognized the value of broader health care that has a focus on overall health, not just illness, opportunities for occupational therapy consultation in a variety of settings has increased (Gourley, 2001). Occupational therapy practice is establishing a more visible presence in the community, some of which is in programs providing a more holistic, preventive approach to care.

> The shift from a primarily rehabilitative discipline to one that includes a more preventive component has broadened the practice arena for occupational therapists. Practitioners are finding a place in areas such as school violence prevention, ergonomics and home modification, and health and wellness programs. (Gourley, 2001, p. 16)

Although practitioners are being encouraged to work in community settings (considered the practice area of the future), community-based practice has not yet reached its full potential (Baum & Law, 1998; Scaffa, 2001). Occupational therapy can reach this potential only if practitioners become more knowledgeable about community systems; values, cultures, and folkways in specific environments; and the health goals of diverse community consumers (Jaffe, 1980, 1986; Scaffa, 2001). Community-based practice requires a collaborative service model in which practitioner, client, family, consultant, and community members develop communication networks on behalf of the individual consumer of occupational therapy services.

Community-based occupational therapy consultation will continue to grow in new markets. New areas of concern will include poverty, advocacy, and independent living (Marmer, 1995). In addition, the current technology-oriented information society requires consultants to be more knowledgeable with respect to the use of robotics and computers. Occupational therapy consultants may collaborate with other professionals in the community, including with industrial engineers to offer ergonomic consultation and with builders to provide home modification consultation (Gourley, 2001). Having occupational therapy expertise in using occupation as a health determinant and having an understanding of the effect that activity has on health are important assets not only in community-based practice but also in this rapidly changing society.

American consumers currently are more willing to pay for services that give them autonomy over their health care, in particular, using health professionals who provide a variety of services, including alternative methods and preventive care. "It's in these nontraditional areas that direct payment clients can often be found" (Gourley, 2001, p. 16). As more practitioners choose to go into private practice, especially in community-based environments, having multiple sources of revenue becomes increasingly important. Therefore, occupational therapy consultants may need to seek arenas in which clients are willing to pay for services out of pocket.

## Creating a Consultation Business Plan

A decision to own and operate a business is a significant step for any practitioner. The considerations and the complexities of entrepreneurship require major commitments of time, energy, and money. Self-education, risk-taking abilities, and organizational and management skills are important prerequisites (Beich, 1999; Epstein, 1992b). The world of business may be a new and unfamiliar place for the occupational therapy practitioner. Stepping into it requires research, in-depth planning, and professional advice. A broad array of books, periodicals, organizations, and information on the Internet are available as resources to practitioners contemplating this step (see chapter 9).

The prospective consultant should develop a business plan to provide an overall framework for the practice and a basis for decision making. It should include an assessment of the consultation target market, a statement of mission and goals, a business concept, and an organizational plan (see information on business plans in chapter 9). The aspiring entrepreneur should seek guidance from financial and legal advisers. At this important juncture, the knowledge of these experts will be critical in making final decisions with respect to issues such as the pros and cons of self-employment compared with partnership or incorporation and the development of contract formats for use with potential clients.

Being in business for oneself is an exciting and rewarding experience. Although the venture involves many risks, numerous frustrations, and extensive commitments, this model of practice is attracting increasing numbers of practitioners. The satisfaction of building a business, the opportunities offered in new markets, and the freedom of self-direction are among the many dividends (see chapter 9).

## Marketing Consultation Services

Success at consultation is related intimately to successful marketing (see chapter 7). The consultant performs an in-depth analysis of both the market that he or she has targeted and the ability of the business to be responsive. The establishment of an effective marketing mix consists of identifying a needed consultation service (a product) in a particular market; pricing this service competitively, which provides a persuasive proposal to a potential client; and using creative promotional strategies to build a referral base. The consultant must dedicate time, energy, and money to this important aspect of business (Epstein, 1992d).

The promotion plan is based on identification of an area of competence, potential practice environments, and the market plan (see chapter 7). This effort requires knowledge of the target market and the potential for acceptance of the service. In addition, it involves identifying all possible activities that can generate referrals or recommended clients, for example,

- Promoting services through tools such as professional brochures, letters, business cards, and local phone book listings;
- Networking with fellow practitioners, professionals in allied fields, and former clients and agency personnel who are advocates of the consultant's competence; and
- Doing research to gather marketing information from health planning reports, economic indicators of growing health services, local health classified ads, and state department of health listings of potential user agencies and organizations.

The potential consultant must be willing to contribute time and energy to community activities that focus on health concerns. A consultant's visibility can be heightened by providing free lectures, assisting in planning and running special programs, and participating in committees and on boards. These activities also will expand the consultant's knowledge base and resource network. The consultant might offer free information on a subject of interest to potential clients as a sales promotion technique, for example, providing current information on new rulings pertaining to the ADA.

Public relations strategies are important. These include news releases, articles published by the consultant, and lectures at meetings at which potential clients gather.

Consultation is a service product. It is intangible, directly related to the consultant providing the service. Consequently, it is also inseparable from the consultant's perspective and his or her interactions with the client. Consultant services are perishable. If a limited or fluctuating market exists, the consultant can be without work. Therefore, marketing must be a continuous process for the consultant. Indeed, the consultant must integrate consistent and meaningful marketing into his or her management of the consultation practice.

## Developing and Using Resources

To provide effective consultation services, the consultant must develop competence and devote time, money, and creative energy to build up necessary resources. Resources not only are important in a given consultation setting but also provide a natural support system for the consultant, who often practices in isolation. Included in this resource category are people, places, literature, educational experiences, and political and economic concerns. The old saying, "It is not what you know but who you know" needs modification for the consultant: "It is what and whom you know that help make you successful." Experience alone, especially within a sheltered setting, will not expand the consultant's knowledge base for consultation activities. Meeting other professionals within and outside occupational therapy broadens the consultant's perspective. Additionally, networking with local and national professional organizations can heighten the consultant's awareness of important trends, alert the consultant to changes affecting health care practice, and build a natural support system. These affiliations help the consultant develop a roster of experts who can provide needed information, advice, or direction on a specific problem. Membership in community and other professional organizations as well as participation in meetings and committees extend the resource network. Field visits stimulate information sharing and networking as well as help provide broader perspectives on geographic and socioeconomic differences that influence the responses of a given system.

The consultant should be prepared to continue his or her education to keep abreast of trends, changes, emerging issues affecting the health care market, and new information. This effort involves extensively reviewing professional and related literature as well as attending occupational therapy and multidisciplinary conferences and workshops. Additionally, continuing education helps maintain and improve the consultant's competence, and it increases the consultant's familiarity with differences in language usage and terminology in a given system, thus enhancing communication skills.

Economics and politics play major roles in shaping the delivery of health care. Legislation, newly enacted laws, changes in reimbursement methodologies, and revised guidelines for service delivery all have significant implications. The consultant can stay up-to-date with continual review of current publications and special newsletters.

Judicious use of resources helps maintain a broad and well-rounded knowledge base. This expanded perspective, with its related support system, encourages creativity and flexibility. A commitment to continued development of resources allows the consultant and the client to benefit from a comprehensive and current pool of information.

## Conclusion

Consultation is a rapidly expanding area of occupational therapy practice. As the pool of experienced practitioners increases and as settings diversify and proliferate, consultants are playing major roles in shaping future practice. Practitioners at every level of practice should take advantage of opportunities to build and apply their consultation skills. With greater experience, they can attempt more complex consultation tasks. As practitioners increase their visibility, particularly in the community, they must expand their knowledge of consultation, the varied systems in which intervention takes place, and the issues and trends that affect a system's growth. Successful consultation practice is based on maintaining and improving professional competence and developing evidence-based practice opportunities. Experience and competence are hallmarks of the community consultant, who will continue to forge new roles and directions for the profession.

Consulting has emerged as a major force in the health care arena, the business world, and society in general. Occupational therapy's role in prevention of disability and promotion of health will continue to grow with the expansion of consultation services, especially in community-based practice. The ultimate goal of any consultation is to help the client or client system to prevent further problems. The consultant should understand and use prevention principles to achieve preventive outcomes. The consultant model presented in this chapter is based on a human ecology perspective. These concepts will help prepare the practitioners of today and tomorrow to function in a world of rapid change.

## References

Allison, N. (Ed.). (1999). *The illustrated encyclopedia of body–mind disciplines.* New York: Rosen.

American Occupational Therapy Association. (1993a). Occupational therapy roles. *American Journal of Occupational Therapy, 47,* 1087–1099.

American Occupational Therapy Association. (1993b). *1993 member data survey.* Bethesda, MD: Author.

American Occupational Therapy Association. (1995). Concept paper: Service delivery in occupational therapy. *American Journal of Occupational Therapy, 49,* 1029–1031.

American Occupational Therapy Association. (1996). *ROTE: The role of occupational therapy with the elderly.* Bethesda, MD: Author.

American Occupational Therapy Association. (2001). *AOTA 2000 member compensation survey.* Bethesda, MD: Author.

American Occupational Therapy Association. (2002). Occupational therapy practice framework: Domain and process. *American Journal of Occupational Therapy, 56,* 609–639.

Americans with Disabilities Act of 1990, Pub. L. No. 101-336, 104 Stat. 327.

Baum, C., & Law, M. (1998). Community health: A responsibility, an opportunity, and a fit for occupational therapy. *American Journal of Occupational Therapy, 52,* 7–10.

Beich, E. (1999). *The business of consulting: The basics and beyond.* San Francisco: Jossey-Bass/Pfeiffer.

Bender, M., & Davidson, D. (2002). Freedom through technology. *Technology Special Interest Section Quarterly, 12*(1), 1, 2, 4.

Best, K., Noblitt, M., Synold, S., & Hughes, B. (2001). What are you fit for? Emerging practice areas for occupational therapists. *Advance for Occupational Therapy Practitioners, 17*(15), 30–33.

Croser, M. D. (2002). Word from Washington. *Journal of Mental Retardation, 40,* 168–177.

Dettner, P., Dyck, N., & Thurston, L. (1999). *Consultation, collaboration, and teamwork for students with special needs* (3rd ed.). Boston: Allyn & Bacon.

Diffendal, J. (2000). Community re-entry: Blazing new trails. *Advance for Occupational Therapy Practitioners, 16*(17), 10–11.

Dunn, W. (2000). *Best practice occupational therapy in community service with children and families.* Thorofare, NJ: Slack.

Dunn, W., Brown, C., & McGuigan, A. (1994). The ecology of human performance: A framework for considering the effect of context. *American Journal of Occupational Therapy, 48,* 595–607.

Epstein, C. F. (1979). Directions in long-term care. *Gerontology Specialty Section Newsletter, 2*(4), 1, 4.

Epstein, C. F. (1992a). Adult day-care consultation in a rural community. In E. G. Jaffe & C. F. Epstein (Eds.), *Occupational therapy consultation: Theory, principles, and practice* (pp. 419–430). St. Louis, MO: Mosby YearBook.

Epstein, C. F. (1992b). Developing a consultation practice. In E. G. Jaffe & C. F. Epstein (Eds.), *Occupational therapy consultation: Theory, principles, and practice* (pp. 634–649). St. Louis, MO: Mosby/YearBook.

Epstein, C. F. (1992c). Long-term care. In H. L. Hopkins & H. D. Smith (Eds.), *Willard and Spackman's occupational therapy* (8th ed., pp. 816–821). Philadelphia: Lippincott.

Epstein, C. F. (1992d). Marketing: A continuous process. In E. G. Jaffe & C. F. Epstein (Eds.), *Occupational therapy consultation: Theory, principles, and practice* (pp. 650–674). St. Louis, MO: Mosby/YearBook.

Gallessich, J. (1982). *The profession and practice of consultation.* San Francisco: Jossey-Bass.

Gilfoyle, E. M. (1992). Future directions: Vital connections. In E. G. Jaffe & C. F. Epstein (Eds.), *Occupational therapy consultation: Theory, principles, and practice* (pp. 777–783). St. Louis, MO: Mosby/YearBook.

Gourley, M. (2001). Consumers recognize the value of occupational therapy. *Occupational Therapy Practice, 6*(7), 15–18.

Grady, A. P. (1992). Technology adoption: Linking through communication. In E. G. Jaffe & C. F. Epstein (Eds.), *Occupational therapy consultation: Theory, principles, and practice* (pp. 581–590). St. Louis, MO: Mosby/YearBook.

Grady, A. P. (1995). Building inclusive community: A challenge for occupational therapy (1994 Eleanor Clarke Slagle Lecture). *American Journal of Occupational Therapy, 49,* 300–310.

Grossman, J. (1977). Preventive health care and community programming (nationally speaking). *American Journal of Occupational Therapy, 31,* 351–354.

Hoelscher, D., & Taylor, S. (2000). Ergonomics consultation: An opportunity for occupational therapists. *Occupational Therapy Practice, 5*(1), 16–18, 19.

Idol, L., Paolucci-Whitcomb, P., & Nevin, A. (1994). *Collaborative consultation* (2nd ed.). Austin, TX: PRO-ED.

Individuals with Disabilities Education Act, Final Regulations, Pub. L. 1205-17, 34 C.F.R. Part 300 (1999).

Jaffe, E. G. (1980). The role of the occupational therapist as a community consultant: Primary prevention in mental health programming. *Occupational Therapy in Mental Health, 1*(2), 47–62.

Jaffe, E. G. (1986). Prevention, "an idea whose time has come": The role of occupational therapy in disease prevention and health promotion. *American Journal of Occupational Therapy, 40,* 749–752.

Jaffe, E. G. (1992a). Health education consultation in the workplace. In E. G. Jaffe & C. F. Epstein (Eds.), *Occupational therapy consultation: Theory, principles, and practice* (pp. 461–477). St. Louis, MO: Mosby/YearBook.

Jaffe, E. G. (1992b). Preparation for consultation. In E. G. Jaffe & C. F. Epstein (Eds.), *Occupational therapy consultation: Theory, principles, and practice* (pp. 118–134). St. Louis, MO: Mosby/YearBook.

Jaffe, E. G. (1992c). Theoretical concepts of consultation. In E. G. Jaffe & C. F. Epstein (Eds.), *Occupational therapy consultation: Theory, principles, and practice* (pp. 15–54). St. Louis, MO: Mosby/YearBook.

Jaffe, E. G. (1996). Occupational therapy consultation in a managed care environment. *OT Practice, 1*(3), 26–31.

Jaffe, E. G., & Epstein, C. F. (Eds.). (1992a). *Occupational therapy consultation: Theory, principles, and practice.* St. Louis, MO: Mosby/YearBook.

Jaffe, E. G., & Epstein, C. F. (1992b). The process of consultation. In E. G. Jaffe & C. F. Epstein (Eds.), *Occupational therapy consultation: Theory, principles, and practice* (pp. 135–166). St. Louis, MO: Mosby/YearBook.

Jaffe, E. G., & Epstein, C. F. (1992c). Toward a theoretical model of occupational therapy consultation. In E. G. Jaffe & C. F. Epstein (Eds.), *Occupational therapy consultation: Theory, principles, and practice* (pp. 676–713). St. Louis, MO: Mosby/YearBook.

LaGrossa, V., & Saxe, S., (1998). *The consultative approach: Partnering for results!* San Francisco: Jossey-Bass/Pfeiffer.

Lewin, K. (1951). *Theory in social science.* New York: Harper.

Lippitt, G., & Lippitt, R. (1986). *The consulting process in action* (2nd ed.). San Diego: University Associates.

Maddox, G. L. (Ed.). (2001). *Encyclopedia of aging* (3rd ed.). New York: Springer.

Mann, W. (2001). Assistive technology and older adults. *Occupational Therapy Practice, 6*(10), 12–15.

Marmer, L. (1995). Community-based OTs: Short on needed skills? *Advance for Occupational Therapists, 11*(18), 11, 50.

Rainville, E. B., Cermak, S. A., & Murray, E. A. (1996). Supervision and consultation services for pediatric occupational therapists. *American Journal of Occupational Therapy, 50,* 725–731.

Scaffa, M. (2001). *Occupational therapy in community-based practice settings*. Philadelphia: F. A. Davis.

Swinth, Y., & Mailloux, Z. (Eds.). (2002). Addressing sensory processing in the schools. *Occupational Therapy Practice, 7*(2), 8–13.

Technology-Related Assistance for Individuals with Disabilities Act of 1988, Pub. L. No. 100-407, 102 Stat. 1044.

Ticket to Work and Work Incentives Improvement Act of 1999, Pub. L. 106-170.

Ulschak, F. L., & SnowAntle, S. M. (1990). *Consultation skills for health care professionals*. San Francisco: Jossey-Bass.

West, W. L. (1969). The growing importance of prevention. *American Journal of Occupational Therapy, 23*, 226–321.

Wiemer, R. B. (1972). Some concepts of prevention as an aspect of community health. *American Journal of Occupational Therapy, 26*, 1–9.

Williams, M. S., & Shellenberger, S. (2001). *Take five! Staying alive at home and school*. Albuquerque, NM: Therapy Works.

Yerxa, E. J. (1978). The occupational therapist as consultant and researcher. In H. L. Hopkins & H. D. Smith (Eds.), *Willard and Spackman's occupational therapy* (5th ed., pp. 689–693). Philadelphia: Lippincott.

# Leading and Organizing

# CHAPTER 11

# Communication
# in the Workplace

Catherine Nielson, MPH, OTR/L, FAOTA

*"Without credible communication, and a lot of it,
employee hearts and minds are never captured."*

JOHN P. KOTTER

**Catherine Nielson, MPH, OTR/L,
FAOTA,** is professor and director in
the Division of Occupational
Science, Department of Allied
Health Sciences, School of
Medicine, University of North
Carolina at Chapel Hill. She
received her BS in occupational
therapy from the Medical College
of Georgia and her MPH in health
policy and administration from
the School of Public Health,
University of North Carolina. She
has been an administrator in both
clinical and academic settings for
most of her career and considers
administration a specialty area of
practice that requires a unique skills
set and a propensity for problem-
solving and development of ideas
and people.

## Key Terms and Concepts

**Communication method.** The verbal, written, or technological channel for transmitting communication.

**Communication roadblock.** Environmental factors or verbal responses that halt communication.

**Effective workplace communication.** The acquisition, evaluation, and dissemination of information that is used to support daily work and achieve organizational goals while considering the needs of employees, the nature of the work, and the impact of organizational and external factors.

**Nonverbal communication.** The kinesics, paralanguage, touch, proxemics, and other graphic and symbolic means of communication.

**Position power.** The information, authority, and responsibility tied to a position.

**Receiving skills.** The communication skills of observing, listening, and empathizing.

**Sending skills.** The communication skills of questioning, describing, and concluding.

## Learning Objectives

After completing this chapter, you should be able to do the following:

- Explain how communication skills support a manager's successful performance across key responsibility areas.

- Discuss the communication aspects of the transition from clinician to manager.

- Describe fundamental communication skills.

- Identify barriers to effective communication.

- Discuss the application of communication methods to specific management functions.

- Explain an integrated approach to managerial communication.

The ability to communicate effectively is a core skill for managers. In an era when emphasis is often placed on productivity, financial management, and technological abilities, communication skills can be overlooked or undervalued. Yet, the ability of the manager to express information, meaning, and values underlies virtually all other management functions. Success in human resource management, in the acquisition and the management of fiscal resources, and in planning and decision-making are all dependent on the manager's skills in acquiring and sharing information. A manager must be able to understand and use information to build and maintain a cohesive workforce, to create and sustain a supportive workplace, and to represent and make known to other levels of the organization and to the public the work that is accomplished.

The control of information is power in organizations (McCall & Cousins, 1990). Position in the organization provides access to varying amounts and types of information and establishes the authority and responsibility to use the information. However, access to information or organizational authority is not what creates power; what is powerful is the skill in using information to achieve organizational goals. *Communication*—the process that links one's access to information and one's ability to act on that information—defines the successful manager.

The manager's ability (a) to understand communication as a relationship and process and (b) to continually develop and refine fundamental skills in communication is essential to acquiring information from all levels of the organization and to analyzing, disseminating, and using that information. In workplace communication, the manager must understand the use of core communication skills in a managerial context and must see how that context influences the nature, timing, and impact of all communications. Although management communication shares a common skills base with all other communication areas, specific contextual differences shape workplace communications. Issues of power and authority, organizational politics, employee confidentiality, marketplace competition and position, and various legal parameters are examples of the kinds of contextual factors that the manager must acknowledge and incorporate into the communication process while still attending to the use of well-developed communication skills and principles.

*Workplace communication*, then, may be defined as the acquisition, evaluation, and dissemination of information to support daily work and achieve organizational goals. Effective workplace communication occurs when the manager uses well-developed communication skills while showing sensitivity to individual employees and to the nature of their work and acknowledging the impact of organizational culture, the formal organization, and any external parameters and issues. The effective manager recognizes the complexities and demands of workplace communication and views the ongoing development of communication skills as central to his or her managerial role.

The development of effective workplace communication skills is a career-long process as skills are revisited, refined, and used in evolving and changing contexts.

This chapter provides a general overview of communication skills and introduces some of the contextual skills and factors related to workplace communications. Communication skills are easy to simplify or overlook in career development. The complexity of the topic requires the manager to search out and use additional resources that provide more in-depth information on topical areas that are only briefly described in this chapter.

## Communication Aspects of the Transition From Clinician to Manager

The position of supervisor is the first type of management position to which clinicians are promoted that removes them from a primary clinical role. In a managerial career path, this type of position is often the initial step to accepting responsibilities in human resource management and, eventually, in other functional areas of management such as financial management, quality management, and program development. Often overlooked in this transition is the communication skill that is necessary to successfully assume and perform these new responsibilities.

Umiker (1998) maintained that most clinicians are not prepared for this type of advancement and that, in fact, the reason for their promotion is often their clinical competence rather than either supervisory or managerial potential or skills. In making this first move, the clinician is often overwhelmed by the new responsibilities and typically concentrates on developing skills in procedural areas of human resource management such as writing position descriptions, monitoring employee performance, and conducting performance reviews. However, as Umiker emphasized, new supervisors not only must maintain a level of clinical skill but also must learn the technical and procedural skills of their supervisory role while expanding their interpersonal skills and developing a "modicum of political skill" (p. 2). Ultimately, communication skills, which involve integrating interpersonal and political skills, are the core abilities that enable the new supervisor to access information and develop organizational contacts and, thus, gain confidence and skill in the new role. When a person moves from a supervisory position to a management position that involves more diverse responsibilities, these same transition issues often recur.

The development and use of communication skills in the transitional phases of a supervisory position or management career are integral to internalizing the new role and responsibilities and to a gaining a new perspective on the organization as well as on one's position and responsibilities in the organization. Three crucial factors characterize communication in this transition: (a) language, (b) position power, and (c) personal approach or style. First, one must acquire a new language, including the words, meanings, and actions associated with the words. The role of supervisor or manager requires fluency in the languages of other disciplines and functional areas of the organization. Just as professional jargon exists within occupational therapy, professional or organizational jargon occurs across the areas of management responsibility.

For example, in human resource management, the new supervisor must understand terms such as *performance standards, grievance procedures,* and *position justification.* Words are symbols for meaning and action and come to represent rules for a work group; thus, understanding the language includes knowing and performing the actions and responsibilities that are linked to the word (McCall & Cousins, 1990). A first step in the transition process is to acquire the language so responsibilities and procedures are clear and so the new supervisor can translate accurately back and forth between occupational therapy and other departments.

The second crucial factor of communication during this time is an understanding of position power and organizational hierarchy as well as of the effect these concepts have on communication. Developing this understanding is one of the most difficult aspects of transitioning from a clinical role to a managerial role. A promotion to a supervisory or management position places the individual in a position of greater authority and responsibility. Suddenly, the new manager has access to more complex and sensitive information and is expected to use that information in making decisions that affect the work lives of former peers. Information, authority, and responsibility that are tied to a position are known collectively as *position power.* The supervisor now speaks and acts not as a peer colleague but as the person with the title, authority, and responsibility of the position. Words, statements, and casual comments take on different meanings as staff members attribute them to the position rather than to the person. At this point in the transition, the new supervisor must begin to accept and assume the full responsibility of the role, including the changes in relationships and communication patterns with former peers.

Finally, communication in the transition phase involves the merging of language and position power into a repertoire of communication skills and approaches—a personal communication style that is consistent with the new role. New supervisors, often uncomfortable with their role and unsuspecting of the change in how they are being interpreted, can be caught off guard when confronted with the impact of their words. After initially realizing this change in communication with former peers (i.e., new subordinates), new supervisors in transition typically adopt a single approach to handing all communications. One supervisor may take an exclusively authoritarian approach to staff communications while another supervisor may try to share all information and involve staff members in all decisions. The exclusive use of any approach is dangerous because situational nuances vary and affect the optimal communication style for the situation.

McCall and Cousins (1990) described various approaches that the supervisor can take in managing superior–subordinate communication. The approaches integrate the skills of telling, listening, asking, and problem-solving in various combinations that enable a supervisor to relay information to and work with subordinates by matching the situation, individuals, and skill mix. The important point is that, during and after the transition to manager, the individual must interpret each communication instance and tailor an approach to the situation. Clearly, the ability to interpret situations is one that develops with attention, reflection, and experience. Nevertheless, a new supervisor will be more effective more quickly when he or she has a base of awareness that one's personal communication style must vary with the situation.

Although the acquisition of a new language, the acceptance of position power, and the development of a multifaceted communication style are crucial in the transition from clinician to manager, perhaps the most fundamental communication element during the transition period and throughout the manager's career is the continuous development and use of well-developed communication skills. Communication skills are the core of management performance, but they often are easily taken for granted. All managers need to reflect periodically on their communication skills and be willing to refresh and renew their basic skills. As McCall and Cousins (1990) stated, "The more we know of the process of communication and the more skilled we become in its practice, the less likely we are to misunderstand or be misunderstood" (p. 34).

## Fundamentals of Communication: An Overview

"Eighty percent of the people who fail at work do so for one reason: They do not relate well to other people. One's productivity as a supervisor or manager . . . is greatly enhanced by the ability to communicate well. In fact, it is difficult to think of a single job in which communication is unimportant" (Bolton, 1986, p. 7). Bolton simply and emphatically stated the importance of good communication skills. He went on to discuss the irony that, although communication is the "lifeblood" (p. 6) of all relationships, the ability to communicate is often left to chance development. Experts in communication have agreed that most people, having learned to communicate from parents, teachers, and cultural influences, have a variable mix of effective and dysfunctional ways of communicating (Bolton, 1986; Haskell, 2001; Maurer, 1994; McCall & Cousins, 1990; McLagan & Krembs, 1995; Ribbens & Thompson, 2001; Rozelle, Druckman, & Baxter, 1997). Additionally, they agreed that communication skills could be improved on and developed at any point in one's life or career.

The communication literature abounds with models, approaches, and perspectives on the development of effective communication skills. This section is not meant to be either an exhaustive review of the communication literature or a model for developing communication skills. Rather, the chapter as a whole is an overview of the communication process and the core skills within that process. Aspiring and experienced managers are encouraged to use this information as a starting point and then search out and use a resource on communication skills that matches their current level and understanding of communication and that challenges their next stage of development.

Communication models describe communication as a reciprocal process, exchange, or relationship (Bolton, 1986; McCall & Cousins, 1990). Commonly, communication skills within the process are categorized as receiving or listening skills and sending or expressive skills (Bolton, 1986; McLagan & Krembs, 1995). Both skill sets address the meaning and purpose of communication to enhance understanding (Bolton, 1986; McCall & Cousins, 1990; McLagan & Krembs, 1995). Communication is acknowledged as having both verbal and nonverbal components and as being contextually influenced (McCall & Cousins, 1990; McLagan & Krembs, 1995; Ribbens & Thompson, 2001; Rozelle et al., 1997). Additional skills are often identified for use in challenging communication situations such as conflict resolution, collaboration, and interactions that require confidentiality or sensitivity (Bolton, 1986).

## Reciprocal Process

Communication first must be recognized as a simultaneous process of (a) sending messages and noting their reception and (b) receiving messages and noting the expressed intent (McCall & Cousins, 1990). Communication depends on a successful blend of the content (i.e., what is said) and the process (i.e., how it is sent, interpreted, refined, and ultimately understood). Effective communication does not simply provide information but engages in a dialogue in which parties exchange and process information until they reach a shared meaning.

Regardless of the number of people involved in the exchange, the hierarchical relationship of the individuals, or the purpose of the communication, the interaction should be viewed as an exchange that links two or more people. One should pay attention to the individuals and how to optimize the relationship and the purpose of the communication. Bolton (1986) articulated this value by stating, "In communication, skills alone are not sufficient" (p. 259). He continued by stressing the need for honesty, acceptance, respect, support, and empathy as fundamental to the communication process.

In many relationships, one participant often assumes a greater responsibility for maintaining the relationship and for ensuring that the intended meanings are understood. In workplace communication, this higher degree of responsibility falls to the manager because of his or her position and responsibility. The manager is responsible not only for the development and use of his or her own communication skills but also for the quality of communication throughout the department, which includes staff development in the area of workplace communication skills. To create a positive environment for reciprocal communication, the manager should be aware of basic communication skills and the aspects of communication that are unique in the workplace. For example, managers should recognize that the hierarchical relationship between the supervisor and employee could affect the employee's comfort and skill in initiating interaction with a superior. In addition, the competing demands for quality and productivity coupled with the intense nature of the work may result in an emotional state for an employee that minimizes his or her ability to articulate concerns or questions. In any situation, the manager must assume responsibility for initiating interaction, coaching the employee, and working to achieve a satisfactory level of understanding.

## Sending and Receiving Skills

At the heart of the communication process are the skill sets of sending and receiving information (Bolton, 1986; McLagan & Krembs, 1995). McLagan and Krembs offered a simple framework for understanding these skills by defining both receptive skills (receiving) and expressive skills (sending). They cautioned that a careful balance is needed between the skill sets for communication to be direct, respectful, and purposeful. Receptive skills include observing, listening, and empathizing. For each skill, McLagan and Krembs provided an outcome that keeps the intent and focus of the skill intact. Observing results in "accurate and specific information about behavior, feelings, patterns of behavior, and results" (p. 29). Listening achieves a common clarity and understanding. Empathizing attends to the relationship to increase trust and rapport. In *People Skills,* Bolton (1986) enhanced understanding and performance of these basic skills sets with a further delineation of some of the skills. He expanded listening into three skills groups—attending, following, and reflecting—and added specific behavioral, nonverbal, and verbal actions to enact the skills (p. 33).

According to McLagan and Krembs (1995), expressive skills are questioning, describing, and concluding. The expressive skills are also defined through outcomes. Questioning "serves to bring relevant information into the discussion and prevent misunderstanding" (p. 34). Describing allows both participants to enhance their common understanding. Concluding is a process of clarifying the positions, decisions, and consequences of the communication. Bolton (1986) again added to an understanding of sending information by emphasizing that communication is effective only when there is a reciprocal process of listening and asserting, or "disclosure to another what the speaker feels, needs, desires" (p. 118). In Bolton's view, assertive communication is a critical expressive skill that blends the speaker's content and emotion into an open and honest message.

In both of these models, the terms that are used to describe the skills of sending and receiving are understandable and simple. The complexity comes in practicing the skills and in changing habitual, perhaps ineffective, ways of receiving and sending information. Bolton (1986) and McLagan and Krembs (1995) described the sending and receiving skill sets as being both active and interactive as well as requiring deliberate attention and practice to achieve mastery. The deceptively simple skills of sending and receiving information are the core of the communication process. However, attention to nonverbal aspects of communication is necessary to add depth of understanding and clarity.

## Nonverbal Communication

In an article that reviews studies of nonverbal communication, Rozelle et al. (1997) provided a thorough review of all aspects of nonverbal communication. As a result of their work, they cautioned against the development of universal principles related to effective nonverbal communication and, instead, advocated that nonverbal behavior should be considered only in a specific context because of the individual, cultural, and situational factors influencing nonverbal behaviors. Knapp (as cited in Rozelle et al., 1997) listed seven types of nonverbal communication behaviors, a list that emphasized the complexity and uniqueness of each individual's pattern of nonverbal communication:

- Kinesics (body language)
- Paralanguage (the way words are spoken)
- Physical contact (touch)
- Proxemics (space between speakers)
- Physical characteristics of the speakers
- Artifacts or adornments of speakers
- Environmental factors.

In examining this list, one can clearly see how the interaction of these nonverbal factors with the spoken exchange can (a) contribute to a more accurate understanding or meaning and purpose or (b) result in misinterpretation and confusion. During the communication process, nonverbal factors must be considered and clarified through the use of verbal skills such as observing, listening, questioning, and concluding.

Ribbens and Thompson (2001) reinforced the importance of body language in communication, equating communication without body language to writing without punctuation. They maintained that less than 10% of the meaning of face-to-face messages occurs through words, whereas tone, posture, and gestures contribute 90% of the meaning. Again, these authors offered a cautionary note about interpreting body language because personal prejudices or cultural differences may influence the interpretation. They advocated considering nonverbal information as further clues to the meaning of the message. Finally, McCall and Cousins (1990) offered a summary note on the importance of nonverbal communication, identifying nonverbal communication as "a host of graphic, olfactory, tactile, spatial, temporal and symbolic means of communication" (p. 45). They stressed the complementary nature of verbal and nonverbal communication and the need to attend to both to clarify the natural ambiguity of words alone.

## Context or Situation

In much of the communication literature, the emphasis is on the individuals and their use of verbal and nonverbal skills. However, communication takes place within specific physical and social environments, and these environments also influence communication. McCall and Cousins (1990) described the concept of situation as encompassing the specific topic that is being talked about, the locale of the conversation, and the relationships of the interacting parties. Any one of these environmental factors will influence the nature, purpose, and meaning of a communication. For example, the interaction between a supervisor and a subordinate at a social gathering is quite different from an interaction between the same two parties in the supervisor's office at the workplace. In addition, one must consider multiple other environmental factors that can have an impact on and influence the communication.

The manager's challenge is to create a shared context within the workplace for all subordinates and, thus, increase the likelihood of common interpretations and productive communication. Multiple discussions of organizational and individual values and of similarities and differences in personal and workplace experiences serve to develop the shared context for the work group. The informal or social aspect of the workplace is an important vehicle for developing a shared context. As coworkers share stories, they more clearly understand individual contexts, they create a common context, and they enhance communications among themselves. The manager must support and participate equally in this process as a means of enhancing context and strengthening communication. The participants must integrate all of the verbal, nonverbal, and situational elements to understand the full meaning within a communication.

## Meaning and Purpose

Parties achieve clarity of meaning, common purpose, and the desired outcomes of communication when they carefully use the receptive and expressive skills in the exchange of ideas, values, and information while also attending to reciprocal nonverbal cues and contextual influences. Relying on words alone can result in miscommunication because words often have different meanings for people that are based on people's life experiences and backgrounds. A common understanding of meaning and purpose occurs when parties carefully listen and check for understanding of the spoken word while they verify the feelings and emotions behind the words.

Clinically, this same skill set contributes to interactive, conditional, and narrative reasoning. Clinicians regularly use these skills to understand a client as a unique individual and to perceive the effect that the client's condition has had (or is having) on his or her everyday life. As clinicians, occupational therapy practitioners naturally look beyond a client's words to other cues to form a complete picture that reveals the depth of the client's reactions. The manager can transfer this skill from the clinic to the manager's office by acknowledging overt expressions of feelings, paying attention to more subtle cues, such as word choice or body language, and by admitting his or her own emotional responses.

Again, the complexity of effective communication is realized not in knowing what has to happen but in using the different skills at the right time; attending to multiple factors simultaneously; and seeing the communication as a process rather than a single, linear event. With time for reflection and practice and acknowledgment of the ongoing development of these basic skills, the manager will build an effective repertoire of basic communication skills.

## Additional Skills for Managers

Although the basic communication skills adequately support most of the manager's communication, some situations require additional skills. In particular, conflict resolution skills and the ability to handle confidential communications are more common in workplace communication than in other areas. In his enduring text on communication skills, Bolton (1986) provided great insight into the area of conflict and the skills that are necessary for preventing, controlling, and resolving conflict in the workplace. Bolton described conflict as an inevitable part of the human experience, which can be either disruptive (or destructive) or beneficial.

The outcome of conflict is determined in part by the manager's ability to evaluate the potential for conflict (or the actual conflict) and to take the appropriate action given the nature of the conflict. An initial distinction must be made between "realistic conflict where there are opposing needs, goals, or values . . . [and] nonrealistic conflict . . . from ignorance, error, historical tradition and prejudice, poor organizational structure, displaced hostility, or the need for tension release" (Bolton, 1986, p. 215). Generally, realistic conflict must be faced and worked through so growth can occur, whereas nonrealistic conflict is either prevented through strategies such as staff development and continuing education or controlled through workplace rules, policies, and procedures. Conflict resolution relies heavily on the ability to use not only basic communication skills but also additional skill in defusing emotions.

Communication issues in the workplace often have an ethical dimension, which is reflected when the speaker decides what information, motives, or feelings to disclose as well as when the listener decides how and when to respond. Confidential information is often expressed in workplace communication. Staff members' compensation and performance evaluations are examples of information the manager must hold in confidence. When a staff member shares personal information, the manager must be an ethical listener. Staff members who come to the manager with personal concerns are taking a risk. The manager should respect that risk. He or she should first decide whether or not to accept the responsibility of receiving personal information. If the manager decides to listen to the information, he or she must consider it privileged. If the manager decides not to engage in a personal exchange, then he or she has a human responsibility to direct the staff member to appropriate support systems.

When staff members share personal information that affects their work, the ethical issues for the manager increase. The manager is in the position of balancing his or her own responsibilities of the organization against a staff member's needs and rights. In most situations that raise ethical issues, there is no right answer. The manager should approach ethical issues in communication just as he or she would approach other ethical issues. A systematic exploration and analysis of the problem can generate options and identify the risks of taking each option. The manager's final decision should be the choice that seems to do the most good with the least amount of harm.

## Barriers to Communication

Communication is a complex activity. Because so many factors are involved in communicating effectively, problems inevitably occur and communication is blocked. Both environmental and personal factors can cause problems (Rakich, Longest, & Darr,

1992). Environmental factors include conditions in both the physical setting and the organizational culture. A chaotic and distracting environment will obviously slow down or sidetrack a conversation. A formal room arrangement can reinforce power and authority and, consequently, intimidate some speakers. An organization with many rules governing communication can stifle the free exchange of ideas and information. Personal factors range from motivation to actual skill in expressing ideas or listening effectively. A high degree of stress can alter a communication. Poor communication skills or inappropriate communication methods can cloud meaning and damage the process. Differences in personal communication styles and conflicting motives can produce barriers (Bolton, 1986; Rakich et al., 1992).

Ideally, the manager recognizes the potential for communication breakdowns to occur and uses good communication skills to prevent them. However, although the use of good communication skills can often prevent breakdowns, it does not provide complete protection. Stressful situations encountered in the workplace can lead to inadvertent responses that, although not intended to be harmful, become so in combination with the emotions surrounding a serious problem or need. If the manager is unaware of the type of responses that can obstruct communication, then he or she can easily make a comment that blocks further conversations, stops problem-solving, or increases the agitation of the situation (Bolton, 1986).

Bolton (1986) considered three categories of responses that can break down communication: (a) judging, (b) providing solutions, and (c) avoiding the expressed concerns. An important point to realize is that none of these responses is used with the intention of stopping communication. In fact, in many instances, they are natural, initial responses to someone in distress. The potential for these kinds of responses to halt communication becomes more apparent when they are studied in comparison to the skills of good communication. The manager may attempt to identify, judge, or label the problem or may attempt to minimize the problem and the subordinate's reactions. In either case, the manager has failed to listen or elicit information and has not read nonverbal cues. He or she has offered an interpretation—a judgment—far too early in the exchange. Providing solutions can range from the benign offer of advice to an authoritative order for an action. By responding with this approach, the manager has failed to use good receiving skills and may compound the original problem or create a new one by failing to understand the problem before trying to solve it. Finally, the manager may stop the conversation by diverting the content or ignoring the emotions of the interaction. In this scenario, the manager violates the concept of the communication as a relationship in which the individual's needs are to be considered with respect and honesty.

In the workplace, these communication shutdowns are as inevitable as conflict. As with conflict, the manager's responsibilities are to prevent breakdowns from occurring and to resolve residual consequences. The consistent use of effective communication skills and the development of subordinates' communication abilities offer the first line of prevention. Given the ease and, therefore, the prevalence of inadvertent communication roadblocks, prevention is not the only answer, however. Once communication has broken down, then the manager has the responsibility to identify the source of the problem and initiate corrections.

## Gender-Based, Cultural, and Generational Differences in Communication

An awareness of differences in communication that occur because of gender, culture, and generation is the final piece one needs to build a solid base in communication skill (Barna, 1997; Davidhizar & Cramer, 2000; Davidhizar, Dowd, & Giger, 1999; Kupperschmidt, 2000; Zemke, Raines, & Filipczak, 2000). With increasing diversity in the workplace, the effective manager must be able to communicate equally well with superiors and subordinates of different gender, cultural backgrounds, and generations. The use of good communication skills is the starting point for interactions with all individuals of a diverse class. The manager can apply common principles to facilitate communication with anyone of a different gender, cultural background, or generation. These principles include

- Acknowledge and set aside stereotypes; maintain an open mind.
- Get to know the individual as an individual.
- Anticipate differences, and actively and openly pursue discussion of them.
- Use conflict resolution techniques as needed to address differing values.
- Value the differences the individual brings to the workplace; see these as strengths.

The manager uses his or her basic communication skills with heightened awareness and intensity when applying these principles. Communication is approached naturally but with an acknowledgment that inherent differences exist between the parties. The skills and process of communication are directed at understanding those differences and developing a working relationship. The relationship is enhanced if the manager acknowledges the specific differences involved in communicating across gender, culture, or generation.

Gender is a powerful influence on communication because men and women continue to have different life experiences that shape their use and definition of words and implied meanings. In an article that reviewed gendered differences in language, Payne (2001) examined numerous studies of male and female communication styles and concluded that men "use more intensive, aggressive, task-oriented, argumentative language forms," whereas women use "less intense language, show more concern with internal psychological states, and are more gentle and compassionate" (pp. 113–114). Payne also revealed that women will use more argumentative and rational language than men would use when in an aggressive situation. This issue has great significance in a profession such as occupational therapy, which has a majority of women. Female occupational therapy managers often deal with men at higher levels in the organization. Male occupational therapy managers supervise staffs of primarily women. At the staff level, men are a minority presence and must interact with female superiors and coworkers. In all three situations, differences in the ways that men and women relate can break down or delay effective communication.

Cultural diversity and its impact on the workplace are readily acknowledged (Davidhizar et al., 1999). Communication in a culturally diverse work setting is especially vulnerable to misinterpretation or misunderstanding because many of the critical elements of communication are influenced by culture. Vocabulary, grammatical structures, voice quality, intonation, rhythm, rate of speech, pronunciation, silences, touch, facial expression, eye movement, and body posture vary across and among people in a cultural group. The manager must understand the unique communication variables associated with the specific cultural group but, at the same time, not fall into stereotyping or ignoring individual differences in skill and style.

One current area of study focusing on group differences that affect relationships and communication in the workplace is the area of cross-generational differences (Kupperschmidt, 2000; Zemke et al., 2000). The work in this area of study acknowledges the need for individualizing communication but introduces the perspective that understanding generational information can explain conflicting values, ambitions, views, and mind-sets that have an impact on communication in the workplace (Zemke, et al, 2000). Zemke et al. admitted that, although there have always been multiple generations working in organizations, in the past, the generations were "sequestered from each other by organizational stratification" (p. 10). Now, senior staff members often assume positions once occupied exclusively by the youngest employees. With downsizing and the flattening of the administrative structures of organizations, the "more horizontal, more spatially compact workplace has stirred the generations into a mix of much different proportions" (p. 10).

Four distinct generational cohorts work side by side in today's workplace. These cohorts are the "Veterans, 1922–1943; the Baby Boomers, 1943–1960; the Generation Xers, 1960–1980; and the Nexters, those born 1980 and after" (Zemke et al., 2000, p. 18). Each group has had defining life events and has shared life experiences that cross gender, socioeconomic, and cultural boundaries. Additionally, each group shapes views and attitudes toward work that influence performance, relationships, and communication in the workplace. Managers are encouraged to acknowledge and make use of generational differences and strengths rather than ignore the differences or attempt to minimize them and homogenize the staff.

As with the development of basic communication competencies, the manager must not only develop his or her expertise in the area of diversity communication but also must foster the competency of staff members in this area. The manager must be able to advance communication and cooperation within the work group and build competence among the staff members in interacting with coworkers who are of different gender, culture, or generation.

## Fundamentals of Communication: A Summary

As the person responsible for initiating interactions with staff members, the manager has the opportunity to craft his or her approach. The manager can think through the proposed conversation, focus clearly on the message, and choose words carefully to express his or her meaning. Sharing information with staff members, initiating a dialogue, developing understanding among staff members, and encouraging an open communication loop are powerful management tools. The manager must use these skills judiciously to maximize the effectiveness of reciprocal communication.

First, the manager is in the best position to distinguish information from communication. Information is factual, for example, data, news, or announcements. "Communication deals with factors such as feelings, values, expectations, and perceptions, which demand that the individual believe or do something or become a particular kind of person" (Devereaux, 1992, p. 264). The manager must correctly decide whether the situation calls for information sharing or a dialogue among staff members.

Second, the manager must determine whether the communication need is urgent, important, or both. Urgent matters call for a rapid response. Important issues are those that relate clearly to the mission and the purpose of the organization. When a rapid response is necessary, the manager may take action and then inform staff members of the action and the rationale for it. With important issues, the manager should communicate with staff members to ensure a common understanding of the issues and possible actions. When issues are both urgent and important, the manager must first take action and inform staff members and then quickly follow up with an explanation and an opportunity for discussion. An accurate assessment of the nature of the situation will ensure that communication with staff members is efficient and effective.

Finally, the manager must determine the timing of multiple pieces of information. Urgency and importance may overlap in such a way that the manager must communicate simultaneously on several issues. At other times, communication may occur sequentially. In either instance, the manager should attempt to choose the optimal timing to ensure open communication. In all situations, the primary communication objective is to keep staff members adequately informed and appropriately involved in issues but not overwhelmed by a volume of unnecessary information at the wrong time.

## Examples of Communication Skills in the Workplace

Communication methods are conduits for messages. Increasingly, the manager has to consider multiple mechanisms for communicating, from low to high technology. A manager typically uses a mix of communication methods for a single message, depending on the content and the intent of the message as well as the number and types of intended recipients.

Selecting the most appropriate communication method requires an examination of (a) the message, (b) the recipient, and (c) the method. Qualities of each influence the final choice. The sender of a message should evaluate factors such as the need for confidentiality or privacy; the need for dialogue; the importance, the length, the complexity, and the urgency of the message; and the need for a permanent record of the communication. Considerations relative to the recipient include his or her skills and comfort with various communication methods, the hierarchical relationship between the sender and recipient, the familiarity of the sender and the recipient, and the proximity of the recipient. Finally, the sender should evaluate the method used to communicate in terms of reliability, cost in time and money, access, confidentiality, and the skill needed to use the method.

Today's manager has multiple means available for communication. The growth in the communication industry is both overwhelming and exciting. A manager can choose the most effective method of communication for any situation from an array of traditional and technologically based methods. The manager engages in numerous interactions across the workday by using a variety of communication methods. Commonly, methods can be categorized as verbal, written, and technology based. Using the basic communication strategies involves unique considerations in each of the methods.

## Verbal Communication

Verbal communication pulls together all of the communication skills and provides the most robust atmosphere for in-depth communication. Very likely, the majority of the manager's communication occurs in this mode in either one-to-one or group situations.

### One-to-One Interactions

The manager's range of responsibilities across the human resource cycle necessitates ongoing and open exchanges with employees from the interviewing and recruitment stages through supervision and development to evaluation and performance review. At any point in this cycle, problematic interactions can occur, especially when a manager must provide critical performance feedback, disciplinary action, or termination of employment. Human resource management is a series of both positive and negative interactions. In many of these interactions, the employee's livelihood, professional performance, identity, and esteem are the content of the interactions. These situations require a heightened awareness to the individual's needs, to confidentiality, to privacy, and to the manager's comfort level with sensitive issues.

Maurer's (1994) work on providing feedback is a useful reference for managers in the highly sensitive area of communication around performance issues. His tips for giving feedback are a practical, simple set of guidelines:

1. Identify the business reason. Why this feedback important?
2. Focus on improvement for the future and not on past transgressions.
3. Use customer-oriented data and feedback, not just an opinion.

4. Put the feedback in the right context, for example, as being a big issue or minor problem.
5. Be specific and give tangible examples.
6. Make the feedback timely, occurring at or near the time of the event.
7. Find someplace private to share negative feedback.
8. Find someplace public to share praise.
9. Keep feedback simple, and deliver it slowly.
10. Focus on work behavior, not on individual personality traits.
11. Explain the impact in organizational, business, or professional terms.
12. Speak from the heart, and state your feelings.
13. Speak for yourself, using the first person and owning the message.
14. Be spontaneous. Unless you are angry, do not wait to give feedback.
15. Do not force feedback on someone.

These guidelines provide the manager with a starting point for approaching difficult employee situations. The guidelines clearly integrate the fundamental skills of communication to provide the manager with a framework for delivering feedback and for building confidence and skill in this area of one-to-one interactions.

### Group Interactions

Most managers also spend considerable time in verbal interactions with groups of employees. Although these group interactions can and should include informal gatherings and conversations, this aspect of communication in formal meetings can be challenging. With the need for efficiency in any workplace, time spent in meetings must be viewed as productive time that supports the primary functions of the department. The manager is faced with the task of running a "good" meeting. Exactly what constitutes a good meeting has many variables. However, managers can use several basic strategies in group communication that can ease the challenge.

First, the manager must use good communication skills when conducting meetings. Second, the manager must develop a knowledge of group process and the phases of group work. Third, the manager must be explicit with respect to the purpose of a meeting or the different purposes of selected agenda items within the meeting. Various purposes of a meeting or agenda items can include team building, disseminating information, planning, problem-solving, or decision-making (Amann, 2000). Fourth, the manager needs to construct and distribute an agenda with sufficient time for participants to review it and prepare. In preparing the agenda, the manager can be helpful by writing a brief description about the item, including background and the type of action desired at the meeting. This "annotated" agenda becomes a communication tool that supports discussion and focuses communication at the meeting. A meeting can be a powerful tool to foster group cohesion and action when it is well designed and run, but it can be impotent or destructive if attention is not given to the communication aspects of the meeting.

## Written Communication

Managerial communication extends beyond verbal interactions to include written communication, often in the form of memos, letters, and statements of policy and procedure. Many of the principles of good verbal communication also apply to written communication. Good written communication, regardless of form, must be complete, technically accurate, clear, and concise, and it must express the appropriate tone (Visco, 1981).

## Technology-Based Communication

Technology is advancing at such a rapid rate that what is considered advanced today will not be next year. Workplace communication has changed dramatically with the advent of the facsimile machine, voice mail, e-mail, cell phones, teleconferencing, and Internet technology. The exchange of information can occur immediately. Confidentiality and privacy, however, are not guaranteed. Higher-technology communication methods are costly in the purchasing, installation, and replacement phases and often require training and additional skills for the communicator to be proficient.

E-mail is an excellent example of how technological methods can have both advantages and potential hazards (Davidhizar & Shearer, 2001). Wide access to e-mail within and outside of the workplace provides an easy, convenient way to quickly exchange large or small amounts of information. However, the method is not always secure, so privacy and confidentiality are not guaranteed. Unnecessary messages and too much information can result in information overload, causing people to overlook important information. The ease and speed of sending e-mail can allow impulsive and sometimes regrettable or inaccurate messages to be sent. Finally, e-mail can create a false sense of urgency, complicating the manager's realistic evaluation of the importance of a message. With these warnings, Davidhizar and Shearer suggested that managers do not use e-mail for problem-solving, conflict resolution, negative messages, or private issues.

Face-to-face communication will never be replaced as the primary method used between the manager and the staff member. Although alternative methods can supplement personal contact, they will still require the same degree of attention to communication basics to be effective tools. Many of the problems that occur in face-to-face communication also happen in alternative methods; however, when they occur in alternative methods, they can be more difficult to diagnose and correct.

## Integrated Approach to Communication

The effective manager is able to integrate his or her communication skills with organizational expectations and employee needs to create a positive workplace environment. Each interaction is an opportunity to move the work group closer to achieving individual, professional, and organizational standards of quality and effectiveness. Although the development of communication competence is an undertaking that continues throughout one's life and career, the manager should not be overwhelmed or daunted by the communication challenges of the workplace. Very simply, the mandates for a manager's communication fall into one or more of the following functions: to inform, to develop, to advocate, or to inspire. Regardless of the kind of interaction, the starting point of good communication is to identify the function and unique requirements of the interaction, analyze the specifics of the context and the individuals involved, and use the basic skills of receiving and sending information.

## Conclusion

Communication underlies most management functions. Ultimately, the manager's success in many areas of administration depends on an ability to communicate clearly with subordinates, peers, and superiors and, in turn, to interpret messages accurately.

Communication involves the exchange of words, nonverbal information, and cues; the interpretation of meaning; and a cycle of feedback, clarification, and verification that determines the intent of the interchange. Clear and accurate communication can be blocked at any point in the process. Learning to communicate effectively in the workplace requires the valuing of good communication, self-awareness of skills and deficits, and a lifelong commitment to develop and practice good habits and skills.

As practitioners transition into managerial roles, three aspects of communication become crucial. First, the person in transition must acquire the language of the functional areas of management. Second, the person in transition must develop an understanding of position power as well as the impact that the manager's responsibility and authority can have on manager–subordinate interactions. Third, the new manager not only must develop a communication style that is based in the power and authority of his or her position but also must be flexible in response to staff needs.

Meaning and purpose in communication are derived through an interaction of content and context and through the use of both verbal and nonverbal skills. Language is inherently ambiguous and subject to different interpretations that are based on individual or cohort perspectives. Therefore, it is critical for the manager to understand the nuances of communicating with individuals of different gender, culture, and generation. Both the sender and receiver have the responsibility to determine when they have reached a point of common meaning.

The manager needs both basic and advanced communication skills to be adept at recognizing the lapses in skill and environmental factors that can confuse or distort the meaning and stop communication. Additionally, the manager must be prepared to handle difficult communication issues that create ethical dilemmas and that require careful analysis and response.

A manager typically uses a mix of communication methods for a single message. Selecting the appropriate communication methods requires an examination of variables related to (a) the message—for example, the need for confidentiality or privacy and the need for dialogue; (b) the recipient—for example, his or her preferred method of communication as well as his or her skill and comfort with various communication methods; and (c) the method—for example, reliability and cost factors.

Managers have multiple methods available for communicating with employees. Although each method requires unique considerations, good communication always rests on the manager's ability to understand the unique aspects of a particular interaction and to use the basic skills of receiving and sending information.

# References

Amann, M. C. (2000). Combining technology and skill to ensure effective meetings. *AAOHN Journal, 48,* 367–369.

Barna, L. M. (1997). Stumbling blocks in intercultural communication. In L. A. Samovar & R. E. Pater (Eds.), *Intercultural communication: A reader* (8th ed., pp. 370–391). New York: Wadsworth.

Bolton, R. B. (1986). *People skills: How to assert yourself, listen to others, and resolve conflicts* (2nd ed.). New York: Simon & Schuster.

Davidhizar, R., & Cramer, C. (2000). Gender differences in leadership in the health professions. *Health Care Manager, 18*(3), 18–24.

Davidhizar, R., Dowd, S., & Giger, J. N. (1999). Managing diversity in the health care workplace. *Health Care Supervisor, 17*(3), 51–62.

Davidhizar, R., & Shearer, R. (2001). E-Mail triage. *Health Care Manager, 20*(2), 11–17.

Devereaux, E. (1992). Principles of communication. In J. Bair & M. Gray (Eds.), *The occupational therapy manager* (rev. ed., pp. 261–273). Rockville, MD: American Occupational Therapy Association.

Haskell, R. E. (2001). *Deep listening: Uncovering the hidden meanings in everyday conversation.* Cambridge, MA: Perseus.

Kupperschmidt, B. R. (2000). Multigeneration employees: Strategies for effective management. *Health Care Manager, 19*(1), 65–76.

Maurer, R. (1994). *Feedback toolkit: Sixteen tools for better communication in the workplace.* Portland, OR: Productivity Press.

McCall, I., & Cousins, J. (1990). *Communication problem solving: The language of effective management.* West Sussex, England: Wiley.

McLagan, P., & Krembs, P. (1995). *On-the-level: Performance communication that works.* San Francisco: Berrett-Koehler.

Payne, K. E. (2001). *Different but equal: Communication between the sexes.* Westport, CT: Praeger.

Rakich, J. S., Longest, B. B., Jr., & Darr, K. (1992). *Managing health services organizations* (3rd ed.). Baltimore: Health Professions Press.

Ribbens, G., & Thompson, R. (2001). *Understanding body language.* Hauppauge, NY: Barron's Educational Series.

Rozelle, R. M., Druckman, D., & Baxter, J. (1997). Non-verbal behavior as communication. In O. D. W. Hargie (Ed.), *The handbook of communication skills* (pp. 67–102). London: Routlege.

Umiker, W. (1998). From technical professional to group leader. *Health Care Supervisor, 16*(3), 1–8.

Visco, L. J. (1981). *The manager as editor.* Boston: CBI.

Zemke, R., Raines, C., & Filipczak, B. (2000). *Generations at work: Managing the clash of veterans, boomers, Xers, and nexters in your workplace.* New York: American Management Association.

# CHAPTER 12

# Personnel Management: Measuring Performance, Creating Success

Christine M. MacDonell, BS, OTR

*"It's a funny thing about life; if you refuse to accept anything but the best, you very often get it."*

W. SOMERSET MAUGHAM

**Christine M. MacDonell, BS, OTR,** is managing director, Medical Rehabilitation/Emerging Markets, Customer Service Unit: Commission on Accreditation of Rehabilitation Facilities in Tucson, AZ. She is a human services specialist with experience as an occupational therapist, director of a rehabilitation continuum, executive director of vocational state use program, and an accreditation specialist.

## Key Terms and Concepts

**Confidence.** Ability to feel that an ethical, all-around approach based on real data has been used during performance evaluation.

**Evaluation.** A measuring of how well goals/objectives that were established have been met. Measurable objectives have to be used in this process.

**Growth.** Improved performance and willingness to learn.

**Performance.** Expected levels/targets/benchmarks of a job. One rates an employee's level to get to that expected level. This "performance" then is rated (e.g., outstanding, very good, satisfactory, marginal, unsatisfactory).

## Learning Objectives

After completing this chapter, you should be able to do the following:

■   Explain the importance of regular job performance reviews.

■   Define what is involved in a job performance review.

■   Describe successful ways to evaluate job performance.

■   Distinguish the roles of both the supervisor and the employee in a job performance review.

Managing job performance effectively is critical to the success of any organization in today's market. The challenge lies not only in developing a meaningful strategy to reward positive behaviors but also in carrying out that strategy in a dynamic, volatile, changing environment in which managers have to keep up with the needs of the business as well as meet the expectations and desires of their supervisors and employees.

W. Somerset Maugham's quote seems to apply to the discussion of job performance evaluations: "It's a funny thing about life; if you refuse to accept anything but the best, you very often get it." As an occupational therapy manager, what are your expectations for your employees' quality performance? Do you have any expectations? Are the expectations clear and reflected in employee job descriptions? Do your own actions reflect quality performance so employees have a role model?

Job performance reviews allow a manager and an organization to communicate to employees in a structured and measurable fashion how they are expected to perform on the job. A performance review also allows employees the opportunity to state problems they may have in performing their jobs. Most employees want to share ideas, make positive changes, and make suggestions related to how their employer can best help them. Employees also want to know when they have exceeded expectations. At the same time, the manager has a responsibility to also let employees know when they have fallen below expectations in performance which, of course, is a much more difficult task.

By listening to employees, the manager shows that they are respected and valued. In a white paper, *Retention Tactics That Work* (Fyock, 2001), sponsored by the Society for Human Resource Management, the Families and Work Institute asked 3,400 employees what they considered as very important in their current jobs. Open communication was rated as the most important factor for retaining satisfaction in their current job. The second factor was opportunities to balance life, and the third factor was meaningful work, which is an important premise in occupational therapy.

Regular or periodic job performance reviews that are conducted effectively will result in a better functioning organization and a more fulfilled staff. Job satisfaction usually results from recognition of one's skills, ability to use one's skills daily, and having all the necessary skills to perform the job well. A regular job performance review will address all of these areas.

## Components of Job Performance

What should be included in a job performance review? First and foremost, the review should consider the job analysis or job description of an individual's position. This description is the concrete foundation of review. It establishes the necessary competencies and skill sets that the individual is most likely to possess and that are required for the job. In the hiring process, the job description helps to quickly identify the expectations of an employer, how much is expected, and how an employee's job performance will be measured. Without the job description, the process to perform a fair and realistic performance review becomes very difficult. The performance review must reflect on previously established mutual goals that can be measured objectively through means such as patient satisfaction scales; measures determining the quality of patient care; documented achievement of predicted outcomes; evidence of relationship building with other stakeholders, including fellow workers, families, payers, and case managers; and evidence showing the ability to market services, the ability to ask for training to develop needed competencies, the ability to mentor staff members, and the ability to develop new programs and services. The particular combination of performance measures that is used in a review depends on the position being evaluated (Commission on Accreditation of Rehabilitation Facilities, 2002, pp. 27–32).

## Requirements of the Review Process

Two critical components of the review are (a) who does the review and (b) how the input into it is gathered. One type of review that is favored by many organizations is called the *360-degree review* because it includes input from a variety of individuals who interact with the employee, including patients or clients, coworkers, supervisors, and referral sources. In this type of performance evaluation, the reviewer develops a better understanding of how an employee is performing on a variety of levels. It allows a supervisor to view how others, both within and outside the organization, perceive the employee's attitude, actions, and style of work performance.

Readers are cautioned to remember that performance information that is gathered all at once just before a review can produce a skewed perspective. If information is gathered throughout the year and from more than one individual (if possible), then the review will be able to provide a more balanced appraisal of the person's work performance.

Reviews are usually conducted annually, although a new employee will likely also go through a review after his or her probationary period has been completed. Reviews that are done more frequently may not further the actual achievement of stated goals, and less frequent reviews create difficulties in the fast-changing human services arena.

Successful performance reviews require a two-way dialogue between the reviewer and the employee. Often, the review process may take two or three sessions to complete. Employees should be given advance notice about when performance reviews will occur. Scheduling methods vary from planning all employees' reviews to occur during the same time each year to linking reviews with dates of hire or other established time frames.

The review process should be familiar to employees, and they should have the opportunity to ask for clarification of their role and what will be expected from them during the review process. In addition, employees should be clearly informed about whom they will report to and who will perform the evaluation. If these points are not clear, then employees can experience confusion and resentment. Managers who are responsible for giving performance reviews must be trained in the review process, and they must demonstrate competency in reviewing other employees.

One outcome of the performance review that is critical to success is the consensus of both the employee and the reviewer with respect to recommendations or expectations for the next review period. By the end of a successful review, the means to accomplish the goals have been reviewed and are clear to both parties. In addition, training needs will have also been identified. At the completion of the review, an employee should definitely know where he or she is headed and how he or she will achieve the identified performance objectives. The expectations, corrective behaviors, or both should be written, signed by both parties, and filed for future reference.

Successful communication is critical in the review process. An employee's buy-in or commitment to improving work performance depends on meaningful communication and mutual respect. Disastrous situations result when employees feel they are not listened to and when programs, productivity goals, or outcomes are forced on them without communication and buy-in. If the reviewer does not understand or know the employee, then the reviewer will have an inadequate understanding not only of what skill sets are necessary for basic job performance but also of what skills are needed for the creative work of enhancing or establishing new services and programs. All of these factors are intertwined and must be addressed (Eli Research Newsletter, p. 6).

The many beneficiaries of performance improvement include the employee, the employer, coworkers, and the patients or clients and their families. They all reap the benefits of an employee who is dedicated to and working toward success.

A strong performance evaluation process that is conducted on a regular basis with employee involvement will reward employees and the employer with a strong and viable workforce that supports an environment where employees want to stay, learn, and grow. If an individual can understand and appreciate how his or her daily roles help fulfill the mission and core values of an organization, then that employee will have pride and ownership in the job. A mission statement is much more than sentences in the employee handbook. It should intrinsically drive employees' actions within the organization. It should be the organization's goal for all activities. Employees should be able to discern, discuss, and understand their roles in achieving the mission. The mission should motivate employees to do the organization's work. Core values are usually intrinsically important to the employees. These values are guiding principles that require no external justification, for example, a core value such as all individuals will be treated with respect and dignity.

Personnel management is never an easy task, but it can be rewarding and fulfilling to the manager who takes the time to become proficient at conducting performance reviews.

# References

Commission on Accreditation of Rehabilitation Facilities. (2002). *2002 CARF medical rehabilitation standards manual.* Tucson, AZ: Author.

Fyock, C. D. (2001). *Retention tactics that work* [White Paper]. Alexandria, VA: Society for Human Resource Management.

*Eli's Rehab Report.* (Vol. IX, No. 2, p. 6). Chapel Hill, NC: Eli Research.

## Resource

Hay Group. (2000, January 14). *Shifting workplace values are dramatically altering pay strategies* [Press Release]. Philadelphia, PA.

# CHAPTER 13

# Motivating Employees

Kate Hayner, EdD, OTR
Evelyn G. Jaffe, MPH, OTR, FAOTA

*"Motivation will almost always beat mere talent."*

NORMAN R. AUGUSTINE

**Kate Hayner, EdD, OTR,** is currently an assistant professor and acting chair for the Master of Occupational Therapy Department at Samuel Merritt College in Oakland, CA. She has served as the director of occupational therapy in a large sub-acute and skilled nursing facility with Vencor Rehabilitation in San Francisco. She also has three advanced degrees in psychology.

**Evelyn G. Jaffe, MPH, OTR, FAOTA,** is an assistant professor at Samuel Merritt College. She has been a consultant in occupational therapy for over 35 years, specializing in community mental health, high-risk infants, school-age parents, and primary prevention in the workplace. She earned her master's degree from the School of Public Health at the University of Michigan.

## Key Terms and Concepts

**Feedback.** A method of communication through the sharing of information and the giving or receiving of ideas and data that facilitate motivation and human communication.

**Intrinsic factors.** Motivational factors that are internal to a person, such as the feeling of satisfaction from a job well done.

**Extrinsic factors.** Factors that originate outside of a person by external causes, such as receiving praise or a raise from a manager.

**Mentoring.** Counseling in the development of both professional and personal skills.

**Motivation.** The act of putting energy into goal-directed behavior, which satisfies some need for the individual, either intrinsic or extrinsic.

**Progressive discipline.** A systematic method of disciplinary action, gradually increasing in severity of sanctions, used to ensure fair and unbiased treatment of employees.

**Team.** "A group of interdependent individuals who have complementary skills, and are committed to a shared, meaningful purpose and specific goals" (Payne, 2001, p. 99).

**Team building.** "A structured series of activities designed to improve the performance of a team" (Skopec & Smith, 1998, p. 14).

## Learning Objectives

After completing this chapter you should be able to do the following:

- Explain effective motivation.
- Describe the benefits of using teams in motivation.
- Identify effective team characteristics.
- Describe the guidelines for giving and receiving feedback to enhance staff motivation.
- Describe the four essential components of communication for effective motivation.
- Discuss the seven steps in the process of communication.
- Describe the benefits of mentoring in motivation.
- Describe how disciplinary action affects motivation.

The roles and responsibilities of a manager are extremely varied, and one of the major objectives of a good leader is to raise the level of staff motivation (Perinchief, 2003). This chapter describes motivation and the leadership and management skills needed to keep employees in occupational therapy satisfied with their jobs and interested in doing them well, especially in these times of constant change. For the purposes of this chapter, *motivation* is defined as putting energy into goal-directed behavior, which will satisfy some need for the individual, either intrinsic or extrinsic. In addition, team building, mentoring, and disciplinary action are discussed as they relate to employee motivation.

## Understanding Motivation

Many textbooks written on effective management skills state that managers cannot motivate staff to be more productive, because motivation is derived from within each individual. Therefore, many authors have argued that self-motivation is what really works (Belker, 1993; Boyd, 1984; Imundo, 1991). Others have argued that managers have many avenues through which they can attempt to motivate employees, based on both intrinsic and extrinsic factors (Lawler, 1994). *Intrinsic factors* are motivational factors that by their nature are internal to a person, such as satisfaction from a job well done. *Extrinsic factors* originate outside of a person by external causes, such as receiving praise or a raise from a manager. Obviously, many factors outside of work can have a direct effect on an individual's motivation. The occupational therapy manager cannot influence these factors but can, at times, address how these factors are affecting the workplace.

Many theories have explained what motivates people; readers may wish to read *Motivation in Work Organizations* by Edward E. Lawler (1994) for an in-depth review of the theories. Briefly, these include Needs Theories, Task Characteristics Theories, Goal Setting Theory, Reinforcement Theory, Equity Theory, and Expectancy Theory.

Of the different Needs Theories, the most familiar is Maslow's Hierarchy of Needs, which hypothesized that within each individual being exists a hierarchy of five needs, and as each becomes satisfied, the next becomes dominant. Task Characteristics Theories identify task characteristics of jobs as well as the relationship of these characteristics to form different jobs and how these relate to employee motivation, satisfaction, and performance. Goal Setting Theory demonstrates that specific goals increase performance, especially more difficult goals that are accepted by the employee, and that feedback lends itself to better employee performance than nonfeedback. Reinforcement Theory is based on behavioral approaches that suggest that reinforcement can condition behavior. Equity Theory looks at the importance of equity within the workplace and how equity influences motivation. This theory recognizes that employees will compare their jobs with those of coworkers and expect equal pay for the same amount of effort and outcome; employees often refer to this as *fairness*. Expectancy Theory suggests that the desire to produce at a given time depends on the person's goals and perception of the relative worth of the performance (Robbins, 1993).

Applying what is known about human behavior in the workplace can assist in learning how to motivate each employee. The following are basic principles to assist in the process:

- Individuals are motivated by different things, so each employee has different motivating factors. What is considered rewarding will increase the likelihood of performing a desired behavior, and what is considered negative will decrease the likelihood of performing a behavior again.
- Leadership style can affect motivation.
- The behavior or goal a manager would like to motivate an employee to change or achieve can be defined in measurable terms.
- Once a goal is determined, it should be clearly defined in relation to rewards for performance.
- The workplace atmosphere should be one of fairness, where all employees are treated equally.

## Determining Individual Motivating Factors

"Large differences clearly exist in the goals and needs people have, and these differences must be considered when viewing individual motivation in organizations" (Lawler, 1994, p. 47). The manager should identify what is rewarding to employees (sometimes referred to as "positive stimuli") and what is not ("negative stimuli") (Craighead, Kazdin, & Mahoney, 1981). Ask about their goals and desires.

Possible motivating factors to consider individually for each employee include

- Appreciation, respect, acceptance, and recognition by managers, peers, or clients;
- Power and competition with peers; and
- Level of job interest and the satisfaction of "a job well done."

More concrete factors may include

- A bonus or pay increase;
- A title change or promotion;
- More or less responsibility;
- Leadership roles and amount of supervision;
- Flextime and other benefits;
- Job security; and
- Perks, such as a well-located parking spot.

## Modeling a Positive Leadership Style

To develop a good rapport with employees, and thus create an environment that will increase employee job satisfaction, managers should provide a positive leadership style to employees. "Satisfied employees have lower rates of turnover and absenteeism than

[do] dissatisfied employees" (Robbins, 1997, p. 44). The following points should be considered by occupational therapy managers to help maintain positive leadership:

- *Recognize that the manager's job is to be a motivator.* Managers often say, "No one ever tells me I am doing a good job." Lack of personal positive feedback should not affect the positive feedback the manager gives to his or her staff.

- *Give credit where credit is due.* Managers who give praise to employees will earn their respect. At the same time, the manager's supervisor will recognize the manager's ability to supervise employees effectively.

- *Show honesty and fairness, and develop good communication skills.* Honesty and fairness are key traits to earning staff respect. It is important that managers remain honest in all communication; if the manager cannot answer a question because of confidentiality issues, he or she should say so. If the manager has not decided on how to proceed with an issue, the manager should communicate this. The manager does not bend the policy for some employees and not for others and must demonstrate that staff can confide in him or her (Robbins, 1997).

- *Listen well.* The skill of listening takes practice and patience, along with a clear understanding of how to be an active listener (using full attention, concentration, and effort while not judging the speaker [Alessandra & Hunsaker, 1993]). McCormack (1984) summed up the concept of listening well when he wrote, "The ability to listen, really to hear what someone is saying, has far greater business implications, of course, than simply gaining insight into people" (p. 8). When the manager uses good listening skills, there are fewer misunderstandings, and therefore, much clearer communication between the manager and employee.

- *Demonstrate confidence* (Robbins, 1997). Managers should exude confidence in their ability to use good communication skills, manage the department well, show respect for others, and use good judgment. Competent management skills earn employees' respect.

- *Manage your space and time well.* Managers should organize their workspaces and schedules (tips for becoming and staying organized are offered in the literature and in consumer publications; see Douglas & Douglas, 1993; Mayer 1990). The manager's daily schedule should be flexible (Douglas & Douglas, 1993) to maintain control over unexpected demands and interruptions and also be accessible to staff.

- *Help manage employees' time.* The manager's job is not only to manage his or her own time well but also to assist other staff members in the department to do the same, which will help them meet their goals. One way to promote good time management skills with employees is for the manager to demonstrate that he or she can and will do as much as is being asked of the staff. For example, if the expectation is for practitioners within the department to treat seven clients in a 4-hour timeframe, the manager occasionally should schedule the same number of clients for his or her own schedule to demonstrate that the task is reasonable and the level of expectations is fair.

- *Learn how to delegate.* Delegating departmental responsibilities has several advantages for both managers and employees. First, employees will learn new skills. Second, employees can feel like vital contributors and, thus, are "inclined to work both harder and smarter" (Fuller, 1998, p. 108). Third, managers benefit, because assigning duties they formerly performed relieves some of the burdens of the job and allows them "to spend more time resolving issues and guiding the group" (p. 108).

## Set Reasonable Goals and Expectations

Managers and their staff should work toward common individual and department or team goals. When goals and departmental decisions are being determined, staff participation and "buy-in" are essential for employee job satisfaction.

Managers should define the behavior they would like the employee to change, or the goal employees are to achieve in measurable or operational terms, so that the employee knows exactly what is expected. Managers should know each employee's abilities, such as the ability to handle multiple tasks, and be reasonable in managing the employee's time, such as intervention time balanced against requests to complete additional evaluations and attend meetings.

## Define Rewards

Managers must define the behavior change or goal clearly in relation to rewards (ranging from private praise to public recognition to bonuses or promotions) for performance. If specific goals are not defined for an individual practitioner but the goals of the department are clear, the manager should determine which factors will motivate employees to implement the department goals.

When giving praise to employees, the following strategies are effective:

- Relate praise to a specific accomplishment (Fuller, 1995), and do not overly praise routine efforts.
- Be timely with giving praise (Fuller, 1995).
- Praise the entire group or department as deserved.
- Be sincere (Boyd, 1984).

## Give Appropriate Feedback

*Feedback,* an essential component of communication in any group experience, is a method of communication through the sharing of information and the giving or receiving of ideas and data that can facilitate motivation. Feedback may be positive or negative, open or closed. *Open feedback* is considered honest, forthright, and clear information, which may provide direction, encouragement, or support. *Closed feedback* is that which does not "tell the whole story," and the speaker may have a hidden agenda or not wish to reveal information or his or her true feelings. A manager usually operates within other people's point of view; therefore, feedback must focus on "constructive openness," based on an intent to help. Sensitivity to staff or the client's method of communication is essential. Ideally, the feedback should be constructive, well-timed, and to the point (Jaffe, 2001).

Although "telling it like it is" is based on the popular assumption that complete honesty is preferred, responding with absolute openness, which may be referred to as "destructive openness,"can be inappropriate, hurtful and, in some cases, harmful. The manager must weigh issues of confidentiality and privileged information, judgment, employee personality traits, and expectations (of the manager, staff, client, or client's family) against what outcomes are desired (Jaffe, 2001).

A more constructive form of feedback that promotes growth in an individual is "strategic openness"; "being *strategically open* implies a responsibility to check out the system carefully, being alert to cues that say to go on and to cues that say stop!" (Pfeiffer & Jones, 1972, p. 198). Openness grows in a nurturing environment; thus, the manager should attempt to open up communications by developing strategies to facilitate trust and willingness to change. Also, managers must be aware that the level of openness may need to be renegotiated over time.

Strategic openness should focus on modifying behavior in a positive manner. For example, an employee is having difficulty completing a proposal on time. Instead of responding negatively, the manager could state quietly and privately, "You've been a little tentative lately with work on your program proposal. Why don't we try to work on it together or have the administrative assistant help you so you can respond a little faster, with more assertiveness?"

Sometimes exchanges can be humorous, if said in good faith or fun, with no malice intended, depending on the kind of communication culture the manager has set up. However, such communication can appear to some people to be too pointed, rude, or disrespectful. Therefore, an important aspect of giving feedback is knowing who is listening (Jaffe, 2001).

Frequently, situations arise in which miscommunication, lack of understanding, or feelings of inhibition (usually because of lack of trust) occur. The resulting misunderstanding could result in the spread of "confusion dust" (Jaffe, 1999), or an atmosphere that precludes expression of feelings. Thus, it is important to use positive feedback to encourage constructive communication, collaboration, and cooperation (Jaffe, 1997).

Communication is a two-way process that involves the sending and receiving of messages. A fundamental concept in motivation is the attainment of good communication skills. Successful communication involves four essential components:

- A sender
- A receiver
- A message
- A response.

The process includes the following steps:

1. The sender formulates the message.
2. The sender translates or encodes the message so it is meaningful to the receiver.
3. The sender transmits the message, which is the communication vehicle (e.g., discussion, lecture, memo, "slap on the hand").
4. The receiver deciphers or encodes the message based on his or her experiences. This is where some communication can get muddy or confused, and "confusion dust" may be spread.
5. The receiver retains only relevant parts of the message ("you hear only what you want to hear!").
6. The receiver responds. All parties must listen carefully.
7. The sender solicits feedback.

This response determines the accuracy or effectiveness of the message. Both manager and employee should follow this process to enhance motivation by the manager and follow-through by the employee.

Guidelines for giving and receiving feedback to encourage positive communication, both for the manager and the employee, include the following:

- Be objective in describing the behavior.
- State specific details, not generalities.
- State positive behaviors before suggesting changes.
- Describe behaviors rather than evaluating them.
- Deal only with changeable behavior.
- Describe the impact of the behavior on the group or individual.
- Provide enough information without overloading the employee.
- Check that the feedback is understood (Jaffe, 1999; Payne, 2001).

Also important are the following guidelines for receiving feedback:

- Keep an open mind; be receptive and willing to hear suggestions for change.
- Avoid judgmental, argumentative, or accusatory statements.
- Listen without interrupting, justifying, or explaining before responding.
- Paraphrase the feedback so that the person who gave it can determine whether the intended message is understood.
- Ask for an example or further explanation to clarify the feedback if the message is not understood.

## Team Building and Motivation

Team building became an important management tool in the social psychology and group dynamics era of the 1960s. Initially, the concept of team building was used to improve group relationships and cohesion. Today, however, team building is ranked among one of the most critical challenges faced by organizations, as it can facilitate the accomplishment of organizational goals and tasks (Payne, 2001).

Payne (2001) defined *team building* as "a vehicle for ensuring that individuals work together harmoniously, productively, and effectively to maximize task accomplishment and goal achievement" (p. 4). Additionally, team building is important for the individual because it facilitates his or her contribution to the organization and helps integrate his or her personal goals with those of the organization, both important aspects of motivation.

Payne (2001) defined a *team* as a group of "interdependent individuals who have complementary skills and are committed to a shared, meaningful purpose and specific goals. They have a common, collaborative work approach, clear roles and responsibilities, and hold themselves mutually accountable for the team's performance" (p. 99). Work or project teams in the occupational therapy department may be interdisciplinary or multidisciplinary. The manager may be responsible for the entire team or only a part of the team, such as only the rehabilitation staff in a multidisciplinary setting that includes occupational therapy practitioners and also physicians, nurses, social workers, respiratory therapists, physical therapists, and speech–language pathologists.

Effective team characteristics include
- A shared mission or purpose
- Specific and measurable goals
- A collaborative approach
- Well-defined roles, responsibilities, and expectations
- Shared responsibility for effective, focused meetings
- Specific skills or expertise to achieve the goals (e.g., interpersonal skills, technical expertise, problem-solving and decision-making skills)
- Mutual responsibility and accountability for the mission and goals of the team
- Enthusiasm, confidence, and passion for the team's purpose and activities (Payne, 2001).

Staff meetings provide a useful opportunity to build essential team skills. Assigning staff to committees to work on specific departmental tasks frequently starts the process of skills building and, if good communication skills are developed, this can create a bond and good working relationships among the team members, both of which can be motivating factors.

Smaller occupational therapy departments may not have a multidisciplinary team but rather an occupational therapy manager supervising individuals (most of them occupational therapists and occupational therapy assistants) who work alongside but are separate from others in the department. But, when the size of the department allows, building teams of differing health care professionals within the department will provide added benefits to the department, including
- Less supervision, because members tend to work toward the norm of the group and any questions often can be answered within the group. For example, an individual within the group will be more likely to complete all necessary paperwork on time if the norm is to have work completed in a timely manner.

- Improved performance of underachievers, as each individual works toward the norm of the group.
- Improved team behaviors, as group members deal directly with undesirable behaviors that interfere with the performance of the whole group (Imundo, 1991).
- Informed decisions made more quickly (Chesla, 2000), as the team can gather the information more rapidly. (But this principle might work in reverse if there are multiple perspectives and a breadth of knowledge involved.)
- Better-informed decisions (Chesla, 2000), because teams can do a better job investigating facts pertinent to decision-making, gathering information, and determining solutions.
- Improved quality of work, because all members critique the performance variables before they are presented to the department.
- Added strengths, as members bring their different expertise to the group, allowing for a large pool of ideas.
- Increased performance, because a team can outperform a single individual (Chesla, 2000).

Traditional reasons for engaging in team building have included staff communication problems and conflict, dysfunctional behaviors, low morale, apathy, and poor execution or lack of commitment to organizational task or goals (Payne, 2001). Other indicators include proposed or actual changes in organizational structure and strategic challenges to organizational goals. Change can create many reactions; to avoid some of the negative behaviors associated with change, the manager can engage his or her staff in team-building activities that include shared decision-making. Thus, they will be more apt to work together to develop strategies to address the change with a positive attitude (Jaffe, 1997).

## Mentoring and Motivation

Mentoring involves counseling in the development of both professional and personal skills. Mentors usually are experienced and trusted managers who take time to work with staff members to improve their skills in the workplace. Murray (1991) gave a definition of *mentoring* as "a deliberate pairing of a more skilled or experienced person with a lesser skilled or experienced one, with the agreed-upon goal of having the lesser skilled person grow and develop specific competencies" (p. xiv). Some of those competencies may include ways to improve intervention techniques, how to give better presentations, ideas for advancement within the organization, how to manage report writing, or program development. Additionally, the areas may address more personal characteristics, such as how to give constructive feedback or improve professional and nonjudgmental attitudes with difficult staff and clients.

The term *counseling* is generally used to refer to the act of supportively guiding an individual through a specific problem or issue. It often encompasses personal problems that may or may not affect the job performance. When help is needed that is beyond the manager's comfort level or expertise, it is best to refer the person to an employee assistance program, a counselor, or a psychologist.

*Coaching* is similar to mentoring and counseling, except that a coach attempts to help employees "clarify their mission, purpose, and goals" (C. Roppel, personal life coach, personal communication, March 8, 2002), and then helps them achieve that outcome by overcoming barriers to top work performance and advancement. "It's not about problems or fixing but rather . . . future vision and taking steps to success" (C. Roppel, personal communication, March 8, 2002).

One of the keys to success in one's career is the opportunity to have a mentor who can guide the development of skills and assist in gaining insight into what is needed for performing a particular job with more success and talent. Wellington (2001) reported that senior male executives stated that "influential mentors were second in importance only to education as a factor in their career success" (p. 159). Wellington further mentioned that the main reason why men tend to rise higher than women in the workplace (among those equally talented) is that men have mentors, and many women do not. In her research on mentoring, Wellington further argued that "Mentors are more important to career success than hard work, more important than talent, more important than intelligence" (p. 3). Although this quote may be a bit biased, it makes the point that mentoring is an important aspect in the development of a professional career.

Managers have the unique ability to hold two roles: that of a manager and also of a mentor. Of course, the manager must have the experience and wisdom as well as the desire to mentor others. A manager can mentor employees by providing guidance and feedback on intervention techniques, clinical skills training, effective approaches to documentation, reporting, supervising others, communicating, and career advancement. As a mentor, the manager should have a predetermined mentoring relationship with the mentee, with the goal of the mentee to gain wisdom and receive feedback.

Mentoring works best when interactions between the two individuals are positive, and there is mutual respect. The mentor does not need to be older than the mentee but does need to be more experienced in the area in which skills are to be developed or enhanced. A mentor is generally most effective if he or she clearly understands not only occupational therapy skills but also the varying dynamics of the organization and system.

Probably the most neglected aspect of the mentor–mentee relationship is that the mentee should give something back to the mentor, which can motivate the mentor to continue the mentoring relationship. Wellington (2001) suggested that the mentee should let the mentor know how much the feedback and guidance mean. The mentee can offer to return any favors when possible.

## Disciplinary Action and Motivation

Taking disciplinary action is probably the one area that managers dislike the most but that can, if done well, be useful in staff motivation and job satisfaction.

However, there are some ways to make the process less distasteful and easier to handle:

- Treat all employees in the same manner and with the same expectations, so there is no indication of favoritism.
- Discuss an issue with an employee before it becomes a serious problem, such as arriving to work late. All employees need to be warned of an undesired behavior or performance before further disciplinary action is taken. Allow the employee to explain the problem and then describe the desired behavior.
- If the problem continues, discuss it with the employee by stating the undesirable behavior and then the desired behavior. For example, "Karen, three of your discharge summaries were completed 1 week late. I want all of your paperwork completed on time." The manager can state that department policy requires that the documents be in on time for reimbursement, as well as to show respect for clients and families, who may need access to records after discharge. Clarify the desired behavior, and ask if the employee wishes assistance to meet the desired goal. If this is a formal verbal warning, say so.
- Schedule a follow-up meeting to assess progress. Remember, "Disciplinary action is used to correct employee behavior or inadequate job performance. Its purpose is not to punish the worker" (Fuller, 1995, p. 182).

It appears to be common practice for managers to attribute personality traits to difficult employees. They may label the employee as *controlling, aggressive,* or even *hostile.* Once labeled, the manager may determine the disciplinary approach based on the label. To help understand the personality traits of individuals, the Myers–Briggs Type Indicators assessment has been the most widely used (Robbins, 1997). Still, it is important to understand that there is no evidence that this test is a valid measure of a person's personality (Robbins, 1997). Yet the assessment does allow for a framework that many organizations use to understand their employees, although not necessarily for responses or strategies related to conflict.

There is additional evidence for the five-factor model of personality, which is different from the Myers–Briggs assessment. "In recent years, an impressive body of research supports that five basic personality dimensions underlie all others" (Robbins, 1997 p. 35): (a) extroversion, (b) agreeableness, (c) conscientiousness, (d) emotional stability, and (e) openness to experience. Although the research has found relationships between these personality traits and job performance (Robbins, 1997), the focus has not been on the best conflict resolution strategies and implementation of discipline for people with specific personality traits.

Most organizations have policies (usually in a manual) outlining the recommended stages of disciplinary action. These stages help ensure fair and unbiased treatment of employees. The following is a disciplinary system outlined by Boyd (1984):

1. *Oral warning.* This first step is given with the assumption that the employee did not understand the seriousness of the incident. The manager explains the departmental policy for performance expectations and states that future misconduct will result in a written warning.

2. *Written warning.* When a second occurrence of a prior wrongdoing occurs, the manager notifies the employee in writing of the undesired behavior and includes desired future conduct.

3. *Disciplinary layoff.* With a third occurrence, the employee is suspended from the job for a set period of time without receiving pay. Generally the disciplinary layoff is from 1 to 5 days and is typically outlined in company policy.

4. *Discharge.* After a fourth occurrence of wrongdoing, the employee may be discharged. There should be no misunderstanding by the employee about the reason for being discharged. By this time, "both the employee and company are best served by complete separation" (p. 212).

All of the above steps should be documented with at least two copies, one for the employee, one for the employee's personnel file. Additionally, all employees need to understand the policies of the organization and that all policies will be enforced consistently, using the organization's stages of disciplinary action.

## Conclusion

The occupational therapy manager's role is to act as a motivator to staff to facilitate best practices and job performance. This motivation is achieved by understanding individual differences and using good communication skills, including listening to the individual and providing constructive feedback. Once an individual's specific motivating factors are known, the manager can use these factors to increase the likelihood of improving performance. Providing positive leadership also helps facilitate strong job satisfaction and increase motivation.

There are many benefits of team building, which can be a strong motivating force through building staff commitment, good interpersonal relationships, effective decision-making, and shared values. Team management requires skills similar to those needed for managing individuals, yet positive communication skills among the team members, including the ability to receive as well as give feedback, are the most critical for effective teamwork. The effective manager enables the team—and an effective team enables the manager—to achieve the organization's goals and purpose.

A key to success in a person's career often is the opportunity to be mentored. Through mentoring, the occupational therapy manager can develop employees' personal and professional skills, allowing for further career advancement and success.

Managing disciplinary actions is usually the most unappealing part of the manager's job. A progressive disciplinary approach is the best method; this gives the occupational therapy manager an outline of steps to take in resolving the wrongdoing, thereby ensuring that employees are given fair and unbiased treatment.

The roles and responsibilities of a manager are extremely varied and include managing personal time; making business and policy decisions, including decisions about employees; delegating departmental responsibilities, and assisting in team building. It is essential for managers to be effective listeners, engage in conflict resolution and disciplinary action when necessary, and inform employees about changes and expectations, thereby providing good organizational leadership. One of the most important roles of managers is to communicate effectively and guide staff, motivating employees to do their best job. Managers have many ways to motivate employees, based on both intrinsic and extrinsic factors. The occupational therapy manager can have an exciting and most gratifying job when his or her employees are satisfied and productive.

# References

Alessandra, T., & Hunsaker, P. (1993). *Communicating at work.* New York: Simon & Schuster.

Belker, L. B. (1993). *The first-time manager* (3rd ed.). New York: Amacom.

Boyd, B. B. (1984). *Management-minded supervision* (3rd ed.). New York: McGraw-Hill.

Chesla, E. (2000). *Successful teamwork.* New York: Learning Express.

Craighead, W. E., Kazdin, A. E., & Mahoney, M. J. (1981). *Behavior modification: Principles, issues, and applications* (2nd ed.). Boston: Houghton-Mifflin.

Douglass, M. E., & Douglass, D. N. (1993). *Manage your time, your work, yourself.* New York: Amacom.

Fuller, G. (1995). *The first-time supervisor's survival guide.* Englewood Cliffs, NJ: Prentice-Hall.

Fuller, G. (1998). *Win–win management: Leading people in the new workplace.* Paramus, NJ: Prentice-Hall.

Imundo, L. V. (1991). *The effective supervisor's handbook* (2nd ed.). New York: Amacom.

Jaffe, E. G. (1997). *Administration/management course lecture.* Unpublished document, Samuel Merritt College, Oakland, CA.

Jaffe, E. G. (1999). *Administration/management course lecture.* Unpublished document, Samuel Merritt College, Oakland, CA.

Jaffe, E. G. (2001). *Administration/management course lecture.* Unpublished document, Samuel Merritt College, Oakland, CA.

Lawler, E. E. (1994). *Motivation in work organizations.* San Francisco: Jossey-Bass.

Mayer, J. J. (1990). *If you haven't got the time to do it right, when will you find the time to do it over?* New York: Simon & Schuster.

McCormack, M. C. (1984). *What they don't teach you at Harvard Business School.* New York: Bantam Books.

Murray, M. (1991). *Beyond the myths and magic of mentoring.* San Francisco: Jossey-Bass.

Payne, V. (2001). *The team-building workshop: A trainer's guide.* New York: Amacom.

Perinchief, J. M. (2003). Documentation and management of occupational therapy services. In E. B. Crepeau, E. S. Cohn, & B. A. Boyt Schell (Eds.), *Williard and Spackman's occupational therapy* (10th ed., pp. 897–905). Baltimore: Lippincott Williams & Wilkins.

Pfeiffer, W. J., & Jones, J. E. (1972). Openness, collusion, and feedback. In *Annual handbook for facilitators* (p. 198). San Diego, CA: University Associates.

Robbins, S. P. (1993). *Organizational behavior: Concepts, controversies, and applications* (6th ed., pp. 203–245). Upper Saddle River, NJ: Prentice-Hall.

Robbins, S. P. (1997). *Essentials of organizational behavior* (5th ed.). Upper Saddle River, NJ: Prentice-Hall.

Skopec, E., & Smith, D. M. (1998). *How to use team building to foster innovation throughout your organization.* Chicago: Contemporary Books.

Wellington, S. (2001). *Be your own mentor—Strategies from the top women on the secrets of success.* New York: Random House.

# From Management to Leadership

Ann P. Grady, PhD, OTR, FAOTA

Leadership: *"No society can continue to evolve without it, no family or neighborhood holds together in its absence, and no institution prospers when it is unavailable."*

HELEN ASTIN AND ALEXANDER ASTIN

**Ann P. Grady, PhD, OTR, FAOTA,** is an assistant professor in pediatrics at the University of Colorado Health Sciences Center in Denver. She is the director of interdisciplinary education at JFK Partners, a university-affiliated program of excellence in developmental disabilities, and she is also responsible for teaching the leadership dialogues course and supervising community-based practicum.

## Key Terms and Concepts

**Leadership.** To inspire, direct, guide, and teach others.

**Management.** To increase efficiency, promote stability, assess situations, and select goals.

**Transactional leadership.** A relationship between leader and follower that involves exchange of promises and actions, rewards or punishments as part of motivation for action.

**Transformational leadership.** A relationship between leaders and followers based on shared values and aspirations by which they raise one another to higher levels of motivation and morality. Their purposes for social action are fused in elevating, inspiring purposes.

## Learning Objectives

After completing this chapter, you should be able to do the following:

- Explain the value of developing leadership practices while developing management skills.
- Compare and contrast characteristics of leadership and management.
- Discuss similarities among contemporary leadership theories.
- Identify the means for recognizing developing leadership practices.

The quest to understand leaders and the practice of leadership has intrigued scholars and citizens for centuries. These groups commonly ask questions that focus on leaders and managers. Are leaders and managers different? Are leaders born or made? Can leadership ability be taught and learned? Do men and women lead differently? The purpose of this chapter is not to substantively answer these questions (except the question about differences between managers and leaders) but, rather, to lay a foundation for understanding the evolution of leadership processes through study of leadership theory and its application to occupational therapy.

Understanding the nature and process of leadership is critical for occupational therapy practitioners in health environments, educational settings, and community venues. Broad social changes are affecting the lives of people who need or potentially need occupational therapy services (Legnini, 1994). For example, challenges emerge from restrictive decisions that are made by payers about the frequency and location of service delivery or about the type of intervention that qualifies for payment. Issues such as these demand leadership for change.

On a more positive note, change already under way is creating new opportunities for leadership. For example, new practice venues have been created as a result of the profession's focus on community-based programs for people who are homeless, families living with abuse, very young mothers, and healthy elderly people living in their communities. This long-awaited change calls for leaders with vision to develop the community-based services. Society's updated views about the nature of disability as a difference, not a deficit, is supported by laws and policies that mandate elimination of barriers to permit full access to the environment for all. The challenge to carry out these laws and policies represents another opportunity for occupational therapists to join with colleagues and clients to make change.

For occupational therapy to grow and flourish, leaders in the field need to emerge to infuse the value of occupation into the systems that promote and restore quality and satisfaction in life. Our society needs systems that support engagement with meaningful occupation coupled with opportunities to live, learn, and work in a community of choice (Grady, 1995).

## Leadership Development

The authors of *Leadership Reconsidered: Engaging Higher Education in Social Change* (Astin & Astin, 2000) asked a question with respect to the future: "Who will lead us?" (p. 2). They answered "We will be led by those we have taught, and they will lead us as we have shown them they should" (p. 2). The responsibility for leadership development in the field begins with identifying individuals who have a desire to create change; who are inspired to lead during their basic education; and who are introduced to opportunities to take social action, engage in academic study of leadership as well as management, and discover opportunities for mentoring and coaching as components of their professional development journey. Fortunately, the profession of occupational therapy has had significant leaders serve in its professional association, the American Occupational Therapy Association, and in its foundation, the American Occupational Therapy Foundation. Effective leaders also have emerged from outside the formal organizations to voice concerns and propose actions for change. Developing leaders in occupational therapy can profit from studying past and present leaders in the field.

Occupational therapy practitioners are philosophically and practically qualified to develop leadership skills and use them for social action to affect the systems surrounding practice and education. Both leadership practice and occupational therapy practice are embedded in values that empower others to act and take responsibility for their own lives. At their best, occupational therapy services empower clients to take charge of their lives, including the process for change in their own capabilities, change in barriers that impede development of their highest potential, or both. The leadership practices proposed by Posner and Kouzes (1996) provide a structure for developing leadership practices in concert with values that are held by the occupational therapy profession.

Kouzes and Posner (1987) described *leadership* as "the art of mobilizing others to want to struggle for shared aspirations" (p. 30). They emphasized that the key to effective leadership rests with the words *want to* in the definition. Leadership achieves meaning through its practice in a community. The practices identified in their study include challenging the process, inspiring shared vision, enabling others to act, modeling the way, and encouraging the heart.

## Challenging the Process

Leaders seek and accept challenging opportunities to test their abilities and to find opportunities for change and innovation. Experimenting and taking risks are part of this practice. Occupational therapy leaders have endless opportunities to challenge (a) systems and organizations that do not include, support, and fund needed services or (b) organizations whose service delivery productivity standards no longer allow time for essential components of the service, for example, communication and education that may empower a client to act independently. Challenging communities to be sure all people are included in work and play is also a way for occupational therapists to take leadership.

## Inspiring Shared Vision

Leaders look to the future to propose what is possible and, through their passion, engage others in pursuing the dream. They make it possible for others who are enrolled in the dream to work together and share the success. Therapists join with clients and families to discover priorities for their everyday routines and activities and, in the process, they create a shared vision for the journey.

## Enabling Others to Act

Through an atmosphere of mutual trust and respect, leaders empower others to contribute their best. When leaders involve followers in empowered relationships, they create opportunities for future leaders to emerge. Enabling others to act is at the heart of occupational therapy's focus to create opportunities for clients and their families to engage in gaining or regaining their own health and meaning in life.

## Modeling the Way

Leaders act consistently on standards and values, setting small accomplishments as a standard and then encouraging followers to consistently meet incremental goals on the path to a vision. Leadership that is put into action by "modeling the way" reminds others of the values that guide individual or collective decisions about social actions or client outcomes. Modeling also inspires and guides emerging leaders in the field.

## Encouraging the Heart

Leaders encourage others to continue toward the goals by visibly recognizing and celebrating accomplishments and by promoting balance as part of the work process. Encouraging the heart gives formal and informal recognition to colleague and client accomplishments. Professional associations formalize the recognition process with celebrations.

# Leadership and Management

Creating vision and providing a voice for change are hallmarks of contemporary leadership practice in professional, organizational, and community environments. Leadership and management are complementary processes for creating change or maintaining stability. Leading is about establishing and supporting effectiveness, especially during periods of change. Managing focuses on increasing and maintaining efficiency by promoting stability (Bennis & Nanus, 1985). Table 14.1 presents characteristics of leaders and managers.

Bennis (1984) interviewed 90 leaders and managers in a wide variety of positions and communities, and he identified four competencies associated with leaders:

1. Management of attention by creating a compelling vision and enrolling others in the vision

### Table 14.1 Characteristics of Leaders and Managers

| Leaders | Managers |
|---|---|
| Innovate | Administer |
| Develop | Maintain |
| Focus on people | Focus on structure and systems |
| Inspire trust | Rely on control |
| Keep an eye on the horizon | Keep an eye on the bottom line |
| Challenge the status quo | Accept the status quo |
| Do the right thing | Do things right |

*Note.* From *Leaders: The Strategies for Taking Charge* (p. 16), by W. Bennis and B. Nanus, 1985, New York: Harper & Row. Copyright by Harper & Row. Adapted with permission.

2. Management of meaning by communicating about change in ways that are meaningful to potential followers

3. Management of trust with its component of reliability and constancy

4. Management of self, which focuses on knowing one's own skills and deploying them effectively.

Competencies for managers included use of structure and systems, dependence on control, attention to the bottom line, and investment in the status quo. From his study, Bennis summarized his observations of leaders and managers by reporting that "leaders do the right thing; managers do things right" (Bennis & Nanus, 1985, p. 21).

In a classical study of leaders and managers, Zaleznik (1977) differentiated between managers and leaders according to both their function and their focus. He referred to people who are "once-born" as those for whom adjustments to life have been relatively straightforward developmental experiences. Their sense of self comes from being in harmony with the environment, including people in the environment. They perceive life as a series of orderly events, much like their own experiences. People who are "twice-born" have life experiences that are marked by struggles to achieve a sense of order. Leaders who deal primarily with change are "twice-born." Their sense of self comes from being separate from others and their environment. They develop their self-concept after experiencing a defining or life-changing experience, which they use to withdraw into themselves and then emerge, prepared to deal with the more circular and less predictable progressions of change. As a result, leaders are often in pursuit of opportunities to change the status quo, whereas managers focus on maintaining the status quo.

Throughout the leadership management literature and research, one finds overlap, fusion, and confusion over concepts and functions of management and leadership. Nevertheless, increased development of a "science of management" along with continuing development of concepts of leadership is supporting the differentiation between the nature and functions of leadership and management. According to Zaleznik (1989), leaders are measured by their ability to anticipate the future and lead the change process to achieve a desirable future. Leadership is concerned with purpose and with the distribution of power to influence direction. Managers are measured by how well they get people to go along with the organization's expectations. Management focuses on a rational assessment of situations as well as systematic selection of goals and purposes through strategic planning, the marshaling and assignment of resources, organizational design, and efficient staffing.

In a report on leadership and higher education that was prepared for the Kellogg Foundation, Astin and Astin (2000) stated, "We believe that effective leadership is an essential ingredient of positive social change" (p. iv). In their experience, the power of leaders and leadership is associated with other expressions of the human spirit—hope, commitment, energy, passion, and the capacity to lead—which are rooted in virtually any individual and in every community. Leadership is the property of culture, and it reflects the stated and operating values of a specific society.

> The process of leadership can serve as a lens through which any social situation can be observed. Leadership, especially the ways in which leaders are chosen, the expectations that are placed on them, and how they manifest their authority, can provide remarkable insights into the community, or group. It can tell us how the group defines itself, who and what matters to the group, how things are done, what stories can be told about the outcomes. Within the last few years, we have come to appreciate that the study of leadership within a social context can open up new possibilities for transformation and change. In this way, leadership can be more be a more active tool than a passive lens, allowing individuals, communities, institutions, and societies to narrow the gap between what they value, what their actions express, recognizing that leadership is an integral part of the drama that plays out between the two. (p. vi)

Heifetz (1994) stated that leadership is taking place every day rather than emanating from the traits of a few or existing as a rare event or a once-in-a-lifetime opportunity.

> Every time we face a conflict among competing values, or encounter a gap between our shared values and the way we live, we face the need to learn new ways. A leader has to engage people in facing the challenge, adjusting their values, changing perspectives, and developing new habits of behavior. (p. 275)

The possibilities for transformation and change through the leadership process distinguish leadership from the more transactional process of management. In times of stability, routine management is effective for maintaining the status quo, but in times of change or when change needs to be instigated, leaders must emerge to create or manage that change (Bennis & Nanus, 1985).

## Leadership Types

According to Burns (1978), the study of leadership is central to the structure and processes of human development and political action. DePree (1989) concurred and stated that leadership is a process, much the same as the process of becoming an integrated human being. Leadership is more than a belief or a set of things to do. Leadership is an art form, not a recipe or a one-minute strategy. Leadership is "a continued unfolding of an individual's capabilities and possibilities. Development, leadership development, whatever—it's a lifelong view" (Chandler, 1996, p. 20). Leadership is a structure for action that engages people throughout all levels and within all niches of society.

Burns (1978) described leadership as being part of the dynamics of conflict and power, linked to collective purpose, and measured by actual social change. He identified two basic types of leadership: (a) transactional leadership in which leaders (or managers) engage followers in action that is based on exchange relationships, usually comprising rewards or punishments, and (b) transformational leadership in which leaders recognize an existing need, motive, or demand of a potential follower and seek to satisfy higher needs by engaging the person fully as a follower.

Burns (1978) described transformational and transactional leadership in terms that support the difference between leadership as a process of relationships and management as the execution of distinct skills. According to Bass (1990), Burns viewed leaders as being either transactional or transformational. The interactions between leaders and followers take on these two fundamentally different forms. Bass, however, proposed that transformational leadership augments the effects of exchange relationships (characterized by transactional leadership) to influence the efforts, satisfaction, and effectiveness of followers. The result is a relationship of mutual stimulation and elevation.

## Transactional Leadership

Transactional leadership involves the exchange of valued things. Exchange may be economic, political, or psychological in nature. Each person is aware of the resources held by the other person and of their common, although perhaps temporary, connection. Transactional leadership involves the exchange of promises or actions between leaders and followers, which are often based on self-interests, for example, performance in exchange for pay or increased performance (or additional responsibility) in exchange for increased pay. Transactional leadership tends to be associated with maintaining the status quo or moving along with the tide and is characteristic of management approaches to change. Burns developed the transformational–transactional model after reviewing years of research into the difference between management and leadership and after exploring questions about whether leaders are born or made.

## Transformational Leadership

Transformational, or transforming, leadership occurs when one or more people engage with others in such a way that leaders and followers raise one another to higher levels of motivation and morality. Their purposes, which might have started out separate but related (such as in the case of transactional leadership), become fused. Power bases are linked not as counterweights but as mutual support for a common purpose. Various adjectives are used to describe this kind of leadership: elevating, mobilizing, inspiring, exalting, uplifting, exhorting, evangelizing. The relationship can be moralistic, of course. But transforming leadership ultimately becomes moral in that it raises the level of human conduct and ethical aspirations of both the leader and the led and, thus, has a transforming effect on both (Burns, 1978).

Transformational leadership links leaders and followers in a relationship characterized not only by power but also by mutual needs, aspirations, and values—called "moral leadership" by Burns (1978). Moral leadership includes an element of choice on the part of followers. Choice in this concept of leadership means that followers have knowledge of alternative leaders and programs as well as capacity to choose among the alternatives. Leaders take responsibility for their commitments by providing the means to bring about promised change. Moral leadership emerges from and returns to the fundamental wants, needs, aspirations, and values of the followers. Moral leadership can produce the type of social change that satisfies followers' authentic needs.

Leadership, unlike naked power wielding, is inseparable from followers' needs and goals. The essence of the leader–follower relationship is the interaction of people with different levels of motivation and power potential, including skill, in pursuit of a common or, at least, joint purpose. Transformational leadership involves initiating actions and changing the tide or course of events. A transformational leader recognizes the higher level needs of each follower to engage the full person in achieving a greater good. Thus, this kind of leadership results in mutual stimulation and elevation that converts followers into leaders and that may convert leaders into moral agents. Transformational leaders raise consciousness by articulating and modeling clear values and vision (Astin & Astin, 2000), and their leadership relies on effective communication processes.

When Chemers (1997) summarized Bass's earlier work on transformational and transactional leadership, he observed that transformational leadership involves the followers' perceptions of the leader's charisma; inspirational motivation, which elicits commitment; intellectual stimulation, or new ways of thinking; and an equitable, satisfying focus on individual consideration. In contrast, transactional leadership involves providing contingent rewards to reinforce a positive interaction and initiating negative actions to respond when something goes wrong in the leader–follower interaction.

## Leadership Theories

A review of leadership literature reveals a sequence from a focus on individual leader characteristics to consideration for the environment or situation in which the leader functions to the effects of interaction between leader and followers. The following sections present key theories and models that reflect this progression.

### Trait Theory

When Greenwood (1996) summarized what he called "the meandering of leadership theory," he began by noting that early writings about leadership actually came in the form of comments from authors of management literature in the early 1900s. Specific attributions were associated with the industrial role of foreman (or inspector) and, of course, the role of the company owner to describe the background, qualities, or expertise held by the person in charge. These early references to technical and personal aspects of leaders, including the "great man" concept of leadership (Heifetz, 1994), led to one of the first leadership theories, identified in the literature as the trait theory.

The trait theory was popular during the first half of the 20th century and focused on identifying innate qualities of great political, social, and military leaders, or heroes (Northouse, 1997). At the time, the study of leadership concentrated on searching for the traits of great men that separated them from their followers. Multiple traits of leaders were easily identified, but the number of traits was too numerous to support differences between leaders and followers (Bass, 1990). Northouse stated that ideas from the trait approach were incorporated into the leadership theories that followed.

Trait theory, which began by identifying qualities of people in leadership positions, shifted to include the impact of situations that supported or promoted leadership practice. Trait theory was influenced initially by ideas from management, particularly, the emergence of a new theory of leadership developed by Etzioni (1961) from his industrial background. He studied compliance of workers, which he thought involved a combination of (a) the power held by superiors in organizations and (b) the understanding by subordinates of the impact that that power had on their lives. The amount and type of power available to leaders and managers differs. Managers tend to use power that comes from their personal characteristics, the nature of their position, or the relationships they have with others in power. Leaders tend to use power as influence, which brings others along as participants in the change process. Leaders match leadership style with the degree of follower involvement to exact optimal involvement in the organizational mission. Leaders tend to pull through involvement, whereas managers are likely to push (Bennis & Nanus, 1985). Managers tend to exert power through the allocation of resources and use of rewards or punishments to motivate or control followers. The ways in which leaders use power depend on the involvement of followers. Etzioni's approach to workers was a forerunner to the contingency theory of leadership that was proposed by Fiedler (1967).

### Contingency Theory

Fiedler focused on task and relationship behaviors of leaders and followers wherein different situations required different types of task and relationship behaviors to bring about the desired follower outcomes. Fiedler believed that a person's task-oriented and relationship behaviors remain much the same over time (Fiedler, 1967). The task, or the set of relationship-building requirements of a situation, needs to be matched with the leadership behavior of the person in the position. This theory represented a shift in leadership research, which moved from focusing solely on the leader to considering the situation in which the leader practiced (Northouse, 1997). Fielder developed a program called "Leader-Match" and a Least Preferred Coworker Scale in an attempt to modify leadership situations to match personalities (Greenwood, 1996). Fielder's contingency model led to other situationally based attempts to understand the nature and process of leadership.

### Path–Goal Theory

The path–goal theory of leadership proposed by House (1971) is another situationally based leadership theory. The goal of the leader in the path–goal theory is to enhance employee satisfaction and performance by focusing on motivation. The theory states that the motivational functions of a leaders are to ensure that employees achieve personal rewards for accomplishing their goals at work. The leader clarifies the path to success and removes the roadblocks to the goal. The leader also improves potential for satisfaction by showing consideration and support. The complexity of the work task, the degree to which the task is structured, the follower's perceived need for structure, and available support are components of the leader–follower relationship for enhancing motivation.

### Situational Leadership

Hersey, Blanchard, and Natemeyer (1979) developed a model that they first referred to as the life-cycle theory and later as situational leadership. Like the contingency theory, this model was built around the dimensions of task requirements and relationship behaviors associated with the leadership goal. *Task behavior* is defined as the extent to which a leader uses one-way communication to direct people, telling them what to do and how to do it. *Relationship behavior* is the extent to which the leader engages in two-way communication to motivate and guide potential followers. The driving force of the model is the job competency and psychological maturity of the person assigned to accept the challenge. According to Hersey and colleagues (1979), the leader's style changes according to the maturity level of the follower. A lower maturity level in a follower increases the task behavior of the leader. As the follower's maturity increases, the leader's task behavior decreases, and his or her relationship behavior increases. The base of power held by a leader is an integral component of situational leadership, because followers with different levels of maturity are influenced differently by a leader's base of power.

### Leader–Member Exchange Theory

The leader–member exchange theory identified leadership as an interaction between leader and follower in dyad relationships. The theory, developed by Graen and colleagues (Dansereau, Graen, & Haga, 1975), proposes that, within an organization, leaders develop a series of vertical, dyad relationships with subordinates. In one study to explore this theory (Wayne, Liden, & Sparrowe, 1994), subordinates became part of either an in-group or an out-group, depending on unique relationships or exchanges with each person. Members who were interested in negotiating the work with the leader became part of the in-group and, thus, open to opportunities that exceeded their job description. Those who were not interested in additional responsibilities were in the out-group. High-quality, in-group exchanges were based on mutual trust and support, whereas low-quality, out-group exchanges were based on simply meeting employment conditions. Later studies (Graen & Uhl-Bien, 1995) focused on how leader–follower relationships affected organizational effectiveness. If a high-quality leader–member exchange existed, then the organization had less turnover and more promotions, commitment, and positive attitudes about the organization and work assignments. The leader–member exchange theory is a transactional model.

Bargal and Schmid (1989) reviewed theory and research in leadership and developed themes that encompassed the literature identified to date. The leadership themes they identified include the leader as creator of vision; the leader as creator of organizational culture, transactional or transformational leadership styles; and reciprocal leadership–follower relations. The themes relate to (a) internal management tasks of goal setting, motivation, and development of people, as well as maintenance and administration of tasks and to (b) external management goals, including resource mobilization and achievement of legitimacy.

Early leadership theories concentrated on the traits of great men, or heroes, who were vested with power either because of who they were or because of the position they held. In the 1960s, ideas about leadership moved significantly toward consideration of situations that influenced the emergence and practice of leadership. These situational approaches considered interaction a part of leadership. Theorists then began to emphasize interpersonal interaction in leader–member exchange theory. Finally, the concept of leadership as an exchange, or transaction, emerged and expanded to development of transformational leadership, which continues to influence our thinking.

O'Toole (1995) concurred with Burns's concept of moral leadership as it related to values-based leadership. He stated that, when a leader listens to what potential followers say they need and want and when the leader responds thoughtfully, then potential followers feel respected and become engaged in the vision and values proposed by the leader. The vision of the leader becomes a follower's vision because it is based on a foundation of the follower's needs and aspirations. Moral and effective leaders listen to their followers because they respect them and honestly believe that, along with the social changes they envision, the welfare of followers is the true end of leadership. Ultimately, trust, the essential quality in a leader–follower relationship (Kouzes & Posner, 1993), is built on the respect that a leader holds for a follower. Effective leaders set aside any tendency to lead by pushing others and adopt the behavior of always leading by relying on the pull of inspiring values. Values-based leadership is central to the concept of transformational leadership because leaders join with followers in creating jointly held ends and means for the pursuit of a vision. New leaders are frequently created through collaborative efforts of leaders and followers.

According to Heifetz (1994), values in leadership have been hidden in discussions of leadership theories. The great man, or trait, approach put value on a person with great influence, even though the direction of influence may or may not be congruent with others' values. Trait theories emphasize the idea that individuals make a difference in influencing the direction and outcome of group activities. In situational and contingency theories, leaders' influence continues to emphasize methods to control others in decision making; they have, however, added to our understanding of the role of context in leadership activities. Transactional approaches focus on how influence is gained and maintained, which is not as value-neutral as purported. The transactional theories contributed to the idea that authority can be a reciprocal relationship, which depends on the nature of the relationships between leaders and followers.

Heifetz (1994) stated that a definition of leadership must consider values. He defined *leadership* as adaptive work, which consists of the learning that is required to address conflicts in the values that people hold or to diminish the gap between their values and the realities they face. Adaptive work requires a change in values, beliefs, or behavior and frequently is motivated by the conflicts that either exist internally or are observed externally. Adaptive work in human societies involves not only an assessment of reality but also the use of values clarification to reach commonality of purpose.

Terry (1993) was influenced by Heifetz's ideas when he proposed an "action wheel" for carrying out authentic leadership. In the wheel, meaning legitimates and orients mission; mission directs and focuses power; power energizes and modifies structures; structures sustain power, generate new ideas, and move the mission forward; resources equip structures from what is available or potentially available; and existence both limits and expands resources. Terry defined *leadership* as a subset of action, but not all action is considered leadership. Authentic action involves correspondence, consistency, coherence, concealment, conveyance, comprehensiveness, and convergence. Authenticity in leadership involves not only action but also courage, an ability to cope with fear, a sense of common good, and hope. Therefore, leadership is authentic action.

Lipman-Blumen (1996) developed a connective leadership model that contains a set of nine behavioral facets. She sees a new era for leadership, with interdependence and diversity pulling against each other as hallmarks of the new leadership. Her model gives leaders three tools for action. First, leaders identify the most effective leadership strategies that they personally apply in each unique situation. Second, leaders evaluate leadership potential of others and match their behaviors to the demands of the situations. Third, leaders design new structures that fit not only the tasks to be accomplished but also the behavioral preferences of all participants. Lipman-Blumen's tools incorporate some aspects of situational approaches to leadership but also include components involving interaction and adaptability. Her model consists of three major sets of behavioral styles:

1. The direct style in which people like to confront their tasks individually and directly, emphasizing mastery, competition, and power. Direct styles are related to issues of diversity and individualism.
2. The relational styles, which are related to interdependence. People using relational styles contribute to others' ability to accomplish tasks through collaboration, contribution, and mentoring.
3. The instrumental style, which maximizes interaction for both direct and relational styles by empowering, entrusting, and building networks.

According to Lipman-Blumen (1996),

Connective leadership, based on a nine-style Connective Leadership Model, brings "an ethical instrumentation" to bear on the politics of human interaction. But, it does not throw away everything else. It revitalizes traditional leadership behaviors by harnessing individualism and teamwork through the principled deployment of political strategies. (p. 27)

Chemers and Ayman (1993) also proposed building on past leadership theory and research. Leadership is a process of social influence, and effective leadership is the successful application of the influence to mission accomplishment. In other words, effective leaders are able to obtain the cooperation of other people, and to harness the resources provided by that cooperation to the attainment of a goal. (p. 294)

To build a theory of leadership effectiveness, Chemers (1997) identified essential processes of image management, relationship development, and use of resources. His model attempted to integrate individual, dyadic, group, and organizational interactions. The model is divided into three zones. First, the zone of self-deployment is the interface between the leader and the environment. According to Chemers, groups having leaders who match well with followers have higher levels of confidence and optimism. Second, the zone of transactional relationship portrays the dynamics of interaction between leaders and followers. The forces that create the relationship and exchange between them determine the degree of motivation, commitment, and satisfaction of all involved in the relationship. Influences such as a leader's perceptions of individual needs, of desires, and about the prevailing culture as well as the leader's perceptions of individual needs, desires, and expectations of followers are key elements in forming the relationship. Third, the zone of team deployment focuses team effort, persistence, and contribution. Effort describes how hard the team is willing to work; persistence relates to the team's ability to maintain commitment and energy in the face of challenges; contribution is the amount and type of input and degree of participation that determines group actions.

Chemers (1997) stated that team effort and situational demands are governed by contingency principle and are anchored in objective consequences. He maintained that it is not enough to have a satisfied, loyal team that is committed to an enthusiastic leader unless the actions of the leader and team are appropriate to the demands of the task and success is attained. However, a leader's objective success rests with the subjective influences identified in the three zones of Chemers's model.

## Leadership and Communication

The development and use of communication skills as a component of leadership reflects the view that leadership is understood best as a product of human communication. Leadership competence increases with communication competence (Hackman & Johnson, 1991). According to Hackman and Johnson, leadership shares all features of human communication in the sense that leaders use symbols to create reality by the language they choose, the stories they tell, and the rituals they create. Leaders communicate about past and present as a foundation for the vision they put forth for a desirable future. Leaders make conscious use of symbols to reach their goals.

Leadership, like communication, is a continuous, dynamic, ever-changing process by which information and meaning are transacted through the uniquely human use of symbols. Hackman and Johnson (1991) proposed that "leadership is human (symbolic) communication, which modifies the attitudes and behaviors of others to meet group goals and needs" (p. 11). Leadership effectiveness depends on the development of skills in three areas of communication function (Dance & Larson, 1976): (a) linking with other human beings and their environment, (b) developing higher mental processes as a result of symbol usage, and (c) regulating behavior of self and others. The linking function is critical to leadership because relationships between leaders and individuals as well as between leaders and the environment in which they serve are characterized by listening and processing verbal and nonverbal messages, establishing trust, and creating a successful and satisfying environment for effective work groups and teams. The conceptual abilities of thinking and reasoning rely on and enhance higher mental processes. A leader's ability to use the meaning of the leader's ability to interpret information that is gleaned from linking with people to articulate a vision for the future emanates from the leader's ability to create and use symbols. Once vision and direction are established, the communication function of regulating behavior is accomplished through mutual agreement among leaders and followers, which enables them to adhere to the mission and values set forth and adopted by the group.

Hackman and Johnson (1991) summarized the application of human communication functions to leadership practice as follows:

> Linking skills include monitoring the environment, creating a trusting climate, and team building. Envisioning involves creating new agendas or visions out of previously existing elements. Regulation means influencing others by developing credibility and power, using effective verbal and nonverbal communication, creating positive expectations, managing change, gaining compliance, and negotiating. (p. 18)

The development and use of communication for carrying out the linking, mental processing, and regulating functions of communication are essential for leadership and are particularly related to the challenges that require the leader to address issues of values and change. Finding voice, as identified by Helgesen (1990), reflects ways in which communication functions can foster leadership through speaking, listening, organizing, visioning, modeling, instructing, influencing, and persuading.

## Conclusion

The selected contemporary theories, or models, of leadership, such as Chemers's (1997) integrative model of leadership, Heifetz's (1994) values orientation, Terry's (1993) model of authentic leadership, and Lipman-Blumen's (1996) connective leadership model illustrate the extent to which earlier theories have changed. The previously narrow focus on leaders, followers, situations, or transactions has expanded through the integration of those ideas from the past into the demands of new environments and through respect for the interactional components of leadership. Leadership development requires commitment, self-development, and attention to changing environments.

According to Bennis (1990), individuals pursuing leadership development need to include the following commitments and actions in their development plans:

1. Make a commitment to change and lifelong learning.
2. Develop an ability to embrace error, because successful leaders learn from their mistakes.
3. Adopt a willingness to encourage dissent and engage in creative resolution. Followers who are encouraged to raise issues or disagree tend to become leaders.
4. Engage in "reflective backtalk" with a trusted colleague, coach, or mentor with whom ideas can be critiqued in advance and organized for presentation.
5. Be vulnerable (open) to others when they present a different and better idea for your plan. Your vision and plan will be improved, and the contributors will feel included in the process.
6. Generate a bias toward action with a clear and accountable plan for change.
7. Constantly improve the ability to generate and sustain trust.

Contemporary leadership literature describes practices that are imbedded in underlying values of support and empowerment. These values have been part of occupational therapy's philosophy since its inception. If we believe that leaders are mostly made through engaging in a process of leadership development, then occupational therapists already imbued with values of support and empowerment and challenged by social environments that do not always support and empower the people they serve are therefore ideally suited to focus their efforts on developing the leadership practices required for change.

# References

Astin, A., & Astin, H. (2000). *Leadership reconsidered: Engaging higher education in social change.* Battle Creek, MI: W. K. Kellogg Foundation.

Bargal, D., & Schmid, H. (1989). Recent themes in theory and research on leadership and their implications for management of the human services. *Administration in Social Work, 13*(3/4), 37–54.

Bass, B. M. (1990). *Bass and Stogdill's handbook of leadership: Theory, research, and managerial applications* (3rd ed.). New York: Free Press.

Bennis, W. (1984, August). The 4 competencies of leadership. *Training and Development Journal,* pp. 5–10.

Bennis, W. (1990, August). *Leaders and managers.* Symposium conducted at the Cape Cod Institute, Eastham, MA.

Bennis, W., & Nanus, B. (1985). *Leaders: The strategies for taking charge.* New York: Harper & Row.

Burns, J. M. (1978). *Leadership.* New York: Harper & Row.

Chandler, J. B. (1996). An interview: John W. Gardner, leader of leaders. *Journal of Leadership Studies, 3*(1), 17–24.

Chemers, M. M. (1997). *An integrative theory of leadership.* Mahwah, NJ: Erlbaum.

Chemers, M. M., & Ayman, R. (Eds.). (1993). *Leadership theory and research.* San Diego: Harcourt, Brace, Jovanovich.

Dance, F. E. X., & Larson, C. E. (1976). *The functions of human communication: A theoretical approach.* New York: Holt, Rinehart, & Winston.

Dansereau, F., Graen, G., & Haga, W. (1975). A vertical dyad linkage approach to leadership in formal organizations. *Organizational Behavior and Human Performance, 13,* 46–78.

DePree, M. (1989). *Leadership is an art.* New York: Doubleday.

Etzioni, A. (1961). *A comparative analysis of complex organizations.* New York: Free Press.

Fiedler, S. E. (1967). *A theory of leadership effectiveness.* New York: McGraw-Hill.

Grady, A. P. (1995). Building inclusive community: A challenge for occupational therapy. *American Journal of Occupational Therapy, 49,* 300–310.

Graen, G. B., & Uhl-Bien, M. (1995). Relationship-based approach to leadership: Development of leader–member exchange (LMX) theory of leadership over 25 years: Applying a multi-level, multi-domain perspective. *Leadership Quarterly, 6,* 219–247.

Greenwood, R. (1996). Leadership theory: A historical look at its evolution. *Journal of Leadership Studies, 3*(1), 3–16.

Hackman, M. Z., & Johnson, C. E. (1991). *Leadership: A communication perspective.* Project Heights, IL: Waveland Press.

Heifetz, R. A. (1994). *Leadership without easy answers.* Cambridge, MA: Belknap Press.

Helgesen, S. (1990). *The female advantage: Women's ways of leadership.* New York: Doubleday Currency.

Hersey, P., Blanchard, K. H., & Natemeyer, W. E. (1979). Situational leadership, perception, and the impact of power. *Center for Leadership Studies,* pp. 1–6.

House, R. J. (1971). A path–goal theory of leader effectiveness. *Administrative Science Quarterly, 1,* 321–338.

Kouzes, J. M., & Posner, B. Z. (1987). *The leadership challenge: How to keep getting extraordinary things done in organizations.* San Francisco: Jossey-Bass.

Kouzes, J. M., & Posner, B. Z. (1993). *Credibility: How leaders gain and lose it, why people demand it.* San Francisco: Jossey-Bass.

Legnini, M. W. (1994). Developing leaders vs. training administrators in the health services. *American Journal of Public Health, 84,* 1569–1571.

Lipman-Blumen, J. (1996). *The connective edge.* San Francisco: Jossey-Bass.

Northouse, P. G. (1997). *Leadership: Theory and practice.* Thousand Oaks, CA: Sage.

O'Toole, J. (1995). *Leading change: Overcoming the ideology of comfort and the tyranny of custom.* San Francisco: Jossey-Bass.

Posner, B. Z., & Kouzes, J. M. (1996). Ten lessons for leaders and leadership developers. *Journal of Leadership Studies, 3*(3), 3–10.

Terry, R. W. (1993). *Authentic leadership: Courage in action.* San Francisco: Jossey-Bass.

Wayne, S. J., Liden, R. C., & Sparrowe, R. T. (1994). Developing leader–member exchanges. *American Behavioral Scientist, 37,* 697–714.

Zaleznik, A. (1977). Managers and leaders: Are they different? *Harvard Business Review, 55*(3), 67–78.

Zaleznik, A. (1989). Real work. *Harvard Business Review, 67,* 57–64.

# Controlling
# Outcomes

# Evidence-Based Practice

Beatriz C. Abreu, PhD, OTR, FAOTA

*"What is research but learning—and what scientist ever feels that, being complete, his research is now at last finished? The nature of science is such that a scientist goes on learning all his life."*

PETER B. MEDAWAR

**Beatriz C. Abreu, PhD, OTR, FAOTA,** is director of occupational therapy at the Transitional Learning Center, Galveston, TX, and clinical professor at the University of Texas Medical Branch, Galveston.

## Key Terms and Concepts

**Evidence-based practice (EBP).** The use of systematic research review to formally gather and synthesize information from research findings to determine best practice.

**Meta-analysis.** A study that appraises individual studies using appropriate statistical techniques and provides the highest level of evidence in a secondary source.

**Primary publications.** Experimental or observational studies that report original analytical research.

**Randomization.** The procedure used to predetermine the assignment of treatment to participants so that the chances of assignment to a particular treatment are the same for all participants in the study.

**Secondary publications.** Integrative studies that summarize and draw conclusions from primary research or previously published or unpublished studies.

**Statistical power.** An index used to determine the probability that significant changes are due to the treatment rather than to chance.

## Learning Objectives

After completing this chapter, you should be able to do the following:

- Define the role of evidence-based practice (EBP) for managers in Occupational Therapy and list the five EBP steps.

- Identify effective strategies for getting started in EBP.

- Identify examples of how EBP can be applied by a manager in the practice of occupational therapy.

- Reflect on EBP applications to direct care, research, and education.

Today's increasing quality- and efficiency-driven health care system means that a highly competent workforce is vital for achieving good managerial results. Therefore, occupational therapy managers have had to learn how to become more competent problem-solvers and teach staff members this essential skill. Evidence-based practice (EBP) methods are one way to create and sustain a competent environment in the workplace. Managers use evidence in their decision-making to develop and support effective clinical programs as well as efficient assessment and intervention procedures (Tickle-Degnen, 2002a). This chapter contains practical and simplified information that occupational therapy managers can use to support and guide problem-solving decisions.

## What Is EBP?

EBP involves using systematic research review to formally gather and synthesize information from research findings to determine best clinical practice. This method is derived from evidence-based medicine (Law, 2002; Sackett, Straus, Richardson, Rosenberg, & Haynes, 2000). EBP is an evolving process. It has its roots in medical outcomes, which have transformed to evidence-based medicine, expanded into EBP and, more recently, further expanded to the broad area of evidence-based health care (Ottenbacher, 2002). The distinctions, similarities, and relationship of these concepts are not clear and continue to develop. Clinical practice should provide sufficient evidence to establish the effect of occupational therapy services on health outcomes and to demonstrate that occupational therapy interventions are effective, beneficial, and cost effective (Abreu, 1998; Foto, 1996). Every practitioner in the field is responsible for the validation of occupational therapy services. The ability to incorporate research findings into practice is expected and demanded by our institutions (Holm, 2000; Ottenbacher & Hinderer, 2001). However, the manager faces the challenge of searching through and sorting out a dramatic information explosion, which includes not only impressive research advances but also information that has demonstrated limited use of evidence to support clinical practice. Some investigators estimate that only 15% of health care is supported by documented evidence (Baker, 1996).

This chapter describes the five steps involved in the process of carrying out EBP in the workplace. It also identifies examples, strengths, and limitations of EBP. The chapter concludes with implications for research and education.

## Five Steps in EBP

A complete description of the EBP process for managers is too comprehensive for this chapter. Nevertheless, the following sections describe some highlights of the critical five steps needed by managers to use EBP in clinical reasoning and problem solving: (a) formulate the question, (b) search and sort the evidence, (c) critically appraise the evidence, (d) apply to practice (reject or accept), and (e) conduct self-assessment.

## Step 1: Formulate the Question

The first step involves turning the clinical problem into the form of a question. Questions from everyday practice become the basis for examining the research literature evidence. The questions can be in any topic or area related to (a) therapy or prevention, (b) etiology or harm, (c) prognosis, (d) diagnosis, and (e) economic analysis (Sackett et al., 2000). Additionally, knowledge gaps in clinical and community practice as well as in specific client needs may guide the formulation of questions (McKibbon, 1999).

Richardson, Wilson, Nishikawa, and Hayward (1995) proposed not only that a well-built question is a key to EBP methods but also that it must contain four parts: (a) the problem or patient, (b) the intervention or exposure, (c) the comparison intervention or exposure when relevant, and (d) the outcomes of interest. Law (2002) suggested that a sample of an appropriate question that can yield good results might follow the format that follows: For people with condition _____, will treatment _____ be more effective than treatment _____ in leading to outcome or increasing function in outcome ____?

The best outcomes provide the best evidence for practice. The best practice provides occupational therapists and occupational therapy assistants, whether they are service providers or managers, with the opportunity to render better client care, optimal program evaluation, and quality improvement systems. The therapist can frame evidence-based questions related to client care questions in many ways. For example, two types of treatment questions have to do with effectiveness and efficacy. Effectiveness of treatment is the first step the practitioner takes to ensure that occupational therapy interventions produce changes in the client's performance during his or her stay in the treatment setting or in the discharge environment (Ottenbacher & Hinderer, 2001). Effective evidence is provided by positive findings in outcome research, including the use of outcome measures such as the Functional Independence Measure (FIM; Guide, 1993) to study the results of rehabilitation (McKenna et al., 2002). Effectiveness studies answer the questions, Did clients receiving occupational therapy improve? How much did they improve?

In contrast, evidence of treatment efficacy is more difficult to obtain in occupational therapy. This type of evidence examines the relationship between a particular treatment intervention and an outcome measure (or measures) under very controlled or optimal conditions (Clark et al., 1997; Ottenbacher & Hinderer, 2001), and it answers the question, Which treatment made the clients better? Controlled experiments have two or more groups of participants: one group that receives the treatment under investigation and a second group that receives a standard treatment or a placebo intervention (a treatment with no known therapeutic value). Another control measure used in high-quality efficacy studies such as clinical trials involves the allocation of the client in an unsystematic or random fashion that guarantees no selection bias. The single-blind method is another way of controlling for the awareness that study participants may have of the type of treatment they are receiving. In addition, double-blind studies, which control for the participants' awareness of the treatment they are receiving and the investigators' awareness of the treatment they are providing, add another layer of quality control and rigor.

Efficacy evidence requires the use of the most rigorous experimental research designs, randomized controlled trials (RCTs). (Table 15.1 lists experimental research designs according to levels of rigor.) A properly controlled clinical trial is valued as having the most powerful experimental design and evidence for evaluating the effectiveness of a treatment. A *clinical trial* has been defined as a prospective (followed-forward) study comparing the value and the effect of an occupational therapy intervention group against a control group not receiving treatment. An example of an elegant clinical trial in occupational therapy is one published in the *Journal of the American Medical Association* that supported the benefits of occupational therapy as a preventive health program for independent living in older adults (Clark et al., 1997).

Efficacy questions sometimes cannot be answered fully because of methodological barriers such as the ethical issues surrounding clinical trials. Some of the ethical issues contribute to flaws in the research design. An example is a situation in which a clinical trial used by a pharmaceutical company provides financial incentives for primary investigators to recruit participants for the study. Rao (1999) believed that financial gain for recruiting research participants is wrong because it makes controlled randomized trials (CRTs) lucrative and may compromise the care of clients who are not in the trial. The practice of withholding the best treatment in some studies has also been questioned as being unethical. Some trials provide the treatment to the control group after the study has finished. CRTs, which are synonymous with RCTs, are expensive and time-consuming, and they put high demand on people resources. CRTs can be driven by the researcher's interest instead of the client's needs.

Other types of questions can be asked that go beyond occupational therapy treatment and relate to managerial issues of quality improvement. These questions explore areas that support a continuous drive to improve service delivery performance, reduction of costs for services, and elimination of errors (Byers & Beaudin, 2002; Morahan, 2002). In the areas of individualized care, well-trained staff members as well as client and family network involvement in the health care process is essential. Thus, for example, a manager may use EBP to promote changing a policy in the workplace to improve the quality of the health care process. A *policy* is a plan of action or statement of ideas proposed and adopted by the government, an institution, or profession (*Oxford English Dictionary*, 1995). Muir Gray, Haynes, Sackett, Cook, and Guyatt (1997) have reminded us that policies come in many forms, from those that determine funding in health care to public health policies to clinical policies such as pathways, protocols, clinical standards, expert recommendations, and decision analyses that state what should be done in practice. The best policy is built on sound evidence.

**Table 15.1 Primary Publications and Three Grading Systems.**

| Research Design | Evidence |
| --- | --- |
| **RCTs** | Level I |
| Includes two groups: treatment and control. The treatment or experimental group receives the intervention or treatment under investigation. The control group receives no treatment. Participants are assigned to either of the groups in an unbiased manner. Rigor ranges from single- to double-blind. In a double-blind study, neither the participants nor the researchers know which participants are receiving the treatment. In a single-blind study, only the researchers are blinded. | Grade A<br>1a, 1b, 1c (3 levels of rigor) |
| **Cohort Studies** | Level II |
| Observational studies that follow a group of people over time to find out what will happen to them (prospective study) or what has happened to them (retrospective study). In epidemiology, this type of study looks for how risk factors associate with disease development (incidence of disease). | Grade B<br>2a, 2b, 2c (3 levels of rigor) |
| **"Outcome" Research** | – |
| Observational studies that evaluate best practices (evaluation and intervention), resource utilization, functional gains, timelines, and satisfaction with services. | |
| **Low-Quality RCTs** | – |
| Similar to RCTs, but with lower internal and/or external validity. | |
| **Case–Control Studies** | Level III |
| Observational studies that compare the effect of treatment intervention between participants with a particular condition (case) and participants without the condition (control). Participants may be individuals, a group, an event, or a society. | Grade C<br>3a, 3b (2 levels of rigor) |
| **Case Report or Case Series** | Level IV |
| Studies that involve comparison of the treatment effect of a single or several people, cases, or events at initial baseline and after treatment. | Grade D<br>(no levels of rigor) |
| **Poor-Quality Cohort and Case–Controls** | |
| Similar to cohort studies, but with lower internal and/or external validity. | |
| **Expert Opinion Without Explicit Critical Appraisal** | Level V |
| Studies that describe the judgment or belief of a skillful, trained professional; not based on organized research study findings. | Grade E<br>(no levels of rigor) |
| **Qualitative Research** | |
| At this stage in the development of EBP, the focus is only on quantitative research. | |

*Note.* RCT = randomized controlled trial; EBP = evidence-based practice.

The following examples of selected questions examined in occupational therapy are questions to which answers from the evidence are already available:

- What is the effectiveness of cognitive–behavioral interventions in improving occupational performance (function) for people with chronic pain? (The Occupational Therapy Evidence-Based Practice Research Group, 1998, at McMaster University, Ontario, posed this question.)
- What is the effectiveness of activity programs in improving performance skills and contextual factors for older people with dementia? (The Occupational Therapy Evidence-Based Practice Research Group, 1999, at McMaster University, Ontario, posed this question.)
- What is the efficacy of sensory integration in different behavioral domains and for different diagnostic and age groups compared with other interventions? (The Database of Abstracts of Review of Effectiveness addressed this question as it related to Vargas and Camilli's 1999 sensory integration meta-analysis article published in the *American Journal of Occupational Therapy*.)
- What is the effectiveness of occupational therapy in enhancing the psychosocial well-being, daily functioning, and physical health of older people? (The Database of Abstracts of Review of Effectiveness addressed this question as it related to Carlson, Fanchiang, Zemke, and Clark's 1996 occupational therapy meta-analysis article published in the *American Journal of Occupational Therapy*.)
- Does occupational therapy engagement in purposeful activity produce a better quality of movement than concentration on movement per se? (This question appeared in The Database of Abstracts Reviews of Effectiveness as it related to Lin, Wu, Tickle-Degnen, and Coster's 1997 meta-analysis article published in the *Occupational Therapy Journal of Research*.)

## Step 2: Search and Sort the Evidence

The second step in EBP involves searching and sorting the current best evidence. A systematic and explicit search to identify, select, and summarize evidence is a complex and labor-intensive process. EBP does not recommend searching traditional textbooks as sources of evidence because they are not updated yearly, they are lightly referenced, and they often do not provide evidence in support of the statements made in the book (Sackett et al., 2000). I expect that the future will bring evidence-based Internet textbooks that will be continuously updated.

The occupational therapy manager will be challenged in searching and sorting evidence because he or she will lack time, computer availability, and Internet access. Access to certain databases requires user codes, which are readily available to college students and faculty but are less accessible to therapists. One free, public-access database is PubMed (http://www.ncbi.nlm.nih.gov/PubMed/) which, in addition to providing citations, links the user to related Web resources.

### Primary and Secondary Publications

Regardless of the database used, searches for evidence can be conducted using two major publication sources—primary and secondary research sources. Published *primary studies*, also called *primary research* or *primary publications*, refer to those studies that report original analytical research, which can be experimental or observational. Published *secondary studies*, also called *secondary research, secondary publications*, or *systematic reviews*, refer to integrative studies that summarize and draw conclusions from primary research or from previously published or unpublished studies (McKibbon, 1999).

A useful resource for locating high-quality evidence from primary and secondary publications is the Cochrane Collaboration (http://www.cochrane.org), an international organization of health professionals, librarians, and consumers that was founded in 1993 with the goal of helping people make informed decisions about health care by preparing, maintaining, and ensuring the accessibility of systematic reviews of health care interventions. This worldwide network is named in honor of Archibald Leman Cochrane, a British obstetrician and epidemiologist. In the early 1970s, Cochrane identified a lack of RCTs in the field of obstetrics. Through his writings and advocacy for these trials, he promoted the use of evidence in clinical practice. The Cochrane Library is the electronic collection of information that is available from university libraries on the Internet and in CD-ROM format and that has been developed by the Cochrane Collaboration to carry out the goals of helping people make informed decisions about health care. Refer to Exhibit 15.1 to review the Cochrane Library and some other major electronic sources for clinical evidence.

### Outcome Measures

Managers interested in locating effective evidence such as outcome studies can find good information in specific outcome databases. These databases are designed for the sole purpose of collecting evidence about the effectiveness of rehabilitation related to outcomes in the rehabilitation of clients with particular diagnoses. One specific database was started in 1987 and is funded by the U.S. Department of Education's National Institute on Disability and Rehabilitation Research (NIDRR, 2000) to establish the Traumatic Brain Injury (TBI) Model Systems of Care (for more information, access http://www.tbims.org/combi.html). The database first included 17 centers under NIDRR and established the goal to maintain a national database that is easily accessible for innovative analysis of TBI treatment and outcome. Outcomes tracked within this database relate to interventions that span across several disciplines. Occupational therapy participation in this system is minimal and should be encouraged.

A particular benefit of this system is the identification of the evaluation tests and measures used as outcome measures. These measures represent the most accepted standardized tools in the rehabilitation of clients with TBI. The outcome measures included in the model system are the Agitated Behavior Scale, the Coma/Near Coma

## Exhibit 15.1  Major Electronic Sources of Evidence.

**ACP Journal Club (www.acpjc.org)**

A database including original studies and systematic reviews by the American College of Physicians–American Society of Internal Medicine. It is published bimonthly.

**The Cochrane Library (www.cochrane.org)**

A collection of databases that is published quarterly on the Internet or a CD-ROM and is distributed on a subscription basis. Some of the databases and other information include

- Cochrane Controlled Trials Register
  A bibliography of controlled trials that have been identified by experts as an unbiased source of data for systematic reviews. The register of trials listed was searched and specially selected from the world's literature.
- Database of Abstracts of Reviews of Effectiveness
  A collection of structured abstracts from systematic reviews that have been appraised by qualified reviewers.
- Cochrane Database of Systematic Reviews
  Highly structured and systematic full-text summary articles reviewing effects of health care.
- Also included are Cochrane Review Methodology Database, *Handbook on Critical Appraisal, Glossary of Methodological Terms*, and more information on the Cochrane Collaboration

**Cumulative Index to Nursing and Allied Health Literature (www.cinahl.com)**

A commercial database that indexes more than 650 journal titles, audiovisual materials, computer programs, dissertations, books, and book chapters from 1982 to the present. It focuses primarily on allied health topics.

**EMBASE/Excerpta Medica (www.embase.com)**

A database that many consider to be a European version of Medline, with more than 8 million records from 1974 to the present, including pharmacology literature, allied health areas, and, especially, European literature.

**Evidence-Based Medicine Reviews (www.ovid.com/products/clinical/ebmr.cfm)**

A database that searches material from the Cochrane Library's Systematic Reviews section, Best Evidence; full-text resources from the American College of Physicians; and the Database of Abstracts of Reviews of Effectiveness, which is a full-text database that contains critical overviews of systematic reviews from various medical journals.

**Healthstar (www.ovid.com/documentation/user/field_guide/disp_fldguide.cfm?db=hstrdb.htm)**

A database that indexes journal articles, books, meeting abstracts, technical reports, newspapers, and government documents in the fields of health technology as well as administration and research from 1986 to the present.

**MEDLINE (www.nlm.nih.gov)**

A bibliographic database that contains health care literature published in more than 3,600 journals between 1966 and the present. It is produced by the U.S. National Library of Medicine.

**PsycINFO (www.apa.org/psycinfo)**

A database that indexes journal articles, book chapters, and books. This database contains information on psychology, psychiatry counseling, and other mental health topics published between 1974 and the present. It is produced by the American Psychological Association.

**PubMed (www.ncbi.nlm.nih.gov/entrez/query.fcgi)**

A database that provides access to MEDLINE citations from the mid-1960s to the present. It was developed by the National Center for Biotechnology Information at the National Institutes of Health. It has links to full-text articles at journal Web sites and related Web resources.

Scale, the Community Integration Questionnaire, the Disability Rating Scale, the Family Needs Questionnaire, the Functional Assessment Measure, the FIM, the Glasgow Outcome Scale, the Level of Cognitive Functioning Scale, the Mayo Portland Adaptability Inventory, the Neurobehavioral Functioning Inventory, the Patient Competency Rating Scale, and the Supervision Rating Scale (NIDRR, 2000). Many of the outcome measures used are screening tools. Primarily developed within neuropsychology parameters, many of the measures are suitable for occupational therapy assessment.

Managers may want to search topics related to continuous quality improvement (CQI) systems; analysis of work processes; and staff and client involvement in the monitoring, measuring, and analysis of good outcomes. A simple relevant question the manager might ask is, What are the effects of CQI on professional practice and client outcomes? If one has access to an Internet library, he or she can duplicate the following evidence-based search to investigate that question. Go to an affiliated college or university library's database search engine, an example of which is OVID (http://www.ovid.com). Within the search engine, access the Cochrane Database, the ACP (American College of Physicians) Journal Club, and DARE (Database of Abstracts of Reviews of Effectiveness). By following this process and entering the keyword or phrase *quality improvement* in each of the three databases or collections, I found 119 citations at the time of this writing. However, readers will most likely find more citations because the Cochrane Database is updated quarterly and will be updated more than once while this textbook is being published. Note that the occupational therapy manager and staff members need to use the same database and the same keywords or phrases to obtain similar results.

The 119 evidence-based review articles obtained under "quality improvement" do not necessarily address the topic in the same manner. After the systematic reviews are obtained, downloaded, and sorted, significantly fewer than 119 articles will be identified as being helpful to track evidence. The searching and sorting process can be general or specific, depending on the manager's focus of interest.

## Step 3: Critically Appraise the Evidence

The third step is critical appraisal or formal evaluation of the evidence to determine its soundness, magnitude, and usefulness to practice. Levels of evidence and grading guidelines for evidence vary, reflecting the complexity of the research design used during the investigation (Geyman, Deyo, & Ramsey, 2000; McKibbon, 1999; Sackett et al., 2000). The level of evidence in primary research was originally ranked by Sackett using numerical (roman numeral) indexes from I to V or letter indexes from A to D, where roman numeral I or letter A represents the most controlled, deliberate, nonbiased placement of the study participants. The numerical and alphabetical levels of evidence have been modified in a variety of ways, and readers are referred to the Centre for Evidence-Based Medicine (1999) for more detailed appraisal criteria for interventions.

The ranking is based on the research design used, the number of study participants, and the level of external and internal validity. Internal validity represents the extent to which the results of a study can be attributed to the intervention rather than to the flaws in the research design. External validity represents the extent to which the findings of the study are relevant to participants and settings beyond those in the study. The best and most powerful evidence is based on a foundation of support from high-quality, randomized clinical trials, ideally conducted with controlled double-blind study methods, predetermined outcome measures, and a sample size calculated on the basis of a statistical power analysis.

### Primary Publications

Primary publications, or original experimental and observational studies, can be viewed as having a hierarchical level of evidence depending on the rigor of the research design. RCTs would provide the highest level of evidence, followed by cohort studies, case–control studies, and case reports (see Figure 15.1).

### Secondary Publications

Secondary publications also have hierarchical levels of evidence, as shown in Figure 15.1. Secondary publications include the following: meta-analyses, systematic reviews, nonsystematic reviews, and other publications such as editorials and practice guidelines. However, EBP draws only from meta-analyses and systematic reviews. The level of evidence depends on the thoroughness and quality of the evidence provided by the primary research studies included in the secondary source. Meta-analyses, which provide the highest level of evidence in a secondary source, appraise individual studies using appropriate statistical techniques. Specifically, meta-analysis of multiple RCTs provides the most certain evidence because this type of analysis combines a wide array of the strongest, most objective evidence as compared with the results of just one study. Examples of meta-analytic review are present in occupational therapy journals and in evidence-based databases. For example, Carlson and colleagues (1996) from the University of Southern California performed a meta-analysis of the effectiveness of occupational therapy for older people, concluding that occupational therapy represents a worthwhile treatment option for that population.

Other examples of evidence reviews are two recent evidence-review papers written by Trombly and Ma (Ma & Trombly, 2002; Trombly & Ma, 2002) in the *American Journal of Occupational Therapy* as part of an evidence-based project with the American Occupational Therapy Association that was coordinated by Lieberman and Scheer (2002). They summarized the effect of occupational therapy for people with stroke in restoration of roles, tasks, and activities (Trombly & Ma, 2002) and in remediation of impairments (Ma & Trombly, 2002). The first review found that occupational therapy effectively improves participation and activity after stroke. Similarly, the second review, based on the studies selected for review, found that remediation of impairments yielded more tentative results but in general was effective.

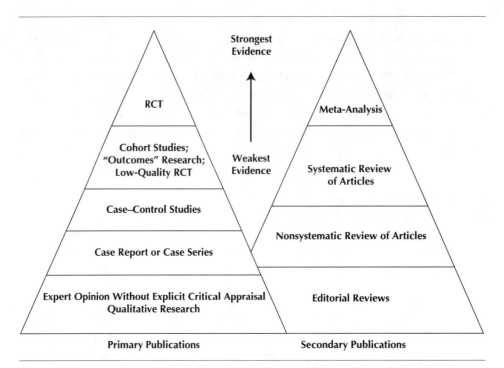

**Figure 15.1  Primary and Secondary Publications Evidence Hierarchies.**

In 1904, Karl Pearson was credited as the first to use formal statistical techniques to combine data from different studies; however, not until 1976 did psychologist Gene V. Glass coin the term *meta-analysis*. Occupational therapists and occupational therapy assistants need to be concerned with meta-analysis, seeing that the traditional narrative review of the literature is prone to bias and error because it does not follow particular guidelines and rules. Meta-analysis is more objective than other types of literature review procedures given that single studies may produce errors and guide the practitioner erroneously (Egger & Smith, 1997).

Meta-analysis can give general information about an intervention so the manager can generalize to individuals beyond the groups used in the studies. These generalizations are greatly dependent upon the similarities and differences of the treatment groups (i.e., the nontreatment and the alternative treatment). Meta-analysis requires statistical analysis and synthesis. The statistical operations required include synthesizing the treatment effect magnitude (the proportion of clients who show positive effect, the difference among the groups in outcomes, the number of clients needed to be treated to achieve a good outcome), the confidence limits (the uncertainty of the measure), and the test of significance (the size of the probability that the treatment effects are not the result of chance alone; Tickle-Degnen, 2002b). The outcome of a meta-analysis depends on the treatment effect found in the researcher's selected studies and the quality of those studies (Cooper & Hedges, 1994).

Meta-analysis also has disadvantages because the selection of the studies chosen for summary, comparison, and criticism (integration) may be valid only for a certain population or for some clients and not for others (Egger & Smith, 1997). For example, a selection bias in a meta-analysis may result from the researcher's selection of high- and low-quality studies that are included in the sample for analysis. Another bias could arise in variations in the approach to the interpretation of the study question. Yet another bias can result from the mixing of study samples, including individual and group studies, which may lead to nonrepresentative estimates of effect. Other potential sources of error include biases in statistical analysis, interpretation of results, and reporting of results. In other words, although meta-analysis is very exciting and promising, it is susceptible to potential Type I (i.e., falsely concluding a treatment effect) and Type II (i.e., falsely concluding no treatment effect) errors (Maxwell & Delaney, 2000).

The other type of secondary publication, the *systematic review*, attempts to summarize published and unpublished written material in every language, including dissertations and special reports. The systematic review is a new type of review article found in evidence-based health care literature that is supported by the evidence in a particular topic rather than based on a hasty and careless literature review that is combined with the author's personal opinion (McKibbon, 1999). Systematic review refers to any type of review that uses objective and orderly methods to avoid bias in the report and synthesis of the research studies (Egger & Smith, 1997).

Two examples of occupational therapy systematic reviews available at the McMaster University Web site (http://www.fhs.mcmaster/ca/rehab/ebp) provide evidence for two types of interventions. One systematic review supports the evidence on cognitive–behavioral interventions in people with chronic pain (Occupational Therapy Evidence-Based Practice Research Group, 1998), and another systematic review critically reviews activity programs for older people (Occupational Therapy Evidence-Based Practice Research Group, 1999). These two examples underscore the easy access and availability of rigorous evidence in occupational therapy using EBP. An example of occupational therapy evidence reviews in the Cochrane Database of Systematic Reviews includes evidence for occupational therapy for arthritis treatment (Steultjens, Dekker, Bouter, van Schaardenburg, van Kuyk, & van den Ende, 2002). Single study reviews are also available. The ACP Journal Club database contains a variety of single study reviews; one of these studies, written by Helewa and colleagues at the University of Western Ontario and published in *Lancet* in 1991 was titled "Effects of Occupational Therapy Home Services on Patients With Rheumatoid Arthritis." The practitioner can choose to quickly read the abstract from the primary study in addition to the abstract and commentary for the ACP Journal Club by Robert A. Hawkins (1991) of Wright State University. Other types of secondary investigations integrate and summarize less explicit and rigorous studies as well as mix the evidence with opinions and, therefore, are not used in the evidence-based process.

Literature reviews are also called *research syntheses*, *research reviews*, and *integrative research reviews*. A more comprehensive research synthesis can be included in literature reviews or stand by themselves as the most objective estimate of support or lack of support for the "best practice" in the area chosen for meta-analysis (Egger & Smith, 1997).

### Qualitative Research

Quantitative research such as meta-analysis is a source of evidence that yields an increased generalizability of studies to clinical practice. In contrast, qualitative research may not be viewed as suitable for generalization (Stevens, Abrams, Brazier, Fitzpatrick, & Lilford, 2001). Although one finds examples of qualitative meta-analysis that refer to the synthesis of research findings into one description model or theory (Paterson, Thorne, Canam, & Jillings, 2001; Stern & Harris, 1985), this method is not highly valued in the process of EBP, which is based on a medical model.

Qualitative research methods explore and describe social phenomena and look beyond statistics, offering access and insight into the health care process (Giacomini, 2001). Occupational therapy has embraced qualitative methodologies in its attempts to better understand the social and personal aspects of heath care (Clark, 1993; Krefting & Krefting, 1991). However, evaluation standards for assessing the rigor of qualitative research methods have not yet been developed (Davies & Dodd, 2002; Whittemore, Chase, & Mandle, 2001). Although occupational therapists and scientists do not agree about how to assess the quality and usefulness of qualitative studies for EBP (Marks, 1999), many of them encourage the use and application of these methods in practice (Abreu, Zhang, Seale, Primeau, & Jones, 2002; Clark, 1993; Krefting & Krefting, 1991). Readers are referred to the guidelines developed by the McMaster University Occupational Therapy Evidence-Based Practice Research Group for a critical review of qualitative studies on the Internet (http://www.fhs.mcmaster/ca/rehab/ebp).

Practitioners traditionally combine the art and science of occupational therapy to determine the quality of clinical care. This integrative perspective requires the use of qualitative studies to help us improve our understanding of occupational therapy and occupational science. *Qualitative methods* best address questions about social meaning, whereas *quantitative research* best addresses questions dealing with biomedical and causal questions (Giacomini, 2001). The contributions to occupational therapy evidence are complemented by both methodologies; they can enhance client and caretaker empowerment and the quality of occupational therapy.

### Degrees of Evidence

Another approach to evidence appraisal is the classification of evidence by the degree of evidence strength found in the research literature. A system introduced by van Tulder,

Cherkin, Berman, Lao, and Koes (2001) used in the Cochrane Library consists of four degrees of strength: strong evidence, moderate evidence, limited evidence, or no evidence. Strong evidence is provided by generally consistent findings in multiple, high-quality RCTs. Moderate evidence is provided by generally consistent findings in one high-quality RCT and multiple low-quality RCTs. Limited evidence is provided by generally consistent findings in one or more lower-quality RCTs. No evidence indicates that either no RCTs were conducted or the results were conflicting.

## Step 4: Apply to Practice

The fourth step is the application of scientific research findings to practice. This step is a culmination of the process of the search. The systematic integration of the evidence with client factors, institution factors, and staff expertise results in either rejection or integration of the research findings into practice.

Decision-making in a variety of settings using EBP is largely based on the quality of quantitative research design rather than the results of statistical calculation. When practitioners look at the best evidence by examining research studies, the following characteristics are examined: the statistical power of the study, the use of randomization techniques in treatment studies, and the clinical significance.

### Statistical Power

The *statistical power* of a study is an index used to determine the probability that significant changes can be attributed to the treatment rather than to chance. For example, Ottenbacher and Maas (1999), after examining 30 studies on the effectiveness of occupational therapy treatment intervention (outcome), found that the majority of the studies were of low statistical power because of their small sample size. To demonstrate occupational therapy effectiveness, studies must carefully account for the appropriate numbers of participants that are statistically required to detect significant changes attributable to the treatment provided.

Interestingly enough, practitioners can end up rejecting a particular occupational therapy treatment because the article they read did not provide evidence to support a treatment effect. A clinical decision made in this way may be incorrect because the study methodology was limited and did not provide statistical power to conclude that the intervention was in fact clinically ineffective. In statistical terms, this kind of error is called a *Type II Error*, a determination falsely concluding that there is no treatment effect. Alternatively, after reading an evidence-based research paper, practitioners can conclude that there is an intervention effect for the technique that is being evaluated. This decision can also be incorrect because the research methodology was limited and may have falsely concluded that there is a treatment effect when, in fact, the treatment was not effective. In statistical terms, this kind of error is called a *Type I Error*.

### Randomization

In addition to the statistical power of study, one must consider the procedure used to determine the assignment of treatment to participants so the chances of assignment to a particular treatment are the same for all participants in the study. This procedure is called *random assignment* or *randomization*. Random assignment is considered the best way to determine the causal relationship between the intervention and the results of treatment. Randomization is the best way to provide an unbiased selection to the treatment that will produce the most valid impact on the results of intervention. However, in occupational therapy research studies, randomization is difficult (e.g., because of financial restraints), unfeasible (e.g., because the study is observational or because it uses a small pool of participants), and sometimes unethical (e.g., because it may involve treatment for some and no treatment for others in situations in which treatment makes a life-altering difference). In occupational therapy, these constraints do not argue against randomization; instead, they support a more flexible research design that enables problem-focused research as compared to methodology-focused research (Ottenbacher, 1992).

### Clinical Significance

A final factor to consider is *clinical significance*, a statistic sometimes provided by the researcher that gives the practitioner a practical meaning for the data. This information is especially important when the results of a study show no statistical significance but show clinical significance. Statistical significance measures the size of the probability that the treatment effects are not attributed to chance alone. The optimal statistical significance of research studies is generally set at a 95% likelihood that a particular effect is related to a particular treatment, with a 5% likelihood that the effect is related to chance alone. Statistical significance is unrelated to clinical effect, but both measures of significance are important (Ottenbacher & Barrett, 1989). Use of a single-subject design and a group comparison design, although considered to have a lower level of evidence under the EBP model, can support clinical significance.

The occupational therapy manager must have a basic clinical and research foundation, clinical experience, motivation, and desire to use this methodology as well as to teach it to the staff. Evidence from scientific studies can persuade and influence any practice. Occupational therapy managers need to remember that EBP is only one way of obtaining evidence. The expertise of practitioners and their practice settings as well as the clients' preferences also need to be considered. The strength of EBP is that it can help in determining best practice by using the most rigorous quantitative research methodology as the highest index for evidence. The occupational therapy manager must weigh the value of conducting research with the quality of service.

As evident from the discussion above, occupational therapy managers who base their practice decisions on evidence-based research must become familiar with research design, methodology, and even inferential or descriptive statistics to become accurate appraisers of the evidence. Although familiarity with research is a practice responsibility, statistical appraisal is not a required practice competence for occupational therapists and occupational therapy assistants. The responsibility to use sound principles of research design rests on those practitioners who are conducting research. The evidence-based databanks supply summary reviews that provide statistical appraisals of the article, thus easing some of the responsibility of the occupational therapist. As occupational therapy continues to develop at higher academic levels, including post-baccalaureate levels and an expansion of clinical doctoral studies, practitioners and managers will become more competent and comfortable using statistical appraisal.

### Step 5: Conduct Self-Assessment

The fifth step is the evaluation of the whole process. This step, not always included in the evidence-based guidelines, is an appraisal of the procedures undertaken in Steps 1–4 and a reflection on the way the occupational therapist or occupational therapy assistant formulated the question, tracked down the evidence, critically evaluated the evidence, and integrated the evidence into practice (McKibbon, 1999; Sackett et al., 2000). Self-assessment is a necessary step to determine the value of using EBP within the occupational therapy workforce.

The value of EBP in highlighting the link between prevention research and the formulation of policy is apparent to those who work in brain injury. For example, evidence-based findings related to prevention can affect governmental actions. These findings include (a) determining the effects of using seat belts and airbags on safe driving and (b) determining the effects of using helmets on safe bicycle riding and other sports. This kind of evidence strengthens the merit of existing laws requiring safety measures.

Once one starts using EBP, the explosion and formidable amount of information can become overwhelming. Therefore, managers and staff members must share this methodology with one another for support and validation. This process requires time and effort to achieve strategies for efficient use of information. The commitment to continuous questioning of clinical practice can become an institutional and personal pledge (Dawes, Davies, Gray, Mant, Seers, & Snowball, 1999).

## Direct Care, Research, and Reflections on Education

Careful consideration of EBP approaches is needed because occupational therapists and occupational therapy assistants often use informal and personal methods in dealing with practice issues. To effectively shape practice policies that successfully manage the complexity and individualistic intervention methods for clients, one must consider solid evidence, client desires, and the art of practice. The shift to EBP modifies the principles that we apply to practice to bring them closer to a more scientific model that includes the best EBPs on studies found in the world's medical literature.

EBP is not a simple or single solution, and although it can promote knowledge and solutions, we must address other implications for occupational therapy practice. Strong evidence has powerful merits when used to enhance problem solving. All of these merits notwithstanding, occupational therapy investigators must use multiple methods of inquiry to address those aspects of practice that fall outside of the scope of problem solving, including the therapeutic relationship, cultural differences, and institutional philosophies and visions. Occupational therapists and occupational therapy assistants must consider client-centered "evidence" alongside evidence generated from population-based research (Egan, Dubouloz, von Zweck, & Vallerand, 1998). Even the most rigorous research must be considered within a holistic context to produce sound interventions (Straus, 1999). A broad-based inquiry beyond EBP is needed to integrate the art and science of occupational therapy practice.

Although we have seen a proliferation of textbooks, articles, and courses at the local, national, and international levels in EBP, the evidence generated from occupational therapy practice is limited (Law, 2002; Law & Baum, 1998; Taylor, 1997; Tickle-Degnen, 1998). The process of imparting and acquiring knowledge about EBP in occupational therapy practice is in its early stages.

Many organizations frequently lack a research culture and the time for research because of the heavy direct care service commitments in the practice setting or heavy teaching responsibilities in the academic setting. In addition, the field has only a limited number of role models who are teaching and applying EBP. As a result, the attention to investigating and disseminating evidence of relevant studies is limited. As occupational therapy moves toward a post-baccalaureate level, research will be more integrated in educational institutions. Canada's McMaster University has contributed to the understanding of EBP. As mentioned earlier in this chapter, the occupational therapy department's Web site at McMaster has helped in the dissemination of information, providing forms to be used to appraise research publications for evidence.

Managers, direct care practitioners, and educators need to overcome barriers to teaching, learning, and carrying out EBP. Four problems for health care professionals have been identified as resistance factors that interfere with teaching and learning EBP: time factors, the practitioner's rudimentary research skills, the limited high-quality research evidence available, and the doubts about the authenticity of this approach. These factors generate criticism or resistance to practice and growth in this area (Davies, 1999).

In the United States, Boston University continues to contribute to the understanding of EBP by promoting the Faculty Summer Institute in teaching EBP in rehabilitation professional curricula (Tickle-Degnen, 2002b) at Sargent College of Health. Additionally, Linda Tickle-Degnen has edited an Evidence-Based Practice Forum in the *American Journal of Occupational Therapy* since September 1999 (Tickle-Degnen, 1999). This forum has increased the awareness and understanding of this methodology.

Direct care practitioners' perceptions of EBP have been investigated through questionnaires. In the United Kingdom, McColl, Smith, White, and Field (1998) obtained a response from 302 practitioners and found that respondents appreciated and agreed that the practice of EBP improves client care. Yet the practitioners reported the lack of personal time to devote to EBP, and only about 40% knew of the Cochrane Database of Systematic Reviews. Two studies found in the *American Journal of Occupational Therapy* investigated therapists' perceptions of EBP. The investigators in the first study, using semistructured interviews to explore the respondents' perception, found that occupational therapists believed EBP was a research process looking for understanding and that it was viewed as a threat to practice (Dubouloz, Egan, Vallerand, & von Zweck, 1999). The second investigation was a single-subject design of three therapists' experience attempting to use a Cochrane review. The investigators found that the experience was not an easy one and that the three experienced therapists were unfamiliar with the Cochrane Database of Systematic Reviews (Gervais, Poirier, Van Iterson, Egan, & Tickle-Degnen, 2002).

The studies appear to indicate that promoting and improving access to summaries of evidence and educating practitioners is needed to encourage the use of EBP. More recently, Dysart and Tomlin (2002), using a survey research methodology, examined the way U.S. occupational therapists accessed and used evidence. They found that therapists are engaging in a modest amount of EBP and that research was considered to have poor applicability to clinical practice. Identifying the barriers to using EBP as well as expanding and clarifying the benefits of using this methodology will continue to be a challenge to occupational therapy managers, occupational therapists, and occupational therapy assistants alike.

The occupational therapy manager's competence in research is necessary because it contributes to the development of better practice, the profession, and the organization within which the manager practices (Abreu, Peloquin, & Ottenbacher, 1998). The occupational therapy manager can establish connections with researchers in the workplace or affiliated university to develop a strategic approach to the use of research and management of data. Allocating to the staff a regularly scheduled time for searches and reading the literature can assist in the use of EBP in the clinic. In addition, the occupational therapy manager can help in the creation of an EBP reference databank that is dedicated to and focused on the particular clients' occupational performance issues as well as staff and organizational priorities. The manager can also assist with the dissemination of research evidence to occupational therapists by producing and distributing summaries and continuing education opportunities for the staff.

The application of EBP is promising. However, substantial work needs to be conducted to improve and identify best practice and clinical decision benefits through this methodology of clinical reasoning. Although occupational therapists are expected to incorporate research findings into their practice and be accountable to their clients and institutions, occupational therapists often lack the research knowledge and workplace support to carry out EBP approaches. In addition, we need to build bridges to connect occupational therapists providing services, researchers, and academicians and to promote more rigorous research activities toward establishing a body of evidence that supports the effectiveness of occupational therapy interventions.

## Acknowledgment

To Kenneth J. Ottenbacher, PhD, OTR, FAOTA, for his numerous writings and help as a resource person offering guidelines for analysis and critique of data interpretation even before EBP emerged. To Joanne Jones, OTR, and the TLC research team for their research and editorial help. This project was partially supported by NIH grant 3R01A617638-01A1S1.

## References

Abreu, B. C. (1998). Additional uses for data. In J. Hinojosa & P. Kramer (Eds.), *Occupational therapy evaluation: Obtaining and interpreting data* (pp. 213–234). Bethesda, MD: American Occupational Therapy Association.

Abreu, B. C., Peloquin, S. M., & Ottenbacher, K. (1998). Competence in scientific inquiry and research. *American Journal of Occupational Therapy, 52,* 751–759.

Abreu, B. C., Zhang, L., Seale, G., Primeau, L., & Jones, J. (2002). Interdisciplinary meetings: Investigating the collaboration between persons with brain injury and treatment teams. *Brain Injury, 16,* 691–704.

Baker, M. (1996). Challenging ignorance. In M. Baker & S. Kirk (Eds.), *Research and development for the NHS* (pp. 19–26). London: National Association for Health Authorities and Trusts.

Byers, J. F., & Beaudin, C. L. (2002). The relationship between continuous quality improvement and research. *Journal of Healthcare Quality, 24,* 4–8.

Carlson, M., Fanchiang, S.-P., Zemke, R., & Clark, F. (1996). A meta-analysis of the effectiveness of occupational therapy in older persons. *American Journal of Occupational Therapy, 50,* 89–98.

Centre for Evidence-Based Medicine. (1999). *Levels of evidence and grades of recommendations.* Retrieved March 21, 2002, from http://cebm.jr2.ox.ac.uk

Clark, F. (1993). Occupation embedded in a real life: Interweaving occupational science and occupational therapy. 1993 Eleanor Clarke Slagle Lecture. *American Journal of Occupational Therapy, 47,* 1067–1078.

Clark, F., Azen, S. P., Zemki, R., Jackson, J., Carlson, M., Mandel, D., et al. (1997). Occupational therapy for independent-living older adults: A randomized controlled trial. *Journal of the American Medical Association, 278,* 1321–1326.

Cooper, H., & Hedges, L. V. (Eds.). (1994). *The handbook of research synthesis.* New York: Russell Sage Foundation.

Davies, D., & Dodd, J. (2002). Qualitative research and the question of rigor. *Qualitative Health Research, 12,* 279–289.

Davies, P. (1999). Teaching evidence-based health care. In M. Dawes, P. Davies, A. Gray, J. Mant, K. Seers, & R. Snowball (Eds.), *Evidence-based practice: A primer for health care professionals* (pp. 223–242). New York: Churchill Livingstone.

Dawes, M., Davies, P., Gray, A., Mant, J., Seers, K., & Snowball, R. (Eds.). (1999). *Evidence-based practice: A primer for health care professionals.* New York: Churchill Livingstone.

Dubouloz, C.-J., Egan, M., Vallerand, J., & von Zweck, C. (1999). Occupational therapists' receptions of evidence-based practice. *American Journal of Occupational Therapy, 53,* 445–453.

Dysart, A. M., & Tomlin, G. S. (2002). Factors related to evidence-based practice among U.S. occupational therapy clinicians. *American Journal of Occupational Therapy, 56,* 275–284.

Egan, M., Dubouloz, C.-J., von Zweck, C., & Vallerand, J. (1998). The client-centered evidence-based practice of occupational therapy. *Canadian Journal of Occupational Therapy, 65,* 136–143.

Egger, M., & Smith, G. D. (1997). Meta-analysis: Potentials and promise. *British Medical Journal, 315,* 1371–1374.

Foto, M. (1996). Nationally speaking: Outcome studies: The what, why, how, and when. *American Journal of Occupational Therapy, 50,* 87–88.

Gervais, I. S., Poirier, A., Van Iterson, L., Egan, M., & Tickle-Degnen, L. (2002). Evidence-based practice forum: Attempting to use a Cochrane review: Experience of three occupational therapists. *American Journal of Occupational Therapy, 56,* 110–113.

Geyman, J. P., Deyo, R. A., & Ramsey, S. D. (Eds.). (2000). *Evidence-based clinical practice: Concepts and approaches.* Boston: Butterworth-Heinemann.

Giacomini, M. K. (2001). The rocky road: Qualitative research as evidence. *ACP Journal Club, 134,* A11–A13.

Glass, G. V. (1976). Primary, secondary, and meta-analysis. *Educational Researcher, 5,* 3–8.

Guide. (1993). *Guide for the Uniform Data Set for medical rehabilitation,* (Adult FIM). Version 4.0 Buffalo, NY: State University of New York at Buffalo.

Hawkins, R. A. (1991). Occupational therapy home service improved rheumatoid arthritis. *ACP Journal Club, 2002*(Nov.–Dec.), 77.

Helewa, A., Goldsmith, C. H., Lee, P., Bombardier, C., Hanes, B., Smythe, H. A., et al. (1991). Effects of occupational therapy home services on patients with rheumatoid arthritis. *Lancet, 337,* 1453–1456.

Holm, H. A. (2000). The 2000 Eleanor Clarke Slagle Lecture. Our mandate for the new millennium: Evidence-based practice. *American Journal of Occupational Therapy, 54,* 575–585.

Krefting, L., & Krefting, D. (1991). Leisure activities after a stroke: An ethnographic approach. *American Journal of Occupational Therapy, 45,* 429–436.

Law, M. (Ed.). (2002). *Evidence-based rehabilitation: A guide to practice.* Thorofare, NJ: Slack.

Law, M., & Baum, C. (1998). Evidence-based occupational therapy. *Canadian Journal of Occupational Therapy, 65,* 131–135.

Lieberman, D., & Scheer, J. (2002). Evidence-based practice forum: AOTA's evidence-based literature review project: An overview. *American Journal of Occupational Therapy, 56,* 344–349.

Lin, K., Wu, C., Tickle-Degnan, L., & Coster, W. (1997). Enhancing occupational performance through occupationally embedded exercise: A meta-analytic review. *Occupational Therapy Journal of Research, 17,* 25–47.

Ma, H-I., & Trombly, C. A. (2002). A synthesis of the effects of occupational therapy for persons with stroke, part II: Remediation of impairments. *American Journal of Occupational Therapy, 56,* 260–274.

Marks, S. (1999). Qualitative studies. In A. McKibbon (with A. Eady & S. Marks) (Eds.), *PDQ: Evidence-based principles and practice* (pp. 187–204). Hamilton, ON: B. C. Decker.

Maxwell, S. E., & Delaney, H. D. (2000). *Designing experiments and analyzing data.* Mahwah, NJ: Erlbaum.

McColl, A., Smith, H., White, P., & Field, J. (1998). General practitioners' perceptions of the route to evidence-based medicine: A questionnaire survey. *British Medical Journal, 316,* 361–365.

McKenna, K., Tooth, L., Strong, J., Ottenbacher, K. J., Connell, J., & Cleary, M. (2002). Predicting discharge outcomes for stroke patients in Australia. *American Journal of Physical Medicine and Rehabilitation, 81,* 47–56.

McKibbon, A., (with Eady, A., & Marks, S.). (Eds.). (1999). *PDQ: Evidence-based principles and practice.* Hamilton, ON: B. C. Decker.

Morahan, S. (2002). Wide application of CQI in home care. *Journal of Nursing Care Quality, 16*(3), 36–49.

Muir Gray, J. A., Haynes, R. B., Sackett, D. L., Cook, D. J., & Guyatt, G. H. (1997). Transferring evidence from research into practice: 3. Developing evidence-based clinical policy. *ACP Journal Club, 126,* A-14.

National Institute on Disability and Rehabilitation Research. (2000). *Traumatic brain injury model systems.* Retrieved August 29, 2000, from http://www.tbims.org

Occupational Therapy Evidence-Based Practice Research Group. (1998). *The effectiveness of cognitive–behavioural interventions with people with chronic pain. A critical review of the literature by the Occupational Therapy Evidence-Based Practice Group.* Hamilton, ON: McMaster University. Retrieved March 21, 2002, from http://www.fhs.mcmaster.ca/rehab/ebp/

Occupational Therapy Evidence-Based Practice Research Group. (1999). *Effectiveness of activity programmes for older persons with dementia. A critical review of the literature by the Occupational Therapy Evidence-Based Practice Research Group.* Hamilton, ON: McMaster University. Retrieved March 21, 2002, from http://www.fhs.mcmaster.ca/rehab/ebp/

Ottenbacher, K. J. (1992). Statistical conclusion validity and Type IV errors in rehabilitation research. *Archives of Physical Medicine and Rehabilitation, 73,* 121–125.

Ottenbacher, K. J. (2002, May). Evidence-based practice in rehabilitation. In Boston University (Ed.), *Faculty Summer Institute: Teaching evidence-based practice in rehabilitation professional curricula* (pp. 1–14). Boston: Boston University.

Ottenbacher, K. J., & Barrett, K. A. (1989). Measures of effect size in rehabilitation research. *American Journal of Physical Medicine and Rehabilitation, 68,* 52–58.

Ottenbacher, K. J., & Hinderer, S. R. (2001). Evidence-based practice: Methods to evaluate individual patient improvement. *American Journal of Physical Medicine and Rehabilitation, 80,* 786–796.

Ottenbacher, K. J., & Maas, F. (1999). How to detect effects: Statistical power and evidence-based practice in occupational therapy research. *American Journal of Occupational Therapy, 53,* 181–188.

*Oxford English Dictionary.* (1995). (5th ed.). Oxford, UK: Oxford University Press.

Paterson, B. L., Thorne, S. E., Canam, C., & Jillings, C. (2001). *Meta-study of qualitative health research: A practical guide to meta-analysis and meta-synthesis* (Vol. 3). Thousand Oaks, CA: Sage.

Pearson, K. (1904). Report on certain enteric fever inoculation statistics. *British Medical Journal, 3,* 1243–1246.

Rao, J. N. (1999). Clinical trials in primary care: Paying doctors for clinical trials is unethical [Letter]. *British Medical Journal, 318,* 1485.

Richardson, W. S., Wilson, M. C., Nishikawa, J., & Hayward, R. S. A. (1995). The well-built clinical question: A key to evidence-based decisions. *ACP Journal Club, 123*, A12.

Sackett, D. L., Straus, S. E., Richardson, W. S., Rosenberg, W., & Haynes, R. B. (2000). *Evidence-based medicine: How to practice and teach EBM* (2nd ed.). New York: Churchill Livingstone.

Stern, P., & Harris, C. (1985). Women's health and the self-care paradox: A model to guide self-care readiness—Clash between client and nurse. *Health Care for Women International, 6*, 151–163.

Steultjens, E. M. J., Dekker, J., Bouter, L. M., van Schaardenburg, D., van Kuyk, M. A. H., & van den Ende, C. H. M. (2002). Occupational therapy for rheumatoid arthritis. *Cochrane Database of Systematic Reviews, 3.*

Stevens, A., Abrams, K., Brazier, J., Fitzpatrick, R., & Lilford, R. (Eds.). (2001). *The advanced handbook of methods in evidence-based healthcare.* Thousand Oaks, CA: Sage.

Straus, S. E. (1999). Evidence-based medicine: Bringing evidence to the point of care. *ACP Journal Club, 4*, 70–71.

Taylor, M. C. (1997). What is evidence-based practice? *British Journal of Occupational Therapy, 60*, 470–473.

Tickle-Degnen, L. (1998). Using research evidence in planning treatment for the individual client. *Canadian Journal of Occupational Therapy, 65*, 152–159.

Tickle-Degnen, L. (1999). Evidence-based forum—Organizing, evaluating, and using evidence in occupational therapy. *American Journal of Occupational Therapy, 53*, 537–539.

Tickle-Degnen, L. (2002a). Communicating evidence to clients, managers, and families. In M. Law (Ed.), *Evidence-based rehabilitation: A guide to practice* (pp. 221–254). Thorofare, NJ: Slack.

Tickle-Degnen, L. (2002b, May). Synthesizing evidence from multiple sources. In Boston University (Ed.), *Faculty Summer Institute: Teaching evidence-based practice in rehabilitation professional curricula* (pp. 1–7). Boston: Boston University.

Trombly, C. A., & Ma, H-I. (2002). A synthesis of the effects of occupational therapy for persons with stroke, part I: Restoration of roles, task, and activities. *American Journal of Occupational Therapy, 56*, 250–259.

Uniform Data System for Medical Rehabilitation. (1993). *Guide for the Uniform Data Set for medical rehabilitation* (Adult FIM, Version 4.0). Buffalo: State University of New York at Buffalo.

van Tulder, M. W., Cherkin, D. C., Berman, B., Lao, L., & Koes, B. W. (2001). *Acupuncture for low back pain* [Review]. *The Cochrane Database of Systematic Reviews, 3*, 1–15.

Vargas, S., & Camilli, G. (1999). A meta-analysis of research on sensory integration treatment. *American Journal of Occupational Therapy, 53*, 189–198.

Whittemore, R., Chase, S. K., & Mandle, C. L. (2001). Validity in qualitative research. *Qualitative Health Research, 11*, 522–537.

# CHAPTER 16

# Documentation of Occupational Therapy Services

Jane D. Acquaviva, OTR/L

*"Documentation is not the most exciting aspect of professional practice, but it is the most critical element in what makes practice 'professional.'"*

JANE ACQUAVIVA

**Jane D. Acquaviva, OTR/L,** has a BS in occupational therapy and is the resource manager at the Visiting Nurse Association of North Carolina in Raleigh. She is a health care manager with significant experience in program development, interdisciplinary management, documentation, and reimbursement mechanisms affecting occupational therapy.

## Key Ideas and Concepts

**Documentation.** The written record of evaluation, intervention, and outcomes of the provided services.

**Long-term goal.** In documentation, a description of the occupational status that a therapist expects a patient or client to have achieved by the end of intervention in a given facility or program; the goal must reflect an area of occupation and must be measurable and objective.

**Short-term goal.** In documentation, a specification of the steps to be taken to achieve a long-term goal; the short-term goal must reflect an area of occupation and must be measurable and objective.

## Learning Objectives

After completing this chapter, you should be able to do the following:

- Describe the elements of effective occupational therapy documentation.

- Identify the various audiences for which the therapist documents.

- Apply information to improve your ability to perform effective documentation.

Occupational therapy documentation is the written record of patient or client evaluation, interventions, and outcomes. That record has multiple audiences such as the physician and the third-party payer. Consequently, it must meet several distinct requirements, which it likely will meet if it is clear and organized and if it reflects the framework provided in this chapter and in related professional resources. Of utmost importance, however, is that documentation must reflect an orientation to results or established measurable goals and to the involvement of the patient in determining those goals. The latter requirement is clearly outlined under Principle 2.A of the *Occupational Therapy Code of Ethics* (American Occupational Therapy Association [AOTA], 1994b): "Occupational therapy personnel shall collaborate with service recipients or their surrogate(s) in determining goals and priorities throughout the intervention process" (p. 1037).

This chapter focuses on the medically oriented record that is typically used in inpatient, outpatient, and community-based practices such as home care and private practice.

## Purpose of Documentation

Effective documentation is a critical responsibility of professionals because it indicates that they are accountable for their actions and that they recognize their obligation to share the product of their efforts with others. The medical record has several particular purposes. It describes the services provided. It also becomes the patient's or client's legal record, a tool for quality improvement audits, a means for determining reimbursement for services, a source of data to demonstrate compliance with accreditation standards, and a potential tool for collecting data for research purposes. Documenting to serve all these purposes is not as difficult as it may seem because each requires essentially the same information.

In general, the documenting professional needs to clearly answer the following questions:

- What was the patient's or client's occupational performance level at the time of evaluation?
- What are the patient's occupational goals?
- Briefly, what interventions were provided?
- Were the patient's occupational goals met?
- What was the patient's occupational performance at the end of treatment?

The medical record has always been the legal documentation of the medical care that was provided. As workers' compensation, personal injury, and malpractice litigation increase, court scrutiny of the record has become more common. Occupational therapists need to remember that documentation may be subject to legal inquiry. This inquiry may involve a court of law, or it could involve an administrative law hearing at which the judge is deciding whether Medicare will pay for the occupational therapy services that are documented in the medical record. The record needs to provide a clear picture of the care that was provided by the occupational therapist, and it needs to reflect the plan of care that the therapist designed.

Occupational therapy documentation also communicates the essence of the role the occupational therapist plays in assisting patients and clients to achieve their goals. Documentation communicates to the referral source, third-party payer, peers, and even the patient or client. Therefore, a therapist's documentation reflects on that therapist and may highlight or diminish that professional's practice, including his or her clinical thinking, ability to develop an appropriate plan, and ability to reach proposed occupational goals.

## References for Documenting Services

Traditionally, practitioners have used their national professional guidelines and the requirements of third-party payers and accrediting agencies to guide documentation. *The Occupational Therapy Practice Framework: Domain and Process* (AOTA, 2002) and the *Elements of Clinical Documentation* (AOTA, 1994a) are AOTA-approved guidelines. These documents reflect current occupational therapy practice and terminology.

In 1990, the Health Care Financing Administration (HCFA) published a description of occupational therapy called "Medical Review (MR) Guidelines for Outpatient OT (Occupational Therapy) Services." This publication is a useful reference for understanding what Medicare and other third-party payers look for when reviewing occupational therapy documentation for the purposes of reimbursement for services. Occupational therapists need to become familiar with this terminology in addition to the terminology used in AOTA official documents.

Other documentation guidelines are specific to the work setting, including the guidelines from the Joint Commission on Accreditation of Healthcare Organizations (JCAHO), which affect numerous health care institutions, and the guidelines from the Commission on Accreditation of Rehabilitation Facilities (CARF), which affect rehabilitation facilities. The JCAHO and CARF guidelines, for instance, require that, when practitioners establish goals, they must indicate a period for achieving the goal. The occupational therapist needs to know and incorporate any additional requirements into his or her documentation that may be associated with the setting where services are provided.

## Evaluation and Intervention Planning

Documentation begins when a person is referred to occupational therapy for evaluation. It is also the beginning of the clinical thinking process. The referral may come from various sources, such as a physician, a community program, a colleague, or a family member of the patient, or it may be a self-referral.

The evaluation process sets the stage for all that follows. Because occupational therapy is concerned with performance in daily life and how performance affects engagement in occupations to support participation, the evaluation process is focused on finding out what the client wants and needs to do and on identifying those factors that act as supports or barriers to performance. The occupational therapist considers performance skills, performance patterns, context, activity demands, and client factors, and determines how each influences performance. (AOTA, 2002, pp. 615–616)

Initially, the practitioner interviews the patient and the patient's family members or caregivers to determine the patient's prior level of occupational performance and the activities that he or she is currently unable to perform. The interview should include the following questions:

- Why is this person seeking services?
- In which occupational areas is the person performing successfully? Which are causing problems?
- What contexts (e.g., physical, cultural, social) inhibit or support the patient's desired goals?
- What is the patient's occupational history (e.g., life experience, values, interests)?
- What are the patient's goals?

At this point, the therapist may develop a working hypothesis with respect to possible reasons for the identified problems and concerns. This hypothesis is not documented but, instead, guides the therapist to consider other factors such as the underlying performance skills required, activity demands, patient routines, and contextual factors. To check the hypothesis, specific tools or instruments will be selected and administered, and the results of those tests will be documented.

The evaluation results will be discussed with the patient and the family, and intervention options will be presented in light of the patient's goals. An intervention plan and functional goals will be developed jointly and documented.

The following checklist provides guidance for documenting the evaluation and intervention planning. Some items are general and administrative, for example, the date of the evaluation; others are specific to the patient.

- Name, age, sex, diagnoses, and date of onset of each diagnosis
- Referral source, date of referral, and date of occupational therapy evaluation
- Relevant medical or educational history, occupational history, and prior level of functioning or occupational performance
- Present levels of functioning or occupational performance
- Other factors affecting performance, for example, deficits in performance skills and patterns, contextual issues or activity demands, and client factors such as motivation
- Specific test results and references to other pertinent reports
- Summary and analysis of evaluation findings

- If intervention is indicated, a statement that the occupational therapist maintains a reasonable expectation that the patient will benefit from occupational therapy services
- Patient or client expectations or goals
- Recommended intervention
- Estimated frequency and duration of intervention
- Measurable, functional goals with a projected time frame that is agreed to by patient, family, and therapist.

## Formulation of Functional Goals

The long-term goals set the direction for the occupational therapy intervention and, therefore, also the documentation. Long-term goals need to reflect expected outcomes at the end of the intervention in the setting where the therapist is treating the patient or client. Some examples follow:

- The patient will be independent in personal activities of daily living (PADL), using assistive devices. (6 weeks)
- The patient will be independent in PADL and in instrumental activities of daily living (IADL), using assistance for shopping, household cleanup, and community mobility. (8 weeks)
- The client will return to work without restriction. (4 weeks)
- The patient will independently care for her infant. (3 months)

To achieve these long-term functional goals in specific areas of occupation, the occupational therapist will develop short-term goals to represent intermediate steps, and intervention will focus on achievement of short-term goals, building toward the long-term goals. Examples of short-term goals follow:

- The patient will maintain sitting balance for 3 minutes as a prerequisite for learning to transfer. (1 week)
- The patient will pick up her infant safely to quiet him. (1 week)
- The patient will gain 20 degrees of metacarpalphalangeal movement in the right dominant hand for grasping grooming devices. (1 week)

The orderly flow of evaluation information, goal development, and outcome reporting in combination with the patient's goals will reflect the therapist's thinking. If the goals and outcomes show a logical progression in which the patient moves toward becoming more independent or in which the caregiver becomes more capable and the patient needs less assistance, then anyone reading them will understand the purpose of the occupational therapy intervention and the progress toward the outcomes.

## Intervention Plan

Documenting a summary of interventions is required, and this summary may change as the patient improves. Documentation of this kind may be written in general terms (as in Exhibits 16.1 and 16.2 that follow) or may include very specific procedures (as in Exhibit 16.3):

1. Intervention will emphasize transfer training, compensatory dressing techniques, and activities to improve right upper extremity movement for independence in PADL.

2. Treatment will emphasize activities to improve group work skills, appropriate social interaction with peers, and grooming and dressing for the work environment to achieve job acquisition.

3. Treatment will initially include the following: teaching patient progressive passive and active range-of-motion modalities to manage swelling; teaching patient compensatory PADL techniques; having patient use a long opponens splint during activities and progress to activities to increase strength and functional use of affected extremity for use in PADL, IADL, and work activities.

## Progress Notes and Weekly or Monthly Summaries

The occupational therapist must periodically review and document the patient's progress to determine whether the long-term goals continue to be realistic, whether the short-term goals accurately reflect ongoing treatment, and whether treatment has been modified without a corresponding change in the goals. The timing of the review will vary with the intensity of the treatment; the setting; and the needs of the referral source, the third-party payer, or the patient–client. For example, in acute care, where the length of stay is relatively short, this review may be daily; in home care, where the patient is treated 2–3 times a week for 2 months, the review may be every 2 weeks.

Every progress note should include the interventions, the patient's response to the interventions, and progress toward goals. Progress in motor, process, or communication skills should be documented even if the patient's functional status has not changed because these improvements contribute to the occupational performance goal.

Many health care settings and third-party payers require a formal summary every 14, 30, or 60 days. Many facilities and programs have specific formats to follow for summarizing progress; however, if none is available, the outline shown in Exhibit 16.1 may be useful for documenting progress. Similarly, Exhibit 16.2 shows a monthly summary using the outline from Exhibit 16.1.

### Exhibit 16.1 Summary of Progress.

| Goal | Outcome |
| --- | --- |
| List short-term goals. | Specify (a) whether goal has been met, modified, or not achieved and why, or (b) why goal is no longer applicable. |
| List any new goals. | |
| Follow this status report with information about the patient's continued rehabilitation potential, frequency, and duration of future occupational therapy intervention and any referrals that will be made or additional resources that the patient will need. | |

**Exhibit 16.2 Monthly Summary.**

| Short-Term Goals | Outcome |
|---|---|
| Patient will be independent in upper body dressing. (2 weeks) | Achieved |
| Patient will transfer from bed to chair with minimal assistance. (2–3 weeks) | Achieved |
| Patient's family will have grab bars installed in bathroom for safe transfers. (2 weeks) | Not achieved. Family unable to schedule work. |
| Patient will use affected (RUE) as gross assist in self-care. | Partially achieved. Patient raises arm during dressing but does not have sufficient grasp for other activities. |

New goals:
- Patient will transfer from bed to chair with verbal cues. (2 weeks)
- Patient will transfer to tub bench with minimal assistance. (2 weeks)

*Note.* RUE = right upper extremity.

The HCFA (1990) guidelines provide uniform descriptions of levels of assistance and are an example of a way to report changes in a person's level of functioning. Using these levels, the practitioner can measure small amounts of improvement even with patients who still need much assistance. Consider the following examples:
- The caregiver transfers the patient using a Hoyer lift.
- Patient transfers with total assistance from one person using sliding board.
- Patient performs sliding board transfer with moderate assistance from one person.

## Discharge Summary

The discharge summary may follow an outline similar to that of the weekly or monthly summaries but will briefly recapitulate the entire treatment process. It states the patient's functional level at the beginning of treatment, restates all the general functional goals for the patient, and indicates the outcome; if the patient did not meet the goals, it gives the reason. Exhibit 16.3 is a sample discharge summary.

## Conclusion

The reader of documentation is usually interested in the outcome of treatment, not just the methods for achieving the outcome. However, if the patient is not reaching the expected outcome, the practitioner should take a careful look at the treatment plan and make a change.

**Exhibit 16.3  Discharge Summary.**

Patient was referred for home care 4 weeks after having a stroke. Initially, the patient required moderate assistance in all self-care activities with the exception of grooming and eating. Patient was seen two times a week for 6 weeks, followed by one time a week for 2 weeks. He made significant progress meeting his goals.

| Long-Term Goals | Outcomes |
| --- | --- |
| Within 6 weeks, patient will dress independently. | Patient was able to dress independently within 6 weeks, using adaptive equipment. |
| Within 5 weeks, patient will bathe with supervision. | Achieved. Patient bathes using tub seat and wall-mounted grab bar, with supervision from his son for safety. |
| Within 6 weeks, patient will prepare breakfast and lunch. | Achieved. Within 4 weeks, patient prepared breakfast independently, but he prefers Meals-on-Wheels for lunch. |
| Within 6 weeks, patient will toilet independently. | Achieved with the use of grab bar on 7th week when family installed bar. |
| Within 6 weeks, patient will use affected RUE as an assist in all ADL. | Achieved. |

Patient will receive assistance with shopping from his son and supervision for showering as needed from his son. Patient plans to return to daily visits to the Senior Center.

This patient has the potential to use his RUE as the dominant extremity. Continued occupational therapy in an outpatient setting was recommended and discussed with the patient and his family and the patient's physician. Information about several outpatient rehabilitation settings was provided to the patient.

*Note.* RUE = right upper extremity.

One of the best ways for a practitioner to improve his or her documentation is to read the documentation of others and ask the following questions:

- Do the evaluation data present a vivid picture of the patient's level of functioning?
- Does the documentation show evidence that the patient is improving in functional activities, or does it show improvement that is apparent in performance skills such as strength, coordination, and attention span?
- Does the documentation provide evidence that the patient, the patient's family, or both were involved in setting goals?
- Are the reasons for any changes in treatment clear?
- Are the treatment methods that are mentioned consistent with the occupational therapy goals?

Learning to document is somewhat like learning a second language. The occupational therapist who initially learns the correct "grammar and spelling" of this language will become competent faster and more easily. Once an occupational therapist has mastered the rules, then documentation simply requires clear logical thinking, involvement of the patient, and an orientation to results.

# References

American Occupational Therapy Association. (1994a). *Elements of clinical documentation.* Bethesda, MD: Author.

American Occupational Therapy Association. (1994b). *The occupational therapy code of ethics.* Bethesda, MD: Author.

American Occupational Therapy Association. (2002). The occupational therapy practice framework: Domain and process. *American Journal of Occupational Therapy, 56,* 609–639.

Health Care Financing Administration. (1990, September). Medical review (MR) guidelines for occupational therapy (OT) outpatient services (DHHS Transmittal No. 1489). In *Medicare intermediary manual* (section 3906 ff., pp. 23–43). Baltimore, MD: Author.

# CHAPTER 17

# Reimbursement

V. Judith Thomas, MGA

*"Now I know my ABCs... ."*

MOTHER GOOSE

**V. Judith Thomas, MGA,** is the director of Reimbursement and Regulatory Policy at the American Occupational Therapy Association, Bethesda, MD. In previous positions, she managed a health care policy branch in the Office of Payment Policy of the Health Care Financing Administration (now the Centers for Medicare and Medicaid), managed a health care consulting company, and provided systems analysis support in the development of a managed health care administrative system. She earned her master's degree from the University of Maryland.

# Key Terms and Concepts

**Beneficiary.** The term applied to a person who has health insurance through the Medicare or Medicaid programs.

**Capitation.** A specified amount of money paid to a health plan or doctor, usually on a monthly basis, for each member of a health plan, regardless of amount of services received.

**Deductible.** The amount that an individual must pay for health care before the health plan begins to pay. Deductibles may be for each benefit period (usually a year), or may be for specific services, or may be for both.

**Durable medical equipment.** Medical equipment such as wheelchairs and walkers that is ordered by a physician for use in the home (Medicare definition).

**Hospice.** Services provided to terminally ill people and their families, including both physical care and counseling. Under Medicare, hospice is a separately defined and paid benefit.

**Prospective payment system.** A method of paying for predefined groups of health care services for a specific illness or injury over a specific duration of time (e.g., per episode, per day).

**Regulation.** A rule or order interpreting a law that is promulgated by a part of the executive branch of the government (e.g., Centers for Medicare and Medicaid, U.S. Department of Defense).

**Third-party payer.** Any payer for health care services (e.g., insurance company) other than the individual receiving care.

# Learning Objectives

After completing this chapter, you should be able to do the following:

- Describe several ways for which occupational therapy services are paid.

- Understand the effects of third-party payer payment policy on a therapist's practice and ethical decisions.

- Understand the relationships among patients' needs and treatment goals, state laws and regulations, employer policy, and payer requirements.

- Describe the most common medical diagnosis and procedure coding systems and discuss the relationship between coding and payment.

- Define types of out-of-pocket payments and explain how these payments affect a person's medical decision making.

- Describe the information occupational therapists should ascertain from health insurance plans about occupational therapy coverage and payment.

- Compare and contrast the Medicare and Medicaid programs.

This chapter examines the major sources of payment that have historically been available for occupational therapy services. It attempts to acquaint readers with payment terminology and concepts that are used by the insurance industry and that should help occupational therapists and managers better understand the fiscal consequences of clinical practice decisions. In addition, it suggests nontraditional practice areas, which are presently rarely reimbursed by third-party payers but may offer future opportunities for occupational therapy practice. Readers are encouraged to refer to the glossary (Appendix 17.A) and abbreviation chart (Appendix 17.B) for clarification of unfamiliar terms.

Although occupational therapy is widely accepted as one of the core rehabilitation therapies, no nationally recognized definitions or standards exist to which health care payers must adhere. Therefore, people often receive occupational therapy services based on a wide variety of coverage and payment criteria that are developed by individual third-party payers and other program administrators.

Occupational therapy services are paid for in a variety of ways, depending on the settings in which therapists work. Although most occupational therapists are employees of or have contractual arrangements with a large health care provider, a school system, or other organization, a growing segment of the profession is opting for private practice. According to the American Occupational Therapy Association's (AOTA's) 2000 compensation survey (AOTA, 2001), approximately 5.5% of occupational therapists work in a private practice. Also, about 1,500 occupational therapists are enrolled with Medicare as private practitioners (Centers for Medicare and Medicaid [CMS], 2002). Regardless of employment status, therapists must understand the effects of payer policies on practice decisions. That is, before initiating treatment, occupational therapists should know what person or entity is paying for the service, what medical or occupational performance outcome is expected, what service or financial limitations apply, and what documentation is required. Occupational therapists today must expect to balance what they determine as the needs and goals of the patient with state practice regulations, employers' priorities, and payer requirements, all within a framework of the ethical standards of the profession.

Most health care in the United States is funded by federal, state, or local programs or is paid for by private insurance plans under contracts with employers, other organizations, and individuals. Individuals are paying for a growing number of health care services out-of-pocket, either because they have no health insurance or because their plans do not cover specific types of services. Table 17.1 shows the distribution in 1999 of the U.S. population with public or private health insurance and the proportion of uninsured people. In 2000, an estimated 14% of the population had no health insurance coverage (U.S. Bureau of the Census, 2001a).

Occupational therapists also provide services in programs that may not be recognized or funded as "medical" coverage. Whether a specific service is considered "medically necessary" often depends on the condition of the individual, the type of

**Table 17.1  Health Insurance Coverage in the United States, 1999.**

| Insurer | % People Insured by Health Plan |
|---|---|
| Government employer | 24.1 |
| Medicare | 13.2 |
| Medicaid | 10.2 |
| Military (Veterans Administration, TRICARE) | 3.1 |
| Employer (private) | 62.8 |
| Any private plan | 71.0 |
| Uninsured | 15.5 |

*Note.* Percentages do not add to 100 due to dual coverage.
*Source.* U.S. Bureau of the Census, Public Information Office, 2001.

third-party payer, or both. These programs, including driving adaptations for older drivers, home modification, and lifestyle redesign or life care management, may receive financial support through grant funding by public agencies, private foundations, or corporations. Additionally, occupational therapy is often provided to individuals who pay out-of-pocket fees for preventive and other services that are not reimbursed by third-party payers.

Public funding for health care is typically available through programs such as Medicare, Medicaid, and workers' compensation or grant-funded programs. These programs may be administered by federal, state, or local organizations. Each insurance program has structured guidelines specifying which services are covered, in what settings, and by whom. Payment mechanisms and amounts differ from payer to payer and within payer programs, depending on site of service, scope of benefits, and other factors. Federally funded grant programs include the Individuals with Disabilities Education Act (1990); the Community Mental Health Centers Act (1963); the Older Americans Act (1965); and Social Security Title XX, the Social Services Block Grant Program (part of the Omnibus Budget Reconciliation Act of 1981). Use of grant money is generally more flexible than insurance programs, allowing private, state, or local entities to provide specially designed programs as long as they meet broad national goals.

Private insurance companies, either proprietary or nonprofit, provide health care benefits under a wide variety of plans, with differing benefits and restrictions. Insurers primarily contract with employers and other organizations to cover employees (or members) and their dependents for a specific array of benefits. Employers may pay all or part of the cost (i.e., premium) of providing health benefits. Additionally, the employee, or policyholder, may be responsible for out-of-pocket copayments and deductibles. Other types of groups (e.g., professional associations) and individuals also may purchase health care coverage from private insurers.

## General Guidelines for Understanding Health Insurance Plans

Occupational therapy is not consistently defined and paid for across plans or even within specific companies. Health care insurance plans, whether publicly or privately funded, consist of contracts that specify the rules or conditions under which they will cover an array of services. The payer also may impose limitations or restrictions on covered services, payment, or both. Some of these coverage and payment rules for individual programs are discussed in more detail later in this chapter. However, a therapist must be able to ascertain the following information about a client's plan to provide the optimal covered care and to assist patients in making decisions about continuing care that their insurance may not cover.

- What is the plan's definition of occupational therapy?
- Are there limitations (or "caps") on the number of visits, the sites at which services may be received, or the yearly costs incurred for occupational therapy services?
- Is there a network of providers from whom patients must obtain services? Can a patient "opt out" of the network, and if so, what financial disincentives exist to control a patient's ability to choose an out-of-network provider?
- Does the plan offer case management services for some conditions?

In addition, to ensure proper payment for services, it is important to know how the payer determines the payment amount and whether the client or secondary payer is responsible for any portion of the cost of services above the insurer's reimbursement. The occupational therapist should ascertain the following:

- Does the plan pay a fee for service, or is payment for occupational therapy "bundled" into a group of services (e.g., a set amount for all rehabilitation services)?
- Does the payer require specific credentials for occupational therapists?
- Does the payer require that the therapist or health care facility or clinic join a provider network?
- Is the client responsible for copayments, deductibles, or other out-of-pocket expenses? Under what circumstances?

## Major Payers and Players

### Medicare

Medicare has been a major influence on both health care and health care spending. In 2000, health care spending grew to $1.3 trillion, up nearly 7% from 1999. Medicare expenditures ($224 billion) account for 17% of this amount (Levit, Smith, Cowan, Lazenby, & Martin, 2002). In 1999, Medicare covered approximately 34 million elderly beneficiaries and more than 5 million beneficiaries with disabilities, making it the single largest health insurance payer in the country. In addition, Medicare payment rules not only directly affect most practice settings in which occupational therapists work but also indirectly affect the policies of Medicaid and private insurance programs that often follow Medicare's lead. Therefore, a basic understanding of Medicare law, regulations, and policy is essential for occupational therapists.

Medicare, established by Congress in 1965 as Title XIII of the Social Security Act, provides health care coverage for people older than age 65, people with disabilities, and people with end-stage renal disease. The Medicare program is administered by the CMS, formerly the Health Care Financing Administration, and consists of the Hospital Insurance Program (Part A) and the Supplementary Medical Insurance Program (Part B).

Together, both parts of Medicare cover services, including occupational therapy, that are provided in hospitals (inpatient and outpatient), skilled nursing facilities (SNFs), home health agencies (HHAs), hospices, and private practices of physicians and occupational therapists. CMS provides interpretation of legislative requirements through regulations, which have the force of law, and manual instructions, which are further interpretations of regulations. The federal regulatory process requires that, before new rules can be implemented, the government should propose changes and allow for public comment. During this comment period, providers, practitioners, and other interested parties have the opportunity to challenge policy and recommend changes, which the federal agency must address but is not obligated to adopt. This process is important as it allows occupational therapists to participate in the development of policy that will affect their practice.

In addition to regulations, CMS disseminates instructions on Medicare requirements through manual transmittals and program memoranda. (Appendix 17.C lists some of the manuals and Web sites from which they can be obtained.) This information provides guidance on national coverage criteria, billing, and documentation required for a claim to be paid. Medicare manuals containing specific coverage information for each delivery setting are available through the U.S. Government Printing Office and may be downloaded from the CMS Web site (see "Additional Resources" section).

Generally, occupational therapy is considered a Medicare-covered service under the following circumstances. Services must be
- Prescribed by a physician and furnished according to a written plan of care approved by the physician
- Performed by a qualified occupational therapist or by an occupational therapy assistant under the supervision of an occupational therapist
- Reasonable and necessary for the treatment of the person's illness or injury.

Under the original Medicare program, CMS contracts with various insurance companies to process Medicare claims and to perform medical review services in accordance with policies promulgated by CMS. Medicare fiscal intermediaries (FIs) process Medicare claims for hospitals, SNFs, comprehensive outpatient rehabilitation facilities (CORFs), HHAs, and rehabilitation agencies. Five regional home health intermediaries oversee HHA claims processing. Medicare carriers adjudicate claims from physicians and occupational therapy private practitioners. Additionally, four durable medical equipment regional carriers (DMERCs) develop policy and process claims for durable medical equipment, prosthetics, orthotics, and supplies (DMEPOS).

Medicare contractors have the authority to develop local medical review policies (LMRPs) to determine coverage for services, except in cases in which a national coverage policy is already in place. Coverage and reimbursement for occupational therapy services will vary by FI or carrier and, sometimes, will vary in each state in which that payer administers claims. LMRPs can be accessed either through the contractor's Web site or by searching a compilation at http://www.lmrp.net.

### Coverage and Payment Policies

The Medicare benefit includes occupational therapy services when they are provided to eligible beneficiaries by all types of "institutional" providers (i.e., hospitals, SNFs, HHAs, free-standing outpatient therapy providers, and hospices). Additionally, Medicare beneficiaries may receive services from occupational therapists who are in private practices or working for physicians. The general coverage guidelines apply to all settings. However, criteria for payment varies from setting to setting, and this variation affects how therapists must provide and document services. This section provides an overview of payment systems for the original Medicare plan. Other Medicare plan options are discussed later in this chapter.

Table 17.2 provides a brief description of the various Medicare payment systems. Occupational therapists working with Medicare beneficiaries must become proficient in securing the specific coverage and payment policies affecting the setting in which they work and the specific benefit under which the patient is receiving services.

### Hospital Inpatient Prospective Payment System

Since October 1983, acute care hospitals have received a prospective, or predetermined, rate per inpatient discharge based on established diagnosis-related groups (DRGs). This per case rate covers all inpatient services, including occupational therapy. Individual hospitals determine the mix of services that is appropriate for each patient. Specialty hospitals and units such as those offering psychiatric, rehabilitation, pediatric, and long-term care services are exempt from the prospective payment system (PPS) that is applicable to acute care hospitals. With the exception of rehabilitation hospitals and units (see below), these specialty facilities and units continue to be paid retrospectively on a reasonable-cost basis with a limit for all covered services. Occupational therapy services are provided to inpatients of psychiatric hospitals or units based on a provision of Medicare Part A that requires hospitals to have a sufficient number of "qualified therapists, support personnel, and consultants" to provide comprehensive therapeutic activities consistent with each patient's treatment program.

*Hospital outpatient PPS.* Outpatient departments provide Part B Medicare services and are paid on the basis of an ambulatory payment classification system, which classifies procedures (by codes) into groups. The hospital is paid an amount that reflects the resources used to provide this group of procedures during a single outpatient visit. Occupational therapy services provided during a day stay in a partial hospitalization program are included in an outpatient prospective payment system (OPPS) per diem rate.

**Table 17.2  Medicare Payment Systems for Therapy in Specific Provider Settings.**

| Provider Type | Payment System |
|---|---|
| Hospital, acute care inpatient | Per episode PPS based on DRG; excludes psychiatric, rehabilitation, alcohol/drug, long-term care hospitals, and distinct-part units |
| Hospice | Cost-related prospective payment, subject to aggregate limit |
| Rehabilitation unit/rehab hospital | Inpatient rehabilitation facility per episode PPS, effective with cost reporting periods beginning in or after January 2001 |
| SNF | Part A benefit: Per diem PPS based on RUG III categories<br>Part B benefit: MPFS |
| HHA | Home health benefit: Per episode (60 days) PPS<br>Outpatient benefit: MPFS |
| Hospital outpatient, CORF, Rehabilitation agency, Occupational therapy private practice | MPFS |
| Partial hospitalization program in hospital or community mental health center | Hospital outpatient PPS |
| Physician's office, Occupational therapy private practice | MPFS |

*Note.* PPS = prospective payment system; DRG = diagnosis-related group; SNF = skilled nursing facility; RUG = resource utilization group; HHA = home health agency; MPFS = Medicare Physician Fee Schedule; CORF = comprehensive outpatient rehabilitation facility.

*Hospital outpatient therapy payment.* Outpatient therapy (i.e., occupational therapy, physical therapy, and speech–language pathology services provided under the hospital outpatient rehabilitation benefit (Part B) are not covered under the OPPS. Payment is made under the Medicare Physician Fee Schedule (MPFS, also known as the Resource Based Relative Value Scale [RBRVS]). Individual procedures, as defined by *Current Procedural Terminology* (CPT) code, are covered according to a formula that represents the resources required to provide the service (see "Outpatient Occupational Therapy" section).

*Inpatient rehabilitation facility PPS.* Beginning in January 2002, rehabilitation hospitals and units are paid under a PPS that classifies patients into categories based on case mix groups (CMGs). The CMGs are derived from scores on a patient assessment instrument, which measures a person's functional (motor and cognitive) abilities. The hospital is paid a single rate per episode of care under the Medicare Part A benefit.

*Skilled nursing facility PPS.* As discussed in the Medicare SNF conditions of participation, occupational therapy is a covered service under Medicare's SNF (Part A) benefit. This benefit provides for 100 days of skilled nursing and therapy care, provided the patient needs these rehabilitation services on a daily basis (defined in Medicare policy as at least 5 days a week). A patient's need for services and the prospective per diem rate are established by a resident assessment instrument (RAI), which classifies patients into resource utilization groups (RUGs). The RAI consists of the Minimum Data Set, a core set of screening, clinical, and functional status assessment elements; the resident assessment protocols; and utilization guidelines (CMS, 1995). The therapy RUGs are based on the number of minutes of therapy per week required by the patient. SNFs also provide Part B Medicare therapy services to residents who do not qualify for Part A coverage. The payment system for all outpatient (including SNF Part B) occupational therapy services is discussed below.

*Home health agency PPS.* To qualify under the home health benefit, a homebound patient must need intermittent skilled nursing care, physical therapy, or speech–language therapy before receiving occupational therapy. However, Medicare patients may continue to receive occupational therapy under the home health benefit after their need for skilled nursing, physical therapy, or speech–language therapy ends (Appendix 17.C). HHAs classify patients using a standard form, the Outcome and Assessment Information Set. An HHA is paid a single rate for each 60 days of services, which is based on the information entered on the assessment. A higher payment is provided if the need for a specific level of therapy is projected and provided. Most services provided under the home health benefit are considered Part A services. HHAs may also provide outpatient therapy (Part B) as indicated below.

*Hospice PPS.* Hospice care is a special Part A benefit for eligible Medicare beneficiaries whom a physician has certified as terminally ill, defined in the regulations as a medical prognosis of fewer than 6 months to live. A patient who elects to receive hospice benefits must waive inpatient Medicare benefits during the election period. Occupational therapy may be provided only to control a patient's symptoms or to enable a patient to maintain activities of daily living and basic functional skills. Hospice benefits are paid on a prospective basis. The rates, which are updated annually, are based on four primary levels of care that correspond to the degree of illness and the amount of care required.

*Outpatient occupational therapy.* Occupational therapy is covered as a Part B outpatient service when furnished by or under (contractual) arrangements with any Medicare-certified provider (i.e., a hospital, an SNF, an HHA, a rehabilitation agency, a clinic, a CORF, or a public health agency). A provider may furnish outpatient occupational therapy services to a beneficiary in the home or in the provider's outpatient facility or, under certain circumstances, to a beneficiary who is an inpatient in another institution. Payment for all outpatient therapy services (i.e., occupational therapy, physical therapy, and speech–language pathology) is made under the MPFS. Medicare pays a provider 80% of the fee schedule amount after the beneficiary has paid a yearly deductible for all Medicare Part B services.

*Occupational therapists in private practice.* Outpatient occupational therapy (Part B) may be furnished to beneficiaries by an occupational therapist in private practice either in the therapist's office or in the patient's home. A therapist in private practice enrolls in the Medicare program as a participating practitioner through the Medicare carrier in much the same way that physicians enroll. Practitioners are paid according to the CPT codes that are billed and at the rates that are established under the MPFS.

*Physicians' offices.* Outpatient occupational therapy services are covered under Medicare (Part B) as incidental to a physician's services when rendered to beneficiaries in a physician's office or in a physician-directed clinic. Occupational therapy services must be directly related to the condition for which the physician is treating the patient, the physician must be on site, and services must be included on the physician's bill to Medicare. The payment amount is determined by the MPFS.

*Payment for DMEPOS.* Expenses incurred by a beneficiary for the rental or purchase of durable medical equipment (e.g., a wheelchair, walker) are reimbursable under Medicare Part B if the equipment is used in the patient's home and is necessary and reasonable to treat an illness or an injury. Medicare defines *durable medical equipment* as that which can withstand repeated use, is primarily and customarily used to serve a medical purpose, and generally is not useful to a person in the absence of illness or injury. Reachers, bathtub grab bars, and most types of adaptive equipment are generally not covered because they are not considered medically necessary. Orthotic devices are defined in regulations as "leg, arm, back and neck braces . . ." and require a prescription and certificate of medical necessity signed by a physician. Orthotics may be provided to beneficiaries in inpatient and outpatient settings.

All medical equipment companies, providers, or practitioners that wish to bill for equipment must apply to become Medicare suppliers. All items classified as durable medical equipment are billed to one of four DMERCs and paid for under a separate durable medical equipment fee schedule. Orthotics and prosthetics also are covered items that are billed in the same manner as durable medical equipment to DMERCs by all providers except hospitals and SNFs, which bill their local FIs for these items.

*Medicare "gap" policies.* Medicare does not pay 100% of the cost of most services but requires that the beneficiary be responsible for deductibles and coinsurance amounts. Many Medicare beneficiaries purchase secondary insurance, often called "Medigap policies," to cover these out-of-pocket expenses. Some companies that sell these types of policies also provide coverage for items and services not covered by Medicare. Bills must be submitted to Medicare before the secondary insurance policy will pay.

*Medicare+Choice.* The CMS certifies and awards contracts to a variety of managed care and fee-for-service entities under the Medicare+Choice program, which was established under the Balanced Budget Act (BBA) of 1997. Approximately 14% of all Medicare beneficiaries are enrolled in one of these alternative Medicare options. CMS pays health maintenance organizations (HMOs) and other Medicare+Choice organizations an amount per enrolled beneficiary based on the individual's county of residence and other factors associated with health care costs. The BBA requires that the county payment rate be determined as the highest of three amounts:

- A minimum 2% increase over the prior year
- A minimum dollar amount, or "floor"
- An amount derived from blending the local rate with a national rate that is based on the historic pattern of Medicare spending.

The Balanced Budget Refinement Act of 1999 and the Medicare, Medicaid, and the State Children's Health Insurance Program [SCHIP] Benefits Improvement and Protection Act of 2000 modified the payment formula, including increasing the minimum to 3%, increasing the floor amount, and establishing bonuses and risk adjustment payments for plans under specific conditions.

Medicare managed care plans typically cover all preventive, acute, and outpatient health services. They must be able to deliver with "reasonable promptness" all medically necessary services that Medicare beneficiaries are entitled to receive and that are available to Medicare beneficiaries who are living in the same geographic area but who are not enrolled in a managed care plan. In addition, many plans offer other health care benefits (e.g., coverage of preventive care and prescriptions) that are not included in traditional Medicare coverage. The standard Medicare Part B premium is always required. Although additional cost-sharing levels vary according to policies established by each plan, the beneficiary is often required to pay a supplemental premium for coverage of deductibles, coinsurance, and services not covered by Medicare.

Another option under Medicare+Choice is enrollment in private fee-for-service (PFFS) plans. Enrollees in a PFFS plan may obtain care from any licensed provider in the United States who can be paid by Medicare and who will accept the PFFS plan's terms of payment. The PFFS plan will pay providers amounts that are derived from the CMS-specified payment methodologies (e.g., DRG payments, MPFS). For cases in which there is no prospectively set payment for a Medicare-covered service, CMS (2000) has approved proxies that result in a payment that is generally equivalent to Medicare payment.

Enrollees in Medicare+Choice plans must adhere to the requirements of the plan, for example, by using a specified network of providers in an HMO plan. Some HMO plans have expanded coverage options to include a point-of-service (POS) option, which permits its HMO enrollees to seek care outside the HMO's provider network. Typically, the HMO imposes higher cost-sharing levels for use of out-of-network providers. Similar to HMOs, Medicare PFFS plans are available to people living in a specific plan area. However, enrollees in PFFS plans may go anywhere in the country to obtain health care services.

## TRICARE Program

The TRICARE Program is the U.S. Department of Defense's (DOD's) health care program for active-duty, retired military, and their eligible family members and survivors younger than age 65. Medical care is provided in Army, Navy, Air Force, and Coast Guard hospitals and clinics located throughout the United States. Additionally, there are Uniformed Services Treatment Facilities operated under a DOD contract. These facilities are former public health hospitals located in Baltimore, MD; Staten Island, NY; Boston, MA; Portland, ME; Cleveland, OH; Houston, TX; and Seattle, WA.

TRICARE offers three plan options: TRICARE Prime, TRICARE Standard (previously CHAMPUS), and TRICARE Extra. TRICARE Prime is an HMO-style plan in which all services must be coordinated through a primary care manager. TRICARE Standard is a fee-for-service program, which allows members to consult a wide choice of providers. It is a higher cost option, requiring annual deductibles and copayments (20% for active-duty family members and 25% for retirees). The third option, TRICARE Extra, is a lower cost version of TRICARE Standard. Members are required to use civilian providers who are part of DOD's preferred provider pool. Deductibles are the same as with TRICARE Standard, but copayments are 5% lower.

As with most public and private plans, preferred or network providers must accept TRICARE's payment and cannot charge the patient. TRICARE will not pay for services from non-network providers if the patient is enrolled in TRICARE Prime or TRICARE Extra. If the member is enrolled in TRICARE Standard, nonparticipating providers will be paid a set amount by TRICARE and may charge the patient the difference to equal their standard fees.

## Veterans' Health Care

As a general rule, to receive medical care from the Veterans Administration (VA), a person must be an honorably discharged veteran (more than 180 days of military service) with a service-connected illness, injury, or disability.

In 1996, Congress passed the Veterans' Health Care Eligibility Reform Act, which mandated that the VA establish and implement a national enrollment system to manage the delivery of health care services. To comply with this law, the VA developed a standard health plan with a single medical benefits package that covers most veterans. Different requirements apply with respect to enrollment, copayments, and other financial liability, depending on the status of the veteran. By law, the VA must submit claims to private health insurance carriers for recovery of the VA's reasonable charges in providing medical care to non-service-connected veterans and to service-connected veterans for non-service-connected conditions. The VA may not request payment from the Medicare program.

In addition to the usual inpatient and outpatient services, the veterans' health plan covers additional needs for some veterans, including nursing home costs, home improvements and structural alterations, alcohol- and drug-dependence treatment, orthotics and prosthetics, and readjustment counseling. The scope of the veterans' health plan varies widely depending on the veteran's status and disability level. Additional information can be found on the Web sites for each VA medical center.

## Federal Employees Health Benefit Program

The Federal Employees Health Benefits (FEHB) Program is administered by the Office of Personnel Management under part 890 of title 5 and chapter 16 of title 48 of the *Code of Federal Regulations*. FEHB is the largest employer-sponsored group health insurance program in the world, covering almost 9 million people, including employees and annuitants as well as their family members and some former spouses and former employees. FEHB offers more than 350 health plans across the United States. Federal employees have a choice of fee-for-service plans, HMOs, and plans offering a POS product. Some plans are available nationwide, and others are available only to employees who are in specific areas or working for specific government agencies. For example, of the 26 FEHB options available in Texas, 10 are nationwide, 9 are available only in certain cities, and 6 apply only to specific groups (U.S. Office of Personnel Management, 2002).

The federal law and regulations governing the scope of benefits that must be offered specify only broad categories such as hospital, surgical, and medical services. Therefore, coverage of individual types of service, such as occupational therapy, and the settings in which they may be provided are determined by each of the private plans with which the government contracts to administer health care services.

The FEHB has historically included insurers such as Blue Cross/Blue Shield (BCBS), PacifiCare, Kaiser, and the Government Employees Hospital Association (GEHA). Each insurer may have more than one plan type with different copayments and deductibles as well as limitations on covered occupational therapy. Most plans cover occupational therapy in some settings; however, scope of coverage, payment, and outpatient visit limitations vary widely. For example, the BCBS plans allow 50 visits per year for occupational therapy, physical therapy, and speech–language pathology combined, whereas the GEHA plan limits members to a combined 60 visits per year for occupational therapy and physical therapy. Kaiser requires precertification of occupational therapy and limits outpatient occupational therapy to 90 days of treatment.

## State and Local Payers

Private insurance companies or public programs that are either funded or administered at the state or local level (or both) pay most health care costs for individuals younger than age 65. This section describes some of the major third-party payers that are regulated or administered primarily by state agencies.

## Medicaid

Medicaid, Title XIX of the Social Security Act (originally enacted in the Social Security Amendments of 1965), is a jointly funded federal–state program that provides health care to poor and medically indigent populations. States must adhere to broad federal guidelines but have great flexibility in the administration of their Medicaid programs. Each state establishes its own eligibility standards; determines the type, amount, duration, and scope of services; and sets the rate of payment for services. Under federal law, states are required to provide Medicaid coverage for most individuals who receive federally assisted income maintenance payments and for other related groups such as recipients of Temporary Assistance to Needy Families, children younger than age 6, pregnant women whose family income is at or below 133% of the federal poverty level, infants born to Medicaid-eligible women, and most beneficiaries of Supplemental Security Income. Additionally, states have the option of covering other "categorically needy" or "medically needy" individuals. Some states have a spend-down provision under which families with moderately high incomes may become eligible for Medicaid when their medical expenses reduce their income below the state standard. Medicaid also is available for some Medicare-eligible beneficiaries who meet specific income level standards to help with out-of-pocket expenses.

Medicaid-covered services fall into two categories: mandatory and optional services. Mandatory services are ones that a state must provide to qualify for federal matching funds. They include hospital services; laboratory work and X-rays; SNF services; physicians' services; early and periodic screening, diagnosis, and treatment (EPSDT) for people younger than age 21; and family planning. States must provide certain services, including occupational therapy, that are necessary to treat a condition identified during an EPSDT assessment. Coverage of these services is required even if they often are not normally covered under the state's Medicaid program. Occupational therapy provided as a free-standing discipline is considered an optional service, along with physical therapy, speech–language therapy, drugs, psychiatric care, and others. Nursing home reforms adopted by Congress in 1987 require Medicaid nursing facilities to provide skilled rehabilitation services, including occupational therapy, to patients who require them.

In 1988, Congress approved legislation to allow school systems to bill Medicaid for certain related services, including occupational therapy, provided to children in schools. Implementation of this rule has resulted in the development of various state methods to determine responsibility and to pay for occupational therapy services provided to school-age children. The seemingly overlapping language of education and Medicaid laws governing the delivery of care for school-age children has given rise to the question of whether services to individual children should be funded as education or health care.

## Medicaid Managed Care

Managed care options under Medicaid have expanded greatly over the past decade. A state may implement a state plan option under Section 1932 of the Social Security Act or apply to the federal government for waivers under Section 1915(b) or 1115, all of which allow states flexibility in types of services provided and delivery methods. For example, under the Section 1932 option, a state may require specific groups of beneficiaries (with exceptions) to enroll with a managed care entity and may restrict the number of providers with whom it contracts to provide services. A Section 1915(b) waiver (of the Social Security Act) allows a state to restrict a beneficiary's choice of provider and is often limited to selected geographic regions within a state. A Section 1115 waiver is a more extensive research-and-demonstration project that is usually granted for 5 years but may be extended for up to 3 additional years under a BBA amendment. Under Section 1115, states are allowed to test major changes in how Medicaid services are delivered. Under most Section 1115 waivers, the existing benefit packages, including occupational therapy benefits, that were available before the waiver was approved continue to be available through a managed care plan contractor. However, the risk of having services limited is increased when authority for case management, coverage decisions, and utilization review is transferred from the state government to a managed care plan.

Because states have a wide range of options in the structure and administration of Medicaid programs, occupational therapists who wish to treat Medicaid recipients or who assist with billing for school systems or health care facilities must understand the specific requirements of their state's plan. Information on Medicaid coverage of occupational therapy may be obtained from state offices of medical assistance.

### Program of All-Inclusive Care for the Elderly
The BBA of 1997 instituted the Program of All-Inclusive Care for the Elderly (PACE) model as a permanent benefit within the Medicare and Medicaid programs and allows states to provide PACE services to Medicaid participants as a state option. PACE is a capitated, managed care program serving Medicare and Medicaid participants who are among the frail elderly population. The mission of the program is to augment the quality of life for older, frail adults who are eligible for nursing home services, enabling them to live in their homes and in their communities for as long as medically and socially possible. PACE organizations employ a multidisciplinary team in a holistic approach to providing medical and social services. Services are provided in adult day care health centers, in participants' homes, and in inpatient facilities.

Each PACE benefit package, regardless of source of payment, must include at a minimum all Medicaid-covered services in the state's Medicaid plan plus other services, including primary care physician services; social work; restorative therapies, including occupational therapy, physical therapy, and speech–language pathology; meals; drugs; DMEPOS; acute inpatient care, including occupational therapy, physical therapy, speech–language pathology, and rehabilitation therapy; and nursing facility care, including occupational therapy, physical therapy, speech–language pathology, and rehabilitation therapy.

For Medicare participants, PACE organizations will receive prospective, capitated monthly payments for each enrolled participant. Because a capitated system program receives a set monthly amount for each enrollee, it assumes some financial risk because the program must provide all covered services for the set amount. This amount is based on the Medicare+Choice payment rates plus a frailty factor and an adjustment factor for PACE participants who have end-stage renal disease. This determination is similar to the methodology used for risk-based HMOs. Separate rates are established for Part A and Part B, and the PACE organization receives payments based on each participant's entitlement to Medicare Parts A and B. Note, however, that PACE is not a Medicare+Choice plan. The two plans are similar in that they are both capitated and risk-based, provide managed care, and are elective options; however, PACE is available only in a limited number of sites, it includes statutory waivers that expand the scope of Medicare-covered services, and it is not available to all beneficiaries (only to defined frail elderly). If Medicare is not the primary payer (e.g., state or federal workers' compensation, self-insured plan), then the PACE organization must coordinate benefits and payment amounts with the primary payer.

For Medicaid-only participants, the state will make prospective monthly capitated payments for each participant eligible under the state plan. The capitation amount will be specified under the PACE program agreement, will consider the frailty of the patient, and will be less than the amount that would have been paid under the state plan if the participant were not enrolled. The payment is based on a blend of the cost of providing nursing home care and community-based care for the frail elderly population. The PACE organization and the state administering agency may renegotiate this rate annually (see http://www.aota.org members only, reimbursement page).

## Payment for Occupational Therapy Services for Children

A large proportion of occupational therapists work with infants and children, either in medical (e.g., neonatal units, children's hospitals) or in educational settings. According to AOTA's 2000 compensation survey (AOTA, 2001), school systems were the number 1 employers (by either salary or contract arrangements) of occupational therapists (24.9%), and the number 2 employers of occupational therapy assistants (22.3%). At least another 6% of occupational therapists and occupational therapy assistants work with children in medical settings or early intervention programs. Many children are covered by private medical insurance as dependents of working parents. However, insurance companies often exclude or restrict services needed by children with chronic conditions and rarely cover "educational" services. The following section describes the primary federal- and state-supported funding sources that are available to low-income children for medical and educational services.

### State Children's Health Insurance Program

The BBA of 1997 established the SCHIP as Title XXI of the Social Security Act, which provides funding for states to expand health care coverage to uninsured, low-income children who do not meet the Medicaid eligibility requirements. A state may create a new program with coverage that (a) is equivalent to one of the following: the standard BCBS preferred provider option offered under the FEHB program, a health benefits plan that is offered and is generally available to state employees, or the HMO plan with the largest commercial enrollment in the state; (b) has an aggregate actuarial value that is at least equivalent to one of the packages listed in (a); (c) is an expansion of an existing comprehensive statewide program (such as Medicaid); or (d) provides appropriate coverage (as determined by the secretary of health and human services) for targeted low-income children. Alternatively, a state may expand eligibility for children under the state's Medicaid program. To be eligible for funds, states must obtain approval for SCHIP from the secretary of health and human services. Information on SCHIP is available from individual state agencies.

### Individuals with Disabilities Education Act

The Education for All Handicapped Children Act of 1975, reenacted in 1990 as the Individuals with Disabilities Education Act (IDEA), provides federal grants to states to ensure that eligible children with disabilities receive a "free, appropriate public education." This statute has been amended over the years to include preschool-age children and additional services such as assistive technology and transition planning. At present, the law outlines the minimum number of services that states must provide to infants, toddlers, children, and youths with disabilities. Part B of IDEA requires that public school systems and other state agencies involved in educating children with disabilities (ages 3–21) provide "a free appropriate public education that includes special education and related services to meet their unique needs" (Education, 1977). Under this program, occupational therapy is considered a related service, playing a supportive role in helping children benefit from special education.

Part C (formerly Part H of IDEA) provides funding to states "to develop and implement a statewide, comprehensive, coordinated, multidisciplinary, interagency program of early intervention services for infants and toddlers with disabilities and their families" (Education, 1989). Under this early intervention program, occupational therapy is considered a primary service for children from the ages of birth through 2 years and can be provided alone or in conjunction with other services. Under Part B and Part C of IDEA, occupational therapy services must be provided according to an individualized education plan or an individualized family service plan, respectively, by a qualified therapist, consistent with state law.

The IDEA Amendments of 1997 were the first major revision to the act in more than 23 years. These amendments and associated regulations strengthen the rights and protections for children with disabilities and emphasize improved educational results for children. Parts C and D of IDEA are scheduled to be reauthorized in the near future. Occupational therapists working with children must monitor subsequent changes in the law, regulations, and state implementation that affect their practice.

## Workers' Compensation

State-based workers' compensation programs provide benefits for employees who have job-related injuries or illnesses. The programs are financed jointly by individual employers or groups of employers and state governments (Burton, 1996). Each state has a workers' compensation governing board or commission that develops policies regulating whether an employer is required to participate, what the financial responsibility of the employer is, what benefits are provided, which workers are covered, and how the insurance is administered. Workers' compensation insurance may be administered through private insurance plans under contract with the state or through individual employers or groups of employers that administer their own programs (a practice known as *self-insuring*). In addition, federal employees are covered either by the Federal Employees' Compensation Act or by the Longshore and Harbor Workers' Compensation Act (Burton, 1996).

Workers' compensation programs provide cash benefits (either to an employee or to survivors) and medical benefits. In reaction to escalating costs in programs from 1985 to 1991, more than half of the state legislatures passed major cost containing amendments to workers' compensation laws during the period from 1989 to 1996. In these jurisdictions, eligibility requirements for benefits became more restrictive, the statutory level of cash benefits was reduced, and managed care concepts were introduced into the health care delivery system (Burton & Spieler, 2001). In 1999, workers' compensation programs paid out more than $43 billion dollars in benefits (Mont, Burton, Reno, & Thompson, 2001).

State statutes vary on whether an employee may select an initial provider of care or change providers during treatment. According to the Workers' Compensation Research Institute, 33 states and the federal government allow employees to choose their primary physicians (with some restrictions) (http://www.workerscompresources.com). In 14 states, the employer or managed care organization makes the selection.

Many states have adopted some type of fee schedule that prescribes payment amounts for all services performed by health care practitioners for workers' compensation patients. Fee schedules vary according to which services are included, what coding scheme is required (see the section "Billing and Coding for Services"), what formulas are used to calculate the actual dollar amounts, which state entity develops and controls the use, and how as well as how often the fee schedules are updated. A relative value system is used in most jurisdictions, but wide state-to-state variations exist in the amount of compensation for individual procedures. Additionally, states have adopted various methods (e.g., fee schedules and discounted charges) to regulate workers' compensation hospital expenditures, often in conjunction with all-payer systems that affect payments to all hospitals. Although some states use the DRG-based Medicare system, many of the DRGs do not apply to the workers' compensation population.

As is true of most public and private insurers today, many states have incorporated various strategies to address the delivery of "unnecessary or inappropriate care," including retrospective claim review, precertification of services, and case management programs. Movement to managed care contracts also has increased by states and employers that self-insure. In this way, workers' compensation programs can take advantage of existing cost containment strategies used by HMOs and preferred provider organizations (PPOs), including case management, utilization review protocols, and return-to-work programs, without having to make incremental changes in state policy. To date, the few research projects designed to determine whether these strategies actually reduce the cost of care are inconclusive.

A more comprehensive approach to the reform of the workers' compensation system is *24-hour coverage*. According to Burton (1996), this term describes

> efforts to reduce or eliminate the distinctions among the medical benefits, income benefits, and disability management services provided to disabled workers for work-related injuries and diseases and . . . [those] provided to disabled workers for non-work-related injuries and diseases. (p. 17)

These attempts to coordinate medical, income, and disability benefits from different payment sources vary greatly in configuration and structure. Additional information may be obtained from individual state workers' compensation boards or commissions or from the International Association of Industrial Accident Boards and Commissions (see "Additional Resources" for contact information).

## Private Insurance

In the United States, a large number of health insurance companies provide benefits to employer and other groups as well as to individual subscribers. Insurers, especially large companies such as BCBS, Aetna, MetLife, and Prudential, have many product lines of health insurance, including managed care options, and often negotiate unique benefit and premium configurations with a single employer. There are 43 local BCBS plans in the United States (http://www.bluecares.com). Each plan has multiple benefit packages that are sold to specific groups. For example, Anthem BCBS offers five HMO or PPO options, offers Medigap coverage, and administers plans for federal employees. In contrast, BCBS of Massachusetts has at least five managed care options, two individual packages, as well as a Medigap and a Medicare+Choice option. It also provides a major medical plan and other traditional insurance. Therefore, an occupational therapist can never make assumptions about a person's coverage by plan name alone. (See Appendix 17.D for general descriptions of insurance plans.)

Many plans enroll a network of participating physicians, nonphysician practitioners, and facility-type providers. Private practitioners must determine whether the patient is required to visit a network provider to have payment for the services reimbursed. If an occupational therapist is not "in the network," the patient may receive a lower reimbursement or be responsible for the total bill as an out-of-pocket expense. In hospitals, clinics, and other large facilities, insurance coverage is generally determined by the business office before the occupational therapist treats the patient.

Because there are no federally mandated requirements for benefits or payment, each state determines the extent of control that it wants to impose on the insurance companies operating within its jurisdiction. Requirements for insurance companies are generally found in the state's insurance regulations. Also, because employers that self-insure health care benefits are governed not by state insurance codes but by the Employee Retirement Income Security Act, practices across the country are widely divergent. In recent years, traditional indemnity insurers, in addition to administrators of managed care organizations, have been introducing managed care principles into their plans.

The following management techniques are often implemented in conjunction with cost-controlling payment strategies, such as use of discounted or capitated rates and preferred provider networks, to manage costs and quality more effectively.

- *Case management.* Especially for long-term or high-cost cases, insurers use case managers, often employed outside the plan, to oversee and designate which group of services will yield the best outcome. Frequently, this decision-making power allows a case manager to approve treatments that a plan might not normally cover. Some insurers use the terms *case management* and *managed care* synonymously.

- *Precertification or preauthorization.* This is the requirement that specific tests, surgical procedures, or categories of services (e.g., occupational therapy, physical therapy, mental health) be authorized before they are allowed. It gives the insurer the opportunity to deny "unnecessary" treatment or substitute lower cost services. Often, precertification allows a specific number of visits within a specific time frame (e.g., 12 visits over 3 months). The provider or patient must then request additional visits if needed.

- *Mandatory second opinion.* Insisting on a second opinion before approval of any or specific types of surgical procedures serves as a check on a physician's decision with respect to the need for surgery. It presents an opportunity for another physician to suggest an alternative, less costly treatment.

- *Third-party administrator.* Insurers may contract with a private company that specializes in management of various administrative functions (e.g., claims) and managed care responsibilities (e.g., utilization review) for a plan or an employer (if self-insured).

## Other State-Based or Community Programs

As stated previously, private insurers are free to negotiate with employers, within the limitations of state law, on types of covered services, exclusions, precertification procedures and other factors affecting health care benefits. Therefore, large groups, such as those including state employees or employers with more than 1,000 employees, may have plans that are very different from other plans offered by the same company.

State and local governments also may fund community programs, which offer to occupational therapists and occupational therapy assistants opportunities for "nontraditional" practice. When exploring these options, therapists should inquire about sources of payment for the program. Although some insurance plans have begun to cover some alternative medicine options, such as acupuncture and biofeedback for specific conditions, most do not consider service such as home modifications or lifestyle redesign programs as "medically necessary." Public or private grants or specific legislative funding may be available to support innovative programs.

## Getting Paid: Practitioner Management and Fiscal Responsibilities

Whether in private practice or as employees, occupational therapists should develop good fiscal management skills as well as clinical expertise. This includes a basic understanding of coverage and claims submission requirements of third-party payers. The following sections introduce the reader to some important aspects of claims management.

### Billing and Coding for Services

To receive payment for services, facilities and individual providers must properly code and complete claim forms. Two common billing forms are (a) the Uniform Bill (UB-92; CMS-1450), used by institutional providers such as hospitals, SNFs, and HHAs and (b) the CMS-1500 claim form, primarily used for practitioner offices such as physicians and occupational therapists in private practice.[1]

Public and private payers usually require health care facilities and practitioners to categorize their services in terms of diagnosis and procedure codes. Readers must remember that not all payers cover the same range of services or permit use of the same codes. In addition, state regulations or payer policies may establish limitations on the amount paid for a specific code or combination of codes. Occupational therapists, whether they are employees of a health care provider or private practitioners, have a fiscal and ethical obligation to ensure that services and documentation, including correct billing information, comply with federal, state, and payer policies.

#### *Diagnosis Codes*

Diagnosis codes describe the patient's condition or the medical reason for the patient's requiring services. They are critical to obtaining a favorable determination of coverage. The *International Classification of Diseases, Ninth Revision, Clinical Modification* (ICD-9-CM, 2001), which is updated annually, is the most frequently used diagnosis-coding system in the United States. Under the ICD coding system, diseases are categorized primarily by anatomical systems. Also, ICD contains supplementary classifications covering (a) factors influencing health status and (b) external causes of injury and poisoning. An additional volume provides a listing of ICD surgical and

---

[1]Insurers generally do not recognize occupational therapy assistants for direct payment because they require supervision and do not perform evaluations.

medical procedures, which are mainly used to code inpatient hospital services. The *Diagnostic and Statistical Manual of Mental Disorders, Fourth Edition, Text Revision* (American Psychiatric Association, 2000) is frequently used by mental health practitioners and providers. This system, which is compatible with ICD-9-CM, groups mental health disorders into 16 major diagnostic classes. The ICD-10 is scheduled to replace these coding systems within the next several years.

### Procedure Codes

Procedure codes describe specific services performed by health care professionals. One of the most widely used procedure-coding systems is the Healthcare Common Procedure Coding System (HCPCS), which includes (a) the CPT, which is updated each year by the American Medical Association (AMA),[2] and is referred to as Level I HCPCS; (b) the CMS-developed alphanumeric codes, referred to as Level II HCPCS; and (c) local codes, referred to as Level III HCPCS, created by Medicare and other carriers as needed when other HCPCS codes do not suffice. Level II HCPCS contains codes for DMEPOS as well as some procedures not found in the CPT system. Few carriers now use local or Level III codes, and this level will become obsolete when all health care providers and payers must be in compliance with the "transaction and code set" regulations required by the Health Insurance Portability and Accountability Act of 1996 (HIPAA). Health plans must comply with these HIPAA rules by October 16, 2003 (H.R. 3323, signed December 27, 2001).

### Current Procedural Terminology

Since 1990, CMS has contracted with the AMA to use the CPT-4 coding system as the basis for the MPFS and to assist with the development of relative value units for each code. In May 1993, the AMA invited nine non-physician-practitioner associations to participate in the CPT Editorial Panel and Relative Value Scale Update Committee processes by forming a Health Care Professionals Advisory Committee (HCPAC). AOTA was included in this initial group along with the American Academy of Physician Assistants, the American Nurses Association, the American Optometric Association, the American Physical Therapy Association, the American Podiatric Medical Association, the American Psychological Association, the American Speech-Language-Hearing Association, and the National Association of Social Workers. In 2002, the HCPAC consisted of advisers from those original organizations plus two added organizations, the American Chiropractic Association and the American Dietetic Association. These associations, individually and as a group, make recommendations to the annual update of CPT and the relative values for work and practice expense.

---

[2]CPT™ is a trademark of the AMA. CPT five-digit codes, two-digit codes, modifiers, and descriptions only are copyrighted (2001) by the AMA. All rights reserved.

The CPT coding system provides a uniform terminology for each of thousands of medical procedures. Occupational therapists in private practice and therapists working in facilities that bill under the outpatient (Part B) Medicare benefit are required to use CPT codes. In addition, most other public and private insurers require CPT for payment. Although occupational therapists most often use codes in the Physical Medicine and Rehabilitation section of CPT, under AMA guidelines, physicians and nonphysician practitioners may select the codes that most accurately identify the services performed. Other than the requirement that the service be within the scope of practice of the practitioner, there are no CPT restrictions for the use of codes in any section.

However, individual payers determine their own rules for coding and billing and may limit the number and range of codes that a specialty may use to bill services. Occupational therapists should request information on allowable codes, service definitions, and documentation policies before billing a new insurer.

## Payment Methods

Payers reimburse for services provided by occupational therapists in a variety of ways. Often, when occupational therapy is performed in a facility or for a large organization that provides many types of health care services, it is not paid for separately but is included as part of a "bundled rate." Table 17.3 describes common methods of payment for health care services.

Regardless of payer, payment denials are inevitable at some time in an occupational therapist's career. It is important that therapists are aware of and are willing to appeal erroneous claims denials. Denials can occur on submission of a claim or when payers review paid claims (a postpayment review, medical review, or audit; Lloyd, 2001). Each insurer must have an administrative process for members, providers, or both to appeal claims. This process differs depending on state law and regulations as well as company policy, so one must ascertain the specific appeal procedures that apply to the insurer that has issued the denial.

Common elements to look for in every appeal process are as follows:
- *Time frames*—How long does the patient or provider have to file an appeal?
- *Levels of appeal*—Generally, more than one opportunity is provided to appeal a denial, and each level must be completed before going to the next. At each level, additional documentation may be submitted. A personal presentation may be possible at some levels, or the payer may allow only a "paper" review. Qualification for some appeal levels may require a minimum-dollar "disputed amount" threshold.
- *Legal rights*—When all administrative appeal options are exhausted, the provider or patient may appeal to an entity outside the payer's purview. In the case of most health insurance plans, this entity would initially be the state department of insurance. After all levels of appeal have failed, state or federal court is the final option.

**Table 17.3  Payment Methods.**

| Payment Method | Description | Examples |
|---|---|---|
| Fee-for-service | Rate per unit of service (e.g., per procedure, per diem); may be a fee schedule (based on CPT code or other designator); may be percentage of charges or other rate-setting methodology | Medicare (RBRVS fee schedule) payment to occupational therapists in private practice<br>State workers' compensation fee schedule |
| Prospective rate | An aggregate payment for groups of services that are necessary for a patient's care for a specific type of injury or illness or over a specific duration (e.g., per case, per episode) | Medicare payment to hospitals for inpatient services, to home health agencies, or to rehabilitation hospitals |
| Capitated rate | Prospectively paid amount, usually on a monthly basis, for each member of a specific population (e.g., members of a health plan or Medicaid beneficiaries), regardless of whether any covered health care service is delivered | HMO payments to primary care providers<br>CMS payments to HMO Medicare+Choice plans |

*Note.* CPT = *Current Procedural Terminology;* RBRVS = Resource Based Relative Value Scale; HMO = health maintenance organization; CMS = Centers for Medicare and Medicaid.

As an example, Table 17.4 shows the appeal rights under the traditional Medicare plan.

To successfully appeal a claims denial, occupational therapists must understand the grounds for denial and the plan's coverage and documentation requirements. They must be able to "demonstrate how services were clinically appropriate, medically necessary, met the profession's standards of care, and were appropriately documented" (Lloyd, 2001, p. 6).

## Conclusion

Occupational therapy services are widely accepted as a major component of rehabilitation and are reimbursed by most third-party payers. However, because the United States has no national health care policy, public and private payer policies differ widely in the scope of occupational therapy coverage, the types of providers that can be paid, and the settings in which they will pay. Occupational therapists, whether they are employees of a health care provider or private practitioners, have a fiscal and ethical obligation to ensure that services and documentation, including correct billing information, comply with federal, state, and payer policies.

The Medicare program, established as Title XIII of the Social Security Act and administered by the CMS, is the single largest health insurance payer in the country, pro-

**Table 17.4 Appeal Rights Under the Medicare Traditional Plan.**

| Appeal Level | Time Frames for Filing Request for Appeal | Required Dollar Amount of the Claims at Issue |
|---|---|---|
| Review | Within 6 months from the date of initial determination | Not a factor |
| HO hearing | Within 6 months from date of the review determination | At least $100 |
| ALJ hearing | Within 60 days from receipt of HO hearing decision | At least $500 ($100 for home health) |
| DAB review | Within 60 days of receipt of ALJ decision | Not a factor |
| Federal court review | Within 60 days of receipt of DAB decision | At least $1,000 |

*Note.* HO = hearing officer; ALJ = administrative law judge; DAB = departmental appeals board.

viding health care to approximately 34 million elderly beneficiaries and more than 5 million beneficiaries with disabilities. Payment for occupational therapy services under the original Medicare plan varies depending on the type of benefit the beneficiary is accessing when services are provided. Under some Medicare benefits, occupational therapy services are paid for according to a fee schedule and under others, according to a PPS. Documentation and billing requirements differ under each payment system. CMS also contracts with private managed care companies to provide health care options to Medicare beneficiaries under Medicare+Choice plans. Other federal agencies that manage health care plans for large groups are DOD (TRICARE) and the Office of Personnel Management (FEHB).

The CMS also oversees the Medicaid program (Title XIX of the Social Security Act) and SCHIP (Title XXI of the Social Security Act), both of which receive federal funding but are administered by individual states. The Medicaid program provides health care to the poor and the medically indigent, and SCHIP was enacted to expand health care coverage to uninsured, low-income children who do not meet the Medicaid eligibility requirements. Eligibility, coverage, and payment requirements differ from state to state.

Other state-directed sources of health care reimbursement include workers' compensation and grant funding under IDEA, which provides federal grants to states to ensure that eligible children with disabilities receive a "free, appropriate public education" (IDEA Amendments of 1997).

Private health insurance companies provide benefits to employers and other groups as well as to individual subscribers. Each company may offer multiple benefit packages within a fee-for-service plan or one of many managed care plan options. Therefore, occupational therapists must consider the individual's coverage and the third-party payer requirements when developing a treatment plan.

In addition to delivering high-quality therapy services, occupational therapists have a fiscal responsibility toward their clients and employers. This responsibility includes becoming familiar with third-party payer policies and understanding coding and billing requirements. Most public and private payers require the use of CPT codes to describe procedures and ICD-9-CM diagnosis codes to describe patient conditions that require occupational therapy. Today's patient services include providing proper documentation and can require submitting appeals to ensure proper reimbursement for services.

In addition to working one-on-one with people in traditional medical and school-based settings, occupational therapists and occupational therapy assistants should see increased career opportunities in community settings and as consultants in areas such as ergonomics, home modifications, and elder driving training. In the future, some nonmedical areas of occupational therapy practice may come under a third-party payer umbrella, and some services will probably remain largely self-pay. Regardless of payer, occupational therapists always should consider the payment source as part of the whole patient picture.

## References

American Medical Association. (2001). *Physicians' current procedural terminology.* Chicago: Author.

American Occupational Therapy Association. (2001). *AOTA 2000 member compensation survey.* Bethesda, MD: Author.

American Psychiatric Association. (2000). *Diagnostic and statistical manual of mental disorders* (4th ed.). Washington, DC: Author.

Balanced Budget Act of 1997, Pub. L. No. 105-33.

Benefits Improvement and Protection Act of 2000, Pub. L. No. 106-554.

Burton, J. (1996). Workers' compensation, twenty-four-hour coverage, and managed care. *Workers' Compensation Monitor, 9*(1), 11–21.

Burton, J., & Spieler, E. (2001). Workers' compensation and older workers. *Health and Income Security for an Aging Workforce, 3,* 1–8.

Education, 34 C.F.R. § 300.1 (1977), redesignated at 45 Fed. Reg. 77368 (1980).

Education, 34 C.F.R. § 303.1 (1989), as amended at 56 Fed. Reg. 54688 (1991).

Education for All Handicapped Children Act of 1975, Pub. L. No. 94-142, 89 Stat. 773.

Education of the Handicapped Amendments of 1990, Pub. L. No. 101-476, 104 Stat. 1103.

Employee Retirement Income Security Act of 1974, Pub. L. No. 93-406, 88 Stat. 829.

Federal Employee Compensation Act, 5 USC 8101 et seq.

Health Insurance Portability and Accountability Act of 1996, Pub. L. No. 104–191.

Individuals with Disabilities Education Act Amendments of 1997, Pub. L. No. 105-17.

*International classification of diseases, 9th revision, clinical modification.* (2001). Salt Lake City, UT: Med-Index Publications; Bethesda, MD: National Center for Health Statistics (Vols. 1–2); Baltimore: Health Care Financing Administration (Vol. 3).

Levit, K., Smith, C., Cowan, C., Lazenby, H., & Martin, A. (2002, January/February). Inflation spurs health spending in 2000. *Health Affairs.*

Lloyd, L. (2001, November). How to fight payment denials. *OT Practice,* p. 6.

Longshore and Harbor Workers' Compensation Act, 33 USC 901-950.

Medicare, Medicaid, and SCHIP Benefits Improvement and Protection Act of 1999, Pub. L. No. 106-113.

Mont, D., Burton, J., Reno, V., & Thompson, C. (2001). *Workers' compensation: Benefits, coverage, and costs. 1999 new estimates and 1996–1998 revisions.* Washington, DC: National Academy of Social Insurance.

Older Americans Act of 1965, Pub. L. No. 89-73, 79 Stat. 218, as amended.

Omnibus Budget Reconciliation Act of 1981, Pub. L. No. 97-35, 95 Stat. 357.

Public Health, 42 C.F.R. § 417.414 (1985), amended at 58 Fed. Reg. 38062 (1993), 60 Fed. Reg. 45673, 45677 (1995).

Rehabilitation Act of 1973, Section 504, Pub. L. No. 93-112, 87 Stat. 355.

Social Security Amendments of 1965, Title XVIII, Medicare, Pub. L. No. 89-97, 79 Stat. 286, as amended.

Social Security Amendments of 1971, Title XIX, Medicaid, Pub. L. No. 92-223, 85 Stat. 802, as amended.

U.S. Bureau of the Census. (2001a). *Current population reports, 2001.* Washington, DC: U.S. Government Printing Office.

U.S. Bureau of the Census. (2001b). Press release about the March 2001 Current Population Survey. Washington, DC: U.S. Government Printing Office.

U.S. Office of Personnel Management. (2002). *Federal Employees Health Benefits (FEHB) Program.* Retrieved from the World Wide Web: http://www.opm.gov/insure/health/

Veterans' Health Care Eligibility Reform Act (1996), Pub. L. 104-262, 38 USC 1710.

## Additional Resources

American Occupational Therapy Association: http://www.aota.org

Blue Cross Blue Shield Association: http://www.bluecares.com

Centers for Medicare and Medicaid: http://cms.hhs.gov
  Medicaid information: http://www.hcfa.gov/medicaid
  Medicare manuals: http://www.cms.gov/manuals/cmstoc.asp

Federal Employees Health Benefits (FEHB) Program, U.S. Office of Personnel Management http://www.opm.gov/insure/health/

International Association of Industrial Accident Boards and Commissions, 714 Vermont Street, Suite 201, Lawrence, KS 66044; (785) 840-9103; http://www.iaiabc.org

John Burton's Workers' Compensation Resources: http://www.workerscomp-resources.com

National Association of Insurance Commissioners link to insurance commissioners in all states: http://www.naic.org/1regulator/usamap.htm

State Medicaid Offices: http://medicaid.aphsa.org/members.htm

TRICARE: http://www.troa.org/HealthCare/TRICARE.asp

U.S. Department of Labor and *Small Business Handbook:* http://www.dol.gov

U.S. Office of Special Education: http://www.ed.gov/offices/OSERS/Policy/IDEA

U.S. Veterans Administration: http://www.va.gov/elig

## Appendix 17.A    Reimbursement Glossary.

**Act, law, statute**—Interchangeable terms for legislation that is passed by Congress and signed by the president or passed over his veto.

**Actual charge**—The amount a health care provider charges for an item or service.

**Administrative law judge (ALJ)**—A hearings officer who presides over appeal conflicts between Medicare contractors and providers or beneficiaries.

**Advance beneficiary notice**—Under the original Medicare plan, a notice that a physician or other health care provider gives to a beneficiary to sign when the provider believes that Medicare will not pay for the service.

**Assignment**—Under the original Medicare plan, a physician or other private practitioner agrees to accept the Medicare fee as full payment. The beneficiary is still responsible for any coinsurance or deductible.

**Benefits**—The range of services provided by a health care insurance plan.

**Bundled rate**—A payment for a group of related health care services, often over a specific time period (e.g., a rehabilitation hospital stay, 60 days of home health care).

**Carrier**—A private insurance company that contracts with Medicare to pay bills received from physicians, other private practitioners, and suppliers.

**Case management**—A process by which a health care practitioner monitors and directs the utilization of health care services by a single member of a health plan.

**Centers for Medicare and Medicaid (CMS)**—The federal agency that administers the Medicare program and works with states to run Medicaid and the State Children's Health Insurance Programs.

**Coinsurance, copayment**—A fixed dollar amount that an individual pays for each medical service received. Coinsurance pays a percentage of the cost of the service.

**Comprehensive Outpatient Rehabilitation Facility (CORF)**—A facility that provides a variety of outpatient services, including occupational therapy, medical, and social or psychological services.

**Covered charges**—Services or benefits for which the health plan makes either partial or full payment.

**Diagnosis code**—The code or codes that must be included on a bill to describe the health condition for which a person received services. ICD-9-CM is the standard set of codes.

**Employee Retirement Income Security Act (ERISA)**—A federal statute that sets the minimum standards under which employee benefit plans are established and maintained by private sector employers, employee organizations, or jointly by one or more private sector employers and an employee organization.

---

*Note.* These definitions were derived from multiple sources, including the Centers for Medicare and Medicaid (http://cms.hhs.gov) and the U.S. Office of Personnel Management (Federal Employees Health Benefit Web site, http://www.opm.gov).

**Exclusions**—Items or services that a plan does not cover and for which it will not pay.

**Fee schedule**—A list of fees used by health plans to pay providers.

**Fiscal intermediary**—A private insurance company that contracts with Medicare to pay bills submitted by "institutional" providers.

**Fraud and abuse**—*Fraud:* The act of purposely misrepresenting items or services on a bill (e.g., billing for services not provided, billing an inflated amount for an item). *Abuse:* The act of billing for items or services incorrectly but without fraudulent intent.

**Gatekeeper**—In a managed care plan, the gatekeeper is the primary care provider who coordinates an individual's medical care and referrals.

**Health care provider**—This term is often used to designate any health care practitioner (e.g., physician, occupational therapist) or facility or organization that is licensed to provide health care services (e.g., hospital, nursing home).

**Health Insurance Portability and Accountability Act of 1996 (HIPAA)**—Public Law 104-191, which amends the Internal Revenue Service Code of 1986. This law, which affects all health care insurers and providers, includes requirements for (a) standardization of electronic interchange of health, administrative, and financial data; (b) unique health identifiers for all health plans and health care providers; and (c) protection of the confidentiality and integrity of "individually identifiable health information."

**Intermediary**—See *Fiscal intermediary.*

**Network**—A group of health care practitioners, hospitals, pharmacies, and other health care organizations that are under contract to a health plan to provide services to its members.

**Out-of-pocket expenses**—Health care costs that are not covered by a plan and for which an individual is responsible.

**Participating practitioner or supplier**—A provider who agrees to accept assignment on all claims.

**Procedure**—The treatment provided by a health care practitioner, usually coded using CPT-IV.

**Referral**—An order for services that is written by a physician to allow an individual to see a specialist.

**Risk adjustment**—A method used by insurance companies to set rates based on health status.

**Secondary payer**—An insurance policy or plan that pays after an individual's primary insurance.

## Appendix 17.B    Reimbursement Abbreviations and Acronyms.

| | |
|---|---|
| ALJ | administrative law judge |
| AMA | American Medical Association |
| APC | Ambulatory Payment Classification |
| BBA | Balanced Budget Act |
| BBRA | Balanced Budget Refinement Act |
| BCBS | Blue Cross/Blue Shield |
| BIPA | Benefits Improvement and Protection Act |
| CMG | case mix group |
| CMS | Centers for Medicare and Medicaid |
| CORF | comprehensive outpatient rehabilitation facility |
| CPT | *Current Procedural Terminology* |
| DAB | departmental appeals board |
| DME | durable medical equipment |
| DMEPOS | durable medical equipment, prosthetics, orthotics, and supplies |
| DMERC | durable medical equipment regional carrier |
| DOD | U.S. Department of Defense |
| DRG | diagnosis-related group |
| DSM-IV | *Diagnostic and Statistical Manual of Mental Disorders, Fourth Edition* |
| EPSDT | early and periodic screening, diagnosis, and treatment |
| ERISA | Employee Retirement Income Security Act |
| FEHB | Federal Employees Health Benefits |
| FI | fiscal intermediary |
| GEHA | Government Employees Hospital Association |
| HCFA | Health Care Financing Administration |
| HCPAC | Health Care Professionals Advisory Committee |
| HCPCS | Healthcare Common Procedure Coding System |
| HHA | home health agency |
| HIPAA | Health Insurance Portability and Accountability Act |
| HMO | health maintenance organization |
| HO | hearing officer |
| ICD-9-CM | *International Classification of Diseases, Ninth Revision, Clinical Modification* |
| IDEA | Individuals with Disabilities Education Act |
| IEP | individualized education plan |
| IFSP | individualized family service plan |
| IRF | inpatient rehabilitation facility |
| LMRP | local medical review policy |
| MDS | Minimum Data Set |

| | |
|---|---|
| MPFS | Medicare Physician Fee Schedule |
| OASIS | Outcome and Assessment Information Set |
| OPPS | outpatient prospective payment system |
| OT | occupational therapy |
| OTPP | occupational therapist in private practice |
| PACE | Program of All-Inclusive Care for the Elderly |
| PAI | patient assessment instrument |
| PFFS | private fee-for-service |
| PM&R | Physical Medicine and Rehabilitation |
| POS | point of service |
| PPO | preferred provider organization |
| PPS | prospective payment system |
| PT | physical therapy |
| RAI | resident assessment instrument |
| RAP | resident assessment protocols |
| RBRVS | Resource-Based Relative Value Scale |
| RHHI | regional home health intermediaries |
| RUG | resource utilization group |
| RT | rehabilitation therapy |
| RVU | relative value unit |
| SCHIP | State Children's Health Insurance Program |
| SLP | speech-language pathology |
| SNF | skilled nursing facility |
| USTF | Uniformed Services Treatment Facility |
| VA | Veterans Administration |

## Appendix 17.C  Selected Medicare Manuals and Internet Links.

| Publication No. | Title | Internet Link |
|---|---|---|
| Pub 06 | Coverage Issues Manual | http://www.cms.gov/manual/cmstoc.asp |
| Pub 09 | Outpatient Physical Therapy/CORF Manual | http://www.cms.gov/manual/cmstoc.asp |
| Pub 10 | Hospital Manual | http://www.cms.gov/manual/cmstoc.asp |
| Pub 11 | Home Health Agency Manual | http://www.cms.gov/manual/cmstoc.asp |
| Pub 12 | Skilled Nursing Facility Manual | http://www.cms.gov/manual/cmstoc.asp |
| Pub 13 | Intermediary Manual | http://www.cms.gov/manual/cmstoc.asp |
| Pub 14 | Carrier Manual | http://www.cms.gov/manual/cmstoc.asp |
| Pub 83 | Program Integrity Manual | http://www.cms.gov/manual/cmstoc.asp |
| Pub 86 | Medicare Managed Care Manual | http://www.cms.gov/manual/cmstoc.asp |

## Appendix 17.D    Types of Health Insurance Plans and Options.

The following are examples of organizations and plans that provide health care coverage in the United States.

**Fee-for-service (FFS) or traditional plans**—Health coverage in which doctors and other providers receive a fee for each service such as an office visit, test, procedure, or other health care service. Plan members usually pay a yearly deductible and are responsible for a copayment amount for each service up to a yearly maximum.

**Health maintenance organization (HMO)**—A health plan that provides care through contracted or employed physicians, nonphysician practitioners, hospitals, and other providers located in particular geographic or service areas. All care must be coordinated and referred by a primary care physician.

**Multi-employer group health plan**—A group health plan that is sponsored jointly by two or more employers or by employers and employee organizations.

**Point of service (POS)**—A managed care product that is offered by an HMO or FFS plan that has features of traditional plans and HMOs. In an HMO, the POS product lets the member use providers who are not part of the HMO network. However, there is a greater cost associated with choosing these non-network providers. In an FFS plan, the plan's regular benefits include deductibles and coinsurance, which may be waived if the member uses a POS network of providers similar to what one would find in an HMO.

**Preferred provider organization (PPO)**—A managed care plan that contains a provider network. Members may use physicians, nonphysician practitioners, and other providers outside the network, but using in-network providers results in fewer out-of-pocket expenses.

**Provider-sponsored organization (PSO)**—A group of physicians, hospitals, and other health care providers that is administered by the providers, not an insurance company. PSOs generally contract with Medicare and individual employers.

# Public
# Policy

# Federal Legislative Advocacy

Marcia Goodman-Lavey, JD, OTR/L
Sandee Dunbar, DPA, OTR/L

*"It has been fashionable in many places to look down on politics, on those in Government.... But, however we feel about politics, the arena of Government is where the decisions will be made which will affect not only all our destinies but the future of our children born and unborn."*

ROBERT F. KENNEDY

**Marcia Goodman-Lavey, JD, OTR/L,** is an occupational therapist and attorney. She is also an adjunct assistant professor in the Master of Occupational Therapy Program at Samuel Merritt College in Oakland, CA. Her academic work includes teaching students about the role of the occupational therapy practitioner in advocacy and legislative issues. She has worked in medical or legal positions as a manager, consultant, entrepreneur, and employee. She has served as a pro bono legislative bill reviewer and was chair of the Government Affairs Committee for the Occupational Therapy Association of California. She also was a board member for the American Occupational Therapy Political Action Committee.

**Sandee Dunbar, DPA, OTR/L,** is an assistant professor in the occupational therapy program at Nova Southeastern University in Fort Lauderdale, FL. She has primarily worked with children with special needs and their families in early intervention and hospital-based programs. She recently completed a doctorate in public administration and teaches courses related to management and pediatrics in an occupational therapy graduate program.

## Key Terms and Concepts

**Advocacy.** The "pursuit of influencing outcomes—including public policy and resource allocation decisions within political, economic, and social systems and institutions—that directly affect people's lives" (Advocacy Institute, 2001).

**Public policy.** A purposive course of action by key players related to local, state, or federal government.

## Learning Objectives

After completing this chapter, you should be able to do the following:

- Identify the core values of occupational therapy that influence occupational therapy practitioner participation in advocacy.
- Understand the significance of public policy and its impact on direct service to clients and professional issues.
- Describe the federal legislative process.
- Identify how occupational therapy practitioners can influence the legislative and regulatory process.
- Identify and describe the three levels of advocacy involvement.
- Discuss the unique role of the occupational therapy manager in instilling a sense of obligation in staff members to advocate for the profession.

A udrey, a 68-year-old Medicare beneficiary who lives alone, breaks her arm in an automobile accident. She receives outpatient occupational therapy to regain functional ability to cook and care for herself. In doing so, she reaches the $1,500 annual payment limitation for therapy services as imposed by federal law. Unfortunately, the break in Audrey's arm does not heal properly, and she undergoes surgery during the same year. She now must pay out-of-pocket for additional therapy services or be at risk of not receiving appropriate care.

This scenario is an example of how federal legislation can greatly affect the occupational therapy profession and the people we serve. The connection between legislation and the payment allowance for specific occupational therapy services is best demonstrated by current reimbursement issues affecting patients with Medicare Part B coverage. The Balanced Budget Act of 1997 (BBA) imposed a $1,500 payment cap for outpatient therapy services. Under Medicare, a patient seeking occupational therapy in an outpatient setting other than a hospital (e.g., private practice, rehabilitation agency, outpatient clinic, comprehensive outpatient rehabilitation facility, skilled nursing facility) may receive a maximum of $1,500 worth of therapy per year, without regard to whether the patient might need more than $1,500 worth of direct intervention per year. Advocacy efforts by the American Occupational Therapy Association (AOTA) on behalf of consumers and occupational therapy practitioners was instrumental in delaying implementation of the cap. Absent such advocacy efforts and the grassroots support of occupational therapists, the cap would have remained in effect from 1999 to the present. Under such constraints, occupational therapists, in many cases, are no longer the professionals making the determination of amount and type of direct intervention indicated. Thus, consumers may be deprived of the course of treatment deemed most effective by their occupational therapist practitioner, and the profession as a whole suffers because of inadequate reimbursement resulting in decreased job opportunities for practitioners. For example, the Medicare Payment Advisory Commission "determined that one-third of nonhospital rehabilitation patients would have exceeded the cap using the previous years' services as a measure. Other investigators have indicated that the cap could adversely affect up to 12% of Medicare therapy recipients" (AOTA, 2002a).

Active involvement in federal legislative advocacy on many levels promotes the interests of the profession and assures continued quality care and a good quality of life for occupational therapy clients. Occupational therapy managers are in a unique position to inspire and induce other practitioners to become involved in the advocacy process. Influencing public policy is about sustaining and promoting the profession through forging and nurturing relationships and being a trusted information source for policymakers and regulators.

## Core Values and Advocacy

It is feasible to facilitate occupational therapy practitioners' roles beyond the scope of direct service to address client needs and professional issues more globally. As health care providers and agents of change for optimal balance in an individual's life, occupational therapists and occupational therapy assistants must understand the impact of public policy.

Clients need to have equitable access to health care services and enhanced opportunities for independent living, which makes advocacy a critical role for occupational therapy managers and their staff. The care and compassion that have always been an integral part of the core values within occupational therapy provide a foundation for involvement in advocacy on multiple levels. Advocacy in the political realm gives occupational therapists an opportunity to extend the boundaries of client service. There are multiple ways to ensure that the profession's core values are upheld, reinforced, and enhanced through involvement in public policy. Activities related to advocacy will have a long-term positive impact on clients and the profession in general.

## What Is Public Policy?

*Public policy* is a term with various meanings, including significant decision-making, program development, implementation, and program evaluation. In general, policy is a purposive course of action by key players related to local, state, or federal government. Subsequent decision-making related to the actual implementation of a policy is also an important aspect of policymaking (Walt, 1994). Public policy can be categorized by area of intended impact. For instance, health care policies may affect the welfare of pregnant teenagers or recipients of mental health services. Social policies may influence housing or immigration. Educational policies may deal with class size and state testing of academic skills.

Public policy is created through a legislative process with elected officials; it is subsequently implemented through regulations. Government agency regulatory officials issue rules to ensure that policies (e.g., the $1,500 Medicare annual cap on occupational therapy services) are implemented according to the law.

Occupational therapists practice in a variety of settings directly affected by public policy, including acute care and rehabilitation hospitals, skilled nursing facilities, schools, home health, and outpatient clinics. Each practice area is closely intertwined, with government legislation affecting the type and amount of services provided and the payment for those services.

## The Federal Legislative Process

Key players are responsible for influencing and forming decisions related to public policy and include federal, state, and local government leaders; federal and state agencies; and the decision-makers in court cases. In addition to these government entities, special interest groups and the media play a significant role in influencing policy decision-making.

Initially, an interested party on any of these levels begins the legislative process by approaching a congressional representative or senator. A representative or senator also may initiate the process based on his or her own personal and professional interests that affect his or her constituents. The legislator introduces the bill into the U.S. House of Representatives or Senate and may approach a congressional or senatorial counterpart to do the same. After the bill is introduced, it is referred to the relevant committee with the appropriate jurisdiction. The following committees in the House and Senate deal with issues related to occupational therapists' wider domain of concern:

- Health, Education, Labor, and Pensions
- Small Business
- Veterans' Affairs
- Education and the Workforce
- International Relations
- Science
- Ways and Means
- Budget
- Finance.

The congressional committees are responsible for investigating the merits of the proposed bill and determining whether to take action on the proposal. Subcommittees of the larger committee often are formed to continue the process of assessing the worthiness of the legislation. This is done through hearings that provide an opportunity for members of Congress and others to relay information regarding the proposed legislation. The outcome of the hearings may lead to "mark-up" sessions during which subcommittee members consider amendments (or changes) to the bill. The subcommittee then votes on the proposed legislation. If passed, the bill next goes to the full committee for a similar review and vote.

After passing full committee vote, the bill, with or without amendments, is brought to the full House and Senate for consideration. If the bills are identical and both the House and Senate vote favorably, the bill goes to the president to be enacted into law. If the bills are different, the House and Senate appoint a committee to resolve differences. The revised bill is voted on again by the House and Senate and forwarded to the president if passed by both chambers. The president has 10 days to sign or veto the bill. Once the bill is signed, it is enacted into law. A vetoed bill may return to Congress for a chance at overriding the veto.

Although a bill may become a law on a certain date, the actual enforcement may take several months. Most bills will identify a time for enforcement and have language from Congress about enforcement. The regulatory processes then will be initiated by the government agency with lead responsibility for implementation. For example, a Medicare bill will go to the U.S. Department of Health and Human Services, where its Center for Medicare and Medicaid Services will oversee the law's implementation. The steps in the regulatory process may vary because of requirements in the law, the need for legislative review, or even constituent lobbying. However, the steps usually include the formulation of the proposed regulation, publication of the proposal, public comment, a public hearing, comments from other agencies, legislative review, and issuance of the final regulations (AOTA, 2000).

## Occupational Therapy's Influence on the Legislative and Regulatory Process

Occupational therapists and occupational therapy assistants can be influential in both the policy development and implementation phases of the federal legislative and regulatory process. The public hearing and comment stages offer numerous opportunities for occupational therapy practitioners to express their opinions regarding the proposed regulations. This involvement may have a direct impact on the implementation phase of policy. For example, occupational therapy practitioners and AOTA have rallied to protest the Medicare $1,500 cap legislation. They have been meeting with legislators on Capitol Hill and conducting letter-writing campaigns to persuade legislators to oppose the cap. They succeeded in the short term with the Medicare Payment Advisory Commission recommending that Congress enact a moratorium on the cap until at least July 2003. Advocacy efforts continue to support legislation to permanently repeal the $1,500 cap (AOTA, 2002b).

Vigilant and dynamic advocacy on many levels will promote the interests of the profession and of our clients. Without ongoing advocacy, past legislative successes may be lost, and key opportunities for improved professional status may be missed. The omission of occupational therapy as a qualifying home health service in the original Medicare policies is an example of a missed opportunity. The profession continues to aggressively advocate for occupational therapy to be accepted as a qualifying service under the home health benefit. Successful inclusion of occupational therapy in other arenas related to Medicare and Medicaid is due to involvement in political action and monitoring of legislative and regulatory processes.

The reauthorization of the Individuals With Disabilities Education Act in 1997 (IDEA; Public Law 105–17) is a positive example of early and ongoing advocacy. IDEA guarantees that any child with a disability has the right to a free and appropriate public education and the related services necessary to take advantage of that education. Occupational therapy is defined as an IDEA-related service that may be required for students to enhance educationally relevant functioning in the school setting (Case-Smith, Rogers, & Johnson, 2001), for example, helping children with motor skills such as running, catching, writing, or drawing or with living skills such as feeding or dressing. For more than two decades, occupational therapists and occupational therapy assistants have been involved with school-based programs that are driven by this legislation and the original act that preceded it. These laws have enabled thousands of occupational therapy practitioners to have an impact on the lives of many children and to be employed by school districts. This involvement has supported professional core values, such as equality and fair treatment. Occupational therapy has remained an integral part of service delivery to students, primarily because of strong advocacy on local, state, and national levels. With the anticipated reauthorization of IDEA, advocacy efforts have increased again. Without this effort, the profession's position in the school system may be changed. In addition, the quality of care for children with special needs may be affected. Professional awareness and action are required to maintain the successful gains of the past and create new avenues of occupational therapy involvement for the future.

## Advocacy

Every occupational therapist and occupational therapy assistant must act as an advocate to further the goals of the profession. *Advocacy* is the "pursuit of influencing outcomes—including public policy and resource allocation decisions within political, economic, and social systems and institutions—that directly affect people's lives" (Advocacy Institute, 2001). Practitioners may advocate individually, under the auspices of an organization, or within a special interest group. To influence government representatives to enact health care legislation that is consistent with the needs of the occupational therapy profession, we must be effective advocates.

## The Three "Cs"

Successfully influencing others in the legislative process involves what are referred to as the three Cs: communication, collectivity, and collegiality (Vance, 1985/1993). In politics, occupational therapists and occupational therapy assistants must develop potent *communication* skills to persuade others and to build relationships with legislators. They need to know how to present information to government officials in a manner that induces receptivity and understanding of their message. *Collectivity* is "the foundation of networking, coalition-building, and collaboration" (p. 110). In politics, the collective voice from individuals and local, state, and national organizations is powerful. Collective action within a well-organized professional association and through networks with other organizations advancing the desired goals will create strong groups that can facilitate bargaining power and influence. *Collegiality* is an ideal referring to members of a group sharing similar identification of the problems and goals as well as being loyal to those goals and to each other. A collegial group functions more effectively in influencing others.

## Special Interest Groups

It is important to have a mechanism whereby occupational therapists are united and collectively represented. *Special interest groups* are organizations or associations organized around common professional, economic, labor, or ideological issues. They may be highly organized or informal. Special interest groups vary in their purpose; for example, some groups may be geared toward lobbying, whereas others may focus on carrying out research activities (Burns, Peltason, Cronin, & Magleby, 1998).

## Professional Associations

Professional associations are focused on achieving a specific purpose (Maraldo & Kinder, 1985) of limited scope. They are voluntary and nongovernmental. Professional associations—like AOTA—are a vehicle by which individual members gain strength through numbers. Legislators generally are more receptive to a special interest group that represents 40,000 members than an individual advocating for a specific cause. There are usually more resources available in a special interest group per se than to a loose association of a few people. For example, AOTA employs professional lobbyists who are in constant contact with key legislators. AOTA's Political Action Committee (AOTPAC) raises funds used to help elect candidates to public office. AOTA also organizes and encourages letter-writing campaigns and grassroots activities aimed at elected officials to support the unique interests of occupational therapists and occupational therapy assistants. AOTA's activities in advocating for occupational therapists in the political arena accomplish the following goals (Metzler & Willmarth, 2000):

- *Viability of the profession:* Assure that practitioners attain and maintain professional qualifications, that occupational therapy is included in benefit lists, that services are maintained in payment issues, and that adequate payment levels exist.
- *Relevance of the profession:* Promote attention to outcomes in policy, use of occupational therapy in targeted programs, and new opportunities for use of service.
- *Access:* Assure that managed care does not exclude occupational therapists and occupational therapy assistants, that other protections are guaranteed in the health care system, that occupational therapy is included as a service in specific programs, and that occupational therapy is included in Medicare and Medicaid coverage.

## Levels of Advocacy Involvement

Occupational therapy managers should encourage their staff's involvement in advocacy and offer to them particular levels of involvement and examples of activities in which to engage (see Table 18.1).

### Level 1: Awareness

Knowledge can enhance an individual's ability to deal with issues effectively. Staying abreast of current issues will provide opportunities for a manager to alert staff of upcoming changes that could affect the workplace or client care. Reading professional and media accounts of the issues prepares one to approach change in a more informed manner. An example of Level 1 advocacy is reading *OT Practice* updates on IDEA. To ensure continued services of children with special needs requires an understanding of the importance of this law to everyday practice, including an awareness of the financial and institutional resources that enable intervention to continue.

**Table 18.1 Sample Activities in Levels of Advocacy.**

| Level 1: Awareness | Level 2: Active Concern | Level 3: Involvement |
|---|---|---|
| • Read newspaper and Internet articles on related topics<br>• Discuss pertinent issues among staff members<br>• Attend continuing education workshops on topics related to legislation and political action<br>• Invite speakers into facilities to discuss pertinent legislative issues<br>• Discuss issues with clients and inform them of upcoming legislation<br>• Read professional literature that provides brief summaries of legislative activity, such as *OT Practice* | • Write letters to members of Congress<br>• Develop brochures on key issues and disseminate within the facility and/or in the community<br>• Develop a Web site with updated information on key legislative issues<br>• Attend town hall meetings<br>• Provide a system for informing groups of clients regarding important legislation that may affect them<br>• Offer to speak to interest groups regarding implications of proposed legislation<br>• Provide financial support to supportive members of Congress<br>• Provide financial support to AOTPAC | • Become an active participant in AOTPAC<br>• Become an active member in the governmental affairs aspect of local, state, and national occupational therapy organizations<br>• Participate in congressional visits<br>• Present to fellow workers and/or community members on key issues<br>• Host fundraisers<br>• Volunteer for a candidate<br>• Volunteer for an interest group that advocates for occupational therapy–related interests<br>• Participate in monitoring and analyzing strategies for an occupational therapy organization |

*Note.* AOTPAC = American Occupational Therapy Political Action Committee.

## Level 2: Active Concern

This level incorporates simple tasks that influence the thoughts and actions of others. For example, occupational therapy managers in outpatient or skilled nursing facilities know that the BBA, particularly the $1,500 cap, signified many changes in health care (Healthcare Financial Management Association, 2000). These managers may mobilize their staff and become involved in letter-writing campaigns to ensure proper coverage for clients receiving occupational therapy services. Suggested texts for letters to congresspersons are available on the AOTA Web site (http://www.aota.org; see also Appendix 18.A for a sample letter).

## Level 3: Involvement

This level includes a consistent commitment to advocacy by ongoing involvement on a local, state, or national level. An example of this level is regular participation in AOTPAC which, as part of its mission, educates occupational therapists and occupational therapy assistants on how they can affect the political system and remain updated on current issues (Lee, 1998; see also Appendix 18.B for more information on AOTPAC). At this level, there are many ways to get involved.

## Monitoring Legislative Action and the
## Administrative Agencies Responsible for Implementation

Numerous resources can assist the occupational therapy manager in determining where to become involved. Many relevant information resources are available through AOTA and state associations. Special interest groups, such as the Children's Defense Fund, can also offer information to the public on pending legislation that may affect the lives of occupational therapy clients. Other resources include the media, national associations, professional organizations, and personal contacts. Monitoring may be as simple as reading or as involved as volunteering with an association or interest group. One of the primary roles of the AOTA is to monitor legislative and regulatory issues that could potentially affect the occupational therapy profession (see Appendix 18.B). Two key Internet resource on pending legislation are http://www.aota.org and http://www.thomas.loc.gov.

## Analyzing Proposed Legislation

When advocating for or against specific issues, it is important to understand the proposal's intent. Analysis includes research regarding the impact of the proposal on the occupational therapy profession and our clients. It also entails assessing the cost and benefits of its implementation. Of crucial importance is an awareness of the stage of the proposal in the legislative process to most effectively mobilize resources. The following are key questions a manager may consider when analyzing a proposal:

- How would this proposal affect the occupational therapy profession?
- How would this proposal affect clients who receive occupational therapy services?
- What will the proposed legislation mean to the greater community?
- What other interest groups support the proposal and why?
- Where in the legislative process is the proposal, and what are the opportunities for advocacy?
- What government agency would be responsible for implementation once the proposed legislation becomes law?

Finding the answers to these questions will facilitate more effective involvement in advocacy for fair, equal, and prudent service delivery. It also will enable occupational therapists and occupational therapy assistants the opportunity to network and build relationships with key decision-makers and interested parties who may, in turn, support professional interests.

## Lobbying

Lobbying is a specific type of advocacy used to persuade the government's representatives to act or abstain from taking a particular action. Lobbyists, whether professional or simply volunteer members of a professional association or special interest group, influence policy decisions and positions in the government. Lobbyists may provide legislators with political and substantive information about a particular subject, assist in drafting pieces of legislation and amendments, testify at legislative hearings, and even make recommendations to organizations regarding monetary donations for legislators and campaigns.

Lobbying can influence legislation through either indirect or direct methods of contact. An indirect method of contact would be a letter-writing campaign to members of Congress about a particular issue. A more direct approach is meeting in person with a representative or senator.

### Meeting With Legislators

One of the best ways to have an impact on the legislative issues facing occupational therapy is to meet personally with members of Congress or their staff. Members of Congress are very willing to receive information from constituents that will assist them in making the best decisions. The *Resource Manual on Influencing Public Policy* (AOTA, 2000) has recommended an organized format for congressional visits. The occupational therapy manager can share the following suggestions with staff members interested in participating in a congressional visit:

- Rehearse what you will say, and write notes with specific points to cover during the meeting. Contact the state association and AOTA, as these organizations may have important and useful information that you should be aware of.
- Be on time and willing to wait.
- Begin the meeting with a brief introduction of yourself, including your place of work, position held, and whether you are a constituent. Explain occupational therapy (see Appendix 18.C), and personalize the explanation to yourself and your clientele.
- Discuss the issues clearly and concisely by stating the issue (designate the exact title, number, status of the bill or law), the occupational therapy perspective (support, oppose), and reason for stance.
- Discuss the specific ways the piece of legislation, or lack thereof, affects the occupational therapy client. Include information, if available, from outcome studies; statistics; personal or patient experiences; and views that reflect and represent the occupational therapy profession, not personal opinion.
- Identify the connection to the constituents by giving examples of personal interest related to the occupational therapist's area of expertise.
- Keep in mind that time for the visit is limited, so be sure to allow time for questions.
- Ask for the member of Congress about his or her position as well as for an explanation of that position. Politely refute a differing view if one is presented, but do not argue or condemn the member for his or her point of view. If appropriate, ask for a commitment on a particular issue.
- Thank the member of Congress for his or her time and interest.
- Leave behind informational brochures, handouts with additional details, and your notes of talking points.

## Unique Role of the Occupational Therapy Manager

The occupational therapy manager is instrumental in instilling the professional obligation of advocating for the profession. The manager should become aware of political issues related to the profession and assist staff members in doing the same. The following are suggestions for how the manager can help staff members to become advocates:

- Reserve time at each staff meeting to review pertinent legislation and related developments. Such information can be found on the AOTA Web site (http://www. aota.org) in the Members area under the Federal Affairs, Licensure, and Reimbursement sections and through the Web sites or newsletters of various state occupational therapy organizations.
- Request, provide the opportunity for, and teach practitioners to write letters to legislators on professional issues. The AOTA Web site's Legislative Action Center is a useful resource to assist in this effort.
- Educate staff members on ways to have an impact on the political process.
- Invite legislators and their staff to visit your workplace, see occupational therapy in action, and discuss important issues affecting the profession.
- Attend dinners and fundraising events for political candidates.
- Assist candidates in their campaigns.
- Visit legislators at their local offices.

The voices of occupational therapy therapists and occupational therapy assistants must be heard for the profession to move forward, and legislative and political advocacy must be an integral part of the practitioner's life. Education about the public policy arena is no longer optional; it is imperative for survival. Sending a letter, donating money to AOTPAC or a state association's PAC fund, or attending a fundraiser for a candidate are now a routine part of the occupational therapy practitioner's professional life. Further, the occupational therapy culture now supports advocacy activity. When occupational therapists and occupational therapy assistants move forward in advocacy, not only do they find many benefits on a personal level, but also the profession is enhanced and the needs of clients receiving occupational therapy services are served.

## References

Advocacy Institute. (2001). *What is advocacy?* Retrieved January 6, 2003, from http://www.advocacy.org/definition.htm

American Occupational Therapy Association, American Occupational Therapy Political Action Committee. (2000). *Resource manual on influencing public policy*. Bethesda, MD: Author.

American Occupational Therapy Association. (2002a). *AOTA supports proposed repeal of the Outpatient Rehabilitation Cap; Bipartisan bill would assure Medicare beneficiaries access to critical services* [Press release]. Retrieved from http://www.aota.org/nonmembers/area6/links/link13.asp

American Occupational Therapy Association, Federal Affairs. (2002b). $1,500 caps on Medicare outpatient rehabilitation services. *AOTAction Alert* [Online]. Bethesda, MD: Author. Retrieved September 2002 from http://www.aota.org/members/area1/links/link25.asp?PLACE+/members/area1/links/LINK25.asp [must be an AOTA member to access link]

Balanced Budget Act. (1997). Pub. L. 105–33, 111 Stat. 251.

Burns, J. M., Peltason, J. W., Cronin, T. E., & Magleby, D. B. (1998). *Government by the people, national version* (17th ed.). Englewood Cliffs, NJ: Prentice-Hall.

Case-Smith, J., Rogers, J., & Johnson, J. H. (2001). School-based occupational therapy. In J. Case-Smith (Ed.), *Occupational therapy for children* (4th ed., pp. 758–759). St. Louis, MO: Mosby.

Healthcare Financial Management Association. (2000). Clinton signs bill providing BBA relief. *Healthcare Financial Management, 54*(1), 9–10.

Lee, S. S. (1998). The American Occupational Therapy Political Action Committee: Twenty years of influencing public policy. *American Journal of Occupational Therapy, 53*, 1085–1086.

Maraldo, P., & Kinder, J. (1985). Politics and the professional organization. In D. J. Mason & S. W. Talbott (Eds.), *Political action handbook for nurses: Changing the workplace, government, organizations, and community* (pp. 60–61). Philadelphia: Saunders.

Metzler, C., & Willmarth, C. (2000, April). *Public policy 101.* Course presented at the Annual Conference of the American Occupational Therapy Association, Seattle, WA.

Reauthorization of the Individuals With Disabilities Education Act. (1997). Pub. L. 105–17, 20 U.S.C. § 1400 *et seq.*

Vance, C. N. (1993). Political influence: Building effective interpersonal skills. In D. J. Mason, S. W. Talbott, & J. K. Leavitt (Eds.), *Policy and politics for nurses: Action and change in the workplace, government, organizations, and community* (2nd ed., pp. 105–117). Philadelphia: Saunders. (Original work published 1985)

Walt, G. (1994). *Health policy: An introduction to process and power.* Johannesburg, South Africa: Witwatersrand University Press.

## Appendix 18.A    Sample Letter to Members of Congress.

Repeal of $1,500 Caps on Medicare Part B Outpatient Rehabilitation

(Insert Date)

The Honorable Bob Graham and The Honorable Bill Nelson
United States Senate
Washington, DC 20510

Dear Senators Graham and Nelson:

I am writing to you about my grave concern regarding a provision in the Balanced Budget Act of 1997 (BBA) that remains a problem. *(Personalize here, i.e., "I am a constituent and an occupational therapy student or occupational therapist working with Medicare Part B patients.")*

I urge you to cosponsor S. 1394, The Medicare Access to Rehabilitation Services Act of 2001, introduced by Sen. John Ensign (R-NE) on September 4, 2001.

The BBA placed a cap of $1,500 annually on the amount of outpatient occupational therapy services an individual can receive under Medicare Part B. The Balanced Budget Refinement Act (BBRA) and Benefits Improvement and Protection Act (BIPA) placed a moratorium on the cap until 2003. But the cap was and is bad policy.

As an *(occupational therapy practitioner or occupational therapy student)*, I know how important completing an adequate course of treatment is for full recovery and prevention of further costly treatment. For instance, an average stroke patient requires a substantial amount of therapy to regain function or learn to live safely with limitations. If inadequate amounts of therapy are provided the patient may be subject to falls, need more substantial home care, or develop other injuries or conditions. All of this will cost more money.

In addition, this provision puts the government squarely between the patient and his or her medical caregiver. Such interference in medical decision-making is exactly the wrong direction for the Medicare program.

Moratoriums on the cap are not enough. I urge you to work to permanently repeal the cap and put in place a system that allows patients access to the full Medicare occupational therapy benefit from providers of their choosing. Policy must move to a more efficient, patient-centered manner of controlling usage of therapy services.

Sincerely,
*(Include your name and address so that they can easily identify you as a constituent. Members of Congress usually do not reply to nonconstituents. This holds true for faxes and e-mail messages and telephone messages to Congress as well.)*

# Appendix 18.B   AOTA/AOTPAC Fact Sheet.

### What Is a PAC?

A political action committee (PAC) is the legally sanctioned vehicle through which organizations, such as the American Occupational Therapy Association, Inc. (AOTA), can engage in otherwise prohibited political action and work to influence the outcome of federal elections.

The Federal Election Commission (FEC) Act of 1971 recognized that corporations and professional and trade associations have a vital and legitimate interest in the operation of government. A PAC is the only legal and ethical way a profession can unite behind the candidates of its choice.

### What Is AOTPAC?

The American Occupational Therapy Political Action Committee (AOTPAC) is a voluntary, nonprofit, unincorporated committee of members of AOTA. AOTPAC was authorized by the Representative Assembly in 1976 and has been operational since the spring of 1978. The purpose of AOTPAC is to further the legislative aims of the Association by influencing or attempting to influence the selection, nomination, election, or appointment of any individual to any federal public office, and of any occupational therapist, registered, certified occupational therapy assistant, or occupational therapy student member of AOTA seeking election to public office at any level. The committee is not affiliated with any political party.

### Why Does AOTA Need a PAC?

AOTA standing alone cannot contribute even a token amount to a candidate. Through a PAC, AOTA can solicit and direct the flow of contributions from its members and provide important assistance to individual candidates for election to federal office.

Decisions of Congress can and do have a direct, long-range effect on the occupational therapy profession. When individuals with mutual interests unite and support candidates who share those interests, steps toward favorable action can be encouraged. The candidates who support the profession need our professional support.

Since its establishment, AOTPAC has made political contributions to candidates for election to both the U.S. House of Representatives and the U.S. Senate in almost every state. This political involvement has enabled the Association to broaden its contacts in the legislative and executive branches. Through AOTPAC, occupational therapy practitioners have a collective voice that will be heard in the debates over the ever-expanding number of health care issues that come before the Congress.

### Who Controls AOTPAC's Money?

Decisions regarding which candidates will receive AOTPAC support are made by a five-member Board of Directors. The Board members are appointed for a 3-year term by the Executive Board of AOTA, and each one represents a specific region of the United States.

By law AOTA is allowed to fund AOTPAC's operating expenses. Through a budgeted allowance, the Association assumes the expenses of office space, supplies, postage, printing, publications, and fundraising. Existing national office staff and office space are used to support AOTPAC activities. The money that the Association provides for expenses is known as "soft" dollars. This money will be made available by the Association as long as the profession is committed to the concept of political action, but it cannot be used to support candidates.

All funds which are raised by AOTPAC are used to their fullest potential as campaign contributions. This money, "hard" dollars, must be placed in a separate segregated fund and is provided by individual contributions.

### Is AOTPAC Ethical?

Yes. A campaign contribution through AOTPAC is not a means of buying votes. It is a "no strings attached" way of ensuring that responsible and dedicated legislators who understand and support the occupational therapy profession remain in or are elected to office.

To ensure the money is well protected and properly spent, many detailed reports are required by the FEC and from both AOTPAC and the candidates it supports. Both must account for the sources of their funds and the purposes for which these funds are spent.

Many professions, including physicians, dentists, nurses, medical laboratory technologists, optometrists, and physical therapists have made the concept of a PAC part of their government affairs efforts, all working within the system to their better advantage.

### What Criteria Determine Which Candidates Are Supported?

Among the factors relied upon by the AOTPAC Board on reaching decisions regarding which candidates will receive AOTPAC support are the recommendations of Association members and officers, the leadership of state associations, and the advice of the Government Relations Department (GRD) staff. GRD staff analyze and interpret congressional voting records and pinpoint who's who in the area of health legislation and who supports the profession of occupational therapy.

Among the criteria used to determine which candidates to support, the AOTPAC Board of Directors considers the following factors:

- Is the candidate sympathetic to the goals of the occupational therapy profession? Has the candidate supported specific proposals or policies advanced by the profession?

- If an incumbent, does the candidate hold a key position of responsibility (i.e., chair or member of important committee or subcommittee; member of majority or minority leadership)?
- If a challenger, will the candidate pursue assignment to a key committee or subcommittee or be likely to be in a position to assist the profession?

AOTPAC makes financial contributions to candidates for Federal office regardless of party affiliation.

### What Is AOTPAC's Record?
In the 1996 federal elections, contributions were used to support 175 candidates across the country. The success rate was 90%, with 158 of the 175 candidates supported being elected or reelected to office.

### How Does AOTPAC Raise Money?
The majority of money raised by AOTPAC is through direct AOTA member contributions. On the application for AOTA membership a space is provided to include a contribution to the PAC. Telemarketing efforts and mail solicitations are conducted at least once per year. Commemorative coffee mugs are distributed at the AOTA Annual Conference in exchange for a PAC contribution. The AOTPAC also provides an evening of entertainment at the conference, the AOTPAC Night.

By becoming politically aware and involved, occupational therapy practitioners can ensure at least some measure of input into the decisions that affect their professional lives so directly. Because of member participation, AOTPAC continues to make a difference, but it can only be as successful as we choose to make it. Remember, the candidates who support our profession need our professional support.

## Additional Resources
GRD of AOTA
AOTPAC video presentation available from GRD

## Related Links
Federal Affairs
Reimbursement and Regulatory Policy
State Policy
Press Center
Write to Congress

Want more information?
E-mail the Federal Affairs Department at FAD@aota.org.

---

## Appendix 18.C   Occupational Therapy: A Vital Link to Productive Living.

*What Is Occupational Therapy?*

*Occupational therapy* is a health profession providing services to people whose lives have been disrupted by physical injury or illness, developmental problems, the aging process, or social and psychological difficulties. The goal of occupational therapy is to assist each individual in achieving an independent, productive, and satisfying life.

*Facts Your Legislator Might Want to Know*

There are numerous facts that your legislator will be eager to learn that you can provide fairly easily. The following list is not all-inclusive, but it does offer a good starting point:

- What is an occupational therapist, occupational therapy assistant? (You might want to use the definition from the *Occupational Therapy Practice Framework: Domain and Process,* p. 610.[a])
- What is the educational background of an occupational therapist or occupational therapy assistant?
- Who are your clients?
- Where do you work?
- How do you relate to other health care providers (i.e., physical therapists, speech therapists, physicians)?
- Are occupational therapy services covered by insurance, workers' compensation, Medicaid, or Medicare?
- How many occupational therapists and occupational therapy assistants are there in United States, your state, and the legislator's district?
- How much do occupational therapists and occupational therapy assistants earn (i.e., salary, per diem, per hour)?
- How are occupational therapists and occupational therapy assistants regulated in your state?
- What is your state organization? Number of members? Legislative concerns, needs, and programs?

---

*Note.* Adapted and reprinted with permission from the Occupational Therapy Association of California.

[a] American Occupational Therapy Association. (2002). Domain. In *Occupational therapy practice framework: Domain and process* (p. 610). Bethesda, MD: Author.

# CHAPTER 19

# State Regulation of Occupational Therapists and Occupational Therapy Assistants

Karen C. Smith, OT, and Charles Willmarth

*"Occupational therapists are the only people who can and should define our practice, education, ethics, values, and research. We owe this much to society and the people we serve."*

ELIZABETH YERXA

**Karen C. Smith, OT,** is a regulatory associate in the AOTA State Affairs Group, where she monitors state regulations that affect occupational therapy and acts as a liaison to state regulatory boards.

**Charles Willmarth** is manager of AOTA's State Affairs Group and is responsible for monitoring and analyzing public policy in the states and providing consultation and assistance to state occupational therapy associations on legislative and regulatory isssues.

# Key Terms and Concepts

**Certification.** The process by which an agency grants a person permission to use a certain title if that person has attained entry-level competence; may also be nongovernmental.

**Certification by NBCOT.** Recognition by the National Board for Certification in Occupational Therapy, Inc. (NBCOT), that an occupational therapist or occupational therapy assistant has met certain professional requirements and is authorized to use NBCOT's registered certification marks Occupational Therapist Registered (OTR®) or Certified Occupational Therapy Assistant (COTA®).

**Credentialing.** The process of assessing and validating the qualifications of a practitioner according to a predetermined set of standards such as current license, education, training, experience, competence, and professional judgment (O'Leary, 1994, pp. 169–170).

**Legislation.** The making of laws, specifically, the exercise of the power and function of making rules that have the force of authority by virtue of their promulgation by an official organ of the state (*Merriam-Webster's Dictionary of Law*, 1996).

**Licensure.** "The process by which an agency of government grants permission to an individual to engage in a given occupation upon finding that the applicant has attained the minimal degree of competence required to ensure that the public health, safety, and welfare will be reasonably well protected" (U.S. Department of Health, Education, and Welfare, 1977, p. 17).

**Registration.** A formal process by which qualified individuals are listed on an official roster or registry maintained by a government or nongovernmental agency, enabling these people to use a particular title and attesting to employing agencies and individuals that minimum qualifications have been met and maintained (O'Leary, 1994, p. 681).

**Regulation.** 1. The act of regulating or state of being regulated. 2. A rule or order issued by a government agency and often having the force of law. An agency is often delegated the power to issue regulations by the legislation that created it. Regulations must be made in accordance with prescribed procedures such as those set out in the federal or a state administrative procedure (*Merriam-Webster's Dictionary of Law*, 1996).

**Statute.** A law enacted by the legislative branch of a government (*Merriam-Webster's Dictionary of Law*, 1996).

**Sunrise law.** A law requiring that a profession meet certain criteria before licensing is initiated (Young, 1987).

**Sunset law.** A law requiring termination of the enabling legislation by a specific date unless the legislature renews it (Young, 1987).

**Title control ( "trademark act" ).** The process by which an agency grants a person permission to use a certain title if that person has attained entry-level competence.

# Learning Objectives

After completing this chapter, you should be able to do the following:

- Explain the importance of state regulation for occupational therapists and occupational therapy assistants.
- Describe the differences among the various forms of regulation.
- Distinguish between the legal requirements of state law regulating occupational therapy and the requirements of private credentialing organizations such as NBCOT.
- Identify components of an occupational therapy practice act.
- Describe roles and responsibilities of occupational therapy regulatory bodies.

Occupational therapy is regulated in all 50 American states, the District of Columbia, Puerto Rico, and Guam. Different states have various types of regulation that range from licensure, the strongest form of regulation, to title control or trademark act, the weakest form of regulation. The major purpose of regulation is to protect consumers in a state or jurisdiction from unqualified or unscrupulous practitioners.

State laws and regulations significantly affect the practice of occupational therapy. Laws or statutes are enacted by legislators, who are elected public officials. Regulations specifically describe how the intent of the laws will be carried out. These regulations are developed by regulators, who are appointed public officials of various departments in state government. Both kinds of officials make decisions that directly and indirectly affect occupational therapy managers and practitioners. These decisions may include the setting of certain standards, coverage and reimbursement for occupational therapy services, funding for higher education, and the awarding of research grants.

In the United States, the earliest evidence of state regulation of professions was the Virginia Medical Practice Act of 1639 (American Occupational Therapy Association [AOTA], 1996). State licensure activity did not begin in earnest, however, until the late 1800s. "By 1900 most states had licensed attorneys, dentists, pharmacists, physicians, and teachers. Between 1900 and 1960, most states also granted licensure to 20 additional groups, including accountants, nurses, real estate brokers, barbers, chiropractors, and funeral directors" (Shimberg & Roederer, 1994, pp. 1–2).

## Types of Regulation

Although licensure is by far the predominant form of regulation for occupational therapists and occupational therapy assistants, a few states use less-stringent forms of regulation such as certification, registration, and title control. As of 2002 (AOTA, State Affairs Group, 2002a, 2002b), 46 states, the District of Columbia, Guam, and Puerto Rico license occupational therapists; 1 state (Indiana) has certification laws governing occupational therapists; 2 states (Hawaii and Michigan) have registration laws; and 1 state (Colorado) has a trademark law. The form of regulation for occupational therapy assistants is often but not always the same as it is for occupational therapists in a given jurisdiction. The District of Columbia, Guam, Puerto Rico, and 43 states license occupational therapy assistants; 3 states (California, Indiana, and Vermont) have certification laws; and 1 state (Michigan) has a registration law. Virginia, Hawaii, and Colorado do not regulate occupational therapy assistants.

Each form of regulation is authorized by state law, and each is meant to protect the public from harm. Table 19.1 presents these forms in decreasing order of restrictiveness, summarizing their major features and differentiating them according to (a) the level of protection that they afford the public, (b) requirements for practice, and (c) state oversight agency.

**Table 19.1  Major Types of State Regulation of Occupational Therapy Practitioners.**

| Type of Regulation | Description | Requirements for Practice | Oversight Agency |
|---|---|---|---|
| Licensure | Provides highest level of public protection by prohibiting unlicensed persons from practicing occupational therapy or referring to themselves as occupational therapists or occupational therapy assistants. Licensure laws reserve a certain scope of practice for those who are issued a license. | Mandates entry-level competence | Government agency usually delegates authority to occupational therapy board or advisory board, consisting of occupational therapy practitioners, other health professionals, and consumers. |
| Certification[a] (certification as granted by an occupational therapy regulatory board or advisory board–council, to be distinguished from nongovernmental certification such as NBCOT certification) | Protects the public by prohibiting noncertified persons from referring to themselves as occupational therapists or occupational therapy assistants. Unlike licensure, under certain circumstances, individuals who do not have this certification can practice if they do not refer to their services as occupational therapy. Certification laws may provide for definition of occupational therapy. | Mandates entry-level competence | Government agency maintains registry of individuals who successfully complete eligibility requirements. An advisory board may be appointed to advise agency on issues related to occupational therapy. |
| Registration[a] | Protects the public by prohibiting nonregistered persons from referring to themselves as occupational therapists or occupational therapy assistants. Unlike licensure, these individuals can, however, under certain circumstances, practice if they do not refer to their services as occupational therapy. Registration laws may provide for definition of occupational therapy. | Competence standards may be required by the government agency maintaining the register | Government agency maintains registry of individuals who successfully complete eligibility requirements. An advisory board may be appointed to advise agency on issues related to occupational therapy. |
| Title control (sometimes called "trademark act") | Provides the least amount of protection to consumers. Protects the titles of occupational therapist or occupational therapy assistant but not specific occupational therapy interventions and techniques. | Mandates entry-level competence | Government agency maintains registry of individuals who successfully complete eligibility requirements. |

*Note.* NCBOT = National Board for Certification in Occupational Therapy.

[a]The terms *certification* and *registration* are often used interchangeably. Individual states may vary in the types of provisions and protections they include in registration or certification laws.

From "Types of State Regulation for Occupational Therapy Practitioners" [Fact sheet], by American Occupational Therapy Association, State Affairs Group, 2002, April. Copyright 2002 by AOTA, State Affairs Group. Adapted with permission of the author.

*Licensure*, the strongest form of state regulation, is "the process by which an agency of government grants permission to an individual to engage in a given occupation upon finding that the applicant has attained the minimal degree of competence required to ensure that the public health, safety, and welfare will be reasonably well protected" (U.S. Department of Health, Education, and Welfare, 1977, p. 17). A key feature of a *licensure law* is that it legally defines a scope of practice. A licensure law is therefore often referred to as a *practice act*, although certification laws also use that term.

*Certification* and *registration* are less stringent forms of state regulation than licensure and may be defined differently by individual state regulatory boards or councils. Certification in the context of state regulation is not the same as certification granted by the National Board for Certification in Occupational Therapy (NBCOT). Please refer to the section "Nongovernmental Certification" in this chapter. In general, certification and registration protect the public by requiring individuals who use the titles *occupational therapist* or *occupational therapy assistant* to meet specific eligibility requirements, similar to licensure. However, under some circumstances, unlike licensure, individuals who are not certified or registered are allowed to use occupational therapy techniques if they do not refer to their services as occupational therapy. Certification and registration may provide a definition of occupational therapy. However, these forms of regulation do not establish a scope of practice. For example, Indiana, which has certification, has a definition of occupational therapy, although somewhat limited, and does not have language that restricts others from performing some of those services.

*Title control* or *trademark law* provides the least amount of protection to consumers. As the name implies, this form of regulation protects the titles used (occupational therapist or occupational therapy assistant) but not specific occupational therapy interventions and techniques. States with title control or trademark law do not designate scope of practice. Therefore, others without qualifications to practice occupational therapy can claim that they can provide those services. Colorado, the only state with trademark law, does not have a definition of occupational therapy but does prohibit deceptive trade practices in using "occupational therapist" or similar titles without meeting specific education and training criteria.

Generally—unlike certification, registration, and trademark laws—a licensure law defines a lawful scope of practice for occupational therapists and for occupational therapy assistants under the supervision of occupational therapists. Defining a scope of practice legally articulates the domain of occupational therapy practice and provides guidance to facilities, providers, consumers, and major public and private health and education facilities about the appropriate use of occupational therapy services and practitioners. Defining the appropriate scope of occupational therapy practice can further ensure important patient protections, particularly in the investigation and resolution of consumer complaints involving fraudulent or negligent delivery of occupational therapy services. A clearly articulated scope of practice also protects occupational therapy from another profession that may challenge the qualifications of practitioners to provide certain services or that may encroach on occupational therapy's scope of practice through unqualified expansion of its practice.

## Regulatory or Advisory Boards for Regulated Jurisdictions

In the health care professions, the agency of government granting the permission under the various types of regulation is typically the state department of health. Under a licensure system, that department usually delegates its authority to administer regulations to a board that consists of members of the profession (who are regulated); consumers or public members; and in some cases, representatives of related professions. Regulatory boards operate on a continuum from full autonomy to a strictly advisory role to no board at all but only a centralized agency responsible for administration (Shimberg & Roederer, 1994). Most boards have the authority to establish the procedures for licensure, investigate violations of the practice act, and promulgate rules to regulate the profession.

In some states, appointed practitioners serve as part of an occupational therapy advisory council. Councils perform many of the same tasks as an occupational therapy board but are less autonomous and serve to advise the administration's staff on the regulation of occupational therapists and occupational therapy assistants. Some states combine occupational therapy boards or advisory councils with other professions such as physical therapy or athletic training. A handful of states have no occupational therapy board or advisory council and rely on administrative officials to promulgate and enforce regulations for the profession. Several states have placed regulation of occupational therapists and occupational therapy assistants under the state's medical board. In these states, a group made up of occupational therapists and, in some cases, occupational therapy assistants advises the medical board on occupational therapy regulatory issues, but this group has far less power and autonomy than a board (AOTA, 2001, p. 3).

No matter what type of regulatory structure is in place in the state, occupational therapy managers, practitioners, entrepreneurs, and consultants as well as state occupational therapy association leaders need to monitor the activities of the occupational therapy board, medical board, or administrative officials who are responsible for regulating occupational therapy and to maintain an ongoing dialogue on professional issues. Occupational therapy regulatory boards may discuss the need to amend state occupational therapy practice acts or regulations to keep them up-to-date with current practice. This updating process may entail making additions or revisions to scope of practice, continuing competence, supervision, or references to certification bodies or education program accreditation institutions.

Occupational therapists and occupational therapy assistants can give input into these processes in a variety of ways. State occupational therapy associations or individuals can propose changes in the practice act or statutes through legislative amendments. They can also attend hearings and comment on amendments to regulations that are proposed by the state regulatory board or advisory council and work with them to initiate needed changes (AOTA, 2001, p. 3).

State associations should be on the mailing list of the occupational therapy board or the advisory council to receive meeting announcements and minutes, and one or more representatives of the associations should regularly attend public occupational therapy board or council meetings. The positive relationships that state associations can develop with board or council members will enhance the work of both entities and help to ensure competent practice by occupational therapists and occupational therapy assistants. In states where practitioners are regulated by a state agency or a medical board, occupational therapists and especially occupational therapy managers should follow medical board activities and meetings as well as regulations proposed by the agency with jurisdiction over health professions. State legislatures are generally the most active from January through May. Activity levels of boards and agencies do not follow this trend; they make important policy decisions year round (AOTA, 2001, p. 3).

## Components of an Occupational Therapy Practice Act

*Practice acts* refer to laws passed by state legislators that establish regulation for health care professions. The purpose of regulating occupational therapy practice is to safeguard the public health, safety, and welfare; to protect the public from incompetent, unethical, or unauthorized persons; to assure a high level of professional conduct on the part of occupational therapists and occupational therapy assistants; and to assure the availability of high-quality occupational therapy services to people in need of those services (AOTA, 2000a). The practice act provides consumers and others with important information about minimum qualifications for practitioners, protects the titles of practitioners, and defines an appropriate scope of practice. Most practice acts or licensure laws have similar components, including requirements for licensure, renewal, supervision, and referral as well as a defined scope of practice, code of ethics, and disciplinary provisions.

### Scope of Practice

Most states include a definition of occupational therapy or occupational therapy practice in their practice acts. Defining a scope of practice legally articulates the domain of occupational therapy practice and provides guidance to facilities, providers, consumers, and major public and private health and education facilities on the appropriate use of occupational therapy services and practitioners. Most practice acts have specific language that prohibits the unauthorized practice of occupational therapy by individuals who are not qualified occupational therapists or occupational therapy assistants and that allows for prosecution of those individuals.

The scope of practice of a profession should be directly related to the standards for education, training, and clinical application within that profession. Some elements of the scopes of practice for different professions may appropriately overlap, but a practice act should also delineate unique aspects of that scope. For example, even though both the occupational therapy and physical therapy practice acts in a given state may authorize the use of physical agent modalities, the occupational therapy practice act might use the wording "application of physical agent modalities as an adjunct to or in preparation for engagement in occupations" to distinguish the unique focus of occupational therapy on occupation, not on the modality.

Exhibit 19.1 presents AOTA's model practice act definition of occupational therapy. States often adopt this model language related to scope of practice because it reflects the current appropriate scope of practice as articulated by the standard-setting body of the profession. All managers, private practice owners, and practitioners need to be aware of their state's or their jurisdiction's scope of practice and need to ensure

### Exhibit 19.1  Definition of Occupational Therapy Practice for State Regulation.

(A) The "Practice of Occupational Therapy" means the therapeutic use of purposeful and meaningful occupations (goal-directed activities) to evaluate and treat individuals who have a disease or disorder, impairment, activity limitation, or participation restriction which interferes with their ability to function independently in daily life roles, and to promote health and wellness. Occupational therapy intervention may include:
  (1) remediation or restoration of performance abilities that are limited due to impairment in biological, physiological, psychological or neurological processes.
  (2) adaptation of task, process or the environment, or the teaching of compensatory techniques, in order to enhance performance.
  (3) disability prevention methods and techniques which facilitate the development or safe application of performance skills.
  (4) health promotion strategies and practices which enhance performance abilities.

(B) "Occupational therapy services" include, but are not limited to:
  (1) evaluating, developing, improving, sustaining or restoring skills in activities of daily living (ADLs), work or productive activities, including instrumental activities of daily living (IADLs), and play and leisure activities.
  (2) evaluating, developing, remediating, or restoring sensorimotor, cognitive, or psychosocial components of performance.
  (3) designing, fabricating, applying, or training in the use of assistive technology or orthotic devices, and training in the use of prosthetic devices.
  (4) adaptation of environments and processes, including the application of ergonomic principles, to enhance performance and safety in daily life roles.
  (5) application of physical agent modalities as an adjunct to or in preparation for engagement in occupations.
  (6) evaluating and providing intervention in collaboration with the client, family, caregiver, or others.
  (7) educating the client, family, caregiver, or others in carrying out appropriate nonskilled interventions.
  (8) consulting with groups, programs, organizations, or communities to provide population-based services.

that practitioners under their supervision are not performing services that are outside their legal scope of practice.

## Requirements for Licensure or Other Forms of Regulation

Requirements for licensure or other forms of regulation generally include demonstration by the applicant that he or she has successfully completed the academic and fieldwork requirements of an educational program for occupational therapists or occupational therapy assistants that is accredited by AOTA's Accreditation Council for Occupational Therapy Education (ACOTE) and has passed an examination approved by the occupational therapy board (typically, the NBCOT entry-level certification examination). States may have additional requirements for internationally trained therapists to ensure that their education and training is equivalent to the standards in the United States and that their English proficiency is adequate. States may have less complicated requirements for licensure by endorsement for practitioners who are currently licensed or regulated in another state or jurisdiction.

## Licensure Renewal Requirements

States also require renewal of licensure, certification, or registration at specific intervals. For most states, this renewal is required every 1 or 2 years. In New York, the renewal period is 3 years. Increasingly, states are requiring not only a fee and completion of the renewal application but also completion of a specific amount of continuing competence activities.

An important role of state regulatory boards is to protect the public from incompetent practitioners. State regulators are mandating continuing competence requirements in an attempt to ensure that practitioners who are licensed or regulated in their state maintain competence. Some regulatory boards limit acceptable continuing competence activities to those activities directly related to clinical practice. Others recognize the importance of an individual maintaining competence in the varied roles and responsibilities related to occupational therapy throughout his or her career and the important ways that these roles directly and indirectly affect competent practice.

As of April 2002, 36 of the 53 jurisdictions regulating occupational therapy had continuing competence or continuing education requirements (AOTA, State Affairs Group, 2002c). Forces both internal and external to the profession are encouraging states to adopt continuing competence requirements, and the expectation is that the number of states with these requirements will continue to grow. Accrediting organizations such as the Commission on Accreditation of Rehabilitation Facilities (CARF) and the Joint Commission on Accreditation of Healthcare Organizations (JCAHO) address competence-related activities in their standards. In their accreditation reviews, JCAHO and CARF look to see that organizations develop competencies needed by their staff members to perform their duties, that a mechanism is in place to measure the level of competency, and that the required competencies are assessed on an annual basis. In addition, the organizations must make opportunities available to improve the competencies of staff members.

Acceptable activities vary in states or jurisdictions and range from attending or presenting courses to supervising fieldwork students or participating in research. The number of required points or contact hours of continuing education activity also varies widely from state to state, ranging from an average of 6 hours per year to 20 hours per year. Appendix 19.A summarizes the required amount of continuing competence activities for each state and the District of Columbia. For the most up-to-date information on specific state requirements, contact the individual state regulatory board or agency.

## Supervision of Occupational Therapy Assistants and Aides

State regulatory boards address supervision of occupational therapy assistants in different ways. Supervision requirements may be included in the definitions of occupational therapy assistant or in the definitions of types or levels of supervision allowed in that state. In many states or jurisdictions, specific subsections in the regulations address the role and supervision of occupational therapy assistants. Most states look to AOTA's professional standards on supervision such as the "Guide for Supervision of Occupational Therapy Personnel in the Delivery of Occupational Therapy Services" (AOTA, 1999a) to reflect current best practice in the profession.

When clarifying these regulations, regulatory boards also consider problems or issues that arise in their state with respect to the supervision of occupational therapy assistants in specific settings. Some state regulatory boards also address supervision of nonregulated support personnel such as aides. Aides who provide supportive services to occupational therapists or occupational therapy assistants are considered non-licensed or nonregulated personnel. Most states do not mention this level of personnel in their statutes or regulations. However, some states have incorporated regulations about the use and supervision of nonlicensed personnel or aides under rules or regulations that outline the responsibilities of occupational therapists or occupational therapy assistants who supervise these people. The regulations may also list types of activities that aides can and cannot do under the supervision of occupational therapists and occupational therapy assistants. This list is often consistent with AOTA's "Guidelines for the Use of Aides in Occupational Therapy Practice" (AOTA, 1999b), which states that "the role of the aide is strictly to support the occupational therapist or the occupational therapy assistant with specific non-client-related tasks, such as clerical and maintenance activities and preparation of a work area or equipment, or with routine aspects of the intervention session" (p. 595). At least one state, New Hampshire, has included a provision in its practice act that prohibits coercing occupational therapists or occupational therapy assistants into compromising patient safety by requiring them to delegate treatment inappropriately.

Managers, consultants, entrepreneurs, and practitioners who supervise occupational therapy assistants and aides must be familiar with their individual state's or jurisdiction's requirements for supervision because they do vary. Some states may require documentation of supervisory sessions in a supervision log or may limit the number of personnel that an occupational therapist may supervise. The amount and type of supervision also varies from jurisdiction to jurisdiction. Many occupational therapists are not fully aware of an important concept: They are legally responsible for the patient care rendered by occupational therapy assistants and aides under their supervision.

## Disciplinary Action

Boards protect the public by providing consumer information, monitoring regulated practitioners, and investigating complaints. They have the power to discipline practitioners through a variety of sanctions that range from reprimand to revocation of license (or certificate or registration). Revocation removes the practitioner's right to practice in that state and, thus, is used only in extreme cases. Less harsh actions may require peer review of records; educational meetings; supervision with or without a mentor; continuing education; payment of a fine; and suspension of a license, a certificate, or registered status (AOTA, 1996, p. 611). Reports of disciplinary actions taken by state regulatory boards, by NBCOT's Disciplinary Action Committee, or by AOTA's Commission on Standards and Ethics are frequently shared among those three bodies and also may be reported to the National Practitioner Data Bank.

Boards may also adopt a code of ethics that articulates the expected behaviors of those who are regulated by the board. They often adopt AOTA's *Occupational Therapy Code of Ethics* in whole or in part. AOTA's code is a public statement of the common set of values and principles used to promote and maintain high standards of behavior in occupational therapy. The code is a set of principles that applies to occupational therapy personnel at all levels. These principles to which occupational therapists and occupational therapy assistants aspire are part of a lifelong effort to act in an ethical manner. The various roles of practitioner (occupational therapist and occupational therapy assistant), educator, fieldwork educator, clinical supervisor, manager, administrator, consultant, fieldwork coordinator, faculty program director, researcher–scholar, private practice owner, entrepreneur, and student are included in the code's scope (AOTA, 2000b).

## The Future of State Regulation

Some have viewed state regulation of health care professionals critically, believing that more can be done to strengthen the state regulatory framework. Reform has occurred through the appointment of public members to licensing boards, the creation of umbrella agencies to oversee licensing boards, the passing of sunrise and sunset laws, and rulings by the Federal Trade Commission on the anticompetitive aspects of some licensing laws (Young, 1987). Some critics have proposed a system that would encourage consumers to rely on information and on their own judgment with respect to the preparation of health care professionals. Others have proposed programs to modify the state regulatory structure.

In 2000, the governors of Minnesota and Florida proposed budget cuts to streamline government. These cuts included deregulation of occupational therapy along with several other professions in their states. Both of these initiatives were defeated because the occupational therapy practitioners in those states, led by their state associations, strongly objected to the proposed deregulation. They were able to provide information that countered the state's rationale for deregulation and made a strong case for licensure as a way to protect consumers from unqualified practitioners.

In 1994, the Pew Commission assembled the Taskforce on Health Care Workforce Regulation to identify how regulation protects the public's health and to propose recommendations with respect to regulation of the health care workforce that might better serve the public's interest. The task force identified many issues that were crucial elements in regulating health professions to best serve the public's interest, including

- Setting requirements for entry to practice
- Ensuring continuing professional competence
- Standardizing regulatory terms and language
- Evaluating regulatory effectiveness.

The task force called for a system that would be standardized when appropriate; accountable to the public; flexible, to support optimal access to a competent workforce; and effective and efficient in protecting and promoting the public's health, safety, and welfare (Gragnola & Stone, 1997).

The report sparked much debate and comment from professions and other stakeholders. Many were supportive of the report's message that regulatory reform was needed but thought that it did not provide adequate information on how to finance and carry out reform (Gragnola & Stone, 1997). In its fourth and final report, the Pew Health Professions Commission (1998) urged health professionals to continually reconsider how they may best add value to the delivery of health services. The commission cited public representation in the regulatory process, demonstration of continuing competence, and flexibility to practice in those domains of demonstrated competence as the most important elements to consider in the needed restructuring of health care regulation. Some of these recommendations appear to be taking hold within the occupational therapy profession because several state regulatory boards have increased the number of consumer members on their boards, and many boards have added continuing competence requirements over the past 5 years.

## Nongovernmental Certification

Nongovernmental credentialing organizations such as NBCOT recognize through the mechanism of certification those individuals who have attained entry-level competence in broad areas of responsibility within their profession. A person completing this non-governmental certification process is granted a certificate and is also entitled to use a special designation such as "certified" or "registered" with his or her name. Chapter 20 on continuing competency discusses advanced certification, which is a different type of nongovernmental certification that recognizes advanced training or experience in specific areas.

## Entry-Level Certification

In the mid-1930s, AOTA initiated a program of nongovernmental certification for occupational therapists, which it then administered for more than 50 years. In the early years, AOTA called the program for occupational therapists *registration* and granted the designation *registered* to applicants who successfully completed the education, fieldwork, and examination requirements. The association introduced a similar program for occupational therapy assistants in the 1960s. In 1986, AOTA created an independent organization, the American Occupational Therapy Certification Board (AOTCB) and transferred the certification program from AOTA to AOTCB. In 1996, AOTCB changed its name to the National Board for Certification in Occupational Therapy, Inc., or NBCOT (AOTA, 1996, p. 613).

NBCOT is a private, not-for-profit credentialing organization that oversees and administers the entry-level certification examination for occupational therapists and occupational therapy assistants. This examination is what the state regulatory boards use as one of the criteria for licensure (or other forms of regulation). NBCOT uses the examination as one of the criteria for initial NBCOT certification.

NBCOT certifies eligible individuals as Occupational Therapist Registered OTR® (OTR) or Certified Occupational Therapy Assistant COTA® (COTA). The OTR® and COTA® credentials are registered certification marks owned by NBCOT. Certification by NBCOT indicates to the public that the OTR or the COTA has met all of NBCOT's educational, fieldwork, and examination requirements (NBCOT, 2002b).

### *Entry-Level Certification Examination*

NBCOT certifies occupational therapy practitioners on the basis of separate examinations for therapists and assistants. The examinations are objective measures of entry-level competence, each consisting of 200 items in a multiple-choice format. A candidate who has passed the NBCOT examination receives a certificate, which he or she may show to employers and regulatory boards (AOTA, 1996, pp. 613–614).

The NBCOT certification examinations are computer delivered and administered at more than 300 test centers throughout North America, including Puerto Rico and the Virgin Islands. Once candidates have completed the NBCOT certification examination registration process, they will receive an Authorization to Test letter that provides instructions on contacting the testing company to schedule their test date and location (NBCOT, 2002a).

*Requirements for Eligibility to Take the Examination*

Eligibility requirements for NBCOT certification examinations vary depending on the candidate's educational background and the type of certification sought. The requirements must be met before a candidate can take an examination.

For entry-level certification as an OTR, people who were educated in the United States, its territories, or commonwealths must have graduated from an occupational therapist education program accredited by AOTA's ACOTE and must have successfully completed all therapist-level fieldwork required by the education program. Similarly, U.S.-educated applicants for entry-level certification as a COTA must have graduated from an occupational therapy assistant education program that is accredited or approved by AOTA's ACOTE and must have successfully completed all assistant-level fieldwork required by the education program.

Internationally educated occupational therapists must meet certain U.S. Immigration and Naturalization Service and NBCOT requirements. These include the following: (a) having graduated from an entry-level occupational therapy program that is either recognized by the World Federation of Occupational Therapy or determined by NBCOT to be professionally comparable to that of a U.S bachelor's degree program in occupational therapy, (b) having completed at least 1,000 hours of fieldwork, and (c) having passed three English tests (unless exempt) (NBCOT, 2002c).

*NBCOT Certification Renewal*

NBCOT created a certification renewal program in 1997 and added a Phase II of the program that begins in 2002 and includes a professional development requirement (AOTA, 2000a). Maintaining NBCOT certification entitles individuals to the continued use of NBCOT's registered certification marks OTR® or COTA®. Individuals who choose not to renew this certification are required by NBCOT to no longer use its certification marks. State licensure or jurisdiction laws (or other forms of state regulation) generally authorize practitioners who meet their licensure requirements to use a wide variety of professional designations, including OT (occupational therapist), OTA (occupational therapy assistant), OT/L (occupational therapist/licensed), and OTA/L (occupational therapy assistant/licensed), among others.

## Relationship of Nongovernmental Certification to State Regulation, Private or Public Employment, and Third-Party Reimbursement

States or jurisdictions commonly require occupational therapists and occupational therapy assistants to be initially certified (i.e., pass the NBCOT entry-level certification exam) before they can qualify for a license. Most states or jurisdictions, however, do not require practitioners to renew this certification to maintain their licenses to practice.

NBCOT recertification is not a legal requirement to practice occupational therapy unless a state mandates it as a condition of licensure, certification, or registration. Certification renewal status does not affect the ability to be reimbursed by Medicare,

Medicaid, or other third-party payers. Additionally, the JCAHO and CARF do not independently require in their standards that occupational therapists and occupational therapy assistants employed by facilities renew their certification with NBCOT.

### Disciplinary Action by NBCOT

NBCOT undertakes disciplinary action procedures against OTRs, COTAs, and examination candidates who are incompetent, unethical, or impaired (e.g., by substance abuse). The disciplinary action program makes it possible to identify, discipline, and require improvements of those who demonstrate incompetent, unethical, or impaired behavior. Individuals who are not exam candidates or who are not currently certified by NBCOT would not be subject to discipline by NBCOT. However, all occupational therapists and occupational therapy assistants who are regulated by a state are subject to discipline by their state regulatory body, and all members of AOTA are subject to discipline by AOTA's Commission on Standards and Ethics.

## Conclusion

Occupational therapy is regulated in all 50 states, the District of Columbia, Puerto Rico, and Guam. The type of regulation may differ from licensure, the strongest form of regulation, to title control or trademark act, the weakest form of regulation. The purpose of regulation is to protect consumers of that state or jurisdiction from unqualified or unscrupulous practitioners.

State laws and regulations significantly affect the profession of occupational therapy, including the setting of professional standards, coverage and reimbursement for occupational therapy services, funding for higher education, and the awarding of research grants. Most licensure laws or practice acts have similar components, including requirements for licensure and renewal and a defined scope of practice. Each individual is responsible to be aware of and compliant with all statutes and regulations governing the occupational therapy practitioners and practice of occupational therapy.

Authority to administer regulations is generally delegated to a regulatory board that provides consumer information, monitors regulated practitioners, investigates complaints, and disciplines practitioners. Practitioners, managers, entrepreneurs, consultants, and state association leaders can take an active part in shaping appropriate state regulation of occupational therapy practice.

## References

American Occupational Therapy Association. (1996). *The occupational therapy manager* (rev. ed.). Bethesda, MD: Author.

American Occupational Therapy Association. (1999a). Guide for supervision of occupational therapy personnel in the delivery of occupational therapy services. *American Journal of Occupational Therapy, 53*, 592–594.

American Occupational Therapy Association. (1999b). Guidelines for the use of aides in occupational therapy practice. *American Journal of Occupational Therapy, 53*, 595–597.

American Occupational Therapy Association. (2000a, October). *Model occupational therapy practice act.* Bethesda, MD: Author.

American Occupational Therapy Association. (2000b, November/December). Occupational therapy code of ethics. *American Journal of Occupational Therapy, 54*, 614–616.

American Occupational Therapy Association. (2001, October/November). Building relationships. In *AOTA state affairs group news* (p. 3). Bethesda, MD: Author.

American Occupational Therapy Association. (2002). *FAQ about continuing competence and NBCOT certification renewal.* Retrieved April 11, 2002, from http://www.aota.org/nonmembers/area1/links/link217.asp

American Occupational Therapy Association, State Affairs Group. (2002a, June). *Jurisdictions regulating occupational therapists (OTs)* [Fact sheet]. Bethesda, MD: Author.

American Occupational Therapy Association, State Affairs Group. (2002b, June). *Jurisdictions regulating occupational therapy assistants (OTAs)* [Fact sheet]. Bethesda, MD: Author.

American Occupational Therapy Association, State Affairs Group. (2002c, April). *Occupational therapy: Continuing competence requirements—Summary chart.* Bethesda, MD: Author.

Gragnola, C. M., & Stone E. (1997). *Considering the future of health care workforce regulation.* San Francisco, CA: UCSF Center for Health Professions.

*Merriam-Webster's Dictionary of Law.* (1996). Retrieved April 11, 2002, from http://dictionary.lp.findlaw.com/scripts/results.pl?co=dictionary.lp.findlaw.com&topic=a5/a55f826bd0b441136f9ee1d89c8f63f0

National Board for Certification in Occupational Therapy. (2002a). *Certification exams.* Retrieved April 11, 2002, from http://www.nbcot.org/programs/ cert_exams.htm

National Board for Certification in Occupational Therapy. (2002b). *Certification renewal.* Retrieved April 11, 2002, from http://www.nbcot.org/programs/ cert_renewal.htm

National Board for Certification in Occupational Therapy. (2002c). *International.* Retrieved April 11, 2002, from http://www.nbcot.org/programs/ international.htm

O'Leary, M. (1994). *Lexikon: Dictionary of health care terms, organizations, and acronyms for the era of reform.* Oakbrook, IL: Joint Commission on Accreditation of Healthcare Organizations.

Pew Health Professions Commission. (1998). *Recreating health professional practice for a new century.* San Francisco, CA: UCSF Center for Health Professions. Retrieved April 4, 2002, from http://www.futurehealth.ucsf.edu/ publications/index.html

Shimberg, B., & Roederer, D. (1994, April 7). *Questions a legislator should ask* (2nd ed., K. Schmitt, Ed.). Lexington, KY: Council on Licensure, Enforcement and Regulation.

U.S. Department of Health, Education, and Welfare. (1977). *Credentialing health manpower* [Publication No. (OS) 77-50057]. Bethesda, MD: Author.

Young, S. D. (1987). *The rule of experts: Occupational licensing in America.* Washington, DC: Cato Institute.

## Appendix 19.A  Occupational Therapy Continuing Competence Requirements.

| State | Status | Requirements |
|---|---|---|
| Alabama | Mandatory | OT:  3.0 CEUs (or 30 contact hours) biennially |
| | | OTA: 2.0 CEUs (or 20 contact hours) biennially |
| Alaska | Mandatory | OT:  20 contact hours of continuing education biennially |
| | | OTA: 20 contact hours of continuing education biennially |
| Arizona | Mandatory | OT:  20 clock-hours for renewal of a 2-year license period |
| | | OTA: 12 clock-hours for renewal of a 2-year license period |
| Arkansas | Mandatory | OT:  10 contact hours of continuing education each year |
| | | OTA: 10 contact hours of continuing education each year |
| California | No requirements | OT:  No requirements |
| | | OTA: No requirements |
| Colorado | No requirements | OT:  No requirements |
| | | OTA: No requirements |
| Connecticut | Mandatory | OT:  12 units of qualifying continuing competency activity during the preceding registration period, renewed biennially every odd year |
| | | OTA: 9 units of qualifying continuing competency activity during the preceding registration period, renewed biennially every odd year |
| Delaware | Mandatory | OT: |
| | | • 20 hours of continuing education for each license renewed biennially |
| | | • new licensees prorated |
| | | OTA: |
| | | • 20 hours of continuing education for each license renewed biennially |
| | | • new licensees prorated |
| District of Columbia | Mandatory | OT:  24 hours of approved continuing education credit during a 2-year licensure period |
| | | OTA: 12 hours of approved continuing education credit during a 2-year licensure period |
| Florida | Mandatory | OT:  24 hours continuing education + 2 hours HIV/AIDS education = total 26 hours biennially |
| | | OTA: 24 hours continuing education + 2 hours HIV/AIDS education = total 26 hours biennially |

(*continued*)

## Appendix 19.A   *(Continued)*

| State | Status | Requirements |
|---|---|---|
| Georgia | Mandatory | OT: 12 contact hours biennially |
| | | OTA: 12 contact hours biennially |
| Hawaii | No requirements | OT: No requirements |
| | | OTA: No requirements |
| Idaho | Voluntary | OT: |
| | | • No requirements |
| | | • May send in continuing education credit voluntarily with license renewal |
| | | OTA: |
| | | • No requirements |
| | | • May send in continuing education credit voluntarily with license renewal |
| Illinois | Requirements will be in effect when rules are completed. | OT: Minimum of 12 units of continuing competency activities biennially |
| | | OTA: Minimum of 12 units of continuing competency activities biennially |
| Indiana | No requirements | OT: No requirements |
| | | OTA: No requirements |
| Iowa | Mandatory | OT: 30 hours of continuing education each biennium (by birth month) |
| | | OTA: 15 hours of continuing education each biennium (by birth month) |
| Kansas | Mandatory | OT: 40 hours every 2 years (from Jan 1 of odd year until Dec. 31 of even year) |
| | | OTA: 40 hours every 2 years (from Jan 1 of odd year until Dec 31 of even year) |
| Kentucky | No requirements | OT: No requirements |
| | | OTA: No requirements |
| Louisiana | Mandatory | OT: 15 contact hours or 1.5 CEUs annually |
| | | OTA: 15 contact hours or 1.5 CEUs annually |
| Maine | Mandatory | OT: 36 contact hours of study equivalent to 3.6 CEUs, which shall be completed for every biennial license renewal on March 31 of the odd year |
| | | OTA: 36 contact hours of study equivalent to 3.6 CEUs, which shall be completed for every biennial license renewal on March 31 of the odd year |

*(continued)*

## Appendix 19.A (*Continued*)

| State | Status | Requirements |
|---|---|---|
| Maryland | Mandatory | OT:<br>• If licensed for more than 2 years, 24 contact hours of continuing education activities obtained within a 2-year period<br>• If licensed for less than 2 years but more than 1 year, 12 contact hours of continuing education activities required<br>• If licensed less than 1 year, no continuing education required<br>OTA:<br>• If licensed for more than 2 years, 24 contact hours of continuing education activities obtained within a 2-year period<br>• If licensed less than 2 years, 12 contact hours of continuing education activities<br>• If licensed less than 1 year, no continuing education requirements |
| Massachusetts | No requirements | OT: No requirements<br>OTA: No requirements |
| Michigan | No requirements | OT: No requirements<br>OTA: No requirements |
| Minnesota | Mandatory | OT: 24 contact hours of continuing education in the 2-year licensure period<br>OTA: 18 contact hours of continuing education in the 2-year licensure period |
| Mississippi | Mandatory | OT: 20 contact hours accrued during the 2-year licensure period<br>OTA: 20 contact hours accrued during the 2-year licensure period |
| Missouri | No requirements | OT: No requirements<br>OTA: No requirements |
| Montana | Mandatory | OT: 10 contact hours of continuing education annually<br>OTA: 10 contact hours of continuing education annually |
| Nebraska | Mandatory | OT: 20 hours of continuing education for biennial license renewal<br>OTA: 15 hours of continuing education for biennial license renewal |
| Nevada | Mandatory | OT: 10 hours of continuing education at annual renewal on June 30<br>OTA: 10 hours of continuing education at annual renewal on June 30 |

(*continued*)

## Appendix 19.A   *(Continued)*

| State | Status | Requirements |
|---|---|---|
| New Hampshire | Mandatory | OT:<br>• 12 hours of continuing professional education annually; 6 hours need to be in clinical application<br>• 24 hours of continuing professional education biennially; 12 hours need to be in clinical application<br>OTA:<br>• 12 hours of continuing professional education annually; 6 hours need to be in clinical application<br>• 24 hours of continuing professional education biennially; 12 hours need to be in clinical application. |
| New Jersey | No requirements | OT:   No requirements<br>OTA: No requirements |
| New Mexico | Mandatory | OT:   2 CEUs (20 contact hours) will be required (annually) for each year of expired licensure<br>OTA: 2 CEUs (20 contact hours) will be required (annually) for each year of expired licensure |
| New York | No requirements | OT:   No requirements<br>OTA: No requirements |
| North Carolina | Mandatory | OT:   15 contact hours each (annual) renewal year<br>OTA: 10 contact hours each (annual) renewal year |
| North Dakota | No requirements | OT:   No requirements<br>OTA: No requirements |
| Ohio | Mandatory | OT:   20 contact hours of continuing education activities within a 2-year period<br>OTA: 20 contact hours of continuing education activities within a 2-year period |
| Oklahoma | Mandatory | OT:   20 contact hours every 2 years<br>OTA: 20 contact hours every 2 years |
| Oregon | Mandatory | OT:   15 points of continuing education during the year immediately preceding the date of the annual license renewal<br>OTA: 15 points of continuing education during the year immediately preceding the date of the annual license renewal |
| Pennsylvania | No requirements | OT:   No requirements<br>OTA: No requirements |

*(continued)*

## Appendix 19.A  *(Continued)*

| State | Status | Requirements | |
|---|---|---|---|
| Rhode Island | Mandatory | OT: | 20 hours biennially |
| | | OTA: | 20 hours biennially |
| South Carolina | Mandatory | OT: | 16 hours of continuing education each biennial renewal |
| | | OTA: | 16 hours of continuing education each biennial renewal |
| South Dakota | Mandatory | OT: | 12 continuing competency points in 1-year period |
| | | OTA: | 12 continuing competency points in 1-year period |
| Tennessee | No requirements | OT: | No requirements |
| | | OTA: | No requirements |
| Texas | Mandatory | OT: | 30 contact hours of continuing education each biennial renewal |
| | | OTA: | 30 contact hours of continuing education each biennial renewal |
| Utah | No requirements | OT: | No requirements |
| | | OTA: | No requirements |
| Vermont | Mandatory | OT: | 20 hours of continuing education during the preceding 2-year licensure period |
| | | OTA: | 20 hours of continuing education during the preceding 2-year licensure period |
| Virginia | Mandatory | OT: | 20 contact hours of continuing education activities every 2 years plus 160 hours of active practice |
| | | OTA: | No requirements |
| Washington | Mandatory | OT: | 30 hours of continuing education every 2 years |
| | | OTA: | 30 hours of continuing education every 2 years |
| West Virginia | Mandatory | OT: | 12 contact hours of continuing competency activities obtained within 1 year |
| | | OTA: | 12 contact hours of continuing competency activities obtained within 1 year |
| Wisconsin | Mandatory | OT: | 18 points of acceptable continuing education in a 2-year period |
| | | OTA: | 12 points of acceptable continuing education in a 2-year period |
| Wyoming | Mandatory | OT: | 16 contact hours of continuing education per year |
| | | OTA: | 16 contact hours of continuing education per year |

*Note.* OT = occupational therapist, OTA = occupational therapy assistant, CEU = continuing education unit.

Adopted by AOTA's Representative Assembly April 4, 1999.

# Professional
# Standards

# Continuing Competency

Penelope A. Moyers, EdD, OTR, FAOTA
Jim Hinojosa, PhD, OT, FAOTA

*"The most strategic asset a leader has to work with is the competency of his or her staff to perform at a level of excellence."*

KERFOOT, 2002

**Penelope A. Moyers, EdD, OTR, FAOTA,** is professor and dean, School of Occupational Therapy, University of Indianapolis. Dr. Moyers is currently the chairperson of AOTA's Commission on Continuing Competence and Professional Development and was the vice-speaker of the Representative Assembly, serving on AOTA's Board of Directors. Dr. Moyers has written and studied issues related to continuing competence since 1987, studying the factors that support and inhibit occupational therapists and occupational therapy assistants in their professional development.

**Jim Hinojosa, PhD, OT, FAOTA,** is professor and chair, Department of Occupational Therapy, The Steinhardt School of Education, New York University. Dr. Hinojosa has served as chairperson of the Commission on Practice of AOTA, on the Executive Board of AOTA, and on the Board of Directors of the American Occupational Therapy Foundation. Currently, he serves on AOTA's Commission on Continuing Competence and Professional Development. Dr. Hinojosa's long history of addressing the issues of continuing competence began in 1985.

## Key Ideas and Concepts

**Competencies.** Competencies are explicit statements that define specific areas of expertise and are related to effective or superior performance in a job (Spencer & Spencer, 1993).

**Competency.** "Competency focuses on an individual's actual performance in a particular situation" (McConnell, 2001, p. 14). Competency implies a determination that one is competent.

**Competency characteristics.** The capabilities that the person brings to the job task, including motives, traits, self-concept, knowledge, and skills (Spencer & Spencer, 1993).

**Competent.** The ability to successfully perform a behavior or task as measured according to a specific criterion (Hinojosa, 1985).

**Continuing competence.** Involves the development of capacity and competency characteristics needed for the future and ✳ is a component of ongoing professional development or lifelong learning.

**Professional development.** May include a program of continuing competence but also includes a focus on one's career development in terms of achieving excellence or achiev-✳ ing role status as an independent practitioner or expert and in terms of assuming new, more complex roles and responsibilities.

## Learning Objectives

After completing this chapter, you should be able to do the following:

- Define competence, competency, and the elements of a professional development plan.
- Discuss the self-directed learning process to ensure competent practices.
- Identify personal responsibilities and relationships with state regulatory boards, the American Occupational Therapy Association, the National Board for Certification in Occupational Therapy, and other accreditation agencies.
- Describe the purpose and the design of AOTA's Continuing Competence Plan for Professional Development (Hinojosa et al., 2000a).

Occupational therapists and occupational therapy assistants are being asked on a daily basis to demonstrate competency. What does it mean to be competent? Who determines whether someone is competent? And, most important, who is responsible for ensuring whether someone is competent? These questions are of concern because consumers, employers, accreditation agencies, licensure boards, the National Board for Certification in Occupational Therapy (NBCOT), and others require that occupational therapists and occupational therapy assistants verify their competency to provide services within specific contexts. Occupational therapy practice is changing rapidly in response to up-to-date information, knowledge, and technologies. Occupational therapists and occupational therapy assistants are challenged in this changing world of practice to assure the public and consumers of their individual professional competency.

This chapter provides the foundation for understanding competency and continuing competence, and it explores the environmental demands that drive expectations surrounding each process. In this chapter, the continuing competence process is described with an emphasis on developing and maintaining a core belief in occupation. The Standards for Continuing Competence (American Occupational Therapy Association [AOTA], 1999) and the AOTA Continuing Competence Plan for Professional Development (AOTA, 1999) are presented. Learning methods for achieving competency are reviewed with a particular emphasis on those methods that lead to a change in practice and to an ultimate improvement in client service outcomes.

## Understanding Competency and Continuing Competence

The difference between continuing competence and competency is subtle because *competence* "refers to an individual's capacity to perform job [professional] responsibilities" (McConnell, 2001, p. 14), and *competency* "focuses on an individual's actual performance in a particular situation" (p. 14). Capacity to perform one's professional responsibilities results from ongoing professional development or lifelong learning. In contrast, competency implies a determination that one is currently competent to perform a behavior or task as measured against a specific criterion (Hinojosa et al., 2000b).

Both continuing competence (building capacity) and competency (current performance against standards) are necessary if one is to be adequately prepared for the complex demands of practice over time. The evolving nature of the health care, educational, and social services systems leads to changing roles and responsibilities of therapists and assistants. Occupational therapists possess job titles ranging from practitioner to manager, from employee to entrepreneur, and from researcher to scholar. Occupational therapy assistants also hold a variety of positions, depending on the organization, their experience, and levels of advanced education. Job titles and descriptions broadly outline an employee's general duties. When one assumes the job title of occupational therapist or occupational therapy assistant, the expectation is that this person will be competent in managing his or her multiple responsibilities. Occupational therapists and occupational therapy assistants are competent when they have the prerequisite knowledge, skills, and attitudes to provide effective, quality practice. Competent therapists and assistants have particular skills that authorize them to perform restricted activities in a skillful manner that will result in defined outcomes. A restricted activity is one that only someone who is licensed or trained in a given profession or technical trade may perform.

Competencies are explicit statements that define specific areas of expertise or competency. According to Decker (1999), competencies are causally related to effective job performance, which means meeting and exceeding customer outcome expectations. When employees or independent occupational therapy service providers do not meet customer expectations, the result can be a loss of business or an inability of the organization or independent practice to achieve its mission. To delineate the competencies that lead to this expected level of expertise, one needs to determine the required knowledge, the set of complex skills, and the criteria for skillful performance. These underlying requirements on which competencies are based are referred to as *competency characteristics* (Decker, 1999).

Expert knowledge and skills are the most visible competency characteristics to measure and develop because these characteristics involve particular behaviors or activities and have discrete performance criteria. Unfortunately, most continuing education or training programs fail to address other competency characteristics because those characteristics have a less visible nature. In addition, competencies (a) may also depend on the occupational therapist's or the occupational therapy assistant's motivation to change performance; (b) may be more conducive to those therapists and assistants with specific physical and character traits, for example, those with a positive self-concept or self-image; or (c) may depend on having certain attitudes or values (Decker, 1999).

All occupational therapists and occupational therapy assistants have unique competency characteristics and sets of competencies that qualify them to practice occupational therapy. In occupational therapy, basic competency is established when a therapist or assistant successfully completes his or her formal academic education, successfully finishes all required fieldwork experiences, and passes the NBCOT examination. A therapist or assistant who has met these three requirements has established general entry-level competence, or the basic capacity to perform in a given context according to standards. In other words, the person has the minimal qualifications needed to practice as an occupational therapist or as an occupational therapy assistant. This basic, entry-level competence verifies to the public and to consumers that the person is qualified to perform selected restricted activities as defined by the profession's scope of practice.

Of concern to employers is how these general competencies are translated into a particular work context with the following variables: a specific client base and corresponding customer expectations, a unique set of institutional policies and protocols for assessment and intervention, a physical environment consisting of limited space and equipment, and prescribed methods for delegating roles and tasks to employees. Accrediting bodies of hospitals and other health care organizations (e.g., Joint Commission on Accreditation of Healthcare Organizations [JCAHO] and CARF . . . the Commission on Accreditation of Rehabilitation Facilities) require competency programs through which employees, when first hired, demonstrate their proficiency in a set of generic and discipline-specific competencies as they relate to the job each is hired to perform (see the discussion of competence assessment in the section "Organizational Accreditations" in this chapter). Employees then must demonstrate their competency periodically thereafter throughout their employment at a given facility (Herringer, 2002).

Even though an employer of occupational therapists and occupational therapy assistants is concerned about the competency of its employees, the AOTA *Code of Ethics* (AOTA, 2000) clearly states that the individual therapist or assistant has the personal responsibility to ensure that he or she is competent to practice. Therefore, therapists and assistants are required by the profession's code of ethics to engage in a lifelong process of self-directed learning to make certain that they are competent to practice occupational therapy. This lifelong process or continuing competence program includes a wide range of learning and educational activities (e.g., academic coursework, continuing education, presentations, publication, research, advanced certification, peer review, work experience) that enhance the knowledge, skills, and attitudes the person will need to practice competently (Thomson et al., 1995).

AOTA has outlined a continuing competence plan (Hinojosa et al., 1999, 2000), which an occupational therapist or occupational therapy assistant may use not only to foster current competency to practice in an area of expertise but also to promote continuing competence for future practice. This plan is based on the belief that continuing competence is a dynamic, multidimensional process in which the individual develops and maintains the knowledge, performance skills, interpersonal abilities, critical reasoning skills, and ethical reasoning skills necessary to perform job-related responsibilities throughout his or her career. The competencies required to practice occupational therapy continually change throughout the therapist or assistant's professional life (Hinojosa & Blount, 1998).

In summary, determination of whether one is competent depends on the set of competencies inherent in one's multiple roles and responsibilities at a given point in time. Competencies are based on a broad range of competency characteristics, including skills, attitudes, abilities, and expertise. All occupational therapists and occupational therapy assistants are challenged to continually maintain competency through a continuing competence plan. Rapidly expanding knowledge, technological advancements, and shifting societal attitudes require that therapists and assistants actively engage in learning activities not only to maintain expertise or competency for current practice but also to prepare for future practice.

# Environmental Demands
## for Competency and Continuing Competence

The following sections discuss how competency demands are influenced by technological advancement, systematic changes, and practice modifications. Rapid changes challenge therapists and assistants to advance their knowledge, skills, and abilities to ensure competent practices. These changes require that all must actively engage in activities to ensure continuing competence for the services they provide.

### Competency: Why Is It So Important? Why Is It Increasing in Importance?

Fostering competency is a strategy to avoid consequences that could occur if services are provided in a less-than-effective manner or if improper service delivery results in client harm. The consequences resulting from incompetent performance could include self-dissatisfaction with respect to one's own performance as well as client and employer dissatisfaction with the performance of the therapist or assistant. Over time, a pattern of ineffectiveness could lead to loss of business and declining revenues, inability to achieve job promotion, loss of job, and difficulty in being hired for other jobs. In extreme cases of provider incompetence resulting in harm, clients may sue for malpractice or negligence, and the occupational therapist or occupational therapy assistant could lose the state license or certification needed to practice in a given jurisdiction. The therapist or assistant could also lose NBCOT certification and AOTA membership. Loss of license or certification in one state and loss of NBCOT certification are reported to other state licensure boards or jurisdictions in which therapists or assistants may relocate, thereby preventing or making it more difficult to practice in the new location.

Occupational therapists and occupational therapy assistants typically are not in a position to cause immediate life-threatening problems for the client as the result of provider incompetence. When one thinks of client harm, the tendency is to associate it only with circumstances in which the occupational therapist or the occupational therapy assistant (a) places the client in a life-threatening situation that could be avoided (e.g., exposing a child with a seizure disorder to aggressive vestibular stimulation), (b) fails to prevent the client's problem from needlessly worsening (e.g., not carrying out a scar management protocol for someone with a burn), or (c) fails to prevent the client from developing secondary complications (e.g., keeping the client's joints immobilized too long without exercise).

With the advent of evidence-based practice (see chapter 15), however, *harm* now can be defined as resulting from (a) using intervention that has been shown by the evidence to be ineffective or (b) using an intervention that is not the most effective in comparison to an alternative intervention. Therefore, harm includes the risks that result when the client misses an opportunity for receiving effective intervention from a competent provider. This kind of harm from ineffective intervention includes the client's (a) incurring increased costs for rehabilitation, (b) being more reliant on durable medical equipment, (c) having to devote more time to the intervention process, and (d) achieving a less-than-expected outcome. Ongoing occupational performance dysfunction may be the result of ineffective intervention, which could cause clients to remain dependent on others or to become dissatisfied with their quality of life. Life dissatisfaction may lead to a range of mental health complications and to a decline in physical function (Moyers, 1999).

## Continuing Competence: Why Is It So Important? Why Is It Increasing in Importance?

In contrast with the obvious need for provider competency, what are the demands for continuing competence or capacity building? "Failing to keep abreast of change or failing to prepare for change can lead to an inability to fulfill professional and organizational expectations" and, thus, ultimately leads to problems of competency in the future (Alsop, 2001, p. 128). The most strategic asset of an organization is the continuing competence or the future capacity of its human resources. The risk for ineffective service delivery increases over time if the occupational therapist or occupational therapy assistant does not engage in an effective continuing competence program. As indicated, with the emphasis on evidence-based practice, the expectation is that the occupational therapist and the occupational therapy assistant will continuously have knowledge (based on the latest evidence) of the most effective assessment tools, intervention methods, and outcome measures. After learning more effective methods, the occupational therapist and occupational therapy assistant are expected to engage in training and other learning activities as necessary to make sure that they possess skills in these more effective methods and techniques. Thus, the competency characteristic that best promotes continuing competence is a positive attitude toward change. "Mastery of change has therefore to be an attribute of all occupational therapists, wherever they practice" (Alsop, 2001, pp. 127–128).

Professions exist to serve society, and because of this function, professions are dynamic and transform as society, knowledge, and technology advance (Kielhofner, 1992; Mosey, 1992). "The delivery of up-to-date healthcare services has to be a continual process of redefining the knowledge needed for practice in a changing environment" (Alsop, 2001, p. 127). Because practitioners of a profession continually adapt, add, change, or discard specific theories and therapeutic practices, the profession is enabled to continually change and maintain its capacity to serve society. In other words, the profession itself cannot grow and change without occupational therapists who build on existing knowledge as well as develop new knowledge and who become "instigators of change" through research, evidence-based practice, and further development or refinement of practice (Alsop, 2001, p. 128).

Because of the role that continuing competence plays in determining the direction of future practice, it cannot be fully abdicated to other stakeholders and remains the responsibility of each occupational therapist and occupational therapy assistant. This responsibility for the future direction of the profession is consistent with Barnett's (1994) view of continuing competence, or a focus on capacity development, as being vital for the growth of a profession. Yerxa (1995) stated, "occupational therapists are the only people who can and should define our practice, education, ethics, values, and research. We owe this to society and the people we serve" (p. 298). The capacity of each occupational therapist and occupational therapy assistant for future practice results in the capacity of the profession to serve society.

## Expectations From Stakeholders

Protection of the consumers of occupational therapy services is the concern of many stakeholders, including the consumer. State regulatory boards, AOTA, and NBCOT share the mission to protect the public and to ensure quality services.

### State Regulatory Boards

State regulatory boards have legal authority to determine whether occupational therapists and occupational therapy assistants have the necessary requirements to practice in a given legal jurisdiction. Typically, the requirements to initially obtain a state license or certification include evidence of passing the NBCOT certification examination, a diploma from an accredited occupational therapy educational program, completion of the required fieldwork, and payment of a state fee. Some states may require fingerprinting to check whether the occupational therapist or occupational therapy assistant has a criminal record. Most jurisdictions require the state license or certification to be renewed periodically on a 2- or 3-year schedule. In addition to payment of a renewal fee, which varies in cost from one state to another, renewal includes attesting to the following: (a) never having been sued for negligence or malpractice or never having an award of negligence or malpractice made against the therapist or assistant or never having a conviction for a crime, (b) never having had one's state license to practice revoked or suspended, and (c) never having had one's practice privileges revoked or suspended by a health care organization. Attesting to an occurrence of disciplinary action will trigger an investigation and requests for more information from the applicant before the board will offer a decision with respect to renewal. The applicant for licensure renewal must attest that the answers to these renewal questions are true. Making untruthful statements on the renewal application leads to disciplinary action and may, in addition to losing the license, include legal action such as a fine and jail term.

The renewal process in 35 states also includes submission of evidence showing that the applicant has participated in continuing education or in other forms of competency programming. The number of continuing education units, or contact hours, required for state licensure renewal varies, with most states requiring approximately 20–30 contact hours biennially. Some states differentiate the number of contact hours that are required from occupational therapists and those that are required from occupational therapy assistants, requiring fewer numbers of contact hours from assistants.

Some states specify how the contact hours may be distributed among program topics, for example, by stating that no more than a third of the contact hours may be in the categories of administration or teaching and that the remainder must be in direct patient care. Some even limit continuing education obtained in specialized areas, requiring a certain portion of the contact hours to be obtained in general occupational therapy practice. In addition, certain topics, including HIV, ethics, medical error detection, and jurisprudence, may be mandatory. Evidence of knowledge about the laws and regulations governing occupational therapy practice or jurisprudence is most often demonstrated through the completion of open-book tests created by the regulatory board.

The continuing education contact hours typically must be obtained through programs approved by the state licensure board, for example, those offered by the state occupational therapy association, AOTA, other professional organizations, and universities. Some states accept contact hours from employer-offered in-service training, excluding those in-services that focus on employee orientation, safety, fire evacuation, and cardiopulmonary resuscitation. If a practitioner obtains continuing education from providers not included in the list of approved providers, then the onus is usually on the occupational therapist or the occupational therapy assistant to seek regulatory board approval for accepting a continuing education provider's course.

States may have a broader interpretation about what constitutes evidence of engagement in a program of continuing competency and may allow professional development activities other than continuing education. In fact, AOTA's *Model Continuing Competence Guidelines for Occupational Therapists and Occupational Therapy Assistants: A Resource for State Regulatory Boards* (AOTA, 2002a) recommends that regulatory boards also accept as evidence of continuing competency learning activities such as independent study, mentorship, fieldwork supervision, peer review activities, publications, presentations, research and grants, and specialty certification. Those states that allow other types of learning activities as evidence of continuing competency often delineate how many contact hours may be obtained in each type of learning activity, giving most of the contact hours for continuing education programming.

Instead of requiring all occupational therapists and occupational therapy assistants within the state to send in documentation of their continuing education or program of continuing competency, most states require therapists and assistants to maintain records that are subject to audit at the request of the regulatory board. What must be maintained in the record documenting continuing education or a program of continuing competency varies from state to state, depending on the type of learning activity. Documentation of continuing education usually involves maintaining a copy of the program title and content; a description of the program sponsor, presenter, or author; a certificate of completion or some other verification of course participation such as a university transcript; location and attendance dates; number of contact hours; and affirmation that the continuing education information is true or correct.

Failure to submit to an audit of documented continuing education is interpreted as grounds for revoking the license to practice in the given jurisdiction because it is viewed as an attempt to obtain a license through misrepresentation. There may be certain exceptions from meeting the continuing education requirements, which could include military service, financial hardship, and illness or disability. A negative audit may be appealed, and ultimate decisions could range from removing the state license or certification to reversing the audit decision to modifying the audit decision. Most states allow therapists and assistants time to correct the problems found in the audit before proceeding with disciplinary action.

### National Board for Certification in Occupational Therapy

NBCOT is a private credentialing body. Both the state regulatory bodies and NBCOT have missions to protect the public; therefore, NBCOT is not a membership organization. As discussed previously, NBCOT is responsible for developing, updating, and administering the initial certification examination used by state regulatory boards in their process to determine whether to initially allow occupational therapists to practice in a given jurisdiction. The initials OTR, to be used by the registered occupational therapist, and COTA, to be used by the certified occupational therapy assistant, are legal trademarks of NBCOT and can be used only when the occupational therapist or the occupational therapy assistant has met the initial certification requirements outlined by NBCOT or has met the renewal requirements for maintaining the certification. This certification renewal program is voluntary and is not required by most state regulatory boards, and it is not required to receive Medicare or Medicaid reimbursement for the delivery of occupational therapy services.

The voluntary certification renewal program of NBCOT includes completing attestation questions similar to those used by state licensure boards, paying a renewal fee, and obtaining 36 professional development units (PDUs) during a 3-year renewal cycle (NBCOT, 2002). NBCOT outlines the type of learning activities that can be counted as PDUs. These learning activities include NBCOT-recognized continuing education along with mentoring, being mentored, volunteering, participating in professional study groups, as well as conducting self-assessment and professional development planning. Additionally, the occupational therapist and the occupational therapy assistant, although not required, are encouraged to select learning activities based on a self-assessment and a professional development plan. Because self-assessment and planning are part of the range of choices among other learning activities, it is not clear how PDUs ensure competency given that the therapist or the assistant may not consider impact on client outcomes when selecting learning activities.

NBCOT selects a random sample of occupational therapists and assistants with each year's renewal population to audit the documentation of their PDUs and to determine whether requirements of what constitutes an acceptable PDU have been met. Failure to meet the renewal requirements leads NBCOT to place the occupational therapist or occupational therapy assistant on inactive status after allowing the individual 6 months to meet the requirements when a problem has been identified.

## Organizational Accreditations

Health care and other service organizations often must go through an organizational accreditation process to qualify for payment or funding from third parties and to represent the organization as a quality service provider. Two organizational accrediting bodies are JCAHO and CARF. As of 1996, JCAHO required hospitals to assess, prove, track, and improve the competence of employees.

Competence assessment must occur before staff members may independently perform their assigned job duties after being hired or after being assigned a new responsibility or technology. Competence then must be ascertained on an ongoing basis at least once during the 3-year accreditation cycle (Herringer, 2002). In addition to validating the performance of staff members on duties described in their job descriptions, competence assessment should also address how staff members incorporate the needs and characteristics of "age-specific" groups. "This doesn't mean that every performed procedure requires the identification of an associated age-related competency. Rather, competence assessment should determine if staff remain knowledgeable about the physical, psychosocial, and emotional characteristics and needs associated with aging, and how these affect care delivery" (Herringer, 2002, p. 22). In other words, staff members are expected to remain competent in working with the age groups for which they are providing service, so if they work only with children, they would not be expected to demonstrate competence in working with older adults. For instance, the fact that older adults may have limitations in vision and in hearing dictates how the therapist will communicate with the older client and how these issues are incorporated within evaluation to adequately assess performance and to determine appropriate interventions to enhance performance.

## The Continuing Competence Process

When an occupational therapist or occupational therapy assistant does not use particular knowledge and skills, he or she becomes less competent in those unused skills and practices. However, the therapist or assistant becomes increasingly competent and skilled in those areas that are the most pertinent to the job and are thus used often in daily practice. Consequently, the process of remaining competent is complex and is complicated by several factors, including difficulties in reaching agreement on (a) which competencies to develop and to measure, (b) the criteria on which competency should be judged, (c) a cutoff point between being competent and incompetent, (d) which competency characteristics are most likely to influence competency, and (e) how best to address other parameters of competency.

## Difficulty in Reaching Agreement on
## Which Competencies to Develop and to Measure

Because the domain of the profession's concern is broad, the context in which practice occurs is varied, and the ability to enact the occupational therapy domain and process depends on a wide range of knowledge and skills, it is almost impossible to come to consensus on the competencies that, when measured, result in a determination of whether one is competent. Professions are dynamic and change focus and practice methods in concert with shifts in society. Therefore, professionals and technicians are always assuming new roles, revising their body of knowledge, and dealing with new problems. Today, occupational therapists might use physical agent modalities, operate computers, and perform job analyses—all of which were not a common part of occupational therapy's practice domain 10 years ago.

Most professions, including occupational therapy, are concerned primarily with methods for judging only entry-level practice competence or the potential capacity to meet the threshold requirements of an entry-level position. Note that entry-level certification from NBCOT and initial state license or certification establishes only that an occupational therapist or occupational therapy assistant is competent for general practice at that point in time. After initial entry-level certification, the profession does not have an agreed-on standard process for ensuring competency over time and for promoting the process of continuing competence.

The problem in creating a national method for ensuring competency beyond an entry level (e.g., NBCOT's voluntary certification renewal program) or in using a state approach for ensuring competency beyond entry level (e.g., in the form of state licensure or certification renewal) is that practice diverges according to the context in which the occupational therapist or occupational therapy assistant works. Statewide and national methods to ensure competency beyond the entry level are based on the assumption that general competencies exist that must be maintained by every occupational therapist and occupational therapy assistant regardless of practice area or regardless of the professional roles one assumes. In fact, these general competencies involve practicing the core of occupational therapy, which is discussed further in a later section in this chapter.

In addition to the general competencies that allow one to call oneself an occupational therapist or an occupational therapy assistant, each provider of occupational therapy develops expertise and advanced skills that are different from the expertise and advanced skills of other therapists and assistants. In fact, advanced practice means that an individual becomes an expert, most often in a specialized area or areas of practice, and becomes less competent in other areas. Because the set of competencies varies greatly from one work setting to another and from one job description to another within the same work setting, the employer or the owner of the independent practice along with each occupational therapist and assistant must take a greater role in ensuring competency and promoting continuing competence. According to Decker and Strader (1997), four types of competencies can be found within a work setting: (a) those that are generic across all jobs in an organization, (b) those that are related to management or supervision roles, (c) those that are threshold or that are the minimum requirements of a job, and (d) those that are specific to a job.

Depending on the organization, generic competencies for all employees might involve demonstrating respect for the client, being accountable for completion of one's job tasks with minimal supervision, using decision-making and problem-solving skills, supporting the organization's values and goals, and demonstrating a customer service orientation (Decker, 1999).

Management competencies relate to managing budgets; developing, marketing, implementing, and revising or discontinuing client programs; hiring, supervising, and training personnel; assigning work and managing workflow; and assessing program outcomes and quality to inform changes in program processes. Management competencies have shifted "from recruitment to reengineering, direct service to multiple service models, department to program management, professional standards to market-driven standards, and single-system to multisystem management" (Schell & Slater, 1998, p. 744). When managing multiple sites of service delivery, other important competencies include the ability to identify and implement flexible staffing, the ability to use communication technologies, and the ability to create service delivery models that are consistent with the core values of the profession.

Threshold or minimum requirements reflect one's license or scope of practice and one's entry-level education as an occupational therapist or occupational therapy assistant. The profession expects that occupational therapists can implement and that assistants can support the occupational therapy process to refer and screen, evaluate, plan interventions, carry out interventions, plan discharges, terminate therapy services, and measure outcomes, each step of which is appropriately focused on the domain of occupational therapy—fostering and supporting engagement in occupations and participation within relevant social and physical contexts (Moyers, 1999). These threshold requirements are modified by the precise nature of the particular job. For example, the occupational therapist in an elementary school setting might need to demonstrate proficiency in competencies addressing the occupational performance needs of children with learning disabilities who demonstrate perceptual–motor problems that interfere with learning.

Within each of these four general categories of competencies, an unlimited number of specific competencies can be generated. Generating the wrong competencies or creating too many competencies leads to frustration and to a view that one is merely satisfying requirements of external stakeholders, and it promotes little understanding of how the competency program is pertinent to practice and truly affects client outcomes. Instead, the goal is for the employer or independent practice owner to select in consultation with the occupational therapists and occupational therapy assistants only those competencies that result in superior client outcomes.

What constitutes a superior client outcome is partially driven by the profession in terms of evidence but also includes specific expectations delineated by the clients themselves (Decker, 1999). Client satisfaction is a source of data about these client expectations, and it indicates the level of respect that the independent practice provider or organization has for meeting client needs. Clients also have expectations related to access, cost, and quality of the services (Decker & Strader, 1997). Quality involves reliability, effectiveness, timeliness, and courtesy (McLaughlin & Kaluzny, 1994).

Competencies generated from expert opinion alone may not improve outcomes the way that competencies arising from a combination of expert opinion and client expectations can improve outcomes. For instance, expert opinion may lead the occupational therapist and occupational therapy assistant to develop skills in delivering a specific intervention method when the client population may not consider that particular method to be a viable intervention option given its expense or the level of commitment it demands from the client in its use.

In addition, competencies are selected only when outcomes are less than what is expected to be achieved. If client outcomes are excellent, then one may assume that the staff is competent (Decker, 1999). If outcomes indicate room for improvement, competencies should be delineated and measured in terms of the key areas that have the potential for improving the client outcomes. Often, these key areas from which competencies are derived involve (a) reducing "high-risk" behaviors that routinely result in poor client outcomes (e.g., incorrectly implementing an often-used evaluation or intervention) or (b) increasing the frequency of "low-volume" behaviors that, when occurring infrequently, lead to poor client outcomes (e.g., infrequent assessment of pain). Decker and Strader (1997) have found that health care organizations with a focus on outcome improvement tend to generate competencies that address whether the provider of client care (a) practices a customer focus (client-centered practice), (b) practices information management, (c) participates in performance improvement, (d) controls costs, (e) protects the rights of clients, (f) satisfies clients and other customers, (g) practices infection control, and (h) practices safety management.

## Difficulty in Reaching Agreement on the Criteria by Which Competency Should Be Judged

Recall that competency is a comparison of current performance with standards. Who sets these standards for judging performance once competencies have been delineated? AOTA sets the standards for entry-level competence, not only in accrediting entry-level educational programs for the occupational therapist and the occupational therapy assistant but also through formulating official documents such as "Standards of Practice for Occupational Therapy" (AOTA, 1998), *Code of Ethics* (AOTA, 2000), *Roles and Responsibilities of the Occupational Therapist and the Occupational Therapy Assistant During the Delivery of Occupational Therapy Services* (AOTA, 2002c), "Guide to Occupational Therapy Practice" (Moyers, 1999), *Occupational Therapy Practice Framework* (AOTA, 2002b), and various practice guidelines. NBCOT, through its practice analysis as well as development and administration of the initial certification examination, reflects and measures knowledge of these standards for entry-level practice. State regulatory boards determine what requirements must be met before one can begin practicing in a given jurisdiction.

However, continuing competence and maintaining competency as one gains expertise and experience involves more than maintaining entry-level, practice-related occupational therapy skills. Continuing competence and ongoing competency must begin with the individual. AOTA recognizes that each therapist and assistant is ultimately responsible for maintaining competence and, thus, has adopted the "Standards for Continuing Competence" (1999), by which one can judge efforts in developing and maintaining a program of continuing competence (see the section in this chapter titled "Competence With a Core Belief in Occupation").

The employer or independent practice owner must work with its occupational therapists and occupational therapy assistants to determine the criteria by which to judge performance on the work-related competencies that are generated from an understanding of client outcomes. This process involves identifying critical behaviors associated with the competencies and establishing methods for validation or evaluation of these critical behaviors (Decker & Strader, 1997). The key to identifying critical behaviors is to select from all the possible behaviors of the occupational therapist and the occupational therapy assistant those behaviors that best exemplify the intent of the competencies. The idea is to develop a narrow list of critical behaviors so one is not needlessly testing all possible tasks implied within the competencies. One should eliminate from this small list of critical behaviors any behaviors that most employees perform adequately because these behaviors will not discriminate between competent and incompetent employees.

Validation of critical behaviors involves a process through which the employer ascertains whether the occupational therapist and the occupational therapy assistant perform the behavior according to standard. Validation may involve the supervisor directly observing the performance of the employee, or it may involve simulation, paper-and-pencil tests, client satisfaction surveys, medical record audits, skills checklists, client case conferences or rounds, or peer reviews. The supervisor, in conjunction with the occupational therapist and the occupational therapy assistant, makes a decision (a) about the best way to determine proof of the critical behavior (e.g., Is the critical behavior best evaluated through medical record audit, or is observation best?) and (b) about the number of or the most effective combination of validation methods needed for measuring each of these competencies (e.g., Should one use observation and medical record audit?).

## Difficulty in Reaching Agreement on the Cutoff Point Between Being Competent and Incompetent

It is not possible to precisely determine an exact point when an error in performance means that one is incompetent. Hansen, Hinojosa, Schroeder, and Sands (1992), when discussing the future of occupational therapy practice, concluded that competency is complex because of its fluid and multidimensional nature. Within the context of one's job, they describe competencies as arising from client outcomes and from evidence generated within the profession's body of knowledge. Obviously, the criteria for determining whether one is competent or incompetent are subjective and depend on the tolerance for error when performing one's job tasks. The supervisor must remember that error-free performance is not consistently possible from all employees. In fact, to raise the average performance of critical behaviors, the supervisor may need to redesign the job to prevent errors. For example, perhaps occupational therapists and occupational therapy assistants would enable the client to progress faster if the assessment instruments available were changed to ones that more sensitively measured small gradations of change and, thus, more quickly triggered a need for modifications in the intervention plan.

Ultimately, the supervisor must decide whether the occupational therapist or occupational therapy assistant possesses the minimal knowledge and skills required for performance on the job. If judged to be incompetent in most of the delineated competencies and their associated critical behaviors, the occupational therapist or the occupational therapy assistant would normally be immediately suspended from duties until the problem could, if possible, be corrected. If the problem were not correctable, then the supervisor would have no choice but to begin the process of disciplinary action, which could lead to firing and to a report of the concern to the state regulatory board and to NBCOT. However, the question remains: How many incompetent ratings for how many observations on how many competencies addressing how many client outcomes lead to a determination of being incompetent? The difficulty in determining incompetence is that the supervisor must balance protection of the client's safety against making sure that the occupational therapist and occupational therapy assistant have been treated fairly by the competency validation process. In some cases, any evidence of missing critical behaviors, especially those associated with threshold competencies, is so significant that there is little tolerance for error.

## Difficulty in Reaching Agreement on Which Competency Characteristics Are Most Likely to Influence Competency

Competency is determined by the person's unique personality, ethics, philosophy, social conscience, intellectual ability, and mental and physical state (Grey, 1997). Obviously, a person's personality will affect whether the person is committed, willing, or prepared to engage in continuing competence activities. Spencer and Spencer (1993) described five types of competency characteristics that involve the following: (a) one's motives to change; (b) one's traits or tendencies to respond in a consistent manner; (c) one's self-concept, including attitudes, values, or self-image; (d) one's knowledge or the information one knows about specific content areas; and (e) one's skills or ability to perform certain physical or mental tasks.

Most organizational accrediting bodies such as JCAHO limit discussion of competency characteristics to knowledge, psychomotor skills, critical thinking, and interpersonal skills (Decker & Strader, 1997). These taxonomies do not include the more hidden competency characteristics involving motives, traits, and self-concept. Knowledge and skill competencies can be developed through training, whereas motives and traits are more difficult to assess and to influence through training. Consequently, during the hiring process, the employer may need to specifically examine who is the most qualified in terms of all the competencies needed, not just in terms of necessary knowledge and skills.

The Civil Rights Act of 1964 (amended 1972, 1991) or the Equal Employment Opportunity Commission's selection or affirmative action guidelines (Decker & Strader, 1997) do not prohibit per se an employer from basing hiring decisions on the possession of all the essential competency characteristics, including motives and attitudes. Discrimination occurs when hiring decisions adversely affect the protected class of employees, those in the minority because of race, ethnicity, religion, gender, and so forth. The employer avoids accusations of discrimination when these hidden competency characteristics are clearly connected with the critical behaviors of interest, especially with respect to how these critical behaviors are representative of the competencies most likely to affect client outcomes. Competencies must be written clearly and the critical behaviors related to them must be measurable to ensure that performance expectations are consistent for all those with specific job responsibilities.

## Difficulty in Reaching Agreement on How Best to Address Other Parameters of Competency

The ability to problem solve and perform is complex and is influenced not only by multiple variables but also by the interaction among those variables. Competency is not always located solely in the person and may arise as an interaction between the person's competency characteristics and a combination of factors within the environment or the organization in which one works (Batalden, 1998). For instance, health care professionals who work together on the same case as a team affect outcomes. Similarly, whether an organization values employee learning as a part of improving client outcomes is specific to the organization and can be ascertained by examining the organization's financial support of its employees' professional development activities and by examining whether leaders support the application of the employees' learning to change systems. Finally, some competency programs may appear to be heavily influenced by the latest management or health care issue rather than result from a focus on systematic change. For example, the generation of multiple nationally sponsored practice guidelines may cause problems when employers base organizational change and new competency expectations solely on this type of expert recommendation rather than determine which competencies would be most relevant and consistent with the organization's mission, more likely supported within the specific organizational context, and therefore more likely able to improve client outcomes.

## Competence With a Core Belief in Occupation

All occupational therapists and occupational therapy assistants share unique occupational therapy knowledge, interpersonal abilities, performance skills, and critical and ethical reasoning skills that become integrated into each professional role and its corresponding responsibilities. In this shared core is knowledge about occupations and human activities as well as their impact on human performance. Additionally, occupational therapists and occupational therapy assistants share unique skills in the areas of activity analysis, activity synthesis, critical problem solving about occupational performance, and ethical reasoning. This core reflects a shared worldview of people as occupational beings who seek to engage and participate in meaningful and purposeful activities. Maintaining competence requires that occupational therapy practitioners continually refine and update their knowledge, skills, and attitudes in those areas that make up the core of occupational therapy.

### AOTA Standards for Continuing Competence
In 1999, AOTA adopted "Standards for Continuing Competence" (Exhibit 20.1). These five standards establish the principal criteria by which each practitioner should examine competence. They should be used with AOTA's "Standards of Practice for Occupational Therapy" (1998) and its *Code of Ethics* (2000). These standards help occupational therapists and occupational therapy assistants build on their understanding of the core of occupational therapy when assessing, maintaining, and documenting competence.

### AOTA Continuing Competence Plan for Professional Development
AOTA's Continuing Competence Plan for Professional Development (Hinojosa et al., 1999, 2000a; see Figure 20.1) is a self-initiated approach that encourages each occupational therapist and occupational therapy assistant to develop an individualized plan to meet his or her own competency and continuing competence learning needs. This plan consists of eight components that together form a dynamic continuum (Figure 20.1): (a) Use triggers to determine need for self-assessment, (b) examine responsibilities, (c) perform a self-assessment, (d) identify needs in light of the "Standards for Continuing Competence," (e) develop a plan for continuing competence, (f) implement the continuing competence plan, (g) document professional development and changes in performance, and (h) implement changes in the plan and demonstrate continuing

## Exhibit 20.1  AOTA's Standards for Continuing Competence.

**Standard 1. Knowledge:** Occupational therapy practitioners shall demonstrate understanding and comprehension of the information required for the multiple roles they assume. The individual must

- integrate mastery of the core of occupational therapy into the multiple roles assumed;
- maintain up-to-date knowledge of appropriate professional Association documents and demonstrate application of this information to practice;
- demonstrate a commitment to lifelong learning;
- document subject matter expertise associated with primary roles;
- demonstrate an understanding of current literature related to primary roles and to the consumer population(s) served; and
- demonstrate knowledge of legislative, legal, and regulatory issues related to practice and the roles assumed.

**Standard 2. Critical Reasoning:** Occupational therapy practitioners shall employ reasoning processes to make sound judgments and decisions within the context of their roles. The individual must

- apply deductive and inductive reasoning in making decisions specific to roles and functions;
- demonstrate problem-solving skills required in assumed roles;
- assess, and when necessary and feasible, modify contextual factors that influence performance;
- integrate information from a variety of sources to formulate actions and to make decisions; and
- reflect on one's own practice to develop revised strategies for action, to make future decisions, and to guide professional development needs.

**Standard 3. Interpersonal Abilities:** Occupational therapy practitioners shall develop and maintain their professional relationships with others within the context of their roles. The individual must

- demonstrate effective communication skills;
- use methods of communication that match the abilities, learning styles, and therapeutic needs of consumers and others;
- demonstrate professional behavior;
- use feedback from consumers, families, supervisors, and colleagues to modify one's professional behavior; and
- collaborate with consumers, families, and professionals to attain consumer outcomes.

**Standard 4. Performance Skills:** Occupational therapy practitioners shall demonstrate the expertise, aptitudes, proficiencies, and abilities to competently fulfill their roles. The individual must

- demonstrate practice grounded in the core of occupational therapy,
- demonstrate the skilled performances required to succeed in roles,
- use resources needed to perform roles,
- evaluate and incorporate technology as appropriate, and
- update performance based on current research and literature.

(*continued*)

**Exhibit 20.1**  *(Continued)*

**Standard 5. Ethical Reasoning:** Occupational therapy practitioners shall identify, analyze, and clarify ethical issues or dilemmas in order to make responsible decisions within the changing context of their roles. The individual must

- understand and adhere to the profession's Code of Ethics as well as other applicable codes of ethics;
- accept responsibility for self-directed learning by defining learning objectives, planning a professional development program, and evaluating progress;
- identify ethical principles and core values and attitudes that are applicable to changing situations and use these principles to resolve ethical dilemmas;
- identify and examine ethical dilemmas using ethical reasoning to guide decisions and actions; and
- reflect on the results of ethical decision making.

*Note.* Adopted by AOTA Representative Assembly, 1999. From "Standards for Continuing Competence," by AOTA, 1999, *American Journal of Occupational Therapy, 53,* pp. 559–560. Copyright 1999 by the American Occupational Therapy Association. Reprinted with permission.

competence. A therapist or assistant can start at any point on the continuum and continue with the process.

### Use Triggers

Triggers are events or circumstances in the job setting that necessitate a person to examine his or her knowledge, skills, or attitudes. Triggers can come from many sources, including changes in the individual, government regulations, marketplace, or the profession itself. Triggers can be gradual or sudden. They can be significant events or minor changes in the system. Triggers are changes beyond the person's control that affect the person's ability to carry out his or her job responsibilities in an efficient and competent manner. Hinojosa and colleagues (2000a) identified six common triggers: "(a) return to clinical practice after years of absence, (b) practice in isolation without a professional support system, (c) employer-mandated productivity that may endanger delivery of safe and effective consumer services, (d) multiple job-site assignments within a short period, (e) an unsatisfactory job performance rating, and (f) personal objectives that may require changes in roles and responsibilities" (p. CE-2).

### Examine Responsibilities

At this point in the process, the occupational therapist, the occupational therapy assistant, or perhaps a supervisor must reflect on the responsibilities and expertise needed to skillfully produce the desired outcomes or performances. This examination of responsibilities begins when the therapist and the assistant reflect on practice and ask several questions, including the following: What are the expectations of the position or role? What are the responsibilities and requirements of the situation? What skills are needed? What advanced knowledge is desirable? What expectations do others have? Have

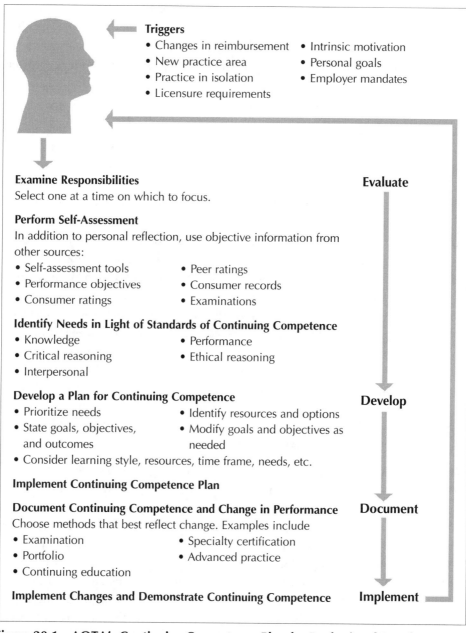

**Figure 20.1   AOTA's Continuing Competence Plan for Professional Development.**

*Note.* From "Self-Initiated Continuing Competence," by Hinojosa, J., Bowen, R., Case-Smith, J., Epstein, C., Moyers, P., & Schwope, C. *OT Practice, 5*(24), (December, 2000), CE1–CE8. Copyright 2000 by AOTA. Reprinted with permission.

changes occurred in technology, consumer expectations, employer demands, systems, community, or my personal life that may affect performance? For example, if a therapist were to be asked to assume responsibilities for supervising occupational therapy students, he or she would have to answer each of these questions in terms of what new responsibilities would be added to his or her job that are related to student learning and supervision of entry-level occupational therapists or occupational therapy assistants.

### Perform a Self-Assessment

Self-assessment provides the means by which occupational therapists and occupational therapy assistants develop goals and plans for professional growth, reassess current goals, assess performance, analyze demands and resources of the work environment, and interpret information about the consumers' outcomes. To develop a continuing competence plan, a therapist or assistant should engage in formalized methods of self-assessment (e.g., self-assessment tools, performance observation, consumer and peer ratings or reports, and intervention records). Using all the information available, a therapist or assistant then synthesizes the information and reflects on his or her assets and limitations in performing expected or assigned responsibilities.

Annual performance evaluations provide a natural opportunity to conduct a self-assessment for development of a continuing competence plan. This annual evaluation provides an opportunity to view a person's responsibilities, skills, and expertise within the context of the institutional goals and expectations. A review of the prior year's plan can validate the existing plan and provide valuable information to the individual and his or her supervisor about how effective selected activities have been in maintaining competence. Realize, however, that triggers, as indicated earlier, may require the plan be updated before the yearly performance evaluation.

### Identify Needs in Light of the Standards for Continuing Competence

The next component of the continuing competence plan is to systemically compare one's learning needs against the "Standards for Continuing Competence" (i.e., knowledge, critical reasoning, interpersonal abilities, performance skills, and ethical reasoning). After defining the responsibilities of one's primary roles in a given employment setting, the therapist or assistant reflects on current performance in each area of responsibility as measured against each of the standards. For instance, is the learning need related to lack of knowledge or to problems in applying knowledge during the critical reasoning process? While reflecting on each standard, the therapist or assistant creates a list of job performance areas in which one's knowledge, critical reasoning, interpersonal abilities, performance skills, and ethical reasoning do not match what is required in one's professional role. Additionally, a therapist or assistant may create a list of areas for growth in one's career.

### Develop a Continuing Competence Plan

Developing a continuing competence plan involves four steps: (a) prioritizing needs based on the self-assessment and the "Standards for Continuing Competence"; (b) reviewing current goals and objectives or developing goals and objectives (expected outcomes); (c) identifying resources and options; and (d) modifying goals and objectives in view of resources, individual learning style, and personal needs.

When selecting resources and options for learning, one not only must focus the learning strategy on evidence-based content but also must use learning strategies that are shown to improve client outcomes. Learning is more likely to translate into a change in practice when it includes interactive components such as role-playing, case discussion, or opportunities to practice skills (Thomson O'Brien et al., 2002). Studies are indicating the importance of using multiple learning activities that are selected specifically to target particular learning needs instead of relying primarily on the traditional continuing education experience that includes workshops, lectures, and conferences (Jordan, 2000). Single learning strategies have little or no effect on translating knowledge into practice (Bero, Grilli, Grimshaw, Oxman, & Thomson, 1998; Davis, Thomson, Oxman, & Haynes, 1995; Oxman, Thomson, Davis, & Haynes, 1995). Particular methods might be better for enhancing knowledge than for affecting interpersonal abilities. Improving interpersonal abilities might require the use of role-playing and video feedback, whereas knowledge acquisition could result from a self-study program of completing readings. Critical and ethical reasoning might be fostered through case studies and discussions (Slater & Cohn, 1991), through reflective writing (Jasper, 1999; Roberts, 2002), and through working either with a mentor (Andrews & Wallis, 1999; Schemm & Bross, 1995; Wilding & Marais-Strydom, 2002) or with a continuing professional development group (Errington & Robertson, 1998; McDonald, 2002). Performance skill development may require practice and demonstration to a rater who judges performance against a criterion (Thomson O'Brien et al., 2002).

### Implement Continuing Competence Plans

A continuing competence plan must be based on desired and realistic outcomes. Further, a continuing competence plan must be administratively feasible, publicly credible, professionally acceptable, legally defensible, and economically feasible (National Council of State Boards of Nursing, 1997). Once a continuing competence plan has been developed and is consistent with these criteria, it needs to be implemented.

An important aspect of the continuing competence plan is identification of the most appropriate methods for assessing and documenting outcomes for each of the specific self-competence goals. The field has no one best system of assessing outcomes. *AOTA's Continuing Competence Plan for Professional Development* recommends three methods: (a) examination (multiple-choice, computer adaptive testing, case simulation), (b) portfolio (see next section for detailed information about portfolios), and (c) outcome education (academic, continuing education). At this point in the process, the therapist or assistant implements the continuing competence plan. This component is not rigid, and any plan should allow for modification or changes in the learning needs to be addressed, the outcome goals, and the learning strategies.

### Document Continuing Competence and Change in Performance

The documentation of the continuing competence plan is important to allow ongoing evaluation of competence and to enable the individual to meet certification and licensure requirements. Some methods of formal assessment and methods for documenting continuing competence activities are multiple-choice examinations, adaptive testing, and case simulation (Grossman, 1997; Hinojosa et al., 1999). These summative evaluations should be used less frequently than the formative, informal methods of self-assessment described earlier.

A highly recommended method of demonstrating continuing competence involves using a portfolio. In a portfolio, the therapist or assistant collects evidence that supports his or her competence. Portfolios contain a person's vita, performance evaluations, consumer reports, documentation of professional accomplishments (e.g., papers, videotapes, articles), and a complete listing of continuing education activities. An individual's vita documents the person's academic record, involvement in professional activities, committee appointments and positions, awards, and honors. Portfolios summarize an individual's career development and are individualized to a person's continuing competence plan. Many credentialing agencies and licensure boards recognize portfolios as an effective method for establishing a person's professional competence.

### Implement Changes and Demonstrate Continuing Competence

Ultimately, an occupational therapist or occupational therapy assistant engages in continuing competence activities to ensure competent practice that should translate into improved client outcomes. However, many factors influence the outcome of any continuing competence plan. Consequently, the process to change practice patterns or behaviors is complex and is best accomplished through a multidimensional approach beyond the efforts of a single occupational therapist or occupational therapy assistant. A change in practice as the result of a continuing competence plan depends on the following: (a) employers recognizing the effect of social systems on change efforts, (b) congruency among employees and employers on the nature of change and its enactment within the organization, (c) participation of occupational therapists and occupational therapy assistants in the design and achievement of practice changes, (d) flexibility of administrative rules (e.g., institutional policies and procedures, standards from organizational accrediting bodies, state licensure renewal processes, voluntary certification renewals), (e) quality of the feedback on the attempts of occupational therapists and occupational therapy assistants to alter practice, and (f) the relationship of financial incentives to demonstration of competency and continuing competence efforts (e.g., promotions, bonuses, awards and recognition, career ladders) (Greco, 1993; Peden, Rose, & Smith, 1990).

## Conclusion

The main point of this chapter is that assessment and maintenance of one's competency to practice as an occupational therapist or as an occupational therapy assistant will gain increasing importance. The issue of competency is complex because of the hidden competency characteristics that involve attitudes and motivations toward change. Thus, professional development and promotion of continuing competence should begin within the academic portion of the occupational therapy curriculum, should be modeled not only by faculty but also by fieldwork supervisors, and should be supported by the employers of those who are maintaining competency. Effective continuing competence management is based on an understanding of how a change in one's own practice patterns best occurs. The changing of practice patterns or behaviors is complex and is best accomplished through a multidimensional approach. Thus, competency and continuing competence depend on the interaction among the competency characteristics of the individual, the nature of the learning needs with respect to affecting client outcomes, the type of learning methods selected, the change process involved when incorporating learning into practice, and the way the change in behavior is supported over time.

# References

Alsop, A. (2001). Competence unfurled: Developing portfolio practice. *Occupational Therapy International, 8,* 126–131.

American Occupational Therapy Association. (1998). Standards of practice for occupational therapy. *American Journal of Occupational Therapy, 52,* 866–869.

American Occupational Therapy Association. (1999). Standards for continuing competence. *American Journal of Occupational Therapy, 53,* 559–560.

American Occupational Therapy Association. (2000). *Code of ethics.* Bethesda, MD: Author.

American Occupational Therapy Association. (2002a). *Model continuing competence guidelines for occupational therapists and occupational therapy assistants: A resource for state regulatory boards.* Bethesda, MD: Author.

American Occupational Therapy Association. (2002). Occupational therapy practice framework: Domain and process. *American Journal of Occupational Therapy,* Bethesda, MD: Author

American Occupational Therapy Association. (2002c). *Roles and responsibilities of the occupational therapist and the occupational therapy assistant during the delivery of occupational therapy services.* Bethesda, MD: Author.

Andrews, M., & Wallis, M. (1999). Mentorship in nursing: A literature review. *Journal of Advanced Nursing, 29,* 201–207.

Barnett, R. (1994). *The limits of competence.* Buckingham, England: Society for Research Into Higher Education/Open University Press.

Batalden, P. (1998). If improvement of the quality and value of health and health care is the goal, why focus on health professional development? *Quality Management in Health Care, 6,* 52–61.

Bero, L., Grilli, R., Grimshaw, H. E., Oxman, D., & Thomson, M. A. (1998). Closing the gap between research and practice: An overview of systematic reviews of interventions to promote the implementation of research findings. *British Medical Journal, 317,* 465–468.

Civil Rights Act of 1964. Pub. L. 88-352, 42 U.S.C., Ch. 21 § 1981–2000.

Davis, D., Thomson, M., Oxman, A., & Haynes, R. (1995). Changing physician performance. A systematic review of the effect of continuing medical education strategies. *Journal of the American Medical Association, 274*, 700–705.

Decker, P. J. (1999). The hidden competencies of healthcare: Why self-esteem, accountability, and professionalism may affect hospital customer satisfaction scores. *Hospital Topics, 77*, 14.

Decker, P. J., & Strader M. K. (1997). Beyond JCAHO: Using competency models to improve healthcare organizations, Part 1. *Hospital Topics, 75*, 23.

Errington, E., & Robertson, L. (1998). Promoting staff development in occupational therapy: A reflective group approach. *British Journal of Occupational Therapy, 61*, 497–503.

Greco, P. J. (1993). Changing physicians' practices. *New England Journal of Medicine, 329*, 1271–1274.

Grey, R. (1997). *Developing and maintaining professional competence.* New York: New York State Society of Certified Public Accountants.

Grossman, J. (1997). *A study of the professions.* White Plains, NY: MAGI Educational Services.

Hansen, R., Hinojosa, J., Schroeder, C., & Sands, M. (1992). *Advanced practice review: A preliminary examination of the practice of experienced occupational therapist registered and certified occupational therapy assistants.* Rockville, MD: American Occupational Therapy Association.

Herringer, J. M. (2002). Once isn't enough when measuring staff competence. *Nursing Management, 33*(2), 22.

Hinojosa, J. (1985). Implications for occupational therapy of a competency-based orientation. *American Journal of Occupational Therapy, 39*, 539–541.

Hinojosa, J., & Blount, M. L. (1998). Nationally speaking: Professional competence. *American Journal of Occupational Therapy, 52*, 699–701.

Hinojosa, J., Bowen, R., Case-Smith, J., Epstein, C., Schwope, C., Moyers, P., et al. (1999). *Professional development for continuing competency.* Bethesda, MD: American Occupational Therapy Association.

Hinojosa, J., Bowen, R., Case-Smith, J., Epstein, C. F., Moyers, P., & Schwope, C. (2000). Self-initiated continuing competence. *OT Practice, 5*(24), CE1–CE8.

Jasper, M. A. (1999). Nurses' perceptions of the value of written reflection. *Nurse Education Today, 19*, 452–463.

Jordan, S. (2000). Educational input and patient outcomes: Exploring the gap. *Journal of Advanced Nursing, 31*, 461–471.

Kielhofner, G. (1992). *Concepts and foundations of occupational therapy.* Philadelphia: F. A. Davis.

McConnell, E. A. (2001). Competence vs. competency. *Nursing Management, 32*(5), 14.

McDonald, R. (2002). Developing a continuing professional development group in a social services setting. *British Journal of Occupational Therapy, 65*, 216–218.

McLaughlin, C. P., & Kaluzny, A. D. (1994). *Continuous quality improvement in healthcare.* Gaithersburg, MD: Aspen.

Mosey, A. C. (1992). *Applied scientific inquiry in the health professions: An epistemological orientation.* Rockville, MD: American Occupational Therapy Association.

Moyers, P. A. (1999). The guide to occupational therapy practice [Special issue]. *American Journal of Occupational Therapy, 53*, 247–322.

National Board for Certification in Occupational Therapy. (2002) *Certification renewal handbook.* Gaithersburg, MD: Author.

National Council of State Boards of Nursing. (1997). *Continued competence and the personal accountability profile.* Chicago: Author.

Oxman, A. D., Thomson, M. A., Davis, D. A., & Haynes, B. (1995). No magic bullets: A systematic review of 102 trials of interventions to improve professional practice. *Canadian Medical Association Journal, 153,* 1423–1431.

Peden, A. R., Rose, H., & Smith, M. (1990). Transfer of continuing education to practice: Testing an evaluation model. *Journal of Continuing Education in Nursing, 21,* 152–155.

Roberts, A. E. K. (2002). Advancing practice through continuing professional education: The case for reflection. *British Journal of Occupational Therapy, 65,* 237–241.

Schell, B. A. B., & Slater, D. Y. (1998). Management competencies required of administrative and clinical practitioners in the new millennium. *American Journal of Occupational Therapy, 52,* 744–750.

Schemm, R. L., & Bross, T. (1995). Mentorship experiences in a group of occupational therapy leaders. *American Journal of Occupational Therapy, 49,* 32–37.

Slater, D. Y., & Cohn, E. S. (1991). Staff development through analysis of practice. *American Journal of Occupational Therapy, 45,* 1038–1044.

Spencer, L. M., & Spencer, S. M. (1993). *Competence at work.* New York: Wiley.

Thomson, L. K., Lieberman, D., Murphy, R., Wendt, E., Poole, J., & Hertfelder, S. D. (1995). *Developing, maintaining, and updating competency in occupational therapy: A guide to self-appraisal.* Bethesda, MD: American Occupational Therapy Association.

Thomson O'Brien, M. A., Freemantle, N., Oxman, A. D., Wolf, F., Davis, D. A., & Herrin, J. (2002). Continuing education meetings and workshops: Effects on professional practice and health care outcomes (Cochrane Review). *The Cochrane Library* (Issue 2). Oxford, England: Update Software.

Wilding, C., & Marais-Strydom, E. (2002). MentorLink: An Australian example of continuing professional development through mentoring. *British Journal of Occupational Therapy, 65,* 224–226.

Yerxa, E. J. (1995). Nationally speaking—Who is the keeper of occupational therapy's practice and knowledge? *American Journal of Occupational Therapy, 49,* 295–299.

# Ethical Dimensions of Occupational Therapy Management

Karin J. Opacich, MHPE, OTR/L, FAOTA

*"Indeed, a concrete understanding of the good life presupposes an ordering, vision, or understanding of goods and harms, as much as any peaceable society presupposes authority from its members. As a consequence, morality in a secular society is the practice of doing the good within the bounds of moral authority across communities with disparate moral vision."*

H. TRISTAM ENGLEHARDT, JR.

**Karin J. Opacich, MHPE, OTR/L, FAOTA,** has a private practice, Opacich Consultative Services, in Chicago. She provides consultation to academic programs in the health care professions in the areas of curriculum development, revision, evaluation, and accreditation. She is completing her doctoral work in public health. Her dissertation research pertains to women with HIV, and it explores the relationship of occupations, health care services, and quality of life.

## Key Terms and Concepts

**Autonomy.** The right to make life decisions on one's own behalf.

**Beneficence.** Actively doing good.

**Confidentiality.** Nondisclosure of personal or privileged information.

**Deliberative justice.** Fairness in conceptualizing and planning programs or services intended to benefit certain people.

**Distributive justice.** Fairness in allocating social benefits.

**Ethical dilemma.** Potentially conflicting responses to an ethical problem.

**Ethical distress.** The result of being compelled to respond to an ethical problem in ways that are incongruent with one's moral code.

**Ethical uncertainty.** Ethically ambiguous situations.

**Fidelity.** Keeping promises.

**Nonmaleficence.** Refraining from causing or perpetuating harm.

**Retributive justice.** Compensation for harm or reallocation of social benefits.

**Social justice.** Fairness in the distribution of societal goods.

**Veracity.** Truthfulness.


## Learning Objectives

After completing this chapter, you should be able to do the following:

- Appreciate the complexity of delivering health care services when providers, payers, and consumers may represent different ethical perspectives and commitments.

- Recognize that all managerial decisions represent an ethical position.

- Delineate the responsibilities of a manager for maintaining the ethical integrity of occupational therapy endeavors.

- Anticipate ethical challenges and develop insight into ethical problem solving.

- Identify the mechanisms and documents within the profession that can provide guidance for ethical decision making.

G iven the complexity and fast pace of modern existence, occupational therapy managers must make decisions expediently. However, contemporary professional life seems to be fraught with ethical challenges. Occupational therapy managers need to recognize ethical content and prepare themselves to consider the impact of their decisions not only in terms of clinical efficacy and fiscal viability but also in terms of ethical integrity. Virtually every managerial decision represents an underlying ethical assumption or commitment.

## Defining the Ethical Enterprise

What is ethics? In short, ethics is the study of collective moral reasoning, a subject of considerable interest to philosophers from ancient to contemporary times. According to Monagle and Thomasma (1998), "*Ethics* is the pattern of values and norms that is 'taken for granted' in a given culture or professional or institutional setting" (p. 567, italics added). *Bioethics* is a term usually applied to ethical practices and tensions that are encountered when providing care and treatment for living beings in various states of physical and mental health. Some examples of bioethical issues are ownership of frozen embryos and criteria for brain death. Health care ethics represents broader ethical concerns related to access and the delivery of care and services. One of the most pressing questions reflecting health care ethics in the United States may be whether health is a right or a privilege. Because access to health care services is tied to economic resources, ethical questions arise about those who might be excluded.

In large part, ethics is about achieving justice, so ethics and laws are inextricably related. Although the law and ethics are not synonymous, managers must be alert to the effect of the law on clinical decisions. Specific legislation may determine the conditions of compliance or noncompliance with codified social ethics, for example, definitions of brain death and concomitant criteria for withdrawing life-sustaining treatment, but that legislation may not be as helpful in identifying ethical priorities for individuals or communities. Although laws enacted by a society primarily address distributive and retributive justice—in other words, who is entitled to what—ethical analysis might also encompass issues of deliberative justice and social justice. Deliberative justice refers to fairness in the recognition and planning phases. Social justice pertains to how members of a society are treated in light of the "natural lottery"—the circumstances of birth that are beyond an individual's control—circumstances such as gender, race, or ethnicity. Both perspectives are important to understand: Not all legal actions are ethical, and not all ethical actions are legal. Some seemingly ethical solutions may not be allowed under the law, and some legal remedies may insufficiently address ethical problems.

By virtue of being a member of the profession, occupational therapy practitioners espouse the values, commitments, and ethical obligations of their discipline. During entry-level professional education, aspiring occupational therapists study and explore the ethics of the profession, which is required in curricula by the *Standards for an Accredited Educational Program for the Occupational Therapist* (Accreditation Council for Occupational Therapy Education [ACOTE], 1998a) and *Standards for an Accredited Educational Program for the Occupational Therapy Assistant* (ACOTE, 1998b). Please refer to http://www.aota.org/nonmembers/area13/links/LINK31.asp. Philosophical statements embedded in the profession's historical documents and contemporary literature serve to guide and shape practice that is consistent with these commitments.

Occupational therapy practitioners commonly participate in both formal and informal ethical deliberations. Occupational therapy managers, in particular, are expected to attend to the interests of the host agency and to safeguard the ethical integrity of the professional discipline, which sometimes results in competing agendas. Consequently, the skills of recognizing, defining, and examining ethical tensions become necessary components of managerial decision making.

## Identifying Ethical Tensions

Affective cues may first alert health care professionals to ethical tensions. For example, a visceral response, a sense of threat to personal integrity, or an awareness of ambivalence about an action could indicate ethical tension. When a person acknowledges that tension exists, he or she must explore the dissonance to discern the underlying ethical causes.

The descriptions of ethical tensions developed by Jameton (1984) help us to identify three kinds of ethical tensions: ethical uncertainty, ethical dilemmas, and ethical distress. Ethical uncertainty occurs when situations are ambiguous and ethical content may be contributing to the confusion. The debate about the ethics of actively killing someone compared to simply letting someone die is a commonly cited example. In the United States, physician-assisted suicide is prohibited, whereas inaction in a case involving previously negotiated DNR (do not resuscitate) documentation is considered acceptable. One experiences ethical dilemmas when potential ethical responses are in conflict. These dilemmas require a reasoned response. And finally, ethical distress results when a person is or feels compelled to respond in ways that are counter to personal moral convictions. In any case, when a source of tension has ethical origins, further analysis is required. Just as clinical problems are rendered understandable by a process of naming and framing, ethical tensions are likewise clarified by the conceptual frames chosen to examine them. In general, responses to ethical tensions can be plotted along a continuum from ethically prohibited to ethically obligatory.

## Ethical Perspectives Applicable to the Health Care Arena

Specific theories and frameworks for analyzing ethical problems can be useful to map an array of ethical responses to a situation just as conceptual models and congruent tests and measures help to illuminate occupational performance problems to design interventions. Pojman (1998), in his comprehensive anthology *Classics of Philosophy*, divides ethical theories into categories, including utilitarianism, deontological (moral obligation) systems, and virtue-based systems. Numerous theories have been postulated within each category, and these can be explored through the literature. These ethical theories provide a perspective from which to evaluate and assess reasonable courses of action. In contrast, theories related to practice lead to specific interventions. The following sections describe four ethical perspectives that occupational therapy managers and practitioners might consider as they engage in ethical reasoning: principle-driven ethics, utilitarian ethics, an ethic of caring, and communitarianism.

## Principle-Driven Ethics

In medical environments, principle-driven ethics most often have been used by physicians and other health care providers to guide actions associated with benefits and burdens of medical interventions, for example, interventions that involve initiating, withholding, or withdrawing life-sustaining treatment and interventions when a person cannot speak on his or her own behalf. Four basic principles have traditionally been interpreted as central to bioethical deliberations: autonomy, beneficence, nonmaleficence, and justice. Many ethicists have provided interpretations of these principles, and *Principles of Biomedical Ethics* (Beauchamp & Childress, 1994) is among the most commonly used references. This resource provides basic definitions and comprehensive explanations that describe the application of these principles in health care.

Furthermore, the *Occupational Therapy Code of Ethics* (American Occupational Therapy Association [AOTA], 2000) is predicated on these universal ethical principles, and the code illustrates the relationship between the principles and the practice of occupational therapy. Please refer to http:// www.aota.org/general/coe.asp. Another important document, "Guidelines to the Occupational Therapy Code of Ethics" (AOTA, 1998), provides additional "statements of morally correct action" (p. 881) that describe the ethical commitments and conduct of practitioners engaging in various aspects of service delivery. A third document, "Core Values and Attitudes of Occupational Therapy Practice" (AOTA, 1993), elaborates on seven values that characterize the moral core of occupational therapy as a discipline and that established the foundation for a professional community constituted around these characteristics. Because the principles of autonomy, beneficence, nonmaleficence, and justice are frequently applied and used in professional literature, they will be briefly summarized in the sections that follow.

### *Autonomy*

*Autonomy* is the principle of self-governance. It pertains to liberty rights, the right to privacy, the right to individual choice, and the right to self-determination. In health care, autonomy is at issue in discussions of decisional competency, informed consent, disclosure of information, and acceptance or refusal of medically indicated treatment. Autonomy becomes more complicated and requires further clarification when care providers are dealing with children, pregnant adults or adolescents, persons with mental impairments or cognitive deficits, and persons who are unable to speak for themselves for any reason.

Many states have enacted legislation addressing autonomy. For instance, in the event that a medical condition impairs a person's autonomy, the law might authorize a surrogate or other health care agent to make decisions on that person's behalf. It is important for occupational therapy managers and the practitioners under their supervision to be aware of laws specific to the states in which they are practicing.

Because occupational therapists and occupational therapy assistants are often involved in team discussions and decisions, they may be called on to contribute observations or other data that reflect a patient's understanding of his or her condition and treatment options. Particularly when discussions ensue about self-defined quality of life, occupational therapy practitioners can contribute the perspective of meaningfulness in living and the way the person expresses it through occupations. In some instances, occupational therapy practitioners have the opportunity to serve on institutional ethics committees (Kyler-Hutchison, 1994). Occupational therapy managers can prepare staff members for these experiences by addressing ethical principles, relevant legislation, and accumulated professional wisdom.

### Beneficence

*Beneficence* refers to actions that benefit others, including acts of mercy, kindness, and charity. It implies both actively "doing good" and considering the potential harm of an action. Paternalism, the presumption that health care professionals know what is best or what will be of greatest benefit for a patient by virtue of their expertise, sometimes results in ethical tension. In today's climate, a patient's or client's participation in the selection of medical or health alternatives is preferred.

Weighing potential good against potential harm, those who analyze options must consider the benefit in light of risk, cost, and burden. Ideally, choices among treatment options are weighed by considering their value to the recipient of service. In the United States, the prevailing reimbursement structure does not always defer to what either providers or the recipients of care might consider most beneficent. Occupational therapy managers and practitioners must recognize that efficacy studies can attest to the outcomes and reflect both the actual and potential benefit of therapy. Making this evidence known increases the likelihood that practitioners will have the opportunity to act beneficently and that the potential good associated with their services will be actualized (Law, Baum, & Dunn, 2001; Mattingly & Fleming, 1994).

### Nonmaleficence

*Nonmaleficence* is inextricably related to beneficence; taken from the Hippocratic tradition, it means "doing no harm." Although debates occur frequently about the extent to which anyone is obligated to prevent or remove harm, the idea is generally accepted that a health care practitioner ought to refrain from inflicting harm. In the extreme, nonmaleficence is debated in relation to withdrawal of burdensome treatment, hastening death by withholding treatment, administering passive and active euthanasia, and making other decisions that affect the length and quality of life. In occupational therapy, ethical tensions relative to nonmaleficence may be less dramatic but nonetheless worthy of note. For instance, an occupational therapy practitioner who is unqualified to use physical agent modalities but who uses these modalities anyway risks inflicting harm and violates the principle of nonmaleficence. More subtly, practitioners who advise the use of techniques that are at the least very unpleasant and that do not demonstrate substantial evidence of any benefit beyond their burden likewise disregard the principle of nonmaleficence.

### Justice

*Justice* is a complex principle that generally relates to issues of equity and fairness. Most familiar to the public are aspects of justice often settled in the courts: (a) *distributive justice,* involving the allocation of property, control, or access to services, and (b) *retributive justice,* involving payment or reallocation of goods or services in light of unfair treatment.

When commodities are limited, as are most health-related resources, allocation is a primary ethical consideration within the perspective of justice. Note that consumers' access to occupational therapy services may be limited by lack of information, cost and reimbursement, location, limited workforce, and other issues inherent in the distribution of health and health-related services. Occupational therapy managers must decide how best to distribute the resources at hand using ethical criteria as well as fiscal and administrative appeals. These decisions explicitly or implicitly reflect notions of distributive justice.

If the services provided (or not provided) result in harm, the person or persons harmed might seek some sort of compensation or retribution, illustrating the notion of retributive justice. Malpractice actions are associated with retributive justice. To expand on these notions, Aday, Quill, and Reyes-Gibby (2001) addressed equity in the delivery of health care as either procedural or substantive, associating these approaches with deliberative, distributive, and social justice paradigms (see Table 21.1). Their model should be of interest to occupational therapy managers because it takes into account policy, organizational characteristics, and issues of access to services.

### Additional Principles Governing Relationships

In addition to the four basic principles described above—and no less important—are several principles governing relationships among health care providers and those receiving care. These principles are critical to establishing trust and form the basis for the covenant between patient and health care practitioners (May, 1975). The right to privacy is subsumed in the principle of autonomy, but the principle of confidentiality

**Table 21.1  Criteria and Indicators of Equity.**

| Dimensions | Criteria | Indicators |
|---|---|---|
| **Procedural Equity** | | |
| *Deliberative Justice* | | |
| Health policy | Participation | • Type and extent of affected groups' participation in formulating and implementing policies and progress |
| *Distributive Justice* | | |
| Delivery system | Freedom of choice | |
| • Availability | | • Distribution of providers |
| • Organization | | • Types of facilities |
| • Financing | | • Sources of payment |
| Realized access | Cost-effectiveness | |
| • Utilization | | • Type and volume of services used |
| • Satisfaction | | • Public opinion, patient opinion |
| *Distributive and Social Justice* | | |
| Population at risk | Similar treatment | |
| • Predisposing | | • Age, sex, race, education, etc. |
| • Enabling | | • Regular source, insurance coverage, income, etc. |
| • Need | | • Perceived, evaluated |
| *Social Justice* | | |
| Environment | Common good | |
| • Physical | | • Toxic, environmental hazards |
| • Social | | • Social capital (family structure, voluntary organizations, social networks) |
| • Economic | | • Human and material capital (schools, jobs, income, housing) |
| Health risks | Need | |
| • Environmental | | • Toxic, environmental exposures |
| • Behavioral | | • Lifestyle, health promotion practices |
| **Substantive Equity** | | |
| Health | Need | |
| • Individuals | | • Clinical indicators |
| • Community | | • Population rates |

*Note.* From *Evaluating the Healthcare System: Effectiveness, Efficiency, and Equity* (2nd ed.), by L. A. Aday, C. E. Begley, D. R. Lairson, and C. H. Slater, 1998, Chicago: Health Administration Press. Copyright 1998 by Health Administration Press. Reprinted with permission.

is often addressed separately as a unique feature of relationships. *Privacy* entails respecting a person's right to limit access to his or her personal sphere, whereas *confidentiality* connotes authorized disclosure or nondisclosure of personal information. Occupational therapy managers are ultimately responsible to see that staff members observe the established guidelines of privacy and confidentiality.

Two additional principles contribute to trusting relationships: veracity and fidelity. *Veracity* reflects a commitment to telling the truth. Whether an occupational therapist or occupational therapy assistant presents information about an individual's performance problems or the evidence of a particular approach's treatment effectiveness, his or her adherence to veracity requires accurate representation. Ethical debate sometimes occurs around the breadth and depth of truth telling as it relates to what a person is able to tolerate and absorb. The principle of *fidelity* invokes a commitment to keeping promises. Promise keeping is an expectation in relationships with patients, clients, and colleagues. Furthermore, keeping faith with the constructs and tenets of the discipline—in this instance, occupational therapy—can also be interpreted as an act of fidelity.

## Utilitarian Ethics

Utilitarian ethics, considered a pragmatic approach to problem solving, subscribes to a commitment to action that yields the greatest good for the greatest number. This model is grounded in liberty rights and is compatible with market-driven health care. Consequently, utilitarian ethics have been applied to many of the economic and business aspects of health care delivery. Rationing health care services is defensible from a utilitarian perspective. For example, the Canadian health care system endeavors to ensure fairness in the distribution of health and health services for Canadian citizens. Depending on the tax base of each province, decisions about health care spending and services are made to promote the best state of health possible for the most citizens given the resources at hand (Wilson, 1995).

## An Ethic of Caring

Each ethical perspective represents a particular priority by which to assess the benefits and the harms connected to a given action. Central to the ethic of caring is this question: Given this set of circumstances, what is the most caring way to respond? Caring involves not only actions to limit suffering but also actions to attend to the concomitant needs of people in distress. Furthermore, an ethic of caring can be particularly useful when crafting policy or programs for marginalized populations such as HIV-positive women. In addressing the shortcomings of other approaches to ethical decision making in health care, Monagle and Thomasma (1998) have synthesized a model of caring predicated on "friendship of an understanding heart" (p. 516) that incorporates caring along with ethical principles.[1] The ethically responsible creativity (ERC) model accommodates the scientific evidence that contributes to understanding of benefit and burden as well as the humanistic issues that lead to ethical actions sensitive to the needs of the suffering individual.

## Communitarianism

Communitarian ethics address the question, What action provides the greatest benefit for this particular community? Community can be a unit as small as a single family or a much larger collection of like-minded members. Individuals are seen in this context as extensions of a larger community, and options are weighed in light of the values, needs, and commitments of the entire community (Blustein, 1998). Ideally, when values are shared and the community functions harmoniously, ethical decisions relative to any individual member reflect the community ethos. This approach to ethical decision making may be particularly useful when addressing public health concerns and allocation of resources for a population-based endeavor (Aday, Begly, Lairson, & Slater, 1998).

## Clarifying Ethical Characteristics and Commitments of a Profession

Before examining the ethical duties and obligations of the occupational therapy manager, let us review three major functions of a profession with respect to ethics:
- Keeping faith with the tenets and principles of the discipline
- Preserving the integrity of the professional community
- Ensuring integrity of individual practitioners.

The following sections clarify ethical characteristics and commitments of the occupational therapy profession with respect to these functions.

## Keeping Faith With the Tenets and Principles of the Discipline

Occupational therapy managers oversee programs and services, and they are in a unique position to ensure that occupational therapy initiatives are consistent with the tenets, principles, and standards of the profession. For instance, occupational therapy managers who remain faithful to the discipline will embrace occupation-based practice in favor of forms of service that may not reflect the constructs central to the profession. Given the stated value of client-centered care, ethical occupational therapists and occupational therapy assistants will include potential consumers in the planning of services (deliberative justice) when they are developing programs. Given the ethical

---

[1]*Friendship* in the ERC model is based on the three levels of friendship described by Aristotle: to chresimon, to hedo, to agathon.

commitment to inclusion, occupational therapy managers will be compelled to consider who would be included and who might be excluded from planned occupational therapy services (social justice).

## Preserving the Integrity of the Professional Community

Because occupational therapists and occupational therapy assistants enter into covenantal relationships with people who by circumstance are vulnerable, the profession must accept a duty to determine the worthiness of those who endeavor to provide care. Professional gatekeeping safeguards the integrity of a profession and establishes criteria for the inclusion of members in the profession. Gatekeeping, or oversight of competency, occurs at points along the career continuum, beginning with admission to a program of study and extending to retirement from professional life. Each juncture poses a unique set of obligations and tensions relative to one or more of the following: (a) getting and maintaining accreditation of academic programs; (b) admitting qualified students to professional education; (c) supervising formative experiences in the field; (d) monitoring academic progress and verifying academic credentials; (e) maintaining professional registration, licensure, or both; (f) monitoring continuing professional competency; and (g) determining and upholding standards of practice. By tacit agreement, occupational therapy managers have a duty to attend to gatekeeping by providing fieldwork opportunities, ensuring professional credentials and competency of staff members, seeking and providing opportunities for staff members to evolve professionally, and ensuring the quality of services provided.

### *Providing Supervision in Fieldwork*

Preparation for virtually all health-related professions includes periods of supervised practice. Although beneficence is the guiding principle in both supervision of students and care of patients, the occupational therapy manager must also consider the potential benefits and harms to the student and the recipients of care in any supervisory arrangement. The 1998 iteration of the standards (ACOTE, 1998a, 1998b) has lifted the constraints on fieldwork to encourage the development of emerging arenas of practice that accentuate the need to consciously establish strategies that benefit all parties. Because the field currently has no formal mechanism for credentialing clinical educators, occupational therapy managers must assume ultimate responsibility for the quality and consistency of clinical education programs within the scope of their authority. However, wide variability exists in aptitude, skill, and commitment to fulfilling the role of clinical educator. Consequently, occupational therapy managers, in collaboration with academic programs, need to consider the realities of their settings and the resources that are necessary to provide beneficial learning opportunities and quality supervision that yield competent, entry-level occupational therapists and occupational therapy assistants.

## Ensuring Integrity of Individual Practitioners

Occupational therapy managers have a responsibility to establish a culture that encourages introspection and self-review as well as invites dialogue and respectful debate. Practitioners are most likely to thrive and grow within this kind of atmosphere. In an open community, members are more likely to hold each other accountable to adhere to high standards. A professional community will more likely build a community of character when it willingly recognizes and analyzes ethical tensions rather than expects clinical and ethical perfection. When tensions and problems do occur, the process of ethical reasoning before action is certainly preferable to the harms that can accrue as a result of ethical infractions. Occupational therapy managers have a duty to encourage staff members to explore their own value systems and broaden the scope of their ethical insights by reading and engaging in meaningful dialogue. Both ethical contemplation and clinical reasoning require perception, understanding, sensitivity, and accountability.

Occupational therapy managers also have a duty to create opportunities for practitioners to grow and cultivate knowledge and expertise. The first line of responsibility for maintaining and expanding professional competencies lies with the individual practitioner. However, members of the professional community may fail to fulfill their roles competently, and in those circumstances, both peers and supervisors must consider their duty to their competent colleagues and to the recipients of services with respect to the failure. Most ethical tensions related to clinical competence are resolved long before disciplinary action is unavoidable. Nevertheless, May (1975) observed long ago, "In professional ethics, the test of moral seriousness may depend not simply upon personal compliance with ethical principles, but upon the courage to hold others accountable" (p. 32).

## Codified Ethical Guidelines

The profession, through AOTA, has codified guidelines and expectations that address its ethical agenda and other agendas. Among the official documents addressing ethics are the following: *Occupational Therapy Code of Ethics* (AOTA, 2000; see http://www.aota.org/general/coe.asp); "Guidelines to the Occupational Therapy Code of Ethics" (AOTA, 1998; see http://www.aota.org/members/area2/links); "Core Values and Attitudes of Occupational Therapy Practice" (AOTA, 1993; see http://www.aota.org/members/area2/links); the *Standards for an Accredited Educational Program for the Occupational Therapist* (ACOTE, 1998a; see http://www.aota.org/nonmembers/area13/links); and the *Standards for an Accredited Educational Program for the Occupational Therapy Assistant* (ACOTE, 1998b; see http://www.aota.org/ nonmembers/area13/links). These documents have been crafted by communities of interest within the profession and represent positions officially adopted and embraced by AOTA. They are intended to guide the actions and endeavors of the membership to be consistent with the values and principles that they put forth. Whether occupational therapists or occupational therapy assistants are managers of people, finances, services, or resources, they all are expected to uphold the values and principles represented by these documents.

## Templates for Unraveling and Resolving Ethical Tensions

The first step in the process of ethical reasoning is to recognize ethical tensions. The second step is to become conversant in the language of ethics and ethical principles, which enables practitioners to articulate ethical tensions clearly and develop cogent arguments when ethical concerns are at stake. Using a systematic approach to unravel ambiguous ethical tension can prevent disproportionate reactions and lead to reasoned responses. The Savage (1990) model of ethical reasoning illustrates a step-by-step process for clarifying content and selecting ethically acceptable responses (see Exhibit 21.1).

**Exhibit 21.1  Savage Facilitation Model of Ethical Contemplation.**

---

1. Ascertain facts, impressions, rumors about situation at hand.
2. Verify information with key players.
3. Identify problems to be solved.
4. Sort decisions to be made (e.g., medical, legal, ethical, educational).
5. Identify range of options.
6. Identify ethical ramifications of those options (e.g., morally obligatory, morally permissible, and morally prohibited).
7. Participate in team discussion to plan conference with parties of interest. (Parties of interest means those who have an investment in the outcomes of the situation. Parties of interest may include patients, relatives, significant others, health care providers, administrators, etc.)
8. Discuss and resolve team conflict, and designate representatives to speak for team.
9. Discuss options with parties of interest.
10. Evaluate ethical soundness of decision.
11. Implement decision; assist with or abide by decision.
12. Reevaluate the decision and process by which the decision was made.
13. Provide support and respect for parties involved.
14. Reflect on your own involvement in the process; incorporate positive aspects into your own decision-making process.

---

*Note.* From *The Underground Role of the Nurse in Ethical Decision-Making,* by T. Savage, 1990, October. Paper presented at the University of Illinois College of Medicine Symposium, "A Time to Live . . . A Time to Die: Medical Ethics in the 90's," Rockford, IL. Copyright 1990 by T. Savage. Adapted with permission.

In evaluating the relative merit of those potential responses, Larry Churchill's (1986) continuum of moral responses can be useful. For any situation, some responses may be ethically prohibited and other responses will be ethically obligatory. Most responses can be plotted somewhere between these two polarities, and these would be considered ethically permissible. Depending on the ethical frame that is used to analyze the situation, some of those permissible responses will be more congruent and will reflect more of the priorities associated with a particular model than others.

Using a template to define ethical problems is especially useful for practitioners who are not primarily ethicists. Additionally, managers should become aware of other resources available to them when wrestling with ethical tensions. These resources can be found in a large, rapidly growing body of literature pertaining to ethics that encompasses ancient classics, publications applicable to health and health care delivery, and literature specific to the discipline. Occupational therapy managers should feel free to consult with ethicists within the discipline (at local, state, or national associations) who may be able to render insightful assistance. Many organizations and institutions have their own ethics consultants or committees designed to assist either formally or informally with ethical problem solving.

Ethical reasoning specific to patient care has become increasingly challenging. The development of elaborate technology, the costs of medical care, fair access to treatment, and cultural beliefs and customs may complicate considerations. Health care practitioners, including occupational therapists, must consider the meaning of the illness experience for the individual and the implications of individual decisions within the larger context of health care. Occupational therapy managers can prepare practitioners for the challenge of clinical ethical problem solving by anticipating and facilitating discussions on relevant topics.

Because personal values and traditions differ, what the major stakeholders consider to be the best option may not be what all team members perceive as the best option. Occupational therapy has at its core moral commitments to honoring patients' values and choices, and these may not always be consistent with those of all stakeholders. Financial stakeholders such as employers, insurance companies, and managed care agencies also influence decisions about the services that are provided to those enrolled in health care plans by funding or denying interventions. Occupational therapy practice that is based on evidence not only ensures the delivery of competent service, but also enhances the credibility of occupational therapy and increases the likelihood that services will be funded by these financial stakeholders. Exhibit 21.2 summarizes the roles and duties of occupational therapy managers in safeguarding ethical integrity.

## Ethical Infractions and Disciplinary Channels

Resolving ethical problems before harms accrue is far preferable to having to take corrective measures. Recourse for ethical infractions may range from a simple apology to legal action. Unethical behavior reflects poorly on individual practitioners and may

**Exhibit 21.2  Roles and Duties of Occupational Therapy Managers in Safeguarding Ethical Integrity.**

Keep faith with the discipline of occupational therapy
Establish program priorities
Provide services fairly
Ensure the quality of services
Attest to integrity of individual practitioners
Facilitate continual professional development

also actually damage the credibility or trustworthiness of the discipline. In some cases, it may be necessary to seek remedy for unethical actions committed by occupational therapists and occupational therapy assistants. When these infractions are considered to be harmful to consumers or damaging to the discipline, formal action may be warranted.

Sanctions can be pursued through state occupational therapy associations, licensing boards, or both as well as through the National Board for Certification in Occupational Therapy and through AOTA. Any manager contemplating this kind of action should check with the appropriate agency about specific requirements and processes for lodging ethical complaints. If the agency determines that unethical behavior has occurred, the person or persons who committed the action may be subject to punitive action. Punitive actions from official bodies generally become a matter of public record.

## Importance of Organizational Context

In his basic book *Ethics in Practice: Managing the Moral Corporation,* Andrews (1989b) emphasized the influence that leaders can have on the moral outlook and the subsequent actions of a company. This influence has become vividly apparent in recent history through the grand jury proceedings pertaining to the demise of Enron. Andrews contends that ethics has been segregated in general and has been removed from its application in the real world. Consequently, managers may be neither exposed to ethical perspectives nor attracted to them until those managers are confronted with serious conflict in the workplace. Connecting ethical reasoning with business endeavors, Andrews (1989a) states,

> Developing it in business turns out to be partly an administrative process involving: recognition of a decision's ethical implications; discussion to expose different points of view; and testing the tentative decision's adequacy in balancing self-interest and consideration of others, its import for future policy, and its consonance with the company's traditional values. (p. 100)

Andrews finds that dereliction in ethical analysis reflects not only failure of individuals but also failure of management, particularly the leaders of an organization. He further purports that managers have as much responsibility to communicate and apply ethical strategies as they do to develop and carry out economic strategies. More recent commentary addressing health care economics and ethical strategies can be useful to occupational therapy managers faced with difficult decisions (Herzlinger, 1997; Loewy & Loewy, 2001).

Another contemporary business ethicist, Marvin T. Brown (1990), has compiled case studies and analyses that reflect the gamut of ethical tensions experienced in the world of work. Some of his examples are specific to health care and can be immensely helpful to managers in illustrating the relationship between business agendas and ethical decision making. Brown also addresses the duties of employees to an organization and the obligations of an organization to its employees. In a society that is dependent on a market-driven economy, health care practitioners may be particularly challenged to honor the ideals and commitments inherent in the health-related professions.

Although the ethics of an institution are not always explicitly stated, they permeate its agendas and actions. Mission and vision statements may reveal the ethical commitments of the agency and lay the foundations of institutional culture. Managers are expected to be agents for the institutions, so their understanding of the organization's ethical platform as it comports with personal ethical commitments is critical to their managerial performance. Employee handbooks describe the particular organizational expectations and guidelines for ethical conduct. Although business acumen is essential for occupational therapy managers, they also must safeguard noble intentions and temper business decisions with ethical conscience.

## Ethics and the Array of Occupational Therapy Endeavors

Because the sociopolitical context of occupational therapy services is subject to change, ethical tensions cannot always be anticipated.

### Special Challenges in Existing Arenas of Practice

In recent years, existing practice settings and especially occupational therapy settings that are aligned with medical organizations have had to respond to tumult in the U. S. health care system. Among the ethical tensions are the documentation requirements that tempt practitioners to portray services in the language preferred by payers. This payer-preferred language has seemed to delimit and constrict the notions of occupation on which occupational therapy is grounded. For instance, occupational therapists who treat neonates in home or early intervention settings have probably had to complete agencies' forms that address range of motions, muscle strength, and other parameters that may not be particularly appropriate or meaningful in describing infant occupation.

As practitioners struggle to deal with external demands, the requirements to meet productivity standards and adhere to pathways have often taken more of their attention than have clinical reasoning and occupation-based services. As health care organizations continue to reorganize and reconfigure the workforce, disappointed practitioners may feel disenfranchised from the profession and may even discourage those aspiring to become occupational therapy practitioners. These forces and circumstances require all of us, especially occupational therapy managers, to reflect on our professional commitments, ethical obligations, and priorities.

### *Special Challenges in Emerging Arenas of Practice*

For many in the occupational therapy field, long-standing practice settings have become less comfortable places in which to work. Consequently, some occupational therapy managers have recognized the need to explore and cultivate other viable settings and mechanisms for delivering occupational therapy services. Among the ethical challenges are those that require occupational therapy managers to find new ways to provide affordable and accessible services to those in need. Ironically, some of the endeavors we call "emerging practice arenas" were actually evident in the early history of the profession. Nevertheless, challenge begets opportunity, and success stories about these alternatives are beginning to appear in the literature.

Furthermore, many of these alternative settings require new knowledge and skills, and entrepreneurial occupational therapy practitioners must commit to rigorous self-assessment and professional development to meet the challenges. The occupational therapists and occupational therapy assistants who are pioneers in emerging arenas of practice also must keep faith with the tenets and principles of occupational therapy while both communicating and demonstrating their value to agencies and individuals.

## Case Examples

The following case examples, although not exhaustive, are designed to reflect situations likely to be experienced by occupational therapy managers. Readers are encouraged to apply the strategies and content contained in the chapter to identify not only the ethical content but also an array of ethically permissible responses. Discussing the cases in small groups may illustrate how different sensitivities and perspectives can lead to varied interpretations and solutions to ethical problems.

## Case Study 1: What Are the Limits of Promise Keeping?

Joan graduated from an occupational therapy program 2 years ago, and she is working as an occupational therapist in an adolescent psychiatry program. She enjoys this population because she is 23 years old and feels that she can easily relate to teenagers and young adults. People in the program are served through an acute inpatient service, a transitional day program, and outpatient groups and services.

While alone one afternoon in the clinic with Joan, one of the girls remarks that she knows a secret about 16-year-old Claire, her roommate in the group home. The girls are known to have a rather contentious relationship. She tells Joan that she has read Claire's journal and that Claire has been writing about suicide. Joan is rather surprised because Claire appeared to be emerging from her depression and to be facing the consequences of her substance abuse. After sharing this information, the young woman tries to extract a promise from Joan not to tell anyone.

Conflicted, Joan meets with the occupational therapy program manager and initiates a conversation about patient–therapist confidentiality.

**Questions:** How might the occupational therapy manager get to the ethical content without prematurely shutting down the dialogue? What are the ethical issues in this scenario? What are the rules concerning confidentiality in this situation? How would you define the ethical priorities in this case?

## Case Study 2: Which Program Gets the Resources?

In a large inner-city health care system, the occupational therapy manager for off-site programs has received requests for service from two programs. However, no additional staff members can be hired without first increasing revenues, so only one program can be served at this time.

The first program under consideration is an executive stress reduction program for middle and higher management personnel in corporate positions who have been identified as being at high risk for heart attacks. Between 5 and 10 people are expected to be enrolled in the program at any given time. The program is requesting a half-time position to offer services at the corporate site, and the services will be handsomely paid from employee enhancement funds.

The second program under consideration targets women with HIV/AIDS. Therapists would meet with the women first at the medical outpatient clinic and later in their homes to develop occupational routines consistent with the health status and abilities of the women. Virtually all of the women are funded through public aid. The program is requesting a half-time position, anticipating that additional program needs will be identified.

**Questions:** What guidelines can the occupational therapy manager use to make a decision about which program to support? What are the ethical considerations associated with each of these programs? How can the manager determine which program is most consistent with the organization's agenda?

## Case Study 3: What Is Wrong With Students These Days?

Harold, an enthusiastic and conscientious student, convinces his academic fieldwork coordinator to allow him to fulfill his Fieldwork II requirement on the acute care service of a large Research I institution. He comes from an academic program that used a problem-based learning approach, and he feels prepared for the challenge. A week before his arrival, his assigned clinical supervisor threatened a miscarriage and is now at home on bed rest for an undetermined period of time. Because the other staff members are very busy, a decision has been made to have staff members share supervisory responsibility for Harold.

During his first week, Harold made a list of topics he needed to better understand and skills that he needed to develop. He was assigned several patients but received little clarification with respect to expectations. When he met with one of his supervisors at the end of the first week, he was told that he asked too many questions and didn't seem to know how to do much. During the second week, he tried not to ask many questions, and he attempted to conduct his assessments and to document treatments according to department protocol. When he met with his second supervisor at the end of the second week, he was told that his documentation was vague and inadequate and that he needed to include measurable outcomes. He was also told that he should have asked more questions.

During the third week, Harold was told he would be running groups that were normally led by the recreation therapist because the program was short staffed and because the group experience would be good for him. He asked whether he was responsible for generating the group treatment plan. He was told that there were group protocols and that he would need to carry out the protocol as planned. Harold communicated that he would rather concentrate on his assigned caseload.

He was shocked and dismayed to receive a call from the academic fieldwork coordinator later that afternoon with respect to his unwillingness to meet the expectations of the fieldwork placement.

**Questions:** What are the conflicting aspects in this scenario? What are the ethical obligations of the student? of the fieldwork setting? of the academic program? What are some of the ethical tensions in this service setting? What issues can the occupational therapy manager raise with the staff about fieldwork? How might the manager promote collaboration with the academic program? What actions and options attend to the student's best interests?

## Case Study 4: Where Is the Evidence?
The managed care company of the majority of clients enrolled in an early intervention program tells an occupational therapy manager that it will no longer reimburse for sensory integration because insufficient evidence is available to show that this treatment is effective. When the manager relays this information to the therapists serving that program, they are outraged. One of the certified occupational therapy assistants declares, "All the preschool teachers say that these kids are doing better. I can't tell you why, I just know it works."

**Questions:** What is the ethical content in this scenario, and how is it related to the scientific content? What are some of the specific concerns and broader issues raised by this situation? What strategies might the manager help staff members to identify to address their concerns? What is the role of research in addressing the ethical tensions in this scenario?

## Case Study 5: You Want Me to Do What?
Rebecca has been an occupational therapist for 6 years, and she consults with several agencies to develop programs and to recruit and supervise staff members. She is contracted to a group of three long-term care facilities for whom she screens new patients, assesses feeding and positioning needs for specified residents, and supervises the full-time certified occupational therapy assistant. She spends one full day a week at each of the three facilities.

The financial officer of the facilities has approached Rebecca requesting that she routinely enroll all residents in feeding groups to be conducted by the certified occupational therapy assistant, who has little experience in treating feeding disorders. Rebecca knows that some of the residents have little chance of benefiting from this intervention and suspects that the underlying motivation is to increase reimbursement for the organization. She senses that, if she protests, she will jeopardize her consultative relationship with the organization.

**Questions:** What are the ethical tensions in this scenario? What are the obligations of the manager (in this case, the consultant) in preserving the integrity of occupational therapy? Might the situation allow ethically permissible compromises?

## Conclusion

This chapter merely taps the ethical enterprise in occupational therapy. Ethical practice is predicated on the recognition of ethical tensions and use of resources to clarify and explore actions consistent with the ethical customs of the profession. The principles, examples, commentary, and resources are intended to be used by occupational therapy managers to promote dialogue and practices that are grounded in occupation and dedicated to improving quality living through meaningful doing. Effective occupational therapy managers are able to recognize and appreciate the ethical aspects of their managerial duties. They also use courage and creativity to address the challenges of designing and delivering ethically responsible occupational therapy services.

## References

Accreditation Council for Occupational Therapy Education (1998a). *Standards for an accredited educational program for the occupational therapist.* Bethesda, MD: American Occupational Therapy Association.

Accreditation Council for Occupational Therapy Education (1998b). *Standards for an accredited educational program for the occupational therapy assistant.* Bethesda, MD: American Occupational Therapy Association.

Aday, L. A., Begley, C. E., Lairson, D. R., & Slater, C. H. (1998). *Evaluating the healthcare system: Effectiveness, efficiency, and equity* (2nd ed.). Chicago: Health Administration Press.

Aday, L. A., Quill, B. E., & Reyes-Gibby, C. (2001). Equity in rural health care. In S. Loue & B. E. Quill (Eds.), *Handbook of rural health* (pp. 45–72). New York: Kluwer Academic/Plenum.

American Occupational Therapy Association. (1993). Core values and attitudes of occupational therapy practice. *American Journal of Occupational Therapy, 47,* 1085–1086.

American Occupational Therapy Association. (1998). Guidelines to the occupational therapy code of ethics. *American Journal of Occupational Therapy, 52,* 881–884.

American Occupational Therapy Association. (2000). *Occupational therapy code of ethics.* Bethesda, MD: Author.

Andrews, K. R. (1989a). Ethics in practice. *Harvard Business Review, 5,* 99–104.

Andrews, K. R. (1989b). *Ethics in practice: Managing the moral corporation.* Cambridge, MA: Harvard Business School Press.

Beauchamp, T. L., & Childress, J. F. (1994). *Principles of biomedical ethics* (4th ed.). New York: Oxford University Press.

Blustein, J. (1998). The family in medical decision making. In J. F. Monagle & D. C. Thomasma (Eds.), *Health care ethics: Critical issues for the 21st century* (pp. 82–91). Gaithersburg, MD: Aspen.

Brown, M. T. (1990). *Working ethics: Strategies for decision making and organizational responsibility.* San Francisco: Jossey-Bass.

Churchill, L. (1986). Moralist, technician, sophist, teacher/learner: Reflections on the ethicist in the clinical setting. *Theoretical Medicine, 7*(1), 3–12.

Herzlinger, R. E. (1997). *Market-driven health care: Who wins, who loses in the transformation of America's largest service industry.* Reading, MA: Persens Books.

Jameton, A. (1984). *Nursing practice: The ethical issues.* Englewood Cliffs, NJ: Prentice-Hall.

Kyler-Hutchison, P. (1994, December 15). Issues in ethics. The role of ethics committees. *OT Week,* pp. 9–10.

Law, M., Baum, C., & Dunn, W. (2001). *Measuring occupational performance: Supporting best practice in occupational therapy.* Thorofare, NJ: Slack.

Loewy, E. H., & Loewy, R. S. (Eds.). (2001). *Changing health care systems from ethical, economic, and cross-cultural perspectives.* New York: Kluwer Academic/Plenum.

Mattingly, C., & Fleming, M. H. (1994). *Clinical reasoning: Forms of inquiry in a therapeutic practice.* Philadelphia: F.A. Davis.

May, W. F. (1975). Code and covenant or philanthropy and contract? *Hastings Center Report, 5*(6), 29–38.

Monagle, J. F., & Thomasma, D. C. (1998). *Health care ethics: Critical issues for the 21st century.* Gaithersburg, MD: Aspen.

Pojman, L. P. (1998). *Classics of philosophy.* New York: Oxford University Press.

Savage, T. (1990, October). *The underground role of the nurse in ethical decision-making.* Paper presented at the University of Illinois College of Medicine Symposium, "A Time to Live . . . A Time to Die: Medical Ethics in the 90's," Rockford, IL.

Wilson, D. M. (Ed.). (1995). *The Canadian health care system.* Edmonton: University of Alberta.

# Accrediting Organizations

# Joint Commission on Accreditation of Healthcare Organizations

Richard W. Scalenghe, MT-BC, CPHQ

*"Occupational therapy practitioners and managers are accountable for their services and should continuously strive to improve the care provided to their patients and families. Practitioners and managers are encouraged to utilize JCAHO standards and surveys as an effective method for accountability and continuous improvement."*

RICHARD W. SCALENGHE

**Richard W. Scalenghe, MT-BC, CPHQ,** has a bachelor's of music therapy from the University of Dayton and his completed course work related to a master's degree in psychopathology from the University of Chicago. He is a private consultant for the Joint Commission on Accreditation of Healthcare Organizations and Joint Commission Resources, Inc. His specialty is behavioral health care; he is certified as a music therapist and is a professional in health care quality.

## Key Terms and Concepts

**Accreditation.** A process by which an institution or an educational organization seeks to demonstrate to an accrediting agency that it complies with generally accepted standards set forth by appropriate professional organizations; also, a kind of status awarded to an organization that demonstrates compliance with standards.

**Function.** A goal-directed, interrelated series of processes (see *process*) such as consumer assessment or human resource management.

**National consensus standards.** Standards based on consensus among providers, consumers, and purchasers of services. National consensus standards are different from standards derived from a research base, such as evidence-based research, that attempts to link standards (descriptions of organizational structures and processes) to demonstrated outcomes.

**Process.** A goal-directed, interrelated series of actions, events, mechanisms, or steps; for example, coordination of care among practitioners.

**Quality of care.** The degree to which health services for individuals and populations increase the likelihood of desired health outcomes and are consistent with current professional knowledge. Dimensions of performance include the following: consumer respect issues; safety within the care environment; and accessibility, appropriateness, continuity, effectiveness, efficacy, efficiency, and timeliness of care.

**Standard.** A statement that defines the performance expectations, structures, or processes that must be substantially in place in an organization to enhance the quality of care.

**Standard of quality.** A generally accepted, objective standard of measurement such as a rule or guideline that is supported through findings from expert consensus and that is based on specific research or documentation in scientific literature against which an individual's or organization's level of performance may be compared.

**Survey.** An on-site visit to an organization seeking accreditation during which an individual or a team assesses the organization's compliance with standards by reviewing documents; by conducting interviews with the people served, the staff members, the purchasers, and other consumers; and by making observations. For purposes of JCAHO accreditation, a survey is conducted by a health care professional who meets the JCAHO surveyor selection criteria and who evaluates standards compliance as well as provides education and consultation about that compliance to surveyed organizations or networks.

## Learning Objectives

After completing this chapter, you should be able to do the following:

■ Explain the importance of the JCAHO for occupational therapy practitioners.

■ Describe the different types of organizations that are accredited by the JCAHO.

■ Describe the role of occupational therapy practitioners in JCAHO standards development and revision.

■ Learn techniques for survey preparation.

The Joint Commission on Accreditation of Healthcare Organizations (JCAHO) is the largest and oldest private agency involved in voluntary accreditation in health care. It dates back to the 1917 formulation of minimum standards for hospitals by the American College of Surgeons and to that group's initiation of on-site inspections of hospitals in 1918. In 1951, the American College of Physicians, the American Hospital Association, the American Medical Association, and the Canadian Medical Association joined with the American College of Surgeons to create the Joint Commission on Accreditation of Hospitals as an independent, not-for-profit organization to provide voluntary accreditation for hospitals. The Canadian Medical Association withdrew in 1959 to start its own accrediting agency. Starting in the 1960s, the Joint Commission expanded to include accreditation for long-term care, mental health, and other areas. The American Dental Association became a governing board member of the Joint Commission in 1979.

Today, the commission's mission is "to continuously improve the safety and quality of care provided to the public through the provision of health care accreditation and related services that support performance improvement in health care organizations." It strives to achieve this mission in the following ways:

- Developing state-of-the-art performance standards
- Providing accreditation services for the full range of mainstream health care and social services organizations
- Ensuring the availability of educational and consultative support for organizations seeking accreditation
- Incorporating outcomes and other performance measures into the accreditation process
- Publicly disclosing organization-specific performance information to interested parties.

In fulfilling its mission, the JCAHO relies on and collaborates with multiple professional and health care organizations and individuals, including the American Occupational Therapy Association (AOTA) and occupational therapy practitioners.

The JCAHO evaluates and accredits nearly 18,000 health care organizations and programs in the United States. The JCAHO's evaluation (AOTA) and accreditation services are provided for the following types of organizations:

- General, psychiatric, children's, and rehabilitation hospitals
- Health care networks, including health maintenance organizations (HMOs), integrated delivery networks (IDNs), preferred provider organizations (PPOs), and managed behavioral health care organizations
- Home care organizations, including those that provide home health services, personal care and support services, home infusion and other pharmacy services, durable medical equipment services, and hospice services
- Nursing homes and other long-term care facilities, including subacute care programs, dementia programs, and long-term care pharmacies

- Assisted living facilities that provide or coordinate personal services, 24-hour supervision and assistance (scheduled and unscheduled), activities, and health-related services
- Behavioral health care organizations, including those that provide mental health and addiction services as well as services to people with developmental disabilities of various ages in various organized service settings
- Ambulatory care providers, including outpatient surgery facilities, rehabilitation centers, infusion centers, and group practices
- Clinical laboratories, including free-standing and organization-based clinical laboratories.

In addition, the Joint Commission established its disease-specific care (DSC) certification in 2002. This optional certification is designed to evaluate disease management and chronic care services that are provided by health plans, disease management service companies, hospitals, and other care delivery settings. The evaluation and resulting certification decision are based on an assessment of

- compliance with consensus-based national standards;
- effective use of established clinical practice guidelines to manage and optimize care; and
- performance measurement and improvement activities.

DSC services that successfully demonstrate compliance in all three areas will be awarded certification for a 1-year period. An extension is granted contingent on the submission of an acceptable assessment of compliance with standards and performance measurement as well as management activities. For more information, access JCAHO's Web page (http://www.jcaho.org).

In 1979, the commission established a professional and technical advisory committee (PTAC) for each field except clinical and pathology laboratories. Advisory committees have also been established for safety fields (e.g. fire safety, occupational health, hazardous waste, health care engineering). PTACs consist of representatives from professional and health care organizations and public representatives relevant to each field. PTACs play a significant role in the development of standards as well as the review and revision of the survey process, and they provide guidance to the JCAHO on future directions. Each PTAC now includes a representative from the Coalition of Rehabilitation Organizations. Created by the Joint Commission for purposes of PTAC representation, the coalition comprises the AOTA, the American Physical Therapy Association, the American Speech-Language-Hearing Association, the American Therapeutic Recreation Association, the National Therapeutic Recreation Society, and the National Coalition of Arts Therapy Associations.

Occupational therapy managers who are interested in affecting JCAHO standards, the survey process, and strategic initiatives are encouraged to communicate with the occupational therapy PTAC representatives. The AOTA can provide information about the occupational therapy practitioner PTACs representing various occupational therapy fields.

Joint Commission Resources, Inc. (JCR), a subsidiary of the Joint Commission, is a global, knowledge-based organization that disseminates information about accreditation, standards development and compliance, good practices, and health care quality improvement. JCR is dedicated to helping health care organizations worldwide to improve the quality of consumer care and to achieve peak performance.

JCR offers a full spectrum of resources for the benefit of any organization in the business of providing or managing health care. Through education programs, publications and multimedia products, the Continuous Survey Readiness initiative, comprehensive health care consulting and custom education, and even accreditation and international consulting for organizations abroad, JCR provides expertise on every aspect of accreditation, performance improvement, and the many other issues that organizations face in a challenging health care environment. The organization's Web site (http://www.jcrinc.com) can provide further information.

Joint Commission International (JCI) extends the Joint Commission's mission worldwide. Through both international consultation and accreditation, JCI helps to improve the quality of consumer care in many nations. JCI has extensive international experience working with public and private health care organizations and with local governments in more than 40 countries.

In response to growing interest in accreditation and quality improvement worldwide, the JCAHO launched its international accreditation program in 1999. JCI accreditation standards are based on international consensus standards, and they set uniform, achievable expectations for structures, processes, and outcomes for hospitals. The accreditation process is designed to accommodate specific legal, religious, and cultural factors within a country. To ensure their international applicability, Joint Commission standards were developed by a 16-member international task force, representing seven major world regions: (a) Western Europe; (b) the Middle East; (c) Latin and Central America; (d) Asia and the Pacific Rim; (e) North America; (f) Central and Eastern Europe; and (g) Africa. The JCR Web site can provide more information (search for "JCI").

## Joint Commission Standards

Survey preparation begins with a knowledge of standards that occupational therapy practitioners need to access the standards manual (or manuals) for the health care field in which they provide services.

### "Functional" Approach to Standards

Joint Commission accreditation is available for seven fields: (a) hospitals, (b) health care networks, (c) home care, (d) long-term care facilities, (e) assisted living, (f) behavioral health care, (g) ambulatory health care providers, and (h) clinical and pathology laboratories. For each of these fields, the Joint Commission publishes a corresponding standards manual. Each manual is available in a "comprehensive" version (which contains accreditation policies, standards, intent statements, scoring guidelines, and aggregation rules) and in a "standards" version (which contains accreditation policies, standards, and intent statements). Every accredited organization receives a complimentary copy of the comprehensive standards manual (or manuals) that applies to its organization.

The Joint Commission also publishes *Perspectives,* a monthly newsletter that reports changes in standards, policies, and procedures and that prints a range of features to improve understanding of accreditation. At the time of the site survey, practitioners are held accountable not only for what is in the current standards manual but also for the changes, the additions, and the corrections noted in *Perspectives.* Every accredited organization receives a complimentary *Perspectives* subscription. Occupational therapy practitioners may purchase standards manuals, the *Perspectives* newsletter, or other JCAHO publications through the JCR Web site.

The format and the content of Joint Commission standards have varied over the years. The commission periodically revises the standards so accreditation can more effectively stimulate health care organizations to demonstrate continuous improvement in performance. These revisions renew the commission's mission to focus on the processes and the functions (both clinical and organizational) that most significantly influence care; to emphasize doing the right things and doing them well; to incorporate significant lessons learned (i.e., adding requirements to promote safety that are based on root cause analyses performed by organizations in response to sentinel events; and to give more attention to what needs to occur than to how it occurs and who does it).

## Structure of the Standards

The current manuals are focused on performance and are structured around functions, with standards organized into two main sections:

1. "Patient [consumer]-Focused Functions," including chapters titled "Rights and Organization Ethics," "Assessment," "Care," "Education," and "Continuum of Care"
2. "Organizational Functions," including chapters titled "Improving Organizational Performance"; "Leadership"; "Management of Information"; "Management of Human Resources"; "Management of the Environment of Care"; and "Surveillance, Prevention, and Control of Infections."

Various manuals may contain additional chapters. For instance, the *Comprehensive Accreditation Manual for Hospitals* (JCAHO, 2002a) contains a third section, "Structures With Important Functions," including chapters titled "Governance" and "Medical Staff" and standards related to the role of the chief executive officer and the nurse executive. Exhibit 22.1 provides an example of a standard from the *Comprehensive Accreditation Manual for Hospitals*.

Occupational therapy practitioners can influence standards either through their AOTA PTAC representation or on an individual basis. Sharing thoughts and suggestions about the standards with the AOTA is important. This information might include feedback about the survey experience, in particular, whether occupational therapy services were sufficiently included in the survey, whether the surveyor or surveyors had adequate knowledge to fairly and thoroughly survey occupational therapy services, and whether the surveyors were professional and consultative.

### Standards Clarifications

Supplementary publications "Standards FAQs," "Standards Revisions," and "Standards Interpretations" are developed by the JCAHO's Standards Interpretation Group when a significant number of organizations have questions that are not clearly addressed in the manuals. These documents generally remain in effect until the information can be incorporated into the standards manual.

"Standards FAQs" can be retrieved by accessing the JCAHO Web page and selecting a health care field (i.e. "hospitals"), then clicking on "standards," then clicking on "FAQs." Standards revisions can by retrieved by accessing the same Web page, selecting a health care field, clicking on "standards," then clicking on "revisions." Occupational therapy practitioners can direct standards interpretation questions to JCAHO's Standards Interpretation Group by phone at 630-792-5900 or by fax at 630-792-5942. A fax inquiry should include the inquirer's full name, name of the health care organization, manual or manuals under which the organization is accredited, full mailing address, phone number (with time and date when the inquirer can be reached by phone), and fax number. Inquiries can also be submitted through e-mail by accessing the commission's Web site, selecting "Contact Us," and then scrolling down to "On-line Question Form."

### Future of Standards

Work has begun to develop "core" standards that are being integrated into all manuals. The goal will be to collapse all the manuals into a core set of standards. A customized set of standards that are based on an organization's application for survey then would be selected from the core set to match the setting (e.g., ambulatory care), the programs (e.g., rehabilitation), and the populations (e.g., geriatric).

## Joint Commission Survey Process

For a successful survey experience, occupational therapy managers and practitioners need to possess an understanding of the survey process as well as commit sufficient preparation time and resources. In 2004, the accreditation process will be significantly changed to a new initiative called "Shared Visions—New Pathways."

**Exhibit 22.1  Sample JCAHO Standard.**

### Standard TX.6.3

An interdisciplinary rehabilitation plan and goals, developed by qualified professionals, in conjunction with the patient and/or his or her family social network, or support system, and based on a functional assessment of patient needs, guide the provision of rehabilitation services, appropriate to the patient's environment.

### Intent of TX.6.3

A collaborative, interdisciplinary approach helps coordinate care and planning to meet patient care goals and achieve optimal outcomes. Based on assessment of the patient's physical, cognitive, emotional, and social status, a written treatment plan is developed that identifies the patient's rehabilitation needs. The rehabilitation plan incorporates, at least

  a. the patient's personal goals for rehabilitation;
  b. rehabilitation goals and objectives related to activities of daily living, learning, and working;
  c. measures and time frames for achievement of rehabilitation goals and objectives; and
  d. factors that may influence use of services or goal achievement.

The rehabilitation plan is designed to provide the skills, support, education, practice, experience, and treatment necessary to help the patient reach reasonable personal rehabilitation goals. The plan describes

  • long-term rehabilitation goals and short-term skill development objectives, in functional terms and developed in collaboration with the patient and family;
  • strategies and time frames for achieving rehabilitation goals;
  • who will help the patient and monitor progress;
  • measures of
    • rehabilitation goal attainment,
    • successful role performance,
    • changes in the patient's level of functioning,
    • efficiency of resource supports;
  • barriers other than the patient's primary problem;
  • criteria for transition to more independent, less restrictive environments and successful adaptation in natural community settings; and
  • patient skill and support requirements for living, learning, and working with optimal independence and choice.

Rehabilitation services are provided to meet patients' needs according to the plan.

### Examples of Evidence of Performance for TX.6.3

  • Interviews with rehabilitation services staff
  • Policies and procedures addressing rehabilitation care planning
  • Medical records

### Scoring for TX.6.3

| 1 | 2 | 3 | 4 | 5 | NA |
|---|---|---|---|---|----|

  a. Are the rehabilitation services for each patient guided by a written plan that addresses the patient's personal goals for rehabilitation?

*(continued)*

**Exhibit 22.1** *(Continued)*

## Scoring for TX.6.3

    b. Are the rehabilitation services for each patient guided by a written plan that addresses reha-
bilitation goals and objectives related to activities of daily living, learning, and working?

    c. Are the rehabilitation services for each patient guided by a written plan that addresses
measures and time frames for achievement of rehabilitation goals and objectives?

    d. Are the rehabilitation services for each patient guided by a written plan that addresses
factors that may influence use of services or goal achievement?

**Score 1**   a. through d. 90% to 100% compliance

**Score 2**   a. through d. 75% to 89% compliance

**Score 3**   a. through d. 50% to 74% compliance

**Score 4**   a. through d. 25% to 49% compliance

**Score 5**   a. through d. Less than 25% compliance

## Examples for TX.6.3

*Rehabilitation Professionals*

The treatment of each patient referred for rehabilitation services is based on the assessment of
the patient's occupational therapy needs. The treatment goal is to maximize the patient's functional occupational independence and may include, but is not limited to, the following areas:

- Activities of daily living: grooming, oral hygiene, bathing or showering, toilet hygiene,
personal device care, dressing, feeding and eating, medication routing, health maintenance, socialization, functional communication, functional mobility, community mobility, emergency responses, and sexual expression;

- Work and productivity activities: home management (clothing, cleaning, meal preparation
and clean-up, shopping, money management, household maintenance, safety procedures),
care of others, educational activities, and vocational activities (vocational exploration, job
acquisition, work or job performance, retirement planning, volunteer participation);

- Play or leisure activities: play or leisure exploration, and play or leisure performance;

- Sensorimotor: sensory (sensory awareness, sensory processing, perceptual), neuromuscu-
loskeletal (reflex, range of motion, muscle tone, strength, endurance, postural control,
postural alignment, soft tissue integrity), and motor (gross coordination, crossing the mid-
line, laterality, bilateral integration, praxis, fine coordination or dexterity, visual–motor
integration, oral motor control);

- Cognitive integration and cognitive components: level of arousal, orientation, recognition, attention span, initiation of activity, termination of activity, memory, sequencing,
categorizing, concept formation, spatial operations, problem solving, learning, and generalization; and

- Psychosocial skills and psychological components: psychological (values, interests, initiation of activity, termination of activity, self-concept), social (role performance, social
conduct, interpersonal skills, self-expression), and self-management (coping skills, time
management, self-control).

*Note.* For more information about how standards are scored, read the chapter in the standards
manual titled "The Accreditation Decision Process and Decision Rules."

From *"Comprehensive Accreditation Manual for Hospitals*, by Joint Commission on Accreditation of Healthcare Organizations, 2002, pp. TX-44a and TX-46. Copyright 2002 by JCAHO.
Reprinted with permission.

## Preparation for a Survey

Occupational therapy managers and practitioners should continuously be in compliance with JCAHO standards. Continuous survey readiness will limit the last-minute rush and anxiety that can be experienced when being surveyed. In addition, continuous readiness will prepare occupational therapy practitioners for "random unannounced," "unscheduled," and "unannounced" surveys.

Occupational therapy managers and practitioners should begin formal preparation for a survey 16 months before the anticipated survey date to be able to demonstrate a 12-month track record of compliance with standards. A 12-month track record is required to receive a score of 1 (substantial compliance). Managers and practitioners must have access to the standards, the scoring guidelines, and the periodical *Perspectives*. The standards promote an interdisciplinary and systems approach to program design, execution, and improvement. To meet the standards, managers and practitioners must collaborate with consumers and consumers' families, their organization's leaders, personnel in other departments and disciplines, and peers.

Staff members need to practice answering sample questions that a surveyor might ask. This practice is crucial and cannot be emphasized enough. A useful resource that assists staff preparation for answering surveyor questions is the series of guide books to the survey process published by the Joint Commission (2002b, 2002c). The hospital version is *The Complete Guide to the 2002 Hospital Survey Process*, the behavioral health services version is *The Complete Guide to the 2001–2002 Behavioral Health Care Survey Process*, and so on.

Sample questions that a surveyor could ask all occupational therapy practitioners may include the following:

- Describe the mechanism used for informing the individual about participation in decisions with respect to his or her care.
- How does the organization ensure that continuing care or discharge needs of the individual are being met?
- What mechanisms are used to identify and prioritize individual needs in determining care delivery?
- How is the care plan updated to reflect consumer progress (or the lack of progress) and changes in the condition of the consumer?
- How is education instruction presented for the consumer and his or her family to address the consumer's health rehabilitation needs?
- What is your role in creating a safe environment for staff members, the consumers, and consumers' families?

Sample questions that a surveyor could ask an occupational therapy manager may include the following:

- How is occupational therapy integrated into the organization (e.g., through strategic planning, budgeting, performance improvement)?

- Give an example of how your organization took action to make an incremental improvement in an existing process.
- Looking at your staffing resources, how did you assess the consumer needs and recommend an adequate number of qualified occupational therapy practitioners?
- Explain what steps you have taken to assess the risks for consumer care and the safety of your organization's buildings, grounds, equipment, occupants, and physical systems.
- Describe how you assess staff members' competence to provide services to various ages of individuals served.
- How have you participated in the organization's information management needs assessment?

Occupational therapy managers can promote improved standards compliance by doing the following:

- Read the standards and their intent, examples of evidence of performance, and examples that are contained in the comprehensive version of the standards manuals.
- Read related publications available through the JCR Web site by selecting "Publications."
- Attend related seminars; a list is available through the JCR Web site by selecting "Education."
- Attend JCAHO-related presentations at occupational therapy conferences.
- Network with other occupational therapy managers and practitioners to see how they are complying with standards.

## Survey Planning

To support survey planning, a representative from the Joint Commission—an account representative—works with each organization before the survey to develop a detailed agenda that tells organization staff members in advance when they will meet with surveyors. Approximately 6 months before the survey, the Joint Commission sends the Application for Survey to the organization to be completed and returned. (A Web-based survey application was initiated in 2002.) This document asks for a description of what services are provided and in which settings. Using the information provided in the document, the Joint Commission's account representative (or, in some instances, the surveyor assigned to survey the organization) assists the organization being surveyed in customizing the survey agenda to the organization's unique structure and characteristics. The account representative (or surveyor) attempts to most efficiently use the time of the organization's staff and surveyor during the survey.

## Surveyor Complement

Depending on the type and size of the organization, one or more surveyors will be assigned to conduct the survey. For instance, "smaller" long-term care, nonhospital, behavioral health, and home care organizations are surveyed by one surveyor. Hospitals typically are surveyed by survey teams, including at minimum a physician, a nurse, and an administrator. In psychiatric hospitals, the physician will be a psychiatrist; in rehabilitation hospitals, a rehabilitation specialist. Hospitals with comprehensive rehabilitation programs may choose to add a physician who is a rehabilitation specialist to the team (organizations making this choice would pay an additional survey fee). Other surveyors are added to the team according to the additional services provided by the organization (e.g., home care, long-term care, addictions, and ambulatory care). The Joint Commission makes every effort to provide surveyors who have experience in the type of organizations that they are surveying.

## Survey Activities

The activities currently used in on-site organization surveys are document review, interviews with the organization's leaders, visits to settings that provide care for consumers, function interviews, review of the organization's processes to assess competence, feedback sessions, and public information interviews. These activities are described in the following sections.

### Document Review

Early on in the survey, the surveyor (or surveyor team) reviews documents that orient him or her (or the team) to how the organization addresses the important functions covered by the standards. The documents that are requested generally describe how the organization has planned for these functions and how it has designed processes to support them. The list of required documents for each accreditation program can be found on JCAHO's Web page by clicking on (a) "Accredited Organizations" and selecting the relevant type of organization, (b) "Preparing for the Survey," and (c) "Guidelines for Document Review." It is important that policies and procedures, plans, and other documents are updated, appropriately approved, and consistent with other units or programs within the organization and that they reflect actual practice. An organization does not need to have separate occupational therapy policies and procedures if sufficient information is contained in organizational policies and procedures.

### Interviews With the Organization's Leaders

The surveyor will conduct several interviews with the organization's leaders that will address the collaboration of leaders in planning, designing, carrying out, and improving consumer care services. Some interviews typically focus on the principal leaders (i.e., the chief executive officer, the medical director), and other leadership interviews include department and service directors (i.e., the occupational therapy director, the rehabilitation director).

### Visits to Settings That Provide Care for Consumers

Much of the survey consists of visits to units and other settings where consumers receive care and services. These visits address how the organization's important functions come together in the care of consumers. Elements of these visits include a discussion with the director, a tour of the setting, a review of open clinical records, and a conversation with or observation of consumers and their significant others. Surveyors may visit only a representative sample of settings that provide care for consumers and, therefore, may not meet with some occupational therapy practitioners.

### Function Interviews

For several interviews, the surveyors gather an interdisciplinary group of the organization's staff members who have important responsibilities relative to a given function or an aspect of it. The interviews follow up on issues identified in the document review and also reflect observations made by surveyors during their visits to various care settings. Issues addressed during the interviews include how the organization measures and assesses its performance of the functions and, when appropriate, improves its performance. Some function interviews relevant to occupational therapy include the clinical and support service interview, the human resources interview, the information management interview, and the performance improvement interview (even though an occupational therapist may not be present at all of these interviews).

### Review of the Organization's Processes to Assess Competence

In a review of the organization's processes to assess competence, surveyors assess the organization's efforts to establish qualifications for staff members with specific responsibilities, to provide education and training pertinent to those responsibilities (or to see that staff members with these responsibilities have all the necessary education and training), and to evaluate staff members specific to their responsibilities. Tips for complying with competence assessment standards include the following:

- Develop job descriptions that are performance based (i.e., that clearly define the knowledge, skills, tasks, and behavior that staff members must demonstrate, including expectations related to assessment, care, consumer education, use of equipment, safety, and role in performance improvement).
- Ensure that new staff members are oriented to their positions and that supervisors document that they assessed the staff members' actual competence through observation before they were permitted to perform care independently.
- Use an approach to competence assessment that is consistent with the organization.
- Assess the competence of contract staff members, a process that may be different from that for regular employees (e.g., job responsibilities might be described in the letter of agreement rather than in a formal job description, and the contract agency might perform the orientation, the assessment, or both, in which case the contract agency needs to document the process and the occupational therapy manager needs to verify it). For more information, access the JCAHO Web site and click on "Standards FAQs."

- Ensure that the competence assessment is consistent with the job description and is based on actual performance. The competence assessment can include observation by the supervisor, demonstration, review of records, and posttests.
- Address in the job description, orientation, and competence assessment the ages of the consumers for whom the occupational therapy practitioner provides care.
- Read about competence assessment in chapter 12.
- Read JCR publications related to competence assessment, including *Assessing Hospital Staff Competence; Management of Human Resources in Hospitals: Examples of Compliance; Meeting Human Resources Challenges in Long-Term Care; Home Care and Hospice Staff Competence: Examples of Compliance;* or *Credentials Review, Clinical Responsibilities, and Competence Assessment: Questions and Answers for Behavioral Health Care Organizations.* For more information, access the JCR Web site and select "Publications."

### Feedback Sessions

Because of the nature of functions that occur throughout an organization, surveyors cannot reach a final score on compliance until they have visited all the scheduled consumer care settings and have conducted all the other survey interviews and activities. However, at the beginning of each day after the first day of the survey, surveyors communicate their observations in briefings.

### Public Information Interviews

Anyone who has information about an organization's compliance with the accreditation standards may request a public information interview. During a triennial survey, the Joint Commission requires an organization to provide an opportunity for consumers and the public as well as staff members of the organization undergoing the survey to present information.

In organizations that provide 24-hour care, the surveyor or surveyors will conduct an off-shift visit during surveys lasting 3 or more days. The surveyor or survey team will not inform the organization as to which unit will be visited or at what time the visit will occur. This practice is an attempt to include more than the "day shift" staff members in the survey process.

## Accreditation Decision Process and Other Issues

At the end of the on-site survey, the surveyor or survey team enter the findings into a laptop computer, print a draft copy of the report, and present it to the organization. The surveyor or survey team then send the findings electronically to the Joint Commission's central office for analysis and review. Professional staff members internally review these results, reach an accreditation decision, and define any necessary follow-up requirements. If the decision falls within established parameters, staff members directly notify the organization of the accreditation decision. Accreditation findings that raise specific concerns are reviewed by the Joint Commission's Accreditation Committee, which then reaches a final decision.

Approximately 45 days after the survey, the organization is sent the official accreditation decision and a report detailing the surveyor's or survey team's findings. This report contains any Type I recommendations pertaining to unsatisfactory compliance that requires correction within a specified time period; supplemental recommendations pertaining to unsatisfactory compliance that must be corrected by the time of the next full survey; the accreditation decision; and the Accreditation Decision Grid, which is a tabular representation of cumulative functional scores. Type I recommendations generate either a focused visit during which one or more surveyors return to check progress toward compliance or a request for a written progress report that the organization will send to the Joint Commission to provide written evidence of compliance.

Most accredited organizations receive one or more Type I recommendations (each of which requires either a visit or a progress report) and supplemental recommendations. For example, if an organization demonstrates good performance in a given area but does not have the essential policies and procedures in place to support this performance over time, it might receive a score of 2 or 3, resulting in a supplemental recommendation that indicates the need to address this issue in the future. If the organization has adequate policies and procedures in place in another area but its performance does not measure up, it might receive a score of 4 or 5, resulting in a Type I recommendation.

Organizations undergo a full survey every 3 years. After being surveyed, they are classified into one of the accreditation categories described in Exhibit 22.2. The only exception is home care agencies seeking deemed status (i.e., recognition of Joint Commission accreditation for the purpose of Medicare reimbursement). These agencies receive visits by Joint Commission surveyors annually. Each annual visit addresses Medicare requirements; every third visit also addresses Joint Commission requirements.

Organizations that are denied accreditation have the right to appeal before a final accreditation decision is made. All other organizations may request a revision of specific recommendations and of the accreditation decision within 30 days of receiving the survey report (with the accreditation decision).

## Exhibit 22.2  Accreditation Categories.

- Accreditation with full standards compliance
- Accreditation with requirements for improvement
- Provisional accreditation (for preliminary on-site evaluation)
- Conditional accreditation
- Preliminary denial of accreditation
- Accreditation denied

## Random Unannounced Surveys

In July 1993, the Joint Commission began conducting annual, unannounced, 1-day surveys at a small, randomly selected sample of accredited organizations. These surveys occurred at the approximate midpoints of the organizations' 3-year accreditation cycles. Conducted by a single surveyor, the survey is limited to five or six "fixed topics" and to "variable topics." Fixed topics are performance areas in which other similar organizations had compliance problems in the previous year. These areas change each year, and they are published in *Perspectives* and are available on JCAHO's Web page (search for "Random"). Variable topics are those performance areas in which the organization had compliance problems during its previous survey. Random unannounced survey results may lead to new Type I recommendations and may even cause a change in the organization's accreditation status.

The rationales for unannounced surveys are as follows:

- To provide for continuing interaction between the Joint Commission and accredited organizations
- To tell the public a highly positive story about the willingness and the ability of health care organizations to maintain good performance on their own cognizance
- To validate the self-sustaining improvement capabilities of continuous quality improvement approaches.

## Unscheduled and Unannounced Surveys

The Joint Commission also may perform an unscheduled or an unannounced survey when it becomes aware of potentially serious issues related to standards compliance, when it becomes aware of care or safety issues, or when it has other valid reasons to survey an accredited organization. Either type of survey can take place at any point in the organization's accreditation cycle. The Joint Commission usually provides the organization with advance notice 24–48 hours before an unscheduled survey. No advance notice is provided for unannounced surveys. Results of any unannounced or unscheduled surveys may generate follow-up activities and can affect an organization's current accreditation status.

## Performance Reports

For surveys conducted in January 1994 and after, the Joint Commission generates Performance Reports, organization-specific accreditation information, which the commission makes available to the public. This access and the information itself have both symbolic and substantive meaning in the new health care environment. Each report contains an overview of the organization; the accreditation date and the decision, including areas with recommendations for improvement, if appropriate; the organization's evaluation level in performance areas that were reviewed during its survey; and a comparison of the organization's evaluation level with that of other organizations. Also included is a two-page commentary from the organization. Each time an organization's Performance Report is requested, the organization is notified of who made the request and when. Performance reports are available to the public by phone or by accessing the JCAHO's Web page (link to "Quality Check").

## Shared Visions—New Pathways

As part of its own continuous improvement initiative, the JCAHO has looked for ways to make the accreditation process better. The culmination of JCAHO's critical look at its services, which included significant input from health care organizations and professionals, is an effort to dramatically redesign and improve the value of its accreditation process. This initiative, "Shared Visions—New Pathways," will be implemented January 2004.

This initiative affects the standards as well as the survey process. The standards will be streamlined and reformatted to more clearly reflect expectations. The survey process will include a greater focus on the actual delivery of clinical care and shift the accreditation-related focus from survey preparations and scores to continuous operational improvement in support of safe, high-quality care and make the accreditation process more continuous. To accomplish this, JCAHO plans on focusing the survey on organization-specific, critical consumer care processes and systems as opposed to rote assessment standards compliance by streamlining the standards and reducing documentation burden to focus more on critical consumer care issues and by having health care organizations conduct a self-assessment midway in the 3-year accreditation cycle. The "new" survey agenda will include the following six basic components: (a) an opening conference; (b) a leadership interview; (c) the validation of the self-assessment results; (d) the focus on actual consumers as the framework for assessing compliance with selected standards; (e) discussion and education on key issues; and (f) a closing conference. In addition, surveyors will develop and apply new skills in systems analysis applicable to clinical care and organization functions. Additional information about standards and the survey process can be retrieved from the JCAHO Web page.

## Use of Outcomes and Other Performance Measures by the Joint Commission

The ORYX initiative, introduced in February 1997, integrates outcomes and other performance measurement data into the accreditation process. This integration is essential to the credibility of any modern evaluation activity for health care organizations. Outcomes and other performance measures supplement and guide the standards-based survey process by providing a more targeted basis for the regular accreditation survey, a basis for monitoring in between surveys, and a basis for guiding and stimulating continuous improvements. It is intended to be a flexible and affordable approach for supporting quality improvement efforts in organizations that are accredited by the Joint Commission and for increasing the value of accreditation.

At present, most accredited hospitals and long-term care, home care, and behavioral health care organizations formally participate in ORYX. Participation includes affiliating with a performance measurement system as well as collecting data and reporting findings on six performance measures. Surveyors assess organizations' use of selected measures in their performance improvement activities during the on-site survey process. For each measure, organizations are expected to demonstrate the ability to collect data reliably, conduct credible analyses of the data, and initiate appropriate system and process improvements.

The ORYX initiative is being carried out in phases, and nationally standardized performance, or core, measures will be identified for each of JCAHO's accreditation programs. In early 1999, the Joint Commission solicited input from a wide variety of stakeholders—clinical professionals, health care provider organizations, health care consumers, and performance measurement experts—about potential focus areas for core measures. Using the input of these stakeholders and recommendations from state hospital associations, the executive committee of the Joint Commission's board of commissioners selected five initial core measurement areas for hospitals:

- Acute myocardial infarction (including coronary artery disease)
- Heart failure
- Community-acquired pneumonia
- Pregnancy and related conditions (including newborn and maternal care)
- Surgical procedures and complications.

Other types of accredited organizations will continue using noncore measures to meet ORYX requirements until core measures are identified for them. Identification of home care core measures will focus on adopting measures derived from Outcome and Assessment Information Set measures for home health agencies, while identification of long-term care core measures will focus on the adoption of measures derived from Minimum Data Set measures. JCAHO is striving to make core measures for home care and long-term care organizations as consistent as possible with Centers for Medicare and Medicaid Services (CMS; formerly the Health Care Financing Administration) requirements to reduce duplication in performance measurement activities. The identification of core measures for behavioral health care organizations that are providing 24-hour care is anticipated to focus on adopting or adapting measures based on field consensus. For more information, go to the JCAHO Web site and click on "Performance Measurement."

### Cooperative Accreditation Initiative

The Joint Commission launched its Cooperative Accreditation Initiative (CAI) in 1995 to reduce redundancy and overlap in the accreditation of health care organizations. The CAI is part of the Joint Commission's national duplication reduction effort to improve the efficiency and reduce the cost of quality oversight activities by enhancing the communication and coordination among various public (i.e., CMS, state licensing bodies) and private sector (i.e., CARF . . . Commission on Accreditation of Rehabilitation Facilities) organizations that have responsibility for these activities. Cooperative agreements permit the Joint Commission to substantially rely on the process, findings, and decisions of other accrediting bodies in circumstances in which the Joint Commission would otherwise conduct potentially duplicative surveys of organizations seeking accreditation.

In 2002, CAI differentiated between two types of agreements—complementary and comparable. Complementary agreements were created because the evaluations conducted by some cooperative partners are not perceived as duplicative of JCAHO surveys; the standards and survey process of these partners focus primarily on technical and clinical functions within a department or unit. Those accrediting bodies that establish complementary agreements with JCAHO will be publicly recognized but will not be required to achieve and maintain comparability with JCAHO policies, standards, and accreditation processes such as random unannounced surveys. However, these organizations will still need to meet basic CAI threshold requirements. Comparable agreements permit the Joint Commission to rely on the process and decisions of the cooperative partner, eliminating the need to conduct duplicative evaluations in organizations seeking JCAHO accreditation because the Joint Commission has found the other accrediting body's standards and policies to be comparable to JCAHO's.

At the time of this publication, JCAHO is in the process of seeking to establish complementary agreements with five current CAI partners: the American Society for Histocompatibility and Immunogenetics, the American College of Surgeons—Commission on Cancer, the American Association of Blood Banks, the American College of Radiology-Radiation Oncology Program, and CARF.

The Joint Commission currently offers a joint survey option to rehabilitation hospitals that choose to have both JCAHO and CARF accreditation. This optional survey is structured in a manner to coordinate many survey activities (i.e., interviews, document reviews) between both sets of surveyors. Note that organizations that choose this survey still maintain separate accreditation decisions from both JCAHO and CARF.

## Conclusion

The JCAHO is the largest and oldest private agency involved in voluntary accreditation in health care. Its mission is to continuously improve the safety and quality of care provided to the public through health care accreditation and related services that support performance improvement in health care organizations.

The JCAHO achieves its mission by developing state-of-the-art performance standards, providing accreditation services for the full range of health care organizations, ensuring the availability of educational and consultative support for organizations seeking accreditation, incorporating outcomes and other performance measures into the accreditation process, and publicly disclosing organization-specific performance information to interested parties. Joint Commission accreditation is available for eight fields: (a) hospitals, (b) health care networks, (c) home care, (d) long-term care facilities, (e) assisted living, (f) behavioral health care, (g) ambulatory health care providers, and (h) clinical and pathology laboratories. A comprehensive standards manual is available for each field. The Joint Commission also publishes the official periodical *Perspectives* that provides key update information related to accreditation. Occupational therapy representatives assist the JCAHO in developing standards and in making recommendations about the survey process and other initiatives. Occupational therapy practitioners who work at organizations accredited by JCAHO need to maintain continuous compliance with the standards.

The focus of the standards and the survey is on the important processes and outcomes affecting customer care and organizational performance, not on specific disciplines such as occupational therapy. Occupational therapy practitioners who provide care in JCAHO-accredited organizations need to become knowledgeable about and continuously comply with the standards. In addition, knowledge about and preparation for the survey process will produce a more favorable survey outcome.

## References

Joint Commission on Accreditation of Healthcare Organizations. (2002a). *Comprehensive accreditation manual for hospitals*. Oakbrook Terrace, IL: Author.

Joint Commission on Accreditation of Healthcare Organizations. (2002b). *The complete guide to the 2001–2002 behavioral health care survey process*. Oakbrook Terrace, IL: Author.

Joint Commission on Accreditation of Healthcare Organizations. (2002c). *The complete guide to the 2002 hospital survey process,* Oakbrook Terrace, IL: Author.

# CHAPTER 23

# CARF . . . Commission on Accreditation of Rehabilitation Facilities

Christine M. MacDonell, BS, OTR

*"Accountability and responsiveness to stakeholders is the key to success for occupational therapy and human service delivery systems. Accreditation offers the foundation of these activities."*

CHRISTINE M. MACDONELL

**Christine M. MacDonell, BS, OTR,** is managing director, Medical Rehabilitation/Emerging Markets, Customer Service Unit, Commission on Accreditation of Rehabilitation Facilities in Tucson, AZ. She is a human services specialist with experience as an occupational therapist, as director of a rehabilitation continuum, as an executive director of a vocational state use program, and as an accreditation specialist.

## Key Terms and Concepts

**Barrier-free environment.** An environment where an individual does not face environmental, architectural, attitudinal, financial, employment, communication, or transportation limitations.

**Carver model.** Results-oriented approach to nonprofit board governance.

**Conformance.** To be in agreement with.

**Continuous improvement.** The activity of measuring against a benchmark and, if met, trying to increase what one is doing to improve performance and always raising the expectation of acceptable performance.

**Field-driven standards.** Considered by an authority as a basis of comparison; a rule or principle used as a basis for judgment.

**Fulfilled lives.** Individuals who are able to participate in society at a level that is acceptable to them.

**Third-party accreditation.** Quality oversight by a private system that has no professional trade or government associations that could overly influence its work.

## Learning Objectives

After completing this chapter, you should be able to do the following:

- Explain the importance of third-party accreditation.

- Define CARF . . . Commission on Accreditation of Rehabilitation Facilities and its major characteristics.

- Describe the CARF accreditation process for review.

- Distinguish between regulatory requirements and accreditation standards.

This chapter provides a description of the CARF . . . Commission on Accreditation of Rehabilitation Facilities, including its history, structure, and processes. In addition, the text explains the importance of accreditation for occupational therapists and what roles they can play in the vital process of accreditation. This process is introduced along with an overview of CARF's accreditation conditions, standards, and outcomes.

## An Overview of CARF

CARF is an international, private, not-for-profit organization that accredits human services organizations with programs and services in the fields of adult day services, assisted living, behavioral health, employment and community services, and medical rehabilitation. CARF was established in 1966 to assist consumers in identifying quality rehabilitation programs and services. Examples of typical programs and services that CARF includes in a review are occupational rehabilitation programs, respite services, criminal justice programs, adult day services, and workforce development programs. CARF develops and maintains relevant and practical standards of quality for human services organizations. The standards address good business practices, the results of services, the process of providing services (e.g., assessment, individual program planning, treatment interventions, and discharge), and specific standards for particular programs and services (e.g., standards for respite care, spinal cord systems of care, community mental health centers, assisted living).

The standards are developed using a field-driven approach. CARF defines the *field* as the persons served, the providers of services, the purchasers of services, and other stakeholders. The process to develop and revise standards includes those members of the field who, from their perspective, have expertise with the standards being developed or revised. Persons served, providers, purchasers, and regulators come together with surveyors, board of trustee members, and CARF staff members to develop a proposed set of standards. This proposed set of standards then goes to the field for review and comment. After careful review and revision, the board gives the final approval for the set of standards. The standards are applied, through a peer review process, to specific programs and services.

CARF is governed by a board of trustees that represents the consumers who receive services, the providers, the payers, and the regulators. The American Occupational Therapy Association (AOTA) applied for and was accepted as a sponsoring member of the board in December 1982. AOTA has been involved in the development and revision of CARF standards and its practices for more than 20 years and plays a vital role in the shaping and ongoing improvement of this accreditation process.

The following information from the *CARF Accreditation Sourcebook* (CARF, 2002a) describes CARF's mission, purpose, vision, and core values. The *Sourcebook* states the mission in the following terms:

The mission of CARF is to promote the quality, value and optimal outcomes of services through a consultative accreditation process that centers on enhancing the lives of the persons served. (p. 3)

CARF's primary purpose is expressed in the following six points:

1. To develop and maintain current, field-driven standards that improve the value and responsiveness of the programs and services delivered to people in need of rehabilitation and other life enhancement services.

2. To recognize organizations that achieve accreditation through a consultative peer-review process and demonstrate their commitment to the continuous improvement of their programs and services with a focus on the needs and outcomes of the persons served.

3. To conduct accreditation research emphasizing outcomes measurement and management, and to provide information on common program strengths as well as areas needing improvement.

4. To provide consultation, education, training, and publications that support organizations in achieving and maintaining accreditation of their programs and services.

5. To provide information and education to consumers and other stakeholders on the value of accreditation.

6. To seek input through a variety of mechanisms (National Leadership Panels, Focus Groups, one-on-one interactions, surveyor interactions) and to utilize the information received to better serve the field and CARF's various stakeholders. (pp. 3–4)

The *Sourcebook* describes CARF's vision in these terms:

Through responsiveness to a dynamic and diverse environment, CARF serves as a catalyst for improving the quality of life of the persons served by CARF-accredited organizations and the programs and services they provide. (p. 3)

Finally, CARF believes in the following core values:

1. All people have the right to be treated with dignity and respect.

2. All people should have access to needed services that achieve optimum outcomes.

3. All people should be empowered to exercise informed choice. (*Informed Choice* is defined in the Glossary of the 2002 CARF Medical Rehabilitation Standards Manual as "A decision made by a person that is based on sufficient experience and knowledge, including exposure, awareness, interactions, or instructional opportunities, to ensure that the choice is made with adequate awareness of the alternatives to and consequences of the options available.") (p. 317)

In 2001, the CARF Board of Trustees identified the moral owners of CARF as being the persons served in the accredited programs and services. *Persons served* are the primary consumers of services, who may be classified as clients, participants, or residents. When these persons are unable to exercise self-representation at any point in the decision-making process, persons served is interpreted to also refer to those persons willing and able to make decisions on behalf of the primary consumers.

CARF's accreditation, research, and educational activities are conducted in accordance with its core values and with the utmost integrity. Some of the most recent activities in this arena are the Performance Indicator Project, the Critical and Discriminatory Standards study, the trend analysis of conformance to standards by program and service level, the revision of surveyor training, and the development of CARF's own performance indicators project that has resulted in a quarterly scorecard with benchmarks and performance improvement activities to reach or exceed the benchmark. In addition, CARF is committed to the following goals:

1. Continuously improving both organizational management and service delivery
2. Achieving diversity and cultural competence in all CARF activities and associations
3. Enhancing the involvement of consumers in all of CARF's activities
4. Involving consumers of services as active participants in the development and application of standards of accreditation
5. Enhancing the meaning, value, and relevance of accreditation to the consumers of services.

## Ends Policies

When the CARF Board of Trustees identified the moral owners of CARF as the persons served, they also established the policies related to the ends for which CARF should be held accountable. The board is using the Carver model of governance policy, a highly effective, results-oriented approach to nonprofit board governance. *Ends* in the Carver governance policy refers to the effect an organization seeks to have on the world outside itself. Ends will cause something to be different for someone at some cost. Ends policies address a threefold concept: an organization's results, the people it serves, and the costs of the results (Carver & Carver 1997). More specifically, ends embrace the following concepts:

- The impact, difference, change, benefit, or outcome to be achieved in the lives of persons served, which also could be called *results*
- The identity, description, or characteristics of the persons served who receive the results of the program or service interventions
- The monetary expense, relative worth, or relative priority of a result or set of results, which is called *cost*.

In many ways, CARF's ends policies also reflect the work of occupational therapy, especially the first end, "Fulfilled Lives." It states

People who receive supports and services in CARF accredited organizations have the opportunity to live fulfilling lives.

A. People live in a barrier-free environment (communications, architectural, attitudinal, mobility, vocational).
B. People live with dignity, respect, and autonomy.
C. People receive supports and services that are culturally relevant.
D. People receive supports and services that are delivered in a safe fashion.
E. People are active participants in decisions that affect their lives.
F. People have access to needed services.
G. People have meaningful work and productive use of time.

    H.  People will have friends and relationships.

    I.  People live in a home of their choice. (CARF, 2002b, p. E1)

As CARF develops and revises standards; develops new strategies to work with professionals, consumers, and payers; and changes its processes, all of the above components of fulfilled lives must be addressed to see whether CARF accreditation continues to affect the lives of persons served through the process of accreditation.

    The second ends policy to which CARF is held accountable is "Competent Service Providers":

    Providers of services shall meet standards for quality that lead to optimal outcomes for persons served.

    A.  There shall be a clear set of standards.

    B.  Best practices will be identified and utilized while developing and revising CARF standards.

    C.  Meeting standards will produce value for accredited programs. Value is defined as quality and cost. The cost of meeting standards should be reasonable and achievable for providers. If they are too costly then there will be limited value and quality will suffer.

    D.  Achievement of the standards will produce acceptable levels of practice.

    E.  Rating scales, consumer reports, and balanced scorecards show that people will choose providers who meet accepted standards.

    F.  Payers/policymakers will choose providers who meet accepted standards. National Committee on Quality Assurance (NCQA); Third party funders; and State departments recognize national accreditation through mandates, acceptances and deemed status. (p. E2)

    The third ends policy to which the CARF Board of Trustees has held CARF accountable is "Successful Service Providers." CARF must assist service providers to achieve organizational success.

    A.  Service providers achieve a positive return on their investment in the accreditation process.

    B.  Service providers learn and grow. (p. 3)

    The ends policies ultimately support many opportunities that CARF offers to providers. These opportunities enable providers to network, learn new skills sets, exchange ideas and best practices, increase their visibility among human services providers, and have a voice in the direction of human services internationally.

## International Aspects

Very few countries have not asked CARF to accredit or consult in the development or enhancement of services for people in need of human services. However, the United States, Canada, and Western Europe have most formally integrated CARF's influence. In March 2002, CARF incorporated in Canada to better address the needs of the Canadian market. CARF CANADA will increase opportunities for human services providers to seek accreditation and participate with CARF by becoming surveyors, associates, and board members. The AOTA's active role and meaningful contributions to CARF will certainly be addressed with its sister organization, the

Canadian Occupational Therapy Association. In 2003–2004, the possibility of a European subsidiary will also be on the drawing board. The Far East and Australia were on the schedule for CARF to begin work with governments, universities, and providers in 2002.

CARF has many ongoing relationships with state agencies and provincial ministries that accept CARF accreditation as a quality review in lieu of or in addition to state or provincial reviews. CARF is also recognized in Europe. Throughout health services industry publications, government studies, consumer advocacy information, and the tort system, evidence from many countries shows that, even with government regulations that address health service workers' competencies and certifications or special recognition of individuals' levels of competencies, many issues related to quality still need attention across the health service delivery systems. These quality issues are a challenge that every government faces and one that creates an excellent opportunity for collaboration with third-party accreditation systems, such as CARF's.

Regulations, which focus more on structural and health or safety issues, seldom address the activities of an organization that involve fiscal responsibility, risk management, ethical behaviors, measurement and management of information and outcomes, involvement of consumers in service planning, or performance improvement. Accreditation systems look at these activities as well as the structural and health or safety issues. CARF offers states, provinces, and other jurisdictions within a country a public–private partnership that gives them more information on the actual performance and more guidance to improve than they have ever had in the past. A collaborative relationship with regulators, providers, and consumers in which all work together to determine how to best protect consumers and improve the results of services for consumers is an excellent step toward more appropriate use of resources and energies of a state agency or payer of services.

Quality oversight by a third-party accreditation system, such as CARF's, is a concept that all occupational therapists should be familiar with and should be applying throughout their careers. This oversight is a systems approach that the occupational therapy profession can use to affect the delivery of quality human services. Occupational therapists have demonstrated leadership in the improvement of human services through their roles as clinicians and educators as well as through their involvement with CARF, through the leadership roles they have accepted with the CARF Board of Trustees, through their participation in advisory committees as recognized and valued health care providers, and through their active participation as surveyors.

## Importance of Accreditation for Occupational Therapists

Over the years, the role of accreditation has dramatically changed. As consumers, payers, regulators, and the general public demand more accountability, the pressure has increased for organizations to disclose information about the actual results they have achieved and how satisfied people have been not only with those results but also with the durability of those results. Third-party quality review has become a tool to differentiate providers. Payers and regulators need many ways to ensure that the organization has identified its risks and has in place a mechanism to reduce risk or, at minimum, share risk with providers. An accredited provider can address how it identifies its own risk and reduces its exposure to loss. Accredited providers can address the results of their services and evaluate their performance using key indicators such as the consumer's satisfaction with services. They can provide information on length, duration, and frequency of services as it relates to the outcomes of services. Accreditation standards establish the framework for business, information, and measurement systems as well as the programmatic components of service delivery. Occupational therapists, whether practicing in a clinic they own themselves or providing services as part of a large team in a health, school, home care, or community system, need to display these same characteristics. The days when providers could say they are good providers without undergoing any outside review or verification are gone. At a minimum, without accreditation, providers must be prepared to fully disclose their activities, services, and the outcomes they produce. Today, the ability to meet an international set of field-driven standards adds to the value and validity of providers.

## Accreditation Process

The process of a CARF survey is based on an on-site review done by peer surveyors. Standards that are developed by consumers, providers, payers, and regulators (i.e., the field) are applied to specific services or programs and to the organization. The emphasis throughout the survey process is always on the persons receiving services and how the provider has provided an individualized program that has achieved predicted outcomes for those individuals. If the predicted outcomes of services for the persons served have not been met or if organizational goals that were established have not been achieved, then performance improvement must demonstrate that performance has been analyzed or that a plan to attain the goal has been created.

### Steps to Accreditation

Achieving accreditation is easier when an organization prepares systematically for the CARF survey. The following 10 steps will clarify what is involved in the process of accreditation. CARF acts a collaborative partner with the organization throughout these steps:

1. An organization contacts the CARF office to ascertain or verify which of the standards manuals it should use for accreditation.
2. The organization conducts a self-study (e.g., by using a Survey Preparation Guide or by using a self-assessment with no written information), which is an evaluation of the organization's conformance to standards.
3. The organization then implements the CARF standards. By the time of the survey, the organization must have been implementing the CARF standards for at least 6 months in the program or service areas for which it is seeking

accreditation. During this time, the organization can actively engage CARF staff members in phone conversations, conference calls, e-mails, and in-person dialogue for technical assistance and standards interpretation.

4. The organization requests an application for the accreditation survey, which it completes and submits a minimum of 3 full months before the month in which it is requesting that the survey take place. The requested survey time should be at least 6 months after the organization has had an opportunity to use the CARF standards in the programs or services for which it is seeking accreditation. The application fee, which is nonrefundable, must accompany the application.

5. After reviewing and approving the application, CARF sends a bill to the organization for the survey fee, which is based on the number of surveyors and days needed to evaluate the organization's programs and services. Organizations outside of the United States and Canada also are charged the cost of airfare for the survey team.

6. CARF selects the survey team based on a match of the surveyors' areas of expertise and the organization's unique needs. As soon as the survey team is selected and at least 30 days before the survey, CARF notifies the organization of the dates of the survey and the names of the team members.

7. The on-site CARF survey is conducted by a peer survey team that evaluates conformance to the standards. The survey comprises interviews with individuals and groups, observations of the service delivery, and review of necessary documentation. Persons served are always interviewed and are an integral part of the survey. At the end of the survey, the survey team holds an exit conference to share its findings and recommendations with the organization. The team submits its findings to CARF in a report. The team neither reports nor makes public the accreditation outcome at the time of the exit conference.

8. CARF evaluates the survey team's findings, and the CARF Board of Trustees renders an accreditation decision from the following options: 3-year accreditation, 1-year accreditation, provisional accreditation, and nonaccreditation. The organization is notified of the accreditation decision and receives a written survey report approximately 8 weeks after the survey.

9. The organization is awarded a Certificate of Accreditation that lists the programs or services that have been included in the rehabilitation process. This certificate is mailed to the organization approximately 4–6 weeks after the survey report is sent.

10. Within 90 days after notification of the outcome, the organization submits a quality improvement plan to CARF outlining the actions that have been taken or will be taken in response to any recommendations of the report. The accreditation conditions require that this document be submitted to retain

accreditation. This quality improvement plan is a detailed, step-by-step process that gives the action plan or plans for each recommendation received during the on-site survey.

For more detailed information please, visit the CARF Web site (http://www.carf.org).

The typical time frame for an organization to prepare for an initial survey is 12–16 months. Accredited organizations should be maintaining conformance to the standards at all times. Preparing for most resurveys takes approximately 6–9 months.

## Accreditation Conditions

In addition to demonstrating substantial conformance to the CARF standards, an organization must also meet the following accreditation conditions to achieve and retain accreditation:

1. For a minimum of 6 months before the site survey, each program or service that is part of the accreditation process should demonstrate
   a. application of CARF's organizational and program standards that are relevant to the program or service and
   b. direct delivery of services to the persons served within the program seeking accreditation.
2. The organization seeking accreditation should provide records and reports as requested by CARF. Note that federal regulations that are being negotiated pursuant to the Health Insurance Portability and Accountability Act (HIPAA) of 1996 define the term *health care operations* to include accreditation activities. This definition means that a health care provider seeking accreditation on or after April 14, 2003, may need to obtain a consumer's consent before using or disclosing protected health information (PHI) to carry out accreditation activities. The organization is expected to make reasonable efforts to limit disclosure of PHI to the minimum necessary information for determining conformance with the standards. Because the federal regulations are not yet finalized, CARF is not able to give definitive answers about how these new regulations will affect the accreditation process. CARF is receiving guidance from HIPAA legal experts.
3. A quality improvement plan (QIP) should be submitted within 90 days after notice of accreditation. This plan will address the organization's future efforts to make ongoing improvements in all areas of the survey report where recommendations are made.

If any of these three conditions is not met, the CARF office will determine the appropriate course of action, which may include denial or withdrawal of an accreditation award.

## CARF Standards

Standards are organized in several categories. Business standards relate to the organization and its leadership; for example, there are standards addressing financial management, risk management, human resources, physical plant, strategic planning, corporate compliance, and corporate citizenship. Standards about information and outcome management focus on performance improvement. Standards about the process of rehabilitation involve how a client enters a program, how he or she is assessed, how his or her needs are identified, how an individual program is established, how a client is discharged, and how follow-up services are conducted. In addition, specific standards address the particular programs or services that are offered. Organizations may choose accreditation for more than 80 possible types of programs and services. Examples are brain injury programs, occupational rehabilitation programs, community mental health programs, respite care services, community assistive technology services, foster family services, assisted living services, adult day services, and crisis intervention services.

The actual site survey is based on a consultative, peer approach that provides feedback on conformance to the standards. The process identifies standard areas that are out of conformance, those that are in partial conformance, and those that are being met in an exemplary fashion. The degree of conformance to the standards determines the accreditation outcome.

## Accreditation Outcomes

To be accredited, an organization should meet each of the CARF accreditation conditions and should demonstrate through a site survey that it meets the standards established by CARF. Although an organization may not be in full conformance with every applicable standard, the accreditation decision will be based on the balance of the organization's strengths with those areas in which the organization requires improvement. Once the organization receives its accreditation outcome, it has 90 days to prepare a QIP and send it to CARF. This plan addresses the standards with which the organization was not in conformance. CARF and the next survey team will use this document throughout the tenure of the accreditation to assist in improvement activities.

Accreditation decisions acknowledge conformance outcomes in four categories: 3-year accreditation, 1-year accreditation, provisional accreditation, and nonaccreditation. CARF's surveyors, staff members, and trustees use the following guidelines to determine each organization's survey outcome.

### Three-Year Accreditation

Guidelines for 3-year accreditation require the organization to meet each of the CARF accreditation conditions and show substantial fulfillment of the standards.

The organization has demonstrated that its services and practices are designed and carried out to benefit the people it serves. Services, personnel, and documentation clearly indicate that present conditions represent an established pattern of total operation and that these conditions are likely to be maintained or improved in the near future.

## One-Year Accreditation

Guidelines for 1-year accreditation require the organization to meet each of the CARF accreditation conditions. Although the organization may demonstrate deficiencies with respect to the standards, the evidence shows the organization's capability and commitment to correct the deficiencies and progress toward their correction. On balance, the services are benefiting those served, and the organization appears to be protecting their health, welfare, and safety.

An organization may be functioning between the level of a 3-year accreditation and that of a 1-year accreditation because of certain conditions. In this instance, accreditation will be awarded for 1 year. An organization may not be awarded a second consecutive 1-year accreditation.

## Provisional Accreditation

The organization is given provisional accreditation if it meets each of the CARF accreditation conditions. Although the organization may demonstrate deficiencies in relation to the standards, the evidence shows the organization's capability and commitment to correct the deficiencies and progress toward conformance. The organization also demonstrates that it is protecting persons served in areas of health, welfare, and safety.

A provisional accreditation may be awarded only once, for a period of 1 year, after an organization has received a 1-year accreditation for the previous site survey. The organization must be functioning at the level of a 3-year accreditation at the end of the tenure of the provisional accreditation or it will receive a survey outcome of nonaccreditation.

## Nonaccreditation

The organization will receive a nonaccreditation decision when (a) it demonstrates major deficiencies in several areas of the standards and serious questions arise as to the benefits of services or the health, welfare, or safety of its clientele; (b) the organization has failed over time to bring itself into substantial conformance with the standards; or (c) the organization has failed to meet any one of the CARF accreditation conditions. A consequence of nonaccreditation could be the loss of funding, the decline in recognition by an outside agency, or a review by a federal or state regulator. Nonaccredited organizations cannot reapply for accreditation for a minimum of 6 months.

## Value of the Accreditation Cycle

The years in between an accreditation cycle are critical. All levels of the organization need to recognize that maintenance of the standards and the ongoing measurement of results as well as improvement of programs and services are important for success. Good business practice strategies and accountable clinicians will assist the human services arena to succeed; however, one must understand that organizations can have human services and accountability and not be accredited. Many overworked organizations are challenged to prepare and master the systems approach to human services delivery, which involves all components of the organization working together toward organizational goals. Accreditation offers an outside review, the tools to do a good job, and guidance for the organization to distinguish itself from other human services organizations. Accreditation is a "good-housekeeping" seal of approval that is recognized by many. CARF accreditation is a value-added benefit to organizations that has become an operational tool for excellence.

## References

Carver, J., & Carver, M. (1997). *Reinventing your board.* San Francisco: Jossey-Bass.

Commission on Accreditation of Rehabilitation Facilities. (2002a, January). *2002 CARF accreditation sourcebook.* Tucson, AZ: Author.

Commission on Accreditation of Rehabilitation Facilities. (2002b, January). *2002 CARF governance policies* (pp. E1–E3). Tucson, AZ: Author.

Commission on Accreditation of Rehabilitation Facilities. (2002c, January). *2002 CARF medical rehabilitation standards manual.* Tucson, AZ: Author.

# CHAPTER 24

# Accreditations Related to Education and Competence

Paula Kramer, PhD, OTR/L, FAOTA
Suzanne Seitz, BA
Barbara Dickson, BA

*"Accreditation of occupational therapy educational programs ensures the quality of the program, by making certain that it meets minimal standards, and by assisting the program with ongoing reflection for the purpose of continuous improvment."*

PAULA KRAMER

**Paula Kramer, PhD, OTR/L, FAOTA,** has been an occupational therapist for 30 years, primarily in pediatrics. She has been an occupational therapy educator for 22 years and has been involved with occupational therapy accreditation since 1985. She has been a member of the Accreditation Council for Occupational Therapy Education since 1996 and its chair since 2001.

**Suzanne Seitz, BA,** is production editor for AOTA Press in Bethesda, MD. She has an editing certificate from George Washington University, Washington, DC. She has written articles and brief columns for *OT Practice.*

**Barbara Dickson, BA,** is editorial assistant for AOTA Press in Bethesda, MD. She served as editor-in-chief of her college newspaper, which under her leadership won the 2000 Pacemaker Award from the Associated Collegiate Press.

## Key Terms and Concepts

**Accreditation.** A formal process to determine if an academic or institutional program is minimally in compliance with a prescribed set of standards.

**Occupational therapy education.** An academic program designed to prepare students to become entry-level occupational therapists.

## Learning Objectives

After completing this chapter, you should be able to do the following:

- Understand the purpose and value of accreditation.

- Appreciate the history of accreditation of occupational therapy educational programs.

- Demonstrate a beginning understanding of the accreditation process for occupational therapy educational programs.

- Articulate the relationship between accreditation and occupational therapy education.

Many types of accreditation are used, including accreditation for hospitals and health care agencies, for colleges and universities, and for specific educational programs. This chapter focuses on the various accreditation processes for these settings. The first section focuses on the accreditation process for occupational therapy education, specifically, the accreditation of educational programs for occupational therapists and occupational therapy assistants. Other sections focus on accreditation processes to ensure quality services for individuals with developmental disabilities (the Council on Quality and Leadership); accreditation of quality home and community health care organizations (the Community Health Accreditation Program, or CHAP); recognition of accredited higher education organizations (the Council for Higher Education Accreditation, or CHEA); representation of specialized accreditation agencies (the Association of Specialized and Professional Accreditors, or ASPA); and processes to ensure quality and fairness in international academic and professional mobility, credentialing, and recognition (the Center for Quality Assurance in International Education, or CQAIE).

Accreditation for specific educational and professional programs is considered specialty accreditation, as compared with the broader based accreditation for colleges and universities in general. Specialty accreditation is a voluntary process and is provided primarily by nongovernmental, independent organizations and professional organizations. Accrediting bodies establish specific criteria, currently referred to as *standards,* that must be met to become an accredited program. These standards identify minimally acceptable criteria. In the past, our standards were called *essentials,* a term that was used by the American Medical Association (AMA), under whom we were initially accredited. The term *standards* is more commonly used today.

## Accreditation for Occupational Therapy Education

The Accreditation Council for Occupational Therapy Education (ACOTE®) is the recognized body that accredits occupational therapy and occupational therapy assistant educational programs. ACOTE is affiliated with the American Occupational Therapy Association (AOTA), housed with the AOTA offices, and supported by the AOTA staff; however, it is an independent body recognized by the U.S. Department of Education (USDE) and the CHEA as the accrediting body for occupational therapy education. The purpose of accreditation is to ensure the quality of the program, ascertaining that it meets minimal standards, and to assist with the ongoing reflection and improvement of the program.

Accreditation of occupational therapy education programs provides a valuable service to several constituency groups: the public, the students, and the institution in which a program is housed. Members of the public value accreditation because it assures them that the program and the institution value external evaluation and that the program meets the standards of the professional field. Accreditation informs the public of those institutions that voluntarily engage in this type of review process, a process that focuses on improving the quality of the program. It identifies programs that are concerned with the continuous improvement of professional services because accreditation standards are modified on an ongoing basis to reflect changes in knowledge and practices in the profession at large (AOTA/ACOTE, 2000).

ACOTE accreditation provides students of occupational therapy and occupational therapy assistant programs with an assurance that the educational program meets professional standards and that, because it meets these standards, it will be able to address the needs of students as future practitioners. Although this assurance cannot guarantee the competence of students as future practitioners, it does ensure that the education that he or she receives is consistent with current knowledge and practice as well as with established criteria.

The accreditation of an occupational therapy program benefits the institution in which the program is housed by providing a stimulus for program self-evaluation and ongoing improvements. This self-evaluation is strengthened both by the external review process and by the consultation that is a part of the process. Accreditation also is viewed positively by the public and, therefore, enhances the reputation of the academic institution (AOTA/ACOTE, 2000).

Accreditation can be seen as a type of gatekeeping. However, the process does not keep individuals out of the profession in the way that one usually expects of gatekeeping; instead, it prevents schools from providing educational programs that do not meet minimum standards, and it identifies areas of strength and areas that require improvement.

## History of Occupational Therapy Education Accreditation

The first standards for occupational therapy education can be traced to about 1923 and appear to have been written in large part by Eleanor Clarke Slagle, one of the founders of the profession (Slagle, 1931). She noted that, a few years after 1923, "the Council of the American Medical Association made a study of the training of workers in occupational therapy and issued a report recommending even higher standards than were in force" (p. 15). Simultaneously, several deans of training schools (as they were called at the time) also recommended that minimal requirements be increased. These changes were adopted. At this time, the accreditation of occupational therapy programs became one of the roles of the AOTA.

In 1933, AOTA requested that the AMA work in cooperation with it to develop and improve educational programs for occupational therapists. The AMA House of Delegates adopted the "Essentials of an Acceptable School of Occupational Therapy" (AOTA/ACOTE, 2000), which was the AMA's first cooperative accreditation activity.

The AOTA Accreditation Committee began approving educational programs for occupational therapy assistants in 1958. At the same time, curriculum directors began a strong movement to again study and increase the requirements for the education of occupational therapists, and they expressed concern that preparation should be more stringent academically, with less technical and medical focus. Some evidence also indicates that the curriculum directors were conflicted about the role of the AMA in regulating occupational therapy education (Colman, 1990).

The collaboration of AOTA (through its Accreditation Committee) and the AMA was officially recognized by numerous private and governmental agencies over the years, including the National Commission on Accreditation, the Federation of Regional Accrediting Commissions of Higher Education, the Council on Post-Secondary Education (COPA), and the USDE. The AMA collaboration with AOTA on accreditation continued under the aegis of AMA's Committee on Allied Health Education and Accreditation (CAHEA). CAHEA was recognized by the USDE as the accrediting body for occupational therapy education. In 1991, based on a request from AOTA, CAHEA began accrediting occupational therapy assistant programs.

The 1990s were a critical period of growth and change for occupational therapy accreditation. In 1994, the Accreditation Committee of the AOTA officially changed its name to the Accreditation Council for Occupational Therapy Education and began to exercise some autonomy. After discussion with various constituency groups, ACOTE began to operate independently from CAHEA. During that same year, ACOTE was recognized by the USDE as the accrediting agency for professional programs in occupational therapy. ACOTE sets the *Standards for an Accredited Educational Program the Occupational Therapist* (ACOTE, 1998a) and the *Standards for an Accredited Educational Program for the Occupational Therapy Assistant* (ACOTE, 1998b). (As of this writing, ACOTE accredits 147 programs at the professional level and 168 occupational therapy assistant programs.)

In 1998, as ACOTE was reviewing draft standards for professional level education, the council adopted a position statement indicating that, because of "the demands, complexity, and a diversity of contemporary occupational therapy practice, ACOTE's position is that the forthcoming educational standards are most likely to be achieved in post-baccalaureate degree programs" (ACOTE, 1998c, p. 1). In April 1999, at the AOTA Annual Conference, the Representative Assembly passed Resolution J, which called for entry-level education for occupational therapist to be at the postbaccalaureate level (AOTA, 1999). ACOTE determined in August 1999 that professional, entry-level education programs "must be offered at the post-baccalaureate entry level by 2007 to receive and maintain ACOTE accreditation status" (ACOTE, 1999, p. i, ii).

## Accreditation Process for Education Programs in Occupational Therapy

ACOTE is made up of 15 occupational therapists and occupational therapy assistants, two public members, and one alternate public member. The council is responsible for setting standards for education for occupational therapists and occupational therapy assistants and for monitoring and regularly reviewing all occupational therapy educational programs. Standards are routinely reviewed, with a formal review process instituted approximately 5 years after each set of standards is revised and accepted.

Programs are routinely required to engage in a self-study process to assess their compliance with the educational standards, a process that is achieved through biennial reports and comprehensive self-study documents. After the completion of a self-study document, representatives of the council conduct a comprehensive on-site visit to meet with all constituency groups involved in the educational process and to verify the information supplied in the report of self-study. On-site visits are conducted by members of ACOTE and members of the Roster of Accreditation Evaluators, a group of occupational therapy educators and practitioners who have been trained to understand the standards and to conduct on-site visits. On-site teams are made up of an educator and a practitioner to adhere to the USDE requirements for accreditation of a practice profession. This requirement is helpful in ensuring that the program is meeting the current standards and reflects current practice.

When a new program applies for ACOTE accreditation, the program must follow a three-step process. First, an application for developing program status must be submitted. This application is reviewed by one member of the council and two members of the Roster. The results of this review are submitted to the council and discussed. After preliminary approval, the program can continue in the process and accept students.

Second, the program subsequently submits an initial report of self-study to the council, describing the program in detail for an initial review. The self-study is comprehensive. Programs must review and comment on all aspects of the educational process included in the standards. This process requires significant time and input from many sources on campus. It is a comprehensive program review that can help the faculty to identify the strengths and potential weaknesses of the program. Once the council has approved this review, programs receive a report and have an opportunity to make improvements.

At this point, the third step in the process, the on-site visit, can take place. After an on-site visit, the council reviews the report and determines the accreditation status of the program. The council report includes a detailed description of compliance with the standards, strengths of the program, suggestions for improvement, and areas of noncompliance. Accreditation status for new programs includes a status of accreditation or of accreditation withheld. Programs being reaccredited may receive a status of accreditation, probationary accreditation, or accreditation withheld.

Once a program has been initially accredited, it must submit biennial reports that provide ongoing information about the program and must assist in determining continuing compliance with educational standards. Accreditation is granted for a period of 5 years after the initial on-site visit and for either 7 or 10 years subsequently. Before an on-site visit, each program must conduct a complete self-study.

## Value of Accreditation for Occupational Therapy Education Programs

Through the development and periodic review of comprehensive standards, the profession can be certain that education is meeting the needs of society. As the profession and its practice grows and changes, the standards are revised to reflect those changes, thus ensuring that future practitioners will have the basic information needed for practice. The standards ensure some degree of uniformity in the education of future occupational therapy practitioners and require educational programs and faculty to remain current and to reflect what is offered for study. This process is valuable to the educational program, its students, and the community it serves.

The schools also benefit from this process. External review validates the quality of the program. Specialty accreditation informs society that the institution cares about the quality of its programs and desires this type of review. Further, programs that receive accreditation status are considered prestigious.

A practitioner's or an educator's involvement in the accreditation process also provides valuable professional experience. Participation requires time and effort, but it is also rewarding. As a member of the Roster of Accreditation Evaluators, one can learn about the education process from a different perspective. One has an opportunity to understand the educational and accreditation processes in more depth and to have some input into the education of future practitioners. This type of service to the profession is highly valued by its members. ACOTE routinely calls for new candidates for the Roster of Accreditation Evaluators in AOTA publications such as *OT Practice*. Experienced Roster members are considered eligible potentially to become ACOTE members.

## Summary: Accreditation for Occupational Therapy Education

The accreditation of occupational therapy educational programs has a long history, beginning in 1920s under the control of the AMA to the present under the ACOTE, an independent specialty accreditation agency that is recognized by the USDE and the CHEA. Ongoing accreditation provides a value to the public, the students, and the institution in which the program is housed. ACOTE is committed to ensuring and maintaining high-quality educational programs that will prepare practitioners to effectively cope with the demands of practice.

# Council on Quality and Leadership

The Council on Quality and Leadership became its own organization in 1969. It was originally part of the Joint Commission on Accreditation of Healthcare Organizations (JCAHO) and became its own organization because of a need to measure the quality of services for people with developmental disabilities.

The Council's mission is to develop quality measures, performance indicators, and evaluation methods that are person centered; to provide consultation, education, and other learning tools to build individual and organizational capacity; to conduct research and to promote the availability of data for decision making and policy development; and to provide access to the latest information, developments, trends, and best practices to consumers, their families, support and service organizations, and governmental organizations (Council on Quality and Leadership, n.d.).

Accreditation activities are managed through the Council's accreditation and evaluation systems division. Its mission is to design and carry out methodologies for the measurement of quality in organizations that provide services to people with disabilities. Methods include accreditation, organization assessment, consultation and technical assistance, third-party evaluation, and research studies (Council on Quality and Leadership, n.d.).

## Accreditation Through the Council on Quality and Leadership

The Council on Quality and Leadership has 85 staff members. Between one and five staff members who are either full-time or part-time conduct any particular accreditation. No peer reviewers conduct accreditation. The staff members who conduct accreditations are usually chosen because their experience in their field matches the organization that will be accredited. For example, the staff member could be a nurse, an occupational therapist, a director, or an insurance specialist (Interview with Cindy Kauffman, Council on Quality and Leadership, March 7, 2002).

The Council accredits only 100 organizations per year, including residential services, employment services, service coordination centers, counseling centers, and other community-based organizations that provide services to people with physical disabilities, mental disabilities, or developmental disabilities. The Council's personal outcomes approach makes the accreditation process a rigorous one for organizations. This approach examines how the organization directly affects individuals. During a review process lasting 3 to 5 days, staff members of the Council conduct personal interviews with people who are receiving services from the organization and with staff members at the organization (Interview with Cindy Kauffman, Council on Quality and Leadership, March 7, 2002). In these interviews, the Council reviewers ask the following questions:

- Are the people who use this organization safe?
- Are their rights protected?
- Do they have access to health care?
- Is the organization fiscally sound?
- Is the organization legally sound?
- Are the organization's policies in place?
- Are supports and training in place?
- How does the organization use the data it receives?
- How does it learn how to fix things from incidents that are reported? (Interview with Cindy Kauffman, Council on Quality and Leadership, March 7, 2002)

## Summary: Council on Quality and Leadership

The Council on Quality and Leadership became its own organization in 1969. It was originally part of the JCAHO. The Council developed because of a need to measure the quality of organizations for people with developmental disabilities, mental disabilities, or physical disabilities. The Council's accreditation process takes 3 to 5 days and uses a personal outcomes approach, which involves Council reviewers asking the people receiving services from the organization and the organization's staff members their opinions of the organization. The Council accredits only 100 organizations per year.

# Community Health Accreditation Program

CHAP was founded in 1965 and is now a subsidiary of the National League for Nursing. CHAP is an independent nonprofit organization that accredits home and community health care organizations, including home health providers, hospice care, public health organizations, home care aide services, primary duty services, supplemental staffing services, home infusion therapy providers, home dialysis services, home medical equipment providers, pharmacy services, day care centers, community nursing centers, and community rehabilitation centers (CHAP, n.d.c).

CHAP's mission is to provide leadership in enhancing the health and well-being of diverse communities. This mission is achieved through the development of standards of excellence that ensure the management of ethical, humane, and competent care in home, community, and public health settings. In addition, the development and dissemination of innovative products, services, and models of care as well as the creation of partnerships further promote this mission (CHAP, n.d.e).

CHAP's four main purposes are (a) to develop standards applicable to providers of home and community health care; (b) to evaluate these providers and accredit the providers who are meeting or exceeding these standards; (c) to provide an external, objective marker for the public, demonstrating that the provider meets national standards of organizational strength and quality; and (d) to provide information to the public to assist in the selection of home and community health services and providers (CHAP, n.d.e).

## Structure of CHAP

Members of the CHAP Board of Directors represent consumers, purchasers, providers, and experts of home and community-based health care services. Each member of the board serves a 3-year term. The board is responsible for determining the mission, purpose, and objectives of CHAP and for evaluating CHAP's performance in how well it meets its purpose (CHAP, n.d.c).

The CHAP Board of Directors authorizes the Board of Review to review and analyze site visit reports and to decide which applicant organizations will be accredited. The Board of Review consists of providers and consumers of home and community-based health care organizations. Each member of the Board of Review serves on the board for 3 years (CHAP, n.d.c).

The Board of Review meets every 2 months, and all members must attend each 2-day session. Four members must be present at each Board of Review session to make an official decision. The site visitor will participate in the review process but will not have the power to vote with the board (CHAP, n.d.c). The Board of Review's responsibilities include (a) reviewing site visit reports and progress reports; (b) analyzing data to see whether those data meet CHAP's standards; (c) making sure that site visit findings are accurate; (d) making objective accreditation decisions based on the site visit team recommendations and the results of the Board of Review process; (e) using survey frequency guidelines to determine time frames for progress reports, focus visits, and annual visits; (f) documenting Board of Review findings in the "Board of Review Summary" for each report reviewed; (g) making recommendations to the Board of Directors and the CHAP administration with respect to accreditation policies, procedures, and practices; and (h) participating in scheduled training programs to remain current with the CHAP process of accreditation (CHAP, n.d.c).

## Accreditation Through CHAP

To start the accreditation process, an organization must send a completed application form along with the application fee to CHAP. The organization will provide the following information on the application form: services offered, number of branches and subsidiaries, annual client visits, and gross revenues. In addition to the application fee, the organization will also need to pay an annual accreditation fee (determined by the organization's gross revenues) and a site visit fee (CHAP, n.d.b).

Next, the organization must complete a self-study report and send it to CHAP. The self-study includes the following information about the organization: the quality of the organization's services and products, the organization's available resources, the organization's financial status, and the organization's attention to consumers (CHAP, n.d.b). The self-study gives the organization an opportunity to evaluate itself and prepare for CHAP's site visit.

The next step in the accreditation process is the site visit. A minimum of two site visitors will attend each site visit. The site visitors will evaluate the organization by making visits to clients who are receiving care at their homes and clients who are receiving care in community-based settings. The site members will also interview staff members as well as governing and advisory board members. They will review documents, policies, procedures, and clinical records (CHAP, n.d.a, n.d.b).

Finally, the Board of Review will review the site visit report as well as other data and make a decision as to whether or not to accredit the organization. If the organization is applying for initial accreditation, the Board of Review may take one of the following three actions: (a) grant full accreditation with or without required actions or recommendations, (b) defer accreditation for a specified time period pending additional information or a focused site visit, or (c) deny accreditation. If an organization is applying for continued accreditation, the board may take one of the following three actions: (a) renew full accreditation with or without required actions or recommendations, (b) submit a notice of formal warning with a specific time period (i.e., 30, 60, or 90 days) given in which the organization must make specific improvements, or (c) withdraw accreditation (CHAP, n.d.b). If an organization is accredited by CHAP, it receives CHAP's Gold Seal of Approval.

### Summary: CHAP

CHAP, an independent nonprofit organization that is also a subsidiary of the National League for Nursing, accredits home and community health care organizations. CHAP's standards ensure that the management of health care will be humane, ethical, and competent. CHAP's latest standards represent a major breakthrough in accreditation and exceed the minimum safety standard set by the federal government (CHAP, n.d.d). CHAP ensures that its standards are met through the process of accreditation, which consists of four steps: (a) the organization completes an application and submits it to CHAP, (b) the organization completes a self-study, (c) CHAP conducts a site visit at the organization, and (d) the Board of Review considers the results of the site visit and other data and determines whether or not the organization will be accredited.

## Council for Higher Education Accreditation

CHEA was founded in 1966. Presidents of American universities and colleges established CHEA to provide recognition of accredited organizations that provide higher education, for example, universities, colleges, schools, and programs. CHEA's mission statement is as follows: "[CHEA] will serve students and their families, colleges and universities, sponsoring bodies, governments, and employers by promoting academic quality through formal recognition of higher education accreditation bodies and will coordinate and work to advance self-regulation through accreditation" (CHEA, n.d.).

Recognition is not accreditation. Accreditation occurs when the faculty, administrators, and staff of an institution (e.g., a college or university) conduct a self-study to see whether they meet the accrediting organization's goals. Then, the accrediting organization conducts on-site visits at the institution and interviews the institution's staff. The accrediting organization reviews the results of the on-site visits and interviews and determines whether or not the institution will be accredited. Recognition involves acknowledging an accrediting organization's high standards of quality performance in its work to accredit organizations and institutions.

For an accrediting organization to be recognized by CHEA, the organization must meet the following five recognition standards: (a) advances academic quality, (b) demonstrates accountability, (c) encourages purposeful change and needed improvement, (d) uses appropriate and fair procedures in decision making, and (e) continually reassesses accreditation practices (CHEA, n.d.). CHEA's first three recognition standards—to advance academic quality, to demonstrate accountability, and to encourage purposeful change and needed improvement—are also its three basic purposes.

## Structure of CHEA

The CHEA Board of Directors appoints members to the CHEA Committee on Recognition according to recommendations by the president of CHEA made in consultation with CHEA-recognized accrediting organizations. The nine-member committee is responsible for the recognition status of new and continuing accrediting organizations. Each member serves a 3-year term. The committee includes members from professional accrediting organizations, colleges and universities, and the public. Public members are people who are not involved with an institution or an accrediting organization. The committee may also consult external readers during the process of recognition. External readers are nonmembers of the committee who will read the organization's application for recognition. The committee advises the 17-member Board of Directors on which organizations are eligible for recognition, and the board makes the final decision (CHEA, n.d.).

## Recognition Process Through CHEA

Usually, the accrediting organization will undergo a recognition review every 10 years, with an interim 5-year report. However, CHEA may decide to review a recognized accrediting organization out of sequence when the organization decides to change its activities or when concerns about the organization have been documented over a period of time.

The steps in the recognition review process are as follows (CHEA, n.d.):

1. The accrediting organization sends a letter of intent to apply for recognition and an application fee to CHEA.
2. CHEA sends the accrediting organization the recognition review materials.
3. The accrediting organization returns the eligibility portion of the application to CHEA, and the committee makes a recommendation on eligibility to the Board of Directors for consideration.
4. The board considers the committee's recommendation and provides the accrediting organization with the opportunity to appear before the board if necessary.
5. The accrediting organization completes the self-study and sends it to CHEA. A self-study should provide evidence that the accrediting organization meets CHEA's five recognition standards.
6. If applicable, CHEA sends a site visitor to the accrediting organization. Site visits are required in any of the following three instances: (a) the accrediting organization is seeking initial recognition, (b) the committee believes that the

material provided by the accrediting organization is insufficient for a fair judgment by the committee, or (c) the committee believes that third-party comments received by the committee are sufficient to raise questions that may be addressed by a site visit.

7. The accrediting organization's response, any reader and site visit reports, and any third-party comments are sent to the CHEA office. An institution's representative, an association's representative, or a member of the general public can make a third-party comment. The third-party comment must relate to the CHEA recognition standards and can be negative or positive. Many third-party comments are testimonials.

8. The accrediting organization gives a public presentation to the committee, and the committee gives a recommendation to the Board of Directors.

9. The accrediting organization responds to any questions the committee has about the public presentation.

10. The Board of Directors considers the committee's recommendation and, if necessary, provides the accrediting organization with an opportunity to appear before the board.

The Board of Directors will consider the recommendations of the committee before making its decisions and will notify accrediting organizations of the board's actions within 30 days after taking any action. If the board recognizes an accrediting organization, the notice will specify the scope of the organization's recognition (including, where indicated, the geographic area, the types of higher education institutions or programs that the organization may accredit, and the degrees and certificates awarded by higher education institutions accredited by the accrediting organization) and the recognition period.

All of the decisions of the Board of Directors with respect to recognition of an accrediting organization will be public knowledge. CHEA will publish the decisions of the board. CHEA may withdraw recognition of an accrediting organization for any sufficient cause, including a determination by CHEA that the organization no longer meets the requirements for eligibility or the standards for recognition (CHEA, n.d.).

## Summary: CHEA

CHEA plays an important role in the accreditation process by formally recognizing accrediting institutions. CHEA was founded in 1966 by presidents of American universities and colleges to strengthen accreditation through recognition. CHEA has five recognition standards: The accrediting institution must advance academic quality, demonstrate accountability, encourage purposeful change and needed improvement, use appropriate and fair procedures in decision making, and continually reassess accreditation practices.

## Association of Specialized and Professional Accreditors

ASPA was formed in the fall of 1993 when COPA dissolved. Accrediting bodies can be divided into two general groups: (a) organizations that accredit colleges and universities as institutions and (b) organizations that deal with professional, specialized, and special-purpose programs (ASPA, n.d.d). Members of COPA, which had authority over specialized accrediting agencies in the United States, created ASPA to act as a voice for accrediting agencies and to provide policy and developmental services (Davenport, 2000). ASPA is the only organization that solely represents specialized accreditation agencies.

ASPA was formed under the District of Columbia Nonprofit Corporation Act for educational, scientific, research, mutual improvement, and professional purposes. ASPA's goals are to maintain and improve the quality of education and to safeguard the public. ASPA's bylaws charge the association with several tasks (ASPA n.d.a):

- Promote quality and integrity in nongovernmental specialized and professional accreditation of postsecondary programs and institutions.
- Provide a forum for discussion and analysis and a mechanism for common action for those concerned with specialized and professional accreditation.
- Address accreditation issues in educational, governmental, and public policy contexts and communicate with the public about accreditation.
- Foster collaboration among programs, institutions, and accreditation organizations.
- Provide a mechanism for individuals and organizations with accreditation responsibility to participate in continuing education.

### Structure of ASPA

ASPA's membership comprises accrediting agencies that adhere to the ASPA member code of good practice. According to ASPA bylaws, voting members review, approve, and amend articles of incorporation; review, approve, and amend bylaws; review and approve proposals for a major reorganization, reorientation, or dissolution of the association; elect a board of directors and officers; and elect the chair and members of the Committee on Nominations.

ASPA's Board of Directors consists of eight members: three chief staff officers from agencies that hold ASPA votes, one chief executive or chief academic officer of an institution holding institutional or programmatic accreditation by at least one voting member of the association, one academic member from programs or institutions accredited by voting members of the association, one practitioner member from among the professions represented by voting members of the association, one member of the public whose vocation is outside the academic and accreditation communities, and APSA's executive director who is ex officio and nonvoting. With the exception of the public member, all board members must have significant experience in accreditation as site visitors, commission or board members, or staff members.

The duties of the Board of Directors, according to the bylaws, are as follows:
- Implement the Bylaws, as approved by the Association.
- Review, approve, and amend *Rules of Practice and Procedure,* policy documents, criteria and procedures for membership, and provisions for recognition following consultation with members of the Association.
- Establish the dues and fees structure(s) of the Association following consultation with members of the Association.
- Review the annual report of the Association's financial position as prepared by official auditors and approve the annual budget.
- Control the funds and properties of the Association, holding and using them on behalf of the Association after consultation with members of the Association.
- Establish and revise testimonial policies and operational guidelines statements of the Association after consultation with members of the Association.
- Elect new members to the Association.
- Establish and oversee an appeals procedure for the recognition process.
- Serve the needs of the membership, recognizing the diversity as well as the common interest of Association members and other constituents of accreditation.
- Appoint the Executive Director of the Association and prescribe his or her duties. (ASPA, n.d.a)

The chair, vice chair, treasurer, and secretary of the Board of Directors as well as the association's executive director form the Executive Committee. The Executive Committee's duties, as prescribed in the bylaws, include the following: be responsible to ASPA and its Board of Directors for carrying out the board's policy decisions and recommendations; monitor the effectiveness of the articles of incorporation, bylaws, provisions for recognition, criteria for membership, code of ethics, as well as other policies and procedures and determine the timing and procedures for revision; function as a finance committee when needed and ensure that ASPA's long-range strategic and financial plan is presented regularly; monitor the effectiveness of all ASPA groups in carrying out their specific missions, goals, objectives, and action plans; and make recommendations to the board concerning the executive director's appointment and duties as well as set his or her salary.

In addition to the Executive Committee, ASPA has three standing committees: (a) the Committee on Membership, (b) the Committee on Recognition, and (c) the Committee on Professional Development. The board, Executive Committee, or chair of the Executive Committee can establish additional committees if needed.

## What ASPA Does

ASPA provides members with a strong national voice on important issues with respect to specialized accreditation. Accrediting agencies that belong to ASPA set national educational standards for entry into approximately 40 specialized disciplines or defined professions (ASPA, n.d.c).

ASPA publishes *ASPA News* twice a year, in January and July. This newsletter provides updates about meetings and conferences, reviews books, and includes articles on issues facing accrediting agencies.

Any accrediting body that wants to join ASPA must demonstrate that its governing body has endorsed the ASPA member code of good practice, which states that the accrediting agency

> pursues its mission, goals, and objectives, and conducts its operations in a trustworthy manner; maximizes service, productivity, and effectiveness in the accreditation relationship; respects and protects institutional autonomy; maintains a broad perspective as the basis for wise decision making; focuses accreditation reviews on the development of knowledge and competence; exhibits integrity and professionalism in the conduct of its operation; and has mechanisms to ensure that expertise and experience in the application of its standards, procedures, and values are present in members of its visiting teams, commissions, and staff. (ASPA, n.d.b)

To be eligible for ASPA membership, accrediting agencies must demonstrate that they meet ASPA's definition of a specialized or professional accrediting body, which is defined as "one with a national scope that accredits higher education programs or institutions that prepare individuals for entry into practice in a specialized discipline or defined profession" (ASPA, n.d.e). ASPA member agencies represent professionals in the nursing, dentistry, education, acupuncture, theater, psychology, and medical education fields.

### Summary: ASPA

ASPA was created to promote quality and integrity in accreditation. ASPA is the only organization that solely represents specialized accrediting agencies. It works to increase the efficiency and effectiveness of accreditation, holding its members to rigorous, comprehensive, and outcome-based standards. Some ASPA member agencies have been accrediting from the earliest years of accreditation and can offer vast knowledge that is beneficial to other agencies, educators, the government, and the public.

## Center for Quality Assurance in International Education

CQAIE was founded in 1991 out of COPA. CQAIE is located at the National Center for Higher Education in Washington, DC, and was created to deal with issues of quality and fairness in international academic and professional mobility, credentialing, and recognition (CQAIE, n.d.c).

CQAIE's purpose is threefold: (a) to assist countries in the development or enhancement of quality assurance systems for higher education; (b) to promote the globalization of the professions; and (c) to monitor quality issues in the transnational movement of higher education. CQAIE fosters communication and collaboration among organizations responsible for quality education and practice within the world's primary professions (CQAIE, n.d.c).

## Structure of CQAIE

An eight-member Board of Directors runs CQAIE. The board comprises the executive directors of the Council for the Accreditation of Counseling and Related Educational Programs, the National Board for Certified Counselors, the Commission on Institutions of Higher Education, the President's Committee on the Arts and the Humanities, and CQAIE. Also serving on CQAIE's Board of Directors are a visiting scholar from CQAIE, the chief executive officer of Teleologic Learning Company, and the vice president for graduate and professional education of the Educational Testing Service (CQAIE, n.d.b).

## What CQAIE Does

CQAIE focuses on the international dimension of accreditation, helping organizations address the growing need for new technology and education about new technology, establishing common standards across borders in the globalization of professions, and handling quality issues as institutions of higher education and accrediting agencies move into other countries.

CQAIE has done extensive work around the world in countries such as Morocco, Indonesia, Japan, Bolivia, Mexico, Estonia, and Romania. It encourages accreditation in these countries by designing legislation or national policy, carrying out training, or evaluating an existing system. In regional meetings that CQAIE convenes, most if not all of the countries of the region participate in developing quality initiatives for that territory (CQAIE, n.d.a).

Thanks to multinational trade agreements and new technology, professions are looking to expand overseas. CQAIE helps professionals who want to move into other countries and assists professions going through the globalization process by working on quality assurance in education and competency assurance in practice (CQAIE, n.d.d). By advising member organizations on issues such as how to identify those countries in which members of a profession wish to practice and how to protect consumers while simultaneously maintaining quality in higher education and practice, CQAIE helps professions learn how to globalize (CQAIE, n.d.d).

In addition to working with foreign countries, CQAIE monitors the quality of education that crosses U.S. borders. Increasingly, U.S. universities are starting programs abroad, but in addition, many foreign schools are establishing campuses within the United States.

CQAIE conducts research to determine the extent of professional globalization and supports research in related fields (e.g., international literacy). The association annually produces a publication for its series *The Trade Agreements and the Globalization of Higher Education and the Professions*. Additionally, periodic newsletters update members on current events and issues.

In response to the needs of these growing professional communities, CQAIE sponsors national and regional meetings. The goals of these meetings include learning about practical issues related to providing higher education in foreign countries, developing principles of good practice, and advocating international trade in education services (CQAIE, n.d.e). CQAIE often sponsors these meetings in conjunction with accrediting agencies.

Member countries of the North American Free Trade Agreement participate in CQAIE's annual conference. Increasingly, members of the European Union, the Asia Pacific Economic Cooperation forum, Mercosur, and the Free Trade Agreement of the Americas also attend the conference (CQAIE, n.d.d). The conference focuses on issues and information related to trade agreements and quality issues in globalization.

### Summary: CQAIE

CQAIE is dedicated to monitoring quality issues with respect to the globalization of higher education and professions and provides assistance in developing and improving quality assurance systems worldwide. CQAIE's programs, its annual publication in *The Trade Agreements and the Globalization of Higher Education and the Professions* series, and its periodic newsletters foster communication and collaboration among the organizations responsible for quality education and practice across many professions.

## References

Accreditation Council for Occupational Therapy Education. (1998a). *Standards for an accredited educational program for the occupational therapist.* Bethesda, MD: American Occupational Therapy Association.

Accreditation Council for Occupational Therapy Education. (1998b). *Standards for an accredited educational program for the occupational therapy assistant.* Bethesda, MD: American Occupational Therapy Association.

Accreditation Council for Occupational Therapy Education. (1998c). *White paper: Educational standards: Foundation for the future.* Bethesda, MD: Author.

Accreditation Council for Occupational Therapy Education. (1999, August 26). ACOTE sets timeline for postbaccalaureate degree programs. *OT Week, 13*(33), i, ii.

American Occupational Therapy Association/Accreditation Council for Occupational Therapy Education. (2000). *Accreditation manual.* Bethesda, MD: Author.

Association of Specialized and Professional Accreditors. (n.d.a). *Association of specialized and professional accreditors bylaws.* Retrieved March 5, 2002, from http://www.aspa-usa.org/ASPABylaws.html

Association of Specialized and Professional Accreditors. (n.d.b). *ASPA—Member code of good practice.* Retrieved March 5, 2002, from http://www.aspa-usa.org/code.html

Association of Specialized and Professional Accreditors. (n.d.c). *ASPA role, function, and purposes.* Retrieved March 5, 2002, from http://www.aspa-usa.org/aspamenu.html

Association of Specialized and Professional Accreditors. (n.d.d). *The importance of specialized accreditation.* Retrieved March 5, 2002, from http://www.aspa-usa.org/publics.html

Association of Specialized and Professional Accreditors. (n.d.e). *Membership info.* Retrieved March 5, 2002, from http://www.aspa-usa.org/meminfo.html

Center for Quality Assurance in International Education. (n.d.a). *Assisting countries in the development of quality assurance systems for higher education.* Retrieved February 8, 2002, from http://www.cqaie.org/Assisting.htm

Center for Quality Assurance in International Education. (n.d.b). *Board of directors.* Retrieved March 13, 2002, from http://www.cqaie.org/board.htm

Center for Quality Assurance in International Education. (n.d.c). *Change agent organization, A.* Retrieved March 5, 2002, from http://www.cqaie.org/welcome.html

Center for Quality Assurance in International Education. (n.d.d). *Globalization of the professions.* Retrieved February 8, 2002, from http://www.cqaie.org/Globalization.htm

Center for Quality Assurance in International Education. (n.d.e). *Transnational education: The globalization of U.S. higher education.* Retrieved February 8, 2002, from http://www.cqaie.org/transnational.htm

Colman, W. (1990). The curriculum directors: Influencing occupational therapy education, 1948–1964. *American Journal of Occupational Therapy, 44,* 357–362.

Community Health Accreditation Program. (n.d.a). *CHAP accreditation process.* Retrieved March 14, 2002, from http://www.chapinc.org/accreditprocess.htm

Community Health Accreditation Program. (n.d.b). *CHAP frequently asked questions.* Retrieved March 14, 2002, from http://www.chapinc.org/chap-faq.htm

Community Health Accreditation Program. (n.d.c). *CHAP introduction: Accreditation process.* Retrieved March 14, 2002, from http://www.chapinc.org/introduction.htm

Community Health Accreditation Program. (n.d.d). *Introduction to the standards of excellence.* Retrieved January 28, 2002, from http://www.chapinc.org/chap-soe.htm

Community Health Accreditation Program. (n.d.e). *Mission, purpose, and objectives.* Retrieved January 28, 2002, from http://www.chapinc.org/chap-mission.htm

Council for Higher Education Accreditation. (n.d.). *CHEA's recognition policy and procedures.* Retrieved February 8, 2002, from http://www.chea.org/About/Recognition.cfm.

Davenport, C. A. (2000). *Recognition chronology.* Chicago: Association of Specialized and Professional Accreditors. (Available from ASPA, 1020 West Byron Street, Suite 8G, Chicago, IL 60613-2987)

Slagle, E. C. (1931). The training of occupational therapists. *Psychiatric Quarterly, 5,* 12–20.

The Council on Quality and Leadership. (n.d.). Retrieved January 28, 2002 from http://www.the council.org/acs/accreditation.html.

# Special Supervision Issues

# CHAPTER 25

# Management of Fieldwork Education

Judith Palladino, MA, OTR/L

*"The challenge to our profession is to begin to strengthen the ties between experienced practitioners, educators, and students. Fieldwork offers a perfect opportunity to create these bonds."*

KOLODNER & HISCHMANN, 2000

**Judith Palladino, MA, OTR/L,** is assistant professor and the academic fieldwork coordinator for the master's in occupational therapy program at Loma Linda University. She coauthored the *Occupational Therapy Manual Assessing Professional Skills*, a text created for fieldwork Level I student assessment and portfolio development. As an active member of the California Occupational Therapy Fieldwork Council, she has developed and conducted many workshops for fieldwork educators and coordinators.

## Key Terms and Concepts

**Academic fieldwork coordinator.** The individual assigned by the college or university to oversee the fieldwork program. The coordinator may be responsible for some or all levels of fieldwork and for other experiences such as observations and community service activities. This individual is considered the occupational therapy program's resource person and expert with respect to fieldwork information.

**Fieldwork coordinator.** The onsite person identified to oversee all activities related to fieldwork. This work generally involves scheduling and coordinating fieldwork and may also include development, delivery, and evaluation of fieldwork education.

**Fieldwork educator.** The occupational therapy practitioner directly responsible for supervising the student. This person may still be referred to as the clinical instructor in some settings.

**Level I fieldwork.** Introduction to the fieldwork experience that involves directed observation and supervised participation. Supervision can be provided by an occupational therapist, occupational therapy assistant, or other professional. The number of experiences or hours will vary with the academic institution.

**Level II fieldwork.** An in-depth experience designed to promote the development of a competent, entry-level generalist occupational therapist or occupational therapy assistant. Supervision is provided by a qualified occupational therapist for occupational therapy students and either a qualified occupational therapist or occupational therapy assistant for occupational therapy assistant students. Each occupational therapy student must complete Level II fieldwork comprising a minimum of 24 weeks of full-time work. Each occupational therapy assistant student must complete Level II fieldwork comprising a minimum of 16 weeks of full-time work.

## Learning Objectives

After completing this chapter, you should be able to do the following:

- Evaluate the readiness of an occupational therapy program for fieldwork education.
- Understand the basics of fieldwork, including the levels of fieldwork and role of the educator.
- Establish the essential framework for a fieldwork education program.
- Understand the student supervisory process, including models, developmental stages, and the effects of culture.
- Understand the need for ongoing evaluation of fieldwork program effectiveness.

S tudents, academic programs, fieldwork educators, and fieldwork sites all benefit from fieldwork education. It is an essential element in the preparation of an individual who is studying to become an occupational therapist or occupational therapy assistant. Fieldwork education also can play an important role in the ongoing quality and quantity of the services provided by the practice setting in which the fieldwork takes place. It maintains the connection between academia and the practice setting. "The challenge to our profession is to begin to strengthen the ties between experienced practitioners, educators, and students. Fieldwork offers a perfect opportunity to create these bonds" (Kolodner & Hischmann, 2000, p. 4).

This chapter provides an overview of the basic elements involved in developing and managing a fieldwork education program. It is divided into five broad sections: (a) "Evaluating Program Readiness for Fieldwork," (b) "Fieldwork Education Basics," (c) "Establishing a Fieldwork Program," (d) "Student Supervision," and (e) "Evaluation of the Fieldwork Program."

An excellent tool that can assist the occupational therapy manager in the development and management of a fieldwork education program is *Meeting the Fieldwork Challenge* (Merrill & Crist, 2000), published by the American Occupational Therapy Association (AOTA). It is a self-paced clinical course that provides a comprehensive overview of occupational therapy fieldwork education. This chapter refers to lessons within that document (Crist, 2000; Hengeveld, 2000; Scott, 2000; Taguchi, 2000; Wells & Hanebrink, 2000) and to other significant AOTA documents. Another excellent resource mentioned throughout this chapter is the academic fieldwork coordinator (AFC). The AFC can play an important role in the development or enhancement of an occupational therapy fieldwork program.

## Evaluating Program Readiness for Fieldwork

When evaluating his or her occupational therapy program's readiness for fieldwork, the occupational therapy manager will need to determine the purpose and philosophy of a fieldwork educator program. A network of support will also need development.

### Determining the Purpose

An occupational therapy manager might want to develop or enhance a fieldwork education program for many reasons, including a desire to maintain or increase practice skills, "payback" for the mentoring that the manager received as a student, the possibility of promotion, pressure from academic institutions, commitment to the occupational therapy profession, as well as enjoyment of teaching and supervising others. Whatever the reasons for pursuing a fieldwork education program, the occupational therapy manager should explore his or her motivations in depth to help determine the purpose and philosophy for establishing it. Hengeveld (2000) suggested a learning exercise that involves considering a master list of reasons. Then, for each reason listed, the manager (and others) can define desired outcomes, costs, and benefits. This activity can be done individually or collaboratively.

In addition to exploring the reasons for a fieldwork program, the occupational therapy manager will need to assess how staffing and clients will affect and be affected by fieldwork education. The number of a program's staff members as well as their productivity capacities, experience levels, and commitment will affect fieldwork education, as will the type and complexity of clients the program serves, the delivery of service, and delivery environments.

The occupational therapy manager will need to identify and build support with the important stakeholders in his or her setting, affirming the known support of some and marketing to or convincing others who are more doubtful about the need or value of a fieldwork education program. Developing positive strategies and plans of action in anticipation of barriers and challenges will help to garner the needed support.

A frequent concern expressed by program administrators is the effect of a student program on staff productivity. Although students should never be viewed as substitute staff members, research supports the positive effects that students have on productivity. Several research articles related to occupational therapy provide valuable cost and benefit information (Chung, Spelbring, & Boissoneau, 1980; Shalik, 1987; Shalik & Shalik, 1988). An important article to review on this subject is by Shalik and Shalik in which the authors suggested that most Level II placements in physical and psychosocial service settings represent a financial benefit to the fieldwork site. Their article provided a method for estimating the amount of financial benefit one can anticipate from a student placement. Hengeveld (2000) also provided an excellent overview of work measurement, including a work measurement tool and study outline. The collaborative fieldwork model, in which the fieldwork educator supervises two or more students at the same time, can boost productivity, especially during the second half of a Level II affiliation (Hengeveld, 2000).

Fieldwork can also be promoted as a potential recruitment tool. Level II placements are an excellent way to evaluate future employment potential and fulfill some of the aspects of a new employee orientation in situations in which a student becomes an employee after completion of a fieldwork experience. Although Level II fieldwork placements appear to be more beneficial financially, Swinehart and Meyers (1993) found that Level I placements also can be viewed as a vehicle for early recruitment.

The purpose of a fieldwork education program should reflect the program's values and goals as well as promote the achievement of the programs' mission. "The mission statement is the common goal that ties all practice arenas and administrative functionaries together" (Hengeveld, 2000, p. 4). Thus, the fieldwork student program can be marketed to management not only as being compatible with the mission but also as being an important tool to achieving it.

## Philosophy

Once the occupational therapy manager has identified the purpose for establishing a fieldwork program, the next important step is to develop a philosophy of fieldwork education. Essentially, this philosophy is a vision statement. According to Hengeveld (2000),

> Your fieldwork philosophy will reflect your beliefs and values about the profession, your facility's vision statement, and your fundamental beliefs about human beings and how they learn. Your philosophy is the theory and logical analysis of principles underlying your conduct, thoughts, knowledge, and the nature of the profession and fieldwork education. (p. 6)

The statement of philosophy needs to be concise but inspirational. Hengeveld (2000) provided several excellent exercises to help managers create this statement. One exercise asks the program manager to examine his or her own fieldwork experiences: exceptional, terrible, or boring. Another exercise asks the manager to remember the most important lessons learned in the areas of practice skills, professional behavior, and personal growth. A third exercise helps managers to then develop a philosophical statement.

## Network, Network, Network

Once the occupational therapy manager has clearly defined the purpose and philosophy of his or her fieldwork education program, he or she can go on to develop a network of support from within and outside the practice setting. This network of administrators, managers, practitioners (both within the profession and from other disciplines), and academic programs can aid in the establishment and growth of the student fieldwork program.

Managers may find established, wonderful fieldwork education programs in the area who are willing to share ideas, resources, strategies, and advice. Workshops and conferences on local, state, and national levels can provide excellent opportunities for training and networking.

AFCs see a major part of their job as being resources and consultants to fieldwork sites. They can help with the development of the fieldwork program and can connect a site with other successful fieldwork education programs. AFCs in many states have established fieldwork councils or consortiums that provide ongoing training and education in student supervision, management of the challenging student, development of critical thinking and professional skills, and other fieldwork education topics.

AOTA operates a special interest section for education (EDSIS), which publishes a quarterly newsletter that covers up-to-date information and topics. AOTA also operates an interactive online fieldwork educators newsgroup that provides an ongoing fieldwork forum to all that subscribe.

## Fieldwork Education Basics

For many years, the terms *clinical education* and *clinical instructor* have been used to describe occupational therapy fieldwork and student supervision, and they are still being used in some settings and by other professions. However, placements have expanded from those predominantly within the medical arena to include placements within a variety of community settings, which has prompted a change of terminology. Clinical education is now referred to as *fieldwork education,* and the clinical instructor is now called a *fieldwork educator.*

Several primary AOTA documents outline the basic information needed with respect to the fieldwork education for both occupational therapy and occupational therapy assistant students. The *Standards for an Accredited Education Program for the Occupational Therapist* (American Council for Occupational Therapy Education [ACOTE], 1999a) and *Standards for an Accredited Education Program for the Occupational Therapist Assistant* (ACOTE, 1999b) specify the requirements for fieldwork within the academic program. Both documents define the goals and purposes of fieldwork education, fieldwork educator requirements, and the minimum amount and type of supervision during fieldwork. They both specify that collaboration between the academic and fieldwork programs, including the development of fieldwork objectives, should be documented.

## Level I Fieldwork

The goal of Level I fieldwork for both occupational therapy and occupational therapy assistant students is "to introduce students to the fieldwork experience, and develop a basic comfort level with and understanding of the needs of clients" (ACOTE, 1999a, 1999b). This fieldwork includes experiences involving directed observation and supervised participation in selected aspects of the occupational therapy process. Independent performance is not the focus of these experiences.

The occupational therapist or occupational therapy assistant student can be supervised by a qualified occupational therapist or occupational therapy assistant or by another professional such as a teacher, nurse, physician assistant, social worker, psychologist, or physical therapist. The academic program should provide the fieldwork site with a method for evaluating and documenting student performance (usually, requirements and forms developed by that academic program).

The *Standards* for both occupational therapy and occupational therapy assistant students do not specify the number of Level I fieldwork experiences a student must complete or the number of hours or weeks each experience should be. Level I experiences cannot be substituted for Level II experiences.

## Level II Fieldwork

The goal of Level II fieldwork for both occupational therapy and occupational therapy assistant students is to develop a competent, entry-level, generalist occupational therapy practitioner. It "shall include an in-depth experience in delivering occupational therapy services to clients, focusing on the application of purposeful and meaningful occupation" (ACOTE, 1999a, 1999b). Ideally, students should be exposed to a variety of settings and to clients of various ages. The fieldwork experience should pro-mote values and beliefs that enable ethical practice as well as development of profes-sional competence and responsibility.

The fieldwork experience for the occupational therapy student should be designed to promote clinical reasoning appropriate to the occupational therapy assistant role. The fieldwork experience for the occupational therapy student should also promote clinical reasoning along with reflective practice and should focus on applications re-lated to research, administration, and management of occupational therapy services. The level of supervision for both occupational therapy and occupational therapy as-sistant students should progress from direct to less direct in nature, depending on the setting, the severity of the client's condition, and the student's ability.

The type and frequency of evaluation is not specified for either occupational ther-apy or occupational therapy assistant students. Generally, fieldwork programs use the current AOTA Fieldwork Level II evaluation documents in conjunction with other re-lated forms developed by the academic setting, the fieldwork setting, or both.

### Occupational Therapy Assistant Fieldwork Student

Occupational therapy assistant students must complete fieldwork that equals a mini-mum of 16 weeks of full-time work. It can be completed on a part-time basis but not less than half-time as defined by the fieldwork setting. Fieldwork can be completed in a minimum of one setting and a maximum of three settings.

The occupational therapy assistant student must be supervised by either a quali-fied occupational therapist or occupational therapy assistant, who is engaged by either the fieldwork site or the academic program. If the setting does not have an occupational therapy practitioner on site, supervision by an off-site supervisor must be provided for a minimum of 6 hours per week, including direct observation of client interaction. This supervisor also must be readily available for communication and consultation during working hours. The educational program must have a documented supervisory plan for the delivery of occupational therapy services for the site (in accordance with any state credentialing requirements). Off-site supervision cannot exceed 8 weeks.

### Occupational Therapy Fieldwork Student

Occupational therapy students must complete fieldwork that equals a minimum of 24 weeks of full-time work. It can be completed on a part-time basis but not less than half-time as defined by the fieldwork setting. Fieldwork can be completed in a mini-mum of one setting and a maximum of four settings.

The occupational therapy student must be supervised by a qualified occupational therapist who is engaged by either the fieldwork site or the academic program. If the setting does not have an occupational therapist on site, supervision by an off-site supervisor must be provided for a minimum of 6 hours per week, including direct ob-servation of client interaction. This supervisor must also be readily available for communication and consultation during working hours. The educational program must have a documented supervisory plan for the delivery of occupational therapy services for the site (in accordance with any state credentialing requirements). Off-site supervision cannot exceed 12 weeks.

## Role of the Fieldwork Educator

In addition to the *Standards* (ACOTE, 1999a, 1999b) documents, another valuable resource for the occupational therapy manager in defining the fieldwork educator role in the practice setting is the AOTA document *Occupational Therapy Roles* (AOTA, 1993). This document describes the following: (a) qualifications; (b) the major function and role; (c) key performance areas, including entry-level, intermediate, and high-proficiency skills; (d) the scope of the role; and (e) fieldwork educator competency.

### Qualifications

To qualify as a fieldwork educator, the occupational therapist or occupational therapy assistant must have received initial certification by the National Board for Certification in Occupational Therapy (NBCOT). He or she also must meet any state regulatory requirements. In addition, this person should have continuing education related to fieldwork education and supervision. Entry-level occupational therapists and occupational therapy assistants can supervise Level I fieldwork students. Occupational therapists with at least 1 year of practice-based experience subsequent to initial certification may supervise occupational therapy and occupational therapy assistant Level II students. Occupational therapy assistants with at least 1 year of practice-based experience subsequent to initial certification may supervise occupational therapy assistant Level II fieldwork students. It is recommended that individuals overseeing fieldwork programs with multiple student supervisors and multiple students have at least 3 years of practice-based experience.

### Major Function and Role

The fieldwork educator manages Fieldwork Level I or II (or both) occupational therapy and occupational therapy assistant students, providing opportunities to practice and carry out practitioner competencies. The role can encompass responsibility for the entire fieldwork program or just one student.

In settings where multiple occupational therapy staff members are supervising multiple students, managers may wish to designate an experienced fieldwork educator as the site fieldwork coordinator. This individual is the main contact person and coordinator for fieldwork placement requests from AFCs. The fieldwork coordinator also can oversee the work done by fieldwork educators and assist the occupational therapy manager in evaluating the effectiveness of individual fieldwork educators and the overall fieldwork program. In addition, the fieldwork coordinator can act as a mediator when challenging issues arise between the student and fieldwork educator and can be the initial contact person for the academic fieldwork coordinator when a student expresses issues of concern directly to the AFC.

### Key Performance Areas

Often, although the new fieldwork educator may have intermediate skills in the practitioner role, he or she will most likely begin at an entry level as a fieldwork educator. Thus, a good starting point for the new fieldwork educator is to mentor Level I fieldwork students. The level at which the fieldwork educator performs in the future will be measured by the successful achievement of higher-level skills. Some occupational therapy staff members may remain as supervisors for Level I students while others may progress to program coordination and oversight.

### Scope of the Role

The fieldwork educator must embrace the role of educator and not fall into the "therapy trap." According to Crist (2000), "when evaluation of student performance is more a report of success in helping the student over personal hurdles than an evaluation of student learning, one is being more of a therapist than an educator" (p. 4).

### Fieldwork Educator Competency

In 1998, AOTA adopted a voluntary self-assessment tool to foster the professional development of fieldwork educators from novice to experienced (AOTA, 1999). It helps the fieldwork educator to assess his or her own levels of competence and to identify areas that need further development or skills building. For sites that include the fieldwork educator role as part of an annual review process, this tool could serve as a supplement.

## Collaboration Between the Occupational Therapy and Occupational Therapy Assistant Students

One way to promote and enhance the understanding between occupational therapists and occupational therapy assistants is to provide collaborative fieldwork learning experiences to both types of students. The teaming of occupational therapist and occupational therapy assistant fieldwork educators to provide training to teams of occupational therapy and occupational therapy assistant students can be an excellent opportunity for these students to understand and build on the similarities and differences in the services that each practitioner provides to the client. This collaboration will also enhance the students' understanding of the supervisory relationship between occupational therapist and occupational therapy assistant.

## Establishing a Fieldwork Program

When establishing a fieldwork program, the occupational therapy manager will need to define essential functions of a fieldwork student, determine behavioral objectives and timelines, and develop relationships with academic programs.

## Defining the Essential Functions of Students

In preparing for a student program, the occupational therapy manager will need to delineate the essential skills and competencies that would be required for a student at his or her site. Establishing these essential fieldwork requirements and functions clarifies those tasks considered to be necessary and fundamental to the performance of the students in the particular setting (Wells & Hanebrink, 2000). This information will guide potential students in assessing their ability to successfully complete their fieldwork experience at a site and in determining the possible need for accommodations. These essential functions should be developed for occupational therapy students, for occupational therapy assistant students, and for all levels of fieldwork. Academic and fieldwork educators can and should be involved in the development of these functions. A good starting point or basis for this fieldwork student "job description" can be the job duties, essential functions, and competencies established for an entry-level practitioner at the site.

Hengeveld (2000) and Wells and Hanebrink (2000) are excellent resources and guides for developing essential functions and tasks for fieldwork students as well as for subsequently determining whether (and if so, what) accommodations might be necessary to assist a student with a disability to perform them. In particular, Wells and Hanebrink provided a helpful resource list of professional documents to review, a clearly defined process for determining a site's essential functions, a description of principles and responsibilities for reasonable accommodation in fieldwork, and case studies through which to further review and define issues involving student disabilities.

## Establishing Behavioral Objectives and Timelines

Once essential functions and tasks have been established, the fieldwork educator and others can then move on to develop behavioral objectives for occupational therapy and occupational therapy assistant students. These objectives can be created with the assistance of the AFC, who often can supply examples of objectives developed by other similar practice sites. These behavioral objectives, once established, are shared with the academic programs that send students and are available for potential students to review before initiating a fieldwork experience.

Timelines that are developed for the achievement of these objectives are generally broken down into weekly segments. According to Hengeveld (2000), pacing is a crucial component in the programming of fieldwork, with learning activities sequenced as follows: planned learning, clarity in communication, variety, repetition, and processing.

Behavioral objectives with timelines become quite important when a student begins to have difficulty. In consultation with the AFC, behavioral objectives and timelines become part of a learning contract that is developed to assist the student in achieving a step-by-step level of competency that will allow him or her to continue in the fieldwork affiliation. They also assist the fieldwork educator in determining whether (and if so, when) termination of the student experience is the best option. McCarron and Crist (2000) provided examples of learning contracts and student supervision forms that incorporate behavioral objectives and timelines.

## Establishing Relationships With Academic Programs

Many factors are involved in the process for deciding with which schools to affiliate. For example, the school might be a manager's alma mater, or it might be a school that is within easy travel distance to the site. The curriculum, philosophy, and theoretical base of a school and its compatibility with the program site are important factors. Some schools train only occupational therapy students; some, only occupational therapy assistants; some, both. If a site wants to provide fieldwork education to occupational therapy and occupational therapy assistant students, it may need to affiliate with several schools. The AFC can be an excellent resource for information about a particular school.

Before accepting and training students from a particular academic program, a contractual agreement or memorandum of understanding needs to be established between the fieldwork site and the academic institution. These legal documents outline the responsibilities and liabilities of each party involved in the fieldwork education of students. ACOTE *Standards* (1999a, 1999b) require that responsibilities of the educational institution and fieldwork site be clearly documented (in a memorandum of understanding) and reviewed at least every 5 years by both parties. These responsibilities are generally divided into those of the facility (fieldwork site), those of the academic program, and joint responsibilities. Fieldwork site obligations usually involve a planned, supervised program; qualified student supervision; periodic evaluations; education schedule; facility insurance and indemnification; and child protection clearance. Academic obligations usually involve a designated AFC, periodic communication or visits by the AFC, student health certificate, student health prerequisites, student health insurance, student liability insurance, academic program liability insurance, and academic program indemnification. Joint responsibilities usually involve a nondiscrimination agreement, a process to remove unacceptable students, guidelines for confidentiality, identification of the student as a nonemployee, and time limits for agreements (Hengeveld, 2000). Taguchi (2000) also provided an in-depth, instructive overview of contract negotiation and maintenance.

## Preparations for the Fieldwork Student

Preparations for the fieldwork student include the placement process, student manual development and maintenance, and student orientation to the facility.

### Setting Up the Fieldwork Placement

Generally, placements are arranged between the AFC and site fieldwork coordinator (or fieldwork educator if the site has no coordinator). Many academic programs will make requests for placement slots in advance (often, by telephone, by e-mail, or by a form that sites complete and return). The AFC will then assign students as they are ready for fieldwork. Once a student is assigned to a fieldwork site and is confirmed by that site (usually by mail or phone), the student is asked to make an initial contact. The initial contact is usually guided by the fieldwork coordinator. It may involve a letter, an e-mail message, a phone call, a shadowing experience, or a face-to-face or phone interview.

The fieldwork coordinator or assigned educator provides introductory information about the fieldwork and answers student questions. It is helpful when the coordinator or educator gives students an overview of the evaluations and interventions used by the setting. Students can be given readings and references to help them prepare before the experience. They also need basic information on dress code, work hours, where to arrive, and so forth. Setting the stage for a positive learning environment will help reduce the student's anxiety.

Before having the student start the fieldwork, the AFC will review fieldwork objectives, policies, and procedures with the student and will send the fieldwork site the student's personal data sheet along with evaluation forms, guidelines, timelines, and supporting documents.

### Student Manual

Although the student manual is typically developed for Level II fieldwork, it can include information that pertains to both fieldwork levels. It should contain clear guidelines for the expectations with respect to professionalism and performance skills. It will also contain specific requirements and assignments (with written expectations for each one). It includes documents that have already been developed: the facility purpose, philosophy, policies, and procedures, and behavioral objectives and timelines. Policies and procedures specific to students are added over time (and are revised as needed). Excellent resources for the development of this manual can include not only the AFC but also cite staff members who can share helpful insights from their own fieldwork experiences. The student manual should be reviewed on an annual basis, and a copy should be made available to prospective students. Hengeveld (2000) provided an example of a typical student manual outline.

### Orientation

The student's orientation to the facility sets the tone for the rest of the fieldwork experience. It needs to be well organized, clearly define expectations and responsibilities, and emphasize mutual respect and collaboration between student and fieldwork educator. Typically, the orientation includes the following: a site tour and introductions to staff members and clients; an explanation of policies and procedures as they pertain to staff members, clients, and students (including basic safety, confidentiality, and acceptable student absences); and an explanation of roles and responsibilities of staff members and students. An orientation form that the student dates and initials is a useful tool for documenting the orientation process.

# Student Supervision

Once the framework for a fieldwork program has been established, the supervisory process should be clarified. The process of student supervision involves overseeing the development of performance skills and fostering the development of professional skills as well as providing feedback on both. A potential aid to this process, according to Crist (2002) and Krupnick, Brown, and Stutz-Tanenbaum (2002), is the new Fieldwork Experience Assessment Tool that has been developed by the Fieldwork Research Team with support from the American Occupational Therapy Foundation and AOTA EDSIS (Atler et al., 2001). This tool is designed to promote the optimal learning environment for the fieldwork experience. It promotes a collaborative effort between the fieldwork educator and student. The fieldwork educator and student, together or individually, reflect on and assess the essential characteristics of three key component areas: (a) environment, (b) fieldwork educator, and (c) student. By discovering and discussing the commonalities and differences in their two perspectives, educator and student can develop strategies for a more balanced fieldwork experience.

In addition, various supervisory approaches can prepare and guide fieldwork educators as they mentor students. The following sections provide a brief overview of these approaches.

## Models of Supervision

Three basic models of supervision typically are used in the supervision of students: (a) formal, (b) informal, and (c) functional.

### Formal

The focus of formal supervision is on the structural components of contact with the student. This kind of supervision involves (a) the amount (and length) of planned contact with the student and (b) written documentation such as supervision feedback and counseling forms, learning contracts, and formal evaluation instruments. According to McCarron and Crist (2000), it "integrates standards for practice, ethical decision making, therapeutic use of self, practice competence, professional empowerment, continuing professional development, and maturation as a competent fieldwork educator" (p. 6).

### Informal

Informal supervision takes place ad hoc. It involves casual conversation and the sharing of thoughts and ideas between sessions, during breaks, or while traveling between appointments or sites. It also involves informal discussions about client care, the student's performance, or both. The more spontaneous nature of informal supervision allows for immediate feedback.

*Functional*

Functional supervision is task specific and focused on competence. For example, the fieldwork educator may arrange for a fellow practitioner with a particular area of expertise and experience to coach or mentor the student in that area.

## Developmental Stages Model

McCarron and Crist (2000) reviewed the four basic stages or phases that the student passes through as he or she progresses toward becoming an entry-level practitioner. The management style that the fieldwork educator uses depends on the developmental phase of the student. Each style will differ on three major dimensions: (a) the amount of supervision provided by the supervisor, (b) the amount of support and encouragement provided by the supervisor, and (c) the extent to which the learner is involved in problem-solving and decision-making. The four phases include (a) the directing phase, in which the supervisor defines, identifies, and specifies for the student, focusing primarily on the student's work and task performance; (b) the coaching phase, in which the supervisor actively guides and directs the student in areas of new learning while the student assumes greater responsibility for his or her own problem-solving and critical thinking; (c) the supporting phase, in which the supervisor focuses more on providing assurance and support as the student takes on more of a lead role in client care; and (d) the delegating phase, in which the supervisor assumes a consulting role that involves monitoring and refining as the student becomes more comfortable working independently.

## Cultural Considerations

An exploration of cultural differences during the first week of the student's orientation will enrich both the student's and the fieldwork educator's experience. Less obvious cultural attributes such as time orientation, learning style, communication style, expectations about space and proximity, as well as values and beliefs are important factors that will affect the course of a fieldwork experience. Understanding cultural differences should improve communication and foster openness; enhance awareness and sensitivity to the student's and the educator's learning, problem-solving, and supervisory styles; and enhance negotiation and management of conflict situations. This approach can be effective also when dealing with a potentially "difficult" or challenging student. Scott (2000) provided a comprehensive overview of cultural and communication issues as well as related legal issues and their effect on fieldwork education.

## Evaluation of the Fieldwork Program

Hengeveld (2000) recommended that a fieldwork program be evaluated for successful outcomes on an annual basis at the least. This evaluation should reveal areas that need improvement and areas of success and achievement. An "intervention plan" that identifies goals and timelines can be developed for those areas needing improvement. Hengeveld also provided a comprehensive list of questions that could be used in analyzing the effectiveness of a fieldwork program.

## Conclusion

Fieldwork education is an essential element of the occupational therapy profession. The development of a fieldwork education program requires the following step-by-step process:

- Evaluate the reasons and potential purpose for a fieldwork program.
- Establish a philosophical base that is compatible with the mission of the site.
- Get support by networking with and marketing to stakeholders and key colleagues.
- Become familiar with and understand the basic components that guide occupational therapy fieldwork education, including the important documents (informative and regulatory), the roles, and the types of fieldwork.
- Establish informal and formal connections with occupational therapy academic programs.
- Establish the framework for a program, including the definition of essential student functions and behavioral objectives.
- Further prepare for the student by setting up placements and by developing a student orientation and manual.
- Understand and enhance the student supervisory process.
- And finally, evaluate the effectiveness of the program.

Managing a fieldwork education program takes time, effort, and commitment. However, the rewards are many. Fieldwork education maintains the connection between practice and academia. Staff members who take on the role of fieldwork educator update and enhance their professional, evaluation, intervention, and documentation skills. The process can open the door to further involvement with academic programs, including continuing education opportunities and guest lectureships. The mentoring of fieldwork students can partially fulfill state regulatory and NBCOT recertification requirements. Fieldwork education can be an effective recruitment tool and can be included as part of an annual assessment of staff skills and commitment.

## References

Accreditation Council for Occupational Therapy Education. (1999a). Standards for the accredited educational program for the occupational therapist. *American Journal of Occupational Therapy, 53,* 575–582.

Accreditation Council for Occupational Therapy Education. (1999b). Standards for the accredited educational program for the occupational therapy assistant. *American Journal of Occupational Therapy, 53,* 583–589.

American Occupational Therapy Association. (1993). Occupational therapy roles. *American Journal of Occupational Therapy, 47*, 1087–1099.

American Occupational Therapy Association. (1999). *Self-assessment for fieldwork educator competency.* Bethesda, MD: Author.

Atler, K., Brown, K., Griswold, L. A., Krupnick, W., Muniz de Melendez, L., & Stutz-Tanenbaum, P. (2001, August). *Fieldwork experience assessment tool.* Retrieved September 28, 2002, from http://www.aota.org/nonmembers/area13/docs/feat.pdf

Chung, Y., Spelbring, L. M., & Boissoneau, R. (1980). A cost–benefit analysis of fieldwork education in occupational therapy. *Inquiry, 17*, 216–229.

Crist, P. A. (2000). Understanding the role of the fieldwork educator in occupational therapy education. In S. C. Merrill & P. A. Crist (Eds.), *Meeting the fieldwork challenge* (pp. 2–53). Bethesda, MD: American Occupational Therapy Association.

Crist, P. A. (2002). Quality fieldwork is quite a FEAT. *Advance for Occupational Therapy, 18,* 5.

Hengeveld, T. (2000). The structural components of the fieldwork program. In S. C. Merrill & P. A. Crist (Eds.), *Meeting the fieldwork challenge* (pp. 2–30). Bethesda, MD: American Occupational Therapy Association.

Kolodner, E. L., & Hischmann, C. L. (2000). The role of fieldwork in occupational therapy practice. In S. C. Merrill & P. A. Crist (Eds.), *Meeting the fieldwork challenge* (pp. 2–20). Bethesda, MD: American Occupational Therapy Association.

Krupnick, W., Brown, K., & Stutz-Tanenbaum, P. (2002). Creating a successful fieldwork experience: The fieldwork experience assessment tool. *OT Practice, 7*, 1–7.

McCarron, K., & Crist, P. A. (2000). Supervision and mentoring. In S. C. Merrill & P. A. Crist (Eds.), *Meeting the fieldwork challenge* (pp. 2–27). Bethesda, MD: American Occupational Therapy Association.

Merrill, S. C., & Crist, P. A. (Eds.). (2000). *Meeting the fieldwork challenge.* Bethesda, MD: American Occupational Therapy Association.

Scott, S. B. (2000). Diversity and fieldwork. In S. C. Merrill & P. A. Crist (Eds.), *Meeting the fieldwork challenge* (pp. 2–16). Bethesda, MD: American Occupational Therapy Association.

Shalik, H. (1987). Cost–benefit analysis of level II fieldwork in occupational therapy. *American Journal of Occupational Therapy, 41*, 638–645.

Shalik, H., & Shalik, L. D. (1988). The occupational therapy Level II fieldwork experience: Estimation of the fiscal benefit. *American Journal of Occupational Therapy, 42*, 164–168.

Swinehart, S., & Meyers, S. K. (1993). Level I fieldwork: Creating a positive experience. *American Journal of Occupational Therapy, 47*, 68–73.

Taguchi, J. (2000). Managing a fieldwork program. In S. C. Merrill & P. A. Crist (Eds.), *Meeting the fieldwork challenge* (pp. 2–28). Bethesda, MD: American Occupational Therapy Association.

Wells, S. A., & Hanebrink, S. (2000). Students with disabilities and fieldwork. In S. C. Merrill & P. A. Crist (Eds.), *Meeting the fieldwork challenge* (pp. 2–27). Bethesda, MD: American Occupational Therapy Association.

## Additional Resources

Alsop, A., & Ryan, S. (1996). *Making the most of fieldwork education: A practical approach.* San Diego, CA: Singular.

Blair, S. E. E., & McLean, J. (2002). Fieldwork education. In J. Creek (Ed.), *Occupational therapy and mental health* (3rd ed., pp. 565–583). Edinburgh, UK: Churchill Livingstone.

Cara, E. (1998). Fieldwork supervision in the mental health setting. In E. Cara & A. MacRae (Eds.), *Psychosocial occupational therapy: A clinical practice* (pp. 609–640). Albany, NY: Delmar.

Kasar, J., & Clark, E. N. (Eds.). (2000). *Developing professional behaviors.* Thorofare, NJ: Slack.

Palladino, J., & Jeffries, R. N. (2000). *The occupational therapy fieldwork manual for assessing professional skills.* Philadelphia: F. A. Davis.

Privott, C. R. (Ed.). (1998). *The fieldwork anthology: A classic research and practice collection.* Bethesda, MD: American Occupational Therapy Association.

Scott, S. S., Wells, S., & Hanebrink, S. (1998). *A guide to reasonable accommodation for OT practitioners with disabilities: Fieldwork to employment.* Bethesda, MD: American Occupational Therapy Association.

Sladyk, K. (Ed.). (2002). *The successful occupational therapy fieldwork student.* Thorofare, NJ: Slack.

Wells, S., & Hanebrink, S. (1997). *Educating college students with disabilities: What academic and fieldwork educators need to know.* Bethesda, MD: American Occupational Therapy Association.

# Occupational Therapy Code of Ethics (2000)

## Preamble

The American Occupational Therapy Association's *Occupational Therapy Code of Ethics (2000)* is a public statement of the common set of values and principles used to promote and maintain high standards of behavior in occupational therapy. The American Occupational Therapy Association and its members are committed to furthering the ability of individuals, groups, and systems to function within their total environment. To this end, occupational therapy personnel (including all staff and personnel who work and assist in providing occupational therapy services, e.g., aides, orderlies, secretaries, technicians) have a responsibility to provide services to recipients in any stage of health and illness who are individuals, research participants, institutions and businesses, other professionals and colleagues, students, and to the general public.

590 THE OCCUPATIONAL THERAPY MANAGER

The *Occupational Therapy Code of Ethics (2000)* is a set of principles that applies to occupational therapy personnel at all levels. These principles to which occupational therapists and occupational therapy assistants aspire are part of a lifelong effort to act in an ethical manner. The various roles of practitioner (occupational therapist and occupational therapy assistant), educator, fieldwork educator, clinical supervisor, manager, administrator, consultant, fieldwork coordinator, faculty program director, researcher/scholar, private practice owner, entrepreneur, and student are assumed. Any action in violation of the spirit and purpose of this Code shall be considered unethical. To ensure compliance with the Code, the Commission on Standards and Ethics (SEC) establishes and maintains the enforcement procedures. Acceptance of membership in the American Occupational Therapy Association (AOTA) commits members to adherence to the Occupational Therapy Code of Ethics (2000) and its enforcement procedures. The *Occupational Therapy Code of Ethics (2000), Core Values and Attitudes of Occupational Therapy Practice* (AOTA, 1993), and the *Guidelines to the Occupational Therapy Code of Ethics* (AOTA, 1998) are aspirational documents designed to be used together to guide occupational therapy personnel.

## Principle 1. Occupational therapy personnel shall demonstrate a concern for the well-being of the recipients of their services. (beneficence)

A. Occupational therapy personnel shall provide services in a fair and equitable manner. They shall recognize and appreciate the cultural components of economics, geography, race, ethnicity, religious and political factors, marital status, sexual orientation, and disability of all recipients of their services.

B. Occupational therapy practitioners shall strive to ensure that fees are fair and reasonable and commensurate with services performed. When occupational therapy practitioners set fees, they shall set fees considering institutional, local, state, and federal requirements, and with due regard for the service recipient's ability to pay.

C. Occupational therapy personnel shall make every effort to advocate for recipients to obtain needed services through available means.

## Principle 2. Occupational therapy personnel shall take reasonable precautions to avoid imposing or inflicting harm upon the recipient of services or to his or her property. (nonmaleficence)

A. Occupational therapy personnel shall maintain relationships that do not exploit the recipient of services sexually, physically, emotionally, financially, socially, or in any other manner.

B. Occupational therapy practitioners shall avoid relationships or activities that interfere with professional judgment and objectivity.

## Principle 3. Occupational therapy personnel shall respect the recipient and/or their surrogate(s) as well as the recipient's rights. (autonomy, privacy, confidentiality)

A. Occupational therapy practitioners shall collaborate with service recipients or their surrogate(s) in setting goals and priorities throughout the intervention process.

B. Occupational therapy practitioners shall fully inform the service recipients of the nature, risks, and potential outcomes of any interventions.

C. Occupational therapy practitioners shall obtain informed consent from participants involved in research activities and indicate that they have fully informed and advised the participants of potential risks and outcomes. Occupational therapy practitioners shall endeavor to ensure that the participant(s) comprehend these risks and outcomes.

D. Occupational therapy personnel shall respect the individual's right to refuse professional services or involvement in research or educational activities.

E. Occupational therapy personnel shall protect all privileged confidential forms of written, verbal, and electronic communication gained from educational, practice, research, and investigational activities unless otherwise mandated by local, state, or federal regulations.

## Principle 4. Occupational therapy personnel shall achieve and continually maintain high standards of competence. (duties)

A. Occupational therapy practitioners shall hold the appropriate national and state credentials for the services they provide.

B. Occupational therapy practitioners shall use procedures that conform to the standards of practice and other appropriate AOTA documents relevant to practice.

C. Occupational therapy practitioners shall take responsibility for maintaining and documenting competence by participating in professional development and educational activities.

D. Occupational therapy practitioners shall critically examine and keep current with emerging knowledge relevant to their practice so they may perform their duties on the basis of accurate information.

E. Occupational therapy practitioners shall protect service recipients by ensuring that duties assumed by or assigned to other occupational therapy personnel match credentials, qualifications, experience, and scope of practice.

F. Occupational therapy practitioners shall provide appropriate supervision to individuals for whom the practitioners have supervisory responsibility in accordance with Association policies, local, state and federal laws, and institutional values.

G. Occupational therapy practitioners shall refer to or consult with other service providers whenever such a referral or consultation would be helpful to the care of the recipient of service. The referral or consultation process should be done in collaboration with the recipient of service.

### Principle 5. Occupational therapy personnel shall comply with laws and Association policies guiding the profession of occupational therapy. (justice)

A. Occupational therapy personnel shall familiarize themselves with and seek to understand and abide by applicable Association policies; local, state, and federal laws; and institutional rules.

B. Occupational therapy practitioners shall remain abreast of revisions in those laws and Association policies that apply to the profession of occupational therapy and shall inform employers, employees, and colleagues of those changes.

C. Occupational therapy practitioners shall require those they supervise in occupational therapy–related activities to adhere to the *Occupational Therapy Code of Ethics (2000)*.

D. Occupational therapy practitioners shall take reasonable steps to ensure employers are aware of occupational therapy's ethical obligations, as set forth in this *Occupational Therapy Code of Ethics (2000)*, and of the implications of those obligations for occupational therapy practice, education, and research.

E. Occupational therapy practitioners shall record and report in an accurate and timely manner all information related to professional activities.

### Principle 6. Occupational therapy personnel shall provide accurate information about occupational therapy services. (veracity)

A. Occupational therapy personnel shall accurately represent their credentials, qualifications, education, experience, training, and competence. This is of particular importance for those to whom occupational therapy personnel provide their services or with whom occupational therapy practitioners have a professional relationship.

B. Occupational therapy personnel shall disclose any professional, personal, financial, business, or volunteer affiliations that may pose a conflict of interest to those with whom they may establish a professional, contractual, or other working relationship.

C. Occupational therapy personnel shall refrain from using or participating in the use of any form of communication that contains false, fraudulent, deceptive, or unfair statements or claims.

D. Occupational therapy practitioners shall accept the responsibility for their professional actions which reduce the public's trust in occupational therapy services and those that perform those services.

### Principle 7. Occupational therapy personnel shall treat colleagues and other professionals with fairness, discretion, and integrity. (fidelity)

A. Occupational therapy personnel shall preserve, respect, and safeguard confidential information about colleagues and staff, unless otherwise mandated by national, state, or local laws.

B. Occupational therapy practitioners shall accurately represent the qualifications, views, contributions, and findings of colleagues.

C. Occupational therapy personnel shall take adequate measures to discourage, prevent, expose, and correct any breaches of the *Occupational Therapy Code of Ethics (2000)* and report any breaches of the *Occupational Therapy Code of Ethics (2000)* to the appropriate authority.

D. Occupational therapy personnel shall familiarize themselves with established policies and procedures for handling concerns about this *Occupational Therapy Code of Ethics (2000),* including familiarity with national, state, local, district, and territorial procedures for handling ethics complaints. These include policies and procedures created by the American Occupational Therapy Association, licensing and regulatory bodies, employers, agencies, certification boards, and other organizations who have jurisdiction over occupational therapy practice.

## References

American Occupational Therapy Association. (1993). Core values and attitudes of occupational therapy practice. *American Journal of Occupational Therapy, 47,* 1085–1086.
American Occupational Therapy Association. (1998). Guidelines to the occupational therapy code of ethics. *American Journal of Occupational Therapy, 52,* 881–884.

## Authors

**The Commission on Standards and Ethics (SEC):**
Barbara L. Kornblau, JD, OT/L, FAOTA, DAAPM, ABDA, CCM, CDMS, *Chairperson*
Melba Arnold, MS, OTR/L
Nancy Nashiro, PhD, OTR, FAOTA
Diane Hill, COTA/L, AP
Deborah Y. Slater, MS, OTR/L
John Morris, PhD
Linda Withers, CNHA, FACHCA
Penny Kyler, MA, OTR/L, FAOTA, *Staff Liaison for the Commission on Standards and Ethics*

*Adopted by the Representative Assembly 2000M15*

*Note:* This document replaces the 1994 document, Occupational Therapy Code of Ethics (*American Journal of Occupational Therapy, 48,* 1037-1038).

Published and copyrighted in 2000 by the American Occupational Therapy Association in the *American Journal of Occupational Therapy, 54,* 614-616.

Edited August 2000

# Occupational Therapy Practice Framework: Domain and Process

## Contents

The *Occupational Therapy Practice Framework*
(Framework), originally appeared in print in the
November/December 2002 issue of *The American
Journal of Occupational Therapy* (*AJOT*).

When citing this document the preferred reference is:

American Occupational Therapy Association. (2002).
Occupational therapy practice framework: Domain and
process. *American Journal of Occupational Therapy, 56,*
609–639.

Occupational therapy is an evolving profession. Over the years, the study of human occupation and its components has enlightened the profession about the core concepts and constructs that guide occupational therapy practice. In addition, occupational therapy's role and contributions to society have continued to evolve. The *Occupational Therapy Practice Framework: Domain and Process* (also referred to in this document as the Framework) is the next evolution in a series of documents that have been developed over the past several decades to outline language and constructs that describe the profession's focus.

The Framework was developed in response to current practice needs—the need to more clearly affirm and articulate occupational therapy's unique focus on occupation and daily life activities and the application of an intervention process that facilitates engagement in occupation to support participation in life. The impetus for the development of the Framework was the review process to update and revise the *Uniform Terminology for Occupational Therapy—Third Edition* (UT-III) (American Occupational Therapy Association [AOTA], 1994). The background for the development of the Framework is provided in a section at the end of this document. As practice continues to evolve, the field should consider the continued need for the *Occupational Therapy Practice Framework: Domain and Process* and should evaluate and modify its format as appropriate.

The intended purpose of the Framework is twofold: (a) to describe the domain that centers and grounds the profession's focus and actions and (b) to outline the process of occupational therapy evaluation and intervention that is dynamic and linked to the profession's focus on and use of occupation. The domain and process are necessarily interdependent, with the domain defining the area of human activity to which the process is applied.

This document is directed to both internal and external audiences. The internal professional audience—occupational therapists and occupational therapy assistants—can use the Framework to examine their current practice and to consider new applications in emerging practice areas. Occupational therapy educators may find the Framework helpful in teaching students about a process delivery model that is client centered and facilitates engagement in occupation to support participation in life. As occupational therapists and occupational therapy assistants move into new and expanded service arenas, the descriptions and terminology provided in the Framework can assist them in communicating the profession's unique focus on occupation and daily life activities to external audiences. External audiences can use the Framework to understand occupational therapy's emphasis on supporting function and performance in daily life activities and the many factors that influence performance (e.g., performance skills, performance patterns, context, activity demands, client factors) that are addressed during the intervention process. The description of the process will assist external audiences in understanding how occupational therapists and occupational therapy assistants apply their knowledge and skills in helping people attain and resume daily life activities that support function and health.

The *Occupational Therapy Practice Framework: Domain and Process* begins with an explanation of the profession's domain. Each aspect of the domain is fully described. An introduction to the occupational therapy process follows with key statements that highlight important points. Each section of the process is then specifically described. Numerous resource materials, including an appendix, a glossary, references, a bibliography, and the background of the development of the Framework are supplied at the end of the document.

## Domain
### The Domain of Occupational Therapy

"A profession's domain of concern consists of those areas of human experience in which practitioners of the profession offer assistance to others" (Mosey, 1981, p. 51). Occupational therapists and occupational therapy assistants focus on assisting people to engage in daily life activities that they find meaningful and purposeful. Occupational therapy's domain stems from the profession's interest in human beings' ability to engage in everyday life activities. The broad term that occupational therapists and assistants use to capture the breadth and meaning of "everyday life activity" is *occupation*. Occupation, as used in this document, is defined in the following way:

> [A]ctivities…of everyday life, named, organized, and given value and meaning by individuals and a culture. Occupation is everything people do to occupy themselves, including looking after themselves…enjoying life…and contributing to the social and economic fabric of their communities…. (Law, Polatajko, Baptiste, & Townsend, 1997, p. 32)

Occupational therapists' and occupational therapy assistants' expertise lies in their knowledge of occupation and how engaging in occupations can be used to affect human performance and the effects of disease and disability. When working with clients, occupational therapists and occupational therapy assistants direct their effort toward helping clients perform. Performance changes are directed to support engagement in meaningful occupations that subsequently affect health, well-being, and life satisfaction.

The profession views occupation as both means and end. The process of providing occupational therapy intervention may involve the therapeutic use of occupation as a "means" or method of changing performance. The "end" of

the occupational therapy intervention process occurs with the client's improved engagement in meaningful occupation.

Both terms, *occupation* and *activity*, are used by occupational therapists and occupational therapy assistants to describe participation in daily life pursuits. Occupations are generally viewed as activities having unique meaning and purpose in a person's life. Occupations are central to a person's identity and competence, and they influence how one spends time and makes decisions. The term *activity* describes a general class of human actions that is goal directed (Pierce, 2001). A person may participate in activities to achieve a goal, but these activities do not assume a place of central importance or meaning for the person. For example, many people participate in the activity of gardening, but not all of those individuals would describe gardening as an "occupation" that has central importance and meaning for them. Those who see gardening as an activity may report that gardening is a chore or task that must be done as part of home and yard maintenance but not one that they particularly enjoy doing or from which they derive significant personal satisfaction or fulfillment. Those who experience gardening as an occupation would see themselves as "gardeners," gaining part of their identity from their participation. They would achieve a sense of competence by their accomplishments in gardening and would report a sense of satisfaction and fulfillment as a result of engaging in this occupation. Occupational therapists and occupational therapy assistants value both occupation and activity and recognize their importance and influence on health and well-being. They believe that the two terms are closely related yet recognize that each term has a distinct meaning and that individuals experience each differently. In this document the two terms are often used together to acknowledge their relatedness yet recognize their different meanings.

The domain of occupational therapy frames the arena in which occupational therapy evaluations and interventions occur. To make the domain more understandable to readers and easier to visualize, the content of the domain has been illustrated in Figure 1. At the top of the page is the overarching statement—Engagement in Occupation to Support Participation in Context or Contexts. This statement describes the domain in its broadest sense. The other terms outlined in the figure identify the various aspects of the domain that occupational therapists and occupational therapy assistants attend to during the process of providing services. The three terms at the bottom of the figure (*context, activity demands,* and *client factors*) identify areas that influence performance skills and patterns. The two terms in the middle of the figure (*performance skills* and *performance patterns*) are used to describe the observed performance that

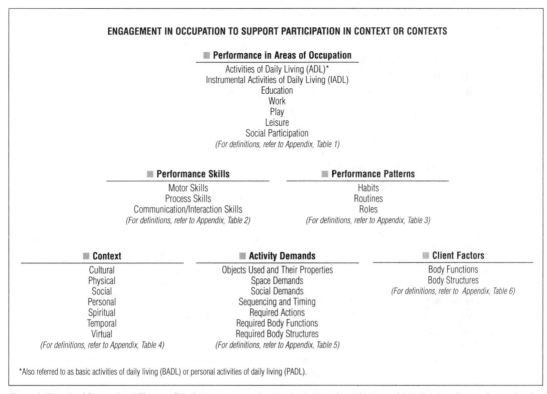

**Figure 1. Domain of Occupational Therapy.** This figure represents the domain of occupational therapy and is included to allow readers to visualize the entire domain with all of its various aspects. No aspect is intended to be perceived as more important than another.

the individual carries out when engaging in a range of occupations. No one aspect outlined in the domain figure is considered more important than another. Occupational therapists are trained to assess all aspects and to apply that knowledge to an intervention process that leads to engagement in occupations to support participation in context or contexts. Occupational therapy assistants participate in this process under the supervision of an occupational therapist. The discussion that follows provides a brief explanation of each term in the figure. Tables included in the appendix provide full lists and definitions of terms.

### Engagement in Occupation to Support Participation in Context

Engagement in occupation to support participation in context is the focus and targeted end objective of occupational therapy intervention. Engagement in occupation is seen as naturally supporting and leading to participation in context.

When individuals engage in occupations, they are committed to performance as a result of self-choice, motivation, and meaning. The term expresses the profession's belief in the importance of valuing and considering the individual's desires, choices, and needs during the evaluation and intervention process. Engagement in occupation includes both the subjective (emotional or psychological) aspects of performance and the objective (physically observable) aspects of performance. Occupational therapists and occupational therapy assistants understand engagement from this dual and holistic perspective and address all the aspects of performance (physical, cognitive, psychosocial, and contextual) when providing interventions designed to support engagement in occupations and in daily life activities.

Occupational therapists and occupational therapy assistants recognize that health is supported and maintained when individuals are able to engage in occupations and in activities that allow desired or needed participation in home, school, workplace, and community life situations. Occupational therapists and occupational therapy assistants assist individuals to link their ability to perform daily life activities with meaningful patterns of engagement in occupations that allow participation in desired roles and life situations in home, school, workplace, and community. The World Health Organization (WHO), in its effort to broaden the understanding of the effects of disease and disability on health, has recognized that health can be affected by the inability to carry out activities and participate in life situations as well as by problems that exist with body structures and functions (WHO, 2001). Occupational therapy's focus on engagement in occupations to support participation complements WHO's perspective.

Occupational therapists and occupational therapy assistants recognize that engagement in occupation occurs in a variety of contexts (cultural, physical, social, personal, temporal, spiritual, virtual). They also recognize that the individual's experience and performance cannot be understood or addressed without understanding the many contexts in which occupations and daily life activities occur.

*Performance in Areas of Occupation*

Occupational therapists and occupational therapy assistants direct their expertise to the broad range of human occupations and activities that make up peoples' lives. When occupational therapists and assistants work with an individual, a group, or a population to promote engagement in occupations and in daily life activities, they take into account all of the many types of occupations in which any individual, group, or population might engage. These human activities are sorted into categories called "areas of occupation"—activities of daily living, instrumental activities of daily living, education, work, play, leisure, and social participation (see Appendix, Table 1). Occupational therapists and occupational therapy assistants under the supervision of an occupational therapist use their expertise to address performance issues in any or all areas that are affecting the person's ability to engage in occupations and in activities. Addressing performance issues in areas of occupation requires knowledge of what performance skills are needed and what performance patterns are used.

*Performance Skills*

Skills are small units of performance. They are features of what one does (e.g., bends, chooses, gazes), versus underlying capacities or body functions (e.g., joint mobility, motivation, visual acuity). "Skills are observable elements of action that have implicit functional purposes" (Fisher & Kielhofner, 1995, p. 113). For example, when observing a person writing out a check, you would notice skills of gripping and manipulating objects and initiating and sequencing the steps of the activity to complete the writing of the check.

Execution of a performance skill occurs when the performer, the context, and the demands of the activity come together in the performance of the activity. Each of these factors influences the execution of a skill and may support or hinder actual skill execution.

When occupational therapists and occupational therapy assistants, who have established competency under the supervision of occupational therapists, analyze performance, they specifically identify the skills that are effective or ineffective during performance. They use skilled observations and selected assessments to evaluate the following skills:
- Motor skills—observed as the client moves and interacts with task objects and environments. Aspects of motor skill include posture, mobility, coordination, strength and effort, and energy. Examples of specific motor performance skills include stabilizing the body, bending, and manipulating objects.
- Process skills—observed as the client manages and modifies actions while completing a task. Aspects of process skill include energy, knowledge, temporal organization, organizing space and objects, and adaptation. Examples of specific process performance skills include maintaining attention to a task, choosing appropriate tools and materials for the task, logically organizing workspace, or accommodating the method of task completion in response to a problem.
- Communication/Interaction skills—observed as the client conveys his or her intentions and needs and coordinates social behavior to act together with people. Aspects of communication/interaction skills include physicality, information exchange, and relations. Examples of specific communication/interaction performance skills include gesturing to indicate intention, asking for information, expressing affect, or relating in a manner to establish rapport with others.

Skilled performance (i.e., effective execution of performance skills) depends on client factors (body functions, body structures), activity demands, and the context. However, the presence of underlying client factors (body functions and structures) does not inherently ensure the effective execution of performance skills. (See Appendix, Table 2, for complete list of performance skills)

*Performance Patterns*

Performance patterns refer to habits, routines, and roles that are adopted by an individual as he or she carries out occupations or daily life activities. Habits refer to specific, automatic behaviors, whereas routines are established sequences of occupations or activities that provide a structure for daily life. Roles are "a set of behaviors that have some socially agreed upon function and for which there is an accepted code of norms" (Christiansen & Baum, 1997, p. 603).

Performance patterns develop over time and are influenced by context (See Appendix, Table 3).

### Context

Context refers to a variety of interrelated conditions within and surrounding the client that influence performance. These contexts can be cultural, physical, social, personal, spiritual, temporal, and virtual. Some contexts are external to the client (e.g., physical context, social context, virtual context); some are internal to the client (e.g., personal, spiritual); and some may have external features, with beliefs and values that have been internalized (e.g., cultural). Contexts may include time dimensions (e.g., within a temporal context, the time of day; within a personal context, one's age) and space dimensions (e.g., within a physical context, the size of room in which activity occurs). When the occupational therapist and occupational therapy assistant are attempting to understand performance skills and patterns, they consider the specific contexts that surround the performance of a particular occupation or activity. In this process, the therapist and assistant consider all the relevant contexts, keeping in mind that some of them may not be influencing the particular skills and patterns being addressed. (See Appendix, Table 4, for a description of the different kinds of contexts that occupational therapists and occupational therapy assistants consider.)

### Activity Demands

The demands of the activity in which a person engages will affect skill and eventual success of performance. Occupational therapists and occupational therapy assistants apply their analysis skills to determine the demands that an activity will place on any performer and how those demands will influence skill execution. (See Appendix, Table 5, for complete list of activity demands.)

### Client Factors

Performance can be influenced by factors that reside within the client. Occupational therapists and occupational therapy assistants are knowledgeable about the variety of physical, cognitive, and psychosocial client factors that influence development and performance and how illness, disease, and disability affect these factors. The occupational therapist and occupational therapy assistant recognize that client factors influence the ability to engage in occupations and that engagement in occupations can also influence client factors. They apply their understanding of this interaction and use it throughout the intervention process.

Client factors include the following:
• Body functions—"physiological function of body systems (including psychological functions)" (WHO, 2001, p. 10). (See Appendix, Table 6, for complete list.) The occupational therapist and occupational therapy assistant under the supervision of an occupational therapist use

knowledge about body functions to evaluate selected client body functions that may be affecting his or her ability to engage in desired occupations or activities.
• Body structures—"anatomical parts of the body such as organs, limbs, and their components" (WHO, 2001, p. 10). (See Appendix, Table 6.) Occupational therapists and occupational therapy assistants under the supervision of an occupational therapist apply their knowledge about body structures to determine which body structures are needed to carry out an occupation or activity.

The categorization of client factors outlined in Table 6 is based on the *International Classification of Functioning, Disability and Health* proposed by the WHO (2001). The classification was selected because it has received wide exposure and presents a common language that is understood by external audiences. The categories include all those areas that occupational therapists and assistants address and consider during evaluation and intervention.

## Process
### The Process of Occupational Therapy: Evaluation, Intervention, and Outcome

Many professions use the process of evaluating, intervening, and targeting intervention outcomes that is outlined in the Framework. However occupational therapy's focus on occupation throughout the process makes the profession's application and use of the process unique. The process of occupational therapy service delivery begins by evaluating the client's occupational needs, problems, and concerns. Understanding the client as an occupational human being for whom access and participation in meaningful and productive activities is central to health and well-being is a perspective that is unique to occupational therapy. Problems and concerns that are addressed in evaluation and intervention are also framed uniquely from an occupational perspective, are based on occupational therapy theories, and are defined as problems or risks in occupational performance. During intervention, the focus remains on occupation, and efforts are directed toward fostering improved engagement in occupations. A variety of therapeutic activities, including engagement in actual occupations and in daily life activities, are used in intervention.

### Framework Process Organization

The *Occupational Therapy Practice Framework* process is organized into three broad sections that describe the process of service delivery. A brief overview of the process as it is applied within the profession's domain is outlined in Figure 2.

Figure 3 schematically illustrates how these sections are related to one another and how they revolve around the col-

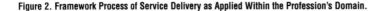

■ **Evaluation**

**Occupational profile**—The initial step in the evaluation process that provides an understanding of the client's occupational history and experiences, patterns of daily living, interests, values, and needs. The client's problems and concerns about performing occupations and daily life activities are identified, and the client's priorities are determined.

**Analysis of occupational performance**—The step in the evaluation process during which the client's assets, problems, or potential problems are more specifically identified. Actual performance is often observed in context to identify what supports performance and what hinders performance. Performance skills, performance patterns, context or contexts, activity demands, and client factors are all considered, but only selected aspects may be specifically assessed. Targeted outcomes are identified.

■ **Intervention**

**Intervention plan**—A plan that will guide actions taken and that is developed in collaboration with the client. It is based on selected theories, frames of reference, and evidence. Outcomes to be targeted are confirmed.

**Intervention implementation**—Ongoing actions taken to influence and support improved client performance. Interventions are directed at identified outcomes. Client's response is monitored and documented.

**Intervention review**—A review of the implementation plan and process as well as its progress toward targeted outcomes.

■ **Outcomes (Engagement in Occupation To Support Participation)**

**Outcomes**—Determination of success in reaching desired targeted outcomes. Outcome assessment information is used to plan future actions with the client and to evaluate the service program (i.e., program evaluation).

**Figure 2. Framework Process of Service Delivery as Applied Within the Profession's Domain.**

laborative therapeutic relationship between the client and the occupational therapist and occupational therapy assistant.

To help the reader understand the process, key statements highlight important points about the process outlined below.

**The process outlined is dynamic and interactive in nature.** Although the parts of the Framework are described in a linear manner, in reality, the process does not occur in a sequenced, step-by-step fashion. The arrows in Figure 3 that connect the boxes indicate the interactive and nonlinear nature of the process. The process, however, does always start with the occupational profile. An understanding of the client's concerns, problems, and risks is the cornerstone of the process. The factors that influence occupational performance (performance skills, performance patterns, context or contexts, activity demands, client factors) continually interact with one another. Because of their dynamic interaction, these factors are frequently evaluated simultaneously throughout the process as their influence on performance is observed.

**Context is an overarching, underlying, embedded influence on the process of service delivery.** Contexts exist around and within the person. They influence both the client's performance and the process of delivering services. The external context (e.g., the physical setting, social and virtual contexts) provide resources that support or inhibit the client's performance (e.g., presence of a willing caregiver) as well as the delivery of services (e.g., limits placed on length of intervention in an inpatient hospital setting). Different settings (i.e., community, institution, home) provide different supports and resources for service

delivery. The client's internal context (personal and spiritual contexts) affects service delivery by influencing personal beliefs, perceptions, and expectations. The cultural context, which exists outside of the person but is internalized by the person, also sets expectations, beliefs, and customs that can affect how and when services may be delivered. Note that in Figure 3, context is depicted as surrounding and underlying the process.

**The term** *client* **is used to name the entity that receives occupational therapy services.** Clients may be

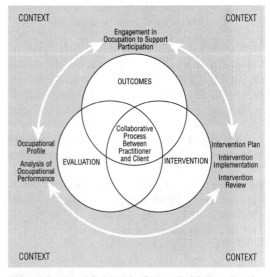

**Figure 3. Framework Collaborative Process Model.** Illustration of the framework emphasizing client–practitioner interactive relationship and interactive nature of the service delivery process.

categorized as (a) individuals, including individuals who may be involved in supporting or caring for the client (i.e., caregiver, teacher, parent, employer, spouse); (b) individuals within the context of a group (i.e., a family, a class); or (c) individuals within the context of a population (i.e., an organization, a community). The definition of *client* is consistent with *The Guide to Occupational Therapy Practice* (Moyers, 1999) and is indicative of the profession's growing understanding that people may be served not only as individuals, but also as members of a group or a population. The actual term used for individuals who are served will vary by practice setting. For example, in a hospital, the person might be referred to as a "patient," whereas in a school, he or she might be called a "student." Clients may be served as individuals, groups, or populations. Although the most common form of service delivery within the profession now involves a direct individual client to service provider model, more and more occupational therapists and occupational therapy assistants are beginning to serve clients at the group and population level (i.e., organization, community). When providing interventions other than in a one-to-one model, the occupational therapist and occupational therapist assistant are seen as agents who help others to support client engagement in occupations rather than as those who personally provide that support. Often, they use education and consultation as interventions. When occupational therapists and occupational therapy assistants are collaborating with clients to provide services at the group or population level, an important point to recognize is that although interventions may be directed to a group or population (i.e., organization, community), the individuals within those entities are the ones who are being evaluated and served. The wants, needs, occupational risks or problems, and performance patterns and skills of individuals within the group or population (i.e., organization, community) are evaluated as an aggregate, and information is compiled to determine group or population occupational issues and solutions.

**A client-centered approach is used throughout the Framework.** The Framework incorporates the value of client-centered evaluation and intervention by recognizing from the outset that all interventions must be focused on client priorities. The very nature of engagement in occupation—which is internally motivated, is individually defined, and requires active participation by the client—means that the client must be an active participant in the process. Clients identify what occupations and activities are important to them and determine the degree of engagement in each occupation. However, in some circumstances the client's ability to provide a description of the perceived or desired occupations or activity may be limited because of either the nature of the client's problems (e.g., autism, dementia) or the stage of development (e.g., infants). When this occurs, the occupational therapist and occupational therapy assistant must then take a broader view of the client and seek input from others such as family or significant others who would have knowledge and insight into the client's desires. By involving the family or significant others, the occupational therapist and assistant can better understand the client's history, developmental stage, and current contexts. Inclusion of others in these circumstances allows the client to be represented in intervention planning and implementation.

The entire process of service delivery begins with a collaborative relationship with the client. The collaborative relationship continues throughout the process and affects all phases of the process. The central importance of this collaboration is noted in Figure 3.

The Framework is based on the belief that the occupational therapist, occupational therapy assistant, and the client bring unique resources to the Framework process. Occupational therapists and occupational therapy assistants bring knowledge about how engagement in occupation affects health and performance. They also bring knowledge about disease and disability and couple this information with their clinical reasoning and theoretical perspectives to critically observe, analyze, describe, and interpret human performance. Therapists and assistants combine their knowledge and skills to modify the factors that influence engagement in occupation to improve and support performance. Clients bring knowledge about their life experiences and their hopes and dreams for the future. Clients share their priorities, which are based on what is important to them, and collaborate with the therapist and assistant in directing the intervention process to those priorities.

**"Engagement in occupation" is viewed as the overarching outcome of the occupational therapy process.** The Framework emphasizes occupational therapy's unique contribution to health by identifying "engagement in occupation to support participation" as the end objective of the occupational therapy process. The profession recognizes that in some areas of practice (e.g., acute rehabilitation, hand therapy) occupational therapy intervention may focus primarily on performance skills or on client factors (i.e., body functions, body structures) that will enable engagement in occupations later in the continuum of care.

## Evaluation Process

The evaluation process sets the stage for all that follows. Because occupational therapy is concerned with performance in daily life and how performance affects engagement in occupations to support participation, the evaluation process is focused on finding out what the client wants and needs to do and on identifying those factors that act as supports or barriers to performance. During the evaluation process, this information is paired with the occupational therapist's knowledge about human performance and the effect that illness, disability, and engagement in occupation have on performance. The occupational therapist considers performance skills, performance patterns, context, activity demands, and client factors and determines how each influences performance. The occupational therapist's skilled observation, use of specific assessments, and interpretation of results leads to a clear delineation of the problems and probable causes. The occupational therapy assistant may contribute to the evaluation process based on established competencies and under the supervision of an occupational therapist.

During the evaluation, a collaborative relationship with the client is established that continues throughout the entire occupational therapy process. The evaluation process is divided into two substeps, the first of which is the occupational profile—the initial step during which the client's needs, problems, and concerns about occupations and daily life activity performance are identified and priorities and values ascertained. The client's background and history in reference to engagement in occupations and in activities are also explored. The second substep of the evaluation process, analysis of occupational performance, focuses on more specifically identifying occupational performance issues and evaluating selected factors that support and hinder performance. Although each subsection is described separately and sequentially, in actuality, information pertinent to both subsections may be gathered during either one. The client's input is central in this process, and the client's priorities guide choices and decisions made during the process of evaluation.

### Occupational Profile

An occupational profile is defined as information that describes the client's occupational history and experiences, patterns of daily living, interests, values, and needs. The profile is designed to gain an understanding of the client's perspective and background. Using a client-centered approach, information is gathered to understand what is currently important and meaningful to the client (what he or she wants and needs to do) and to identify past experiences and interests that may assist in the understanding of current issues and problems. During the process of collecting this information, the client's priorities and desired targeted outcomes that will lead to engagement in occupation to support participation in life are also identified. Only

clients can identify the occupations that give meaning to their lives and select the goals and priorities that are important to them. Valuing and respecting the client's input helps to foster client involvement and can more efficiently guide interventions.

Information about the occupational profile is collected at the beginning of contact with the client. However, additional information is collected over time throughout the process, refined, and reflected in changes subsequently made to targeted outcomes.

*Process.* The theories and frames of reference that the occupational therapist selects to guide his or her reasoning will influence the information that is collected during the occupational profile. Scientific knowledge and evidence about diagnostic conditions and occupational performance problems is used to guide information gathering.

The process of completing the occupational profile will vary depending on the setting and the client. The information gathered in the profile may be obtained both formally and informally and may be completed in one session or over a much longer period while working with the client. Obtaining information through both formal interview and casual conversation is a way of beginning to establish a therapeutic relationship with the client. Ideally, the information obtained through the occupational profile will lead to a more individualized approach in the evaluation, intervention planning, and intervention implementation stages.

Specifically, the following information is collected:

• Who is the client (individual, caregiver, group, population)?
• Why is the client seeking service, and what are the client's current concerns relative to engaging in occupations and in daily life activities?
• What areas of occupation are successful, and what areas are causing problems or risks? (see Figure 1)
• What contexts support engagement in desired occupations, and what contexts are inhibiting engagement?
• What is the client's occupational history (i.e., life experiences, values, interests, previous patterns of engagement in occupations and in daily life activities, the meanings associated with them)?
• What are the client's priorities and desired targeted outcomes (see Appendix, Table 9)?
  – Occupational performance
  – Client satisfaction
  – Role competence
  – Adaptation
  – Health and wellness
  – Prevention
  – Quality of life

After profile data are collected, the therapist reviews the information and develops a working hypothesis regarding possible reasons for identified problems and concerns and identifies the client's strengths and weaknesses. Outcome measures are preliminarily selected.

### Analysis of Occupational Performance

Occupational performance is defined as the ability to carry out activities of daily life, including activities in the areas of occupation: activities of daily living (ADL) [also called basic activities of daily living (BADL) and personal activities of daily living (PADL)], instrumental activities of daily living (IADL), education, work, play, leisure, and social participation. Occupational performance results in the accomplishment of the selected occupation or activity and occurs through a dynamic transaction among the client, the context, and the activity. Improving or developing skills and patterns in occupational performance leads to engagement in one or more occupations (adapted in part from Law et al., 1996, p. 16).

When occupational performance is analyzed, the performance skills and patterns used in performance are identified, and other aspects of engaging in occupation that affect skills and patterns (e.g., client factors, activity demands, context or contexts) are evaluated. The analysis process identifies facilitators as well as barriers in various aspects of engagement in occupations and in daily life activities. Analyzing occupational performance requires an understanding of the complex and dynamic interaction among performance skills, performance patterns, context or contexts, activity demands, and client factors rather than of any one factor alone.

The information gathered during the occupational profile about the client's needs, problems, and priorities guides decisions during the analysis of occupational performance. The profile information directs the therapist's selection of the specific occupations or activities that need to be further analyzed and influences the selection of specific assessments that are used during the analysis process.

*Process.* Using available evidence and all aspects of clinical reasoning (scientific, narrative, pragmatic, ethical), the therapist selects one or more frames of reference to guide further collection of evaluation information. The following actions are taken:

• Synthesize information from the occupational profile to focus on specific areas of occupation and their contexts that need to be addressed.
• Observe the client's performance in desired occupations and activities, noting effectiveness of the performance skills and performance patterns. May select and use specific assessments to measure performance skills and patterns as appropriate.

• Select assessments, as needed, to identify and measure more specifically context or contexts, activity demands, and client factors that may be influencing performance skills and performance patterns.
• Interpret the assessment data to identify what supports performance and what hinders performance.
• Develop and refine hypotheses about the client's occupational performance strengths and weaknesses.
• Create goals in collaboration with the client that address the desired targeted outcomes. Confirm outcome measure to be used.
• Delineate potential intervention approach or approaches based on best practice and evidence.

### Intervention Process

The intervention process is divided into three substeps: intervention plan, intervention implementation, and intervention review. During the intervention process, information from the evaluation step is integrated with theory, frames of reference, and evidence and is coupled with clinical reasoning to develop a plan and carry it out. The plan guides the actions of the occupational therapist and occupational therapy assistant and is based on the client's priorities. Interventions are carried out to address performance skills, patterns, context or contexts, activity demands, and client factors that are hindering performance. Periodic reviews throughout the process allow for revisions in the plan and actions. Again, collaboration with the client is vital in this section of the process to ensure effectiveness and success. All interventions are ultimately directed toward achieving the overarching outcome of engagement in occupation to support participation.

### Intervention Plan

An intervention plan is defined as a plan that is developed based on the results of the evaluation process and describes selected occupational therapy approaches and types of interventions to reach the client's identified targeted outcomes. An intervention plan is developed collaboratively with the client (including, in some cases, family or significant others) and is based on the client's goals and priorities.

The design of the intervention plan is directed by
• the client's goals, values, and beliefs;
• the health and well-being of the client;
• the client's performance skills and performance patterns, as they are influenced by the interaction among the context or contexts, activity demands, and client factors; and
• the setting or circumstance in which the intervention is provided (e.g., caregiver expectations, organization's purpose, payer's requirements, or applicable regulations).

Interventions are designed to foster engagement in occupations and in activities to support participation in life. The selection and design of the intervention plan and goals are directed toward addressing the client's current and potential problems related to engagement in occupations or in activities.

*Process.* Intervention planning includes the following steps:

1. Develop the plan. The occupational therapist develops the plan. The occupational therapy assistant, based on established competencies and under the supervision of the occupational therapist, may contribute to the plan's development. The plan includes the following:
   - Objective and measurable goals with a timeframe
   - Occupational therapy intervention approach or approaches based on theory and evidence (see Appendix, Table 7).
     - Create or promote
     - Establish or restore
     - Maintain
     - Modify
     - Prevent
   - Mechanisms for service delivery
     - Who will provide intervention
     - Types of interventions
     - Frequency and duration of service
2. Consider potential discharge needs and plans.
3. Select outcome measures.
4. Make recommendation or referral to others as needed.

### Intervention Implementation

Intervention is the process of putting the plan into action. Intervention implementation is defined as the skilled process of effecting change in the client's occupational performance, leading to engagement in occupations or in activities to support participation. Intervention implementation is a collaborative process between the client and the occupational therapist and assistant.

Interventions may be focused on changing the context or contexts, activity demands, client factors, performance skills, or performance patterns. Occupational therapists and occupational therapy assistants recognize that change in one factor may influence other factors. All factors that affect performance are interrelated and influence one another in a continuous dynamic process that results in performance in desired areas of occupation. Because of this dynamic interrelationship, dynamic assessment continues throughout the implementation process.

*Process.* Intervention implementation includes the following steps:

1. Determine and carry out the type of occupational ther-

apy intervention or interventions to be used (see Appendix, Table 8).
   - Therapeutic use of self
   - Therapeutic use of occupations or activities
     - Occupation-based activity
     - Purposeful activity
     - Preparatory methods
   - Consultation process
   - Education process
2. Monitor client's response to interventions based on ongoing assessment and reassessment.

### Intervention Review

Intervention review is defined as a continuous process for reevaluating and reviewing the intervention plan, the effectiveness of its delivery, and the progress toward targeted outcomes. This process includes collaboration with the client (including, in some cases, family, significant others, and other service providers). Reevaluation and review may lead to change in the intervention plan. The intervention review process may be carried out differently in a variety of settings.

*Process.* The intervention review includes the following steps:

1. Reevaluate the plan and how it is carried out with the client relative to achieving targeted outcomes.
2. Modify the plan as needed.
3. Determine the need for continuation, discontinuation, or referral.

### Outcomes Process

Outcomes are defined as important dimensions of health that are attributed to interventions, including ability to function, health perceptions, and satisfaction with care (adapted from Request for Planning Ideas, 2001). The important dimension of health that occupational therapists and occupational therapy assistants target as the profession's overarching outcome is "engagement in occupation to support participation." The two concepts included in this outcome are defined as follows:

- Engagement in occupation—The commitment made to performance in occupations or activities as the result of self-choice, motivation, and meaning, and includes the objective and subjective aspects of carrying out occupations and activities that are meaningful and purposeful to the person.
- Participation—"involvement in a life situation" (WHO, 2001, p. 10).

Engagement in occupation to support participation is the broad outcome of intervention that is designed to foster performance in desired and needed occupations or activities. When clients are actively involved in carrying out occupations or daily life activities that they find purposeful and meaningful in home and community settings, participation is a natural outcome. Less broad and more specific outcomes of occupational therapy intervention (see Appendix, Table 9) are multidimensional and support the end result of engagement in occupation to support participation.

In targeting engagement in occupation to support participation as the broad, overarching outcome of the occupational therapy intervention process, the profession underscores its belief that health and well-being are holistic and that they are developed and maintained through active engagement in occupation.

The focus on outcomes is interwoven throughout the process of service delivery within occupational therapy. During the evaluation phase of the process, the client's initial targeted outcomes regarding desired engagement in occupation or daily life activities are identified. As further analysis of occupational performance and development of the treatment plan take place, targeted outcomes are further refined. During intervention implementation and reevaluation, targeted outcomes may be modified based on changing needs, contexts, and performance abilities. Outcomes have numerous definitions and connotations for different clients, payers, regulators, and organizations. The specific outcomes chosen will vary by practice setting and will be influenced by the particular stakeholders in each setting.

*Process.* Implementation of the outcomes process includes the following steps:

1. Select types of outcomes and measures, including, but not limited to occupational performance, client satisfaction, adaptation, role competence, health and wellness, prevention, and quality of life.
   - Selection of outcome measures occurs early in the intervention process (see Evaluation Process, Occupational Profile section).
   - Outcome measures that are selected are valid, reliable, and appropriately sensitive to change in the client's occupational performance, and they match the targeted outcomes.
   - Selection of an outcome measure or instrument for a particular client should be congruent with client goals.
   - Selection of an outcome measure should entail considering its actual or purported ability to predict future outcomes.

2. Measure and use outcomes.
   - Compare progress toward goal achievement to targeted outcomes throughout the intervention process.
   - Assess outcome results and use to make decisions about future direction of intervention (i.e., continue intervention, modify intervention, discontinue intervention, provide follow-up, refer to other services).

## An Overview of the Occupational Therapy Practice Process

Table 10 in the Appendix summarizes the process that occurs during occupational therapy service delivery. The arrow placed between the Occupational Profile and Analysis of Occupational Performance evaluation substeps indicates the interactions between these two. However, a similar interaction occurs among all of the steps and substeps. The process is not linear but, instead, is fluid and dynamic, allowing the occupational therapist and occupational therapy assistant to operate with an ongoing focus on outcomes while continually reflecting and changing an overall plan to accommodate new developments and insights along the way.

## Acknowledgments

The Commission on Practice (COP) would like to thank and acknowledge all those who participated in the review and comment process associated with the development of the *Occupational Therapy Practice Framework: Domain and Process.* The COP has found this process invaluable and enriching. Everyone's input has been carefully reviewed and considered. Often, small comments repeated by many can lead to significant discussion and change. The COP hopes that all those who contributed to this process will continue to do so for future documents and will encourage others to participate. The profession is richer for this process.

The COP would like to thank the following individuals for their significant contributions to the direction and final content of this document: Carolyn Baum, PhD, OTR, FAOTA; Elizabeth Crepeau, PhD, OTR, FAOTA; Patricia A. Crist, PhD, FAOTA; Winifred Dunn, PhD, OTR, FAOTA; Anne G. Fisher, PhD, OTR, FAOTA; Gail S. Fidler, OTR, FAOTA; Mary Foto, OT, FAOTA; Nedra Gillette, SCD (HON), MEd, OTR, FAOTA; Jim Hinojosa, PhD, OT, FAOTA; Margo B. Holm, PhD, OTR, FAOTA; Gary Kielhofner, DRPH, OTR/L, FAOTA; Paula Kramer, PhD, OTR, FAOTA; Mary Law, PhD, OT(C); Linda T. Learnard, OTR/L; Anne Mosey, PhD, OTR, FAOTA; Penelope A. Moyers, EDd, OTR, FAOTA; David Nelson, PhD, OTR, FAOTA; Marta Pelczarski, OTR; Kathlyn L. Reed, PhD, OTR, FAOTA; Barbara Schell, PhD, OTR/L, FAOTA; Janette Schkade, PhD, OTR; Wendy Schoen; Carol Siebert, MS, OTR/L; V. Judith Thomas, MGA; Linda Kohlman Thomson, MOT, OT, OT(C), FAOTA; Amy L. Walsh, OTR/L; Wendy Wood, PhD, OTR, FAOTA; Boston University OT Students mentored by Karen Jacobs, EDd, OTR/L, CPE, FAOTA; and the University of Kansas Occupational Therapy Education Faculty.

# Appendix

## TABLE 1. AREAS OF OCCUPATION

*Various kinds of life activities in which people engage, including ADL, IADL, education, work, play, leisure, and social participation.*

### ■ ACTIVITIES OF DAILY LIVING (ADL)

Activities that are oriented toward taking care of one's own body (adapted from Rogers & Holm, 1994, pp. 181–202)—also called basic activities of daily living (BADL) or personal activities of daily living (PADL).

- **Bathing, showering**—Obtaining and using supplies; soaping, rinsing, and drying body parts; maintaining bathing position; and transferring to and from bathing positions.
- **Bowel and bladder management**— Includes complete intentional control of bowel movements and urinary bladder and, if necessary, use of equipment or agents for bladder control (Uniform Data System for Medical Rehabilitation [UDSMR], 1996, pp. III–20, III–24).
- **Dressing**—Selecting clothing and accessories appropriate to time of day, weather, and occasion; obtaining clothing from storage area; dressing and undressing in a sequential fashion; fastening and adjusting clothing and shoes; and applying and removing personal devices, prostheses, or orthoses.
- **Eating**—"The ability to keep and manipulate food/fluid in the mouth and swallow it (O'Sullivan, 1995, p. 191)" (AOTA, 2000, p. 629).
- **Feeding**—"The process of [setting up, arranging, and] bringing food [fluids] from the plate or cup to the mouth (O'Sullivan, 1995, p. 191)" (AOTA, 2000, p. 629).
- **Functional mobility**—Moving from one position or place to another (during performance of everyday activities), such as in-bed mobility, wheelchair mobility, transfers (wheelchair, bed, car, tub, toilet, tub/shower, chair, floor). Performing functional ambulation and transporting objects.
- **Personal device care**—Using, cleaning, and maintaining personal care items, such as hearing aids, contact lenses, glasses, orthotics, prosthetics, adaptive equipment, and contraceptive and sexual devices.
- **Personal hygiene and grooming**—Obtaining and using supplies; removing body hair (use of razors, tweezers, lotions, etc.); applying and removing cosmetics; washing, drying, combing, styling, brushing, and trimming hair; caring for nails (hands and feet); caring for skin, ears, eyes, and nose; applying deodorant; cleaning mouth; brushing and flossing teeth; or removing, cleaning, and reinserting dental orthotics and prosthetics.
- **Sexual activity**—Engagement in activities that result in sexual satisfaction.
- **Sleep/rest**—A period of inactivity in which one may or may not suspend consciousness.

- **Toilet hygiene**—Obtaining and using supplies; clothing management; maintaining toileting position; transferring to and from toileting position; cleaning body; and caring for menstrual and continence needs (including catheters, colostomies, and suppository management).

### ■ INSTRUMENTAL ACTIVITIES OF DAILY LIVING (IADL)

Activities that are oriented toward interacting with the environment and that are often complex—generally optional in nature (i.e., may be delegated to another) (adapted from Rogers & Holm, 1994, pp. 181–202).

- **Care of others (including selecting and supervising caregivers)**—Arranging, supervising, or providing the care for others.
- **Care of pets**—Arranging, supervising, or providing the care for pets and service animals.
- **Child rearing**—Providing the care and supervision to support the developmental needs of a child.
- **Communication device use**—Using equipment or systems such as writing equipment, telephones, typewriters, computers, communication boards, call lights, emergency systems, braille writers, telecommunication devices for the deaf, and augmentative communication systems to send and receive information.
- **Community mobility**—Moving self in the community and using public or private transportation, such as driving, or accessing buses, taxi cabs, or other public transportation systems.
- **Financial management**—Using fiscal resources, including alternate methods of financial transaction and planning and using finances with long-term and short-term goals.
- **Health management and maintenance**—Developing, managing, and maintaining routines for health and wellness promotion, such as physical fitness, nutrition, decreasing health risk behaviors, and medication routines.
- **Home establishment and management**—Obtaining and maintaining personal and household possessions and environment (e.g., home, yard, garden, appliances, vehicles), including maintaining and repairing personal possessions (clothing and household items) and knowing how to seek help or whom to contact.
- **Meal preparation and cleanup**—Planning, preparing, serving well-balanced, nutritional meals and cleaning up food and utensils after meals.

- **Safety procedures and emergency responses**—Knowing and performing preventive procedures to maintain a safe environment as well as recognizing sudden, unexpected hazardous situations and initiating emergency action to reduce the threat to health and safety.
- **Shopping**—Preparing shopping lists (grocery and other); selecting and purchasing items; selecting method of payment; and completing money transactions.

### ■ EDUCATION

Includes activities needed for being a student and participating in a learning environment.

- **Formal educational participation**—Including the categories of academic (e.g., math, reading, working on a degree), nonacademic (e.g., recess, lunchroom, hallway), extracurricular (e.g., sports, band, cheerleading, dances), and vocational (prevocational and vocational) participation.
- **Exploration of informal personal educational needs or interests (beyond formal education)**—Identifying topics and methods for obtaining topic-related information or skills.
- **Informal personal education participation**—Participating in classes, programs, and activities that provide instruction/training in identified areas of interest.

### ■ WORK

Includes activities needed for engaging in remunerative employment or volunteer activities (Mosey, 1996, p. 341).

- **Employment interests and pursuits**—Identifying and selecting work opportunities based on personal assets, limitations, likes, and dislikes relative to work (adapted from Mosey, 1996, p. 342).
- **Employment seeking and acquisition**—Identifying job opportunities, completing and submitting appropriate application materials, preparing for interviews, participating in interviews and following up afterward, discussing job benefits, and finalizing negotiations.
- **Job performance**—Including work habits, for example, attendance, punctuality, appropriate relationships with coworkers and supervisors, completion of assigned work, and compliance with the norms of the work setting (adapted from Mosey, 1996, p. 342).
- **Retirement preparation and adjustment**—Determining aptitudes, developing interests and skills, and selecting appropriate avocational pursuits.

*(Continued)*

## TABLE 1. AREAS OF OCCUPATION

*(Continued)*

- **Volunteer exploration**—Determining community causes, organizations, or opportunities for unpaid "work" in relationship to personal skills, interests, location, and time available.

- **Volunteer participation**—Performing unpaid "work" activities for the benefit of identified selected causes, organizations, or facilities.

### ▨ PLAY

"Any spontaneous or organized activity that provides enjoyment, entertainment, amusement, or diversion" (Parham & Fazio, 1997, p. 252).

- **Play exploration**—Identifying appropriate play activities, which can include exploration play, practice play, pretend play, games with rules, constructive play, and symbolic play (adapted from Bergen, 1988, pp. 64–65).

- **Play participation**—Participating in play; maintaining a balance of play with other areas of occupation; and obtaining, using, and maintaining, toys, equipment, and supplies appropriately.

### ▨ LEISURE

"A nonobligatory activity that is intrinsically motivated and engaged in during discretionary time, that is, time not committed to obligatory occupations such as work, self-care, or sleep" (Parham & Fazio, 1997, p. 250).

- **Leisure exploration**—Identifying interests, skills, opportunities, and appropriate leisure activities.

- **Leisure participation**—Planning and participating in appropriate leisure activities; maintaining a balance of leisure activities with other areas of occupation; and obtaining, using, and maintaining equipment and supplies as appropriate.

### ▨ SOCIAL PARTICIPATION

Activities associated with organized patterns of behavior that are characteristic and expected of an individual or an individual interacting with others within a given social system (adapted from Mosey, 1996, p. 340).

- **Community**—Activities that result in successful interaction at the community level (i.e., neighborhood, organizations, work, school).

- **Family**—"[Activities that result in] successful interaction in specific required and/or desired familial roles" (Mosey, 1996, p. 340).

- **Peer, friend**—Activities at different levels of intimacy, including engaging in desired sexual activity.

*Note.* Some of the terms used in this table are from, or adapted from, the rescinded *Uniform Terminology for Occupational Therapy—Third Edition* (AOTA, 1994, pp. 1047–1054).

## TABLE 2. PERFORMANCE SKILLS

*Features of what one does, not what one has, related to observable elements of action that have implicit functional purposes (adapted from Fisher & Kielhofner, 1995, p. 113).*

### ▨ MOTOR SKILLS—skills in moving and interacting with task, objects, and environment (A. Fisher, personal communication, July 9, 2001).

- **Posture**—Relates to the stabilizing and aligning of one's body while moving in relation to task objects with which one must deal.

*Stabilizes*—Maintains trunk control and balance while interacting with task objects such that there is no evidence of transient (i.e., quickly passing) propping or loss of balance that affects task performance.

*Aligns*—Maintains an upright sitting or standing position, without evidence of a need to persistently prop during the task performance.

*Positions*—Positions body, arms, or wheelchair in relation to task objects and in a manner that promotes the use of efficient arm movements during task performance.

- **Mobility**—Relates to moving the entire body or a body part in space as necessary when interacting with task objects.

*Walks*—Ambulates on level surfaces and changes direction while walking without shuffling the feet, lurching, instability, or using external supports or assistive devices (e.g., cane, walker, wheelchair) during the task performance.

*Reaches*—Extends, moves the arm (and when appropriate, the trunk) to effectively grasp or place task objects that are out of reach, including skillfully using a reacher to obtain task objects.

*Bends*—Actively flexes, rotates, or twists the trunk in a manner and direction appropriate to the task.

- **Coordination**—Relates to using more than one body part to interact with task objects in a manner that supports task performance.

*Coordinates*—Uses two or more body parts together to stabilize and manipulate task objects during bilateral motor tasks.

*Manipulates*—Uses dexterous grasp-and-release patterns, isolated finger movements, and coordinated in-hand manipulation patterns when interacting with task objects.

*Flows*—Uses smooth and fluid arm and hand movements when interacting with task objects.

- **Strength and effort**—Pertains to skills that require generation of muscle force appropriate for effective interaction with task objects.

*Moves*—Pushes, pulls, or drags task objects along a supporting surface.

*Transports*—Carries task objects from one place to another while walking, seated in a wheelchair, or using a walker.

*Lifts*—Raises or hoists task objects, including lifting an object from one place to another, but without ambulating or moving from one place to another.

*Calibrates*—Regulates or grades the force, speed, and extent of movement when interacting with task objects (e.g., not too much or too little).

*Grips*—Pinches or grasps task objects with no "grip slips."

- **Energy**—Refers to sustained effort over the course of task performance.

*Endures*—Persists and completes the task without obvious evidence of physical fatigue, pausing to rest, or stopping to "catch one's breath."

*Paces*—Maintains a consistent and effective rate or tempo of performance throughout the steps of the entire task.

### ▨ PROCESS SKILLS—"Skills...used in managing and modifying actions en route to the completion of daily life tasks" (Fisher & Kielhofner, 1995, p. 120).

- **Energy**—Refers to sustained effort over the course of task performance.

*Paces*—Maintains a consistent and effective rate or tempo of performance throughout the steps of the entire task.

*(Continued)*

## TABLE 2. PERFORMANCE SKILLS

*(Continued)*

*Attends*—Maintains focused attention throughout the task such that the client is not distracted away from the task by extraneous auditory or visual stimuli.

• **Knowledge**—Refers to the ability to seek and use task-related knowledge.

*Chooses*—Selects appropriate and necessary tools and materials for the task, including choosing the tools and materials that were specified for use prior to the initiation of the task.

*Uses*—Uses tools and materials according to their intended purposes and in a reasonable or hygienic fashion, given their intrinsic properties and the availability (or lack of availability) of other objects.

*Handles*—Supports, stabilizes, and holds tools and materials in an appropriate manner that protects them from damage, falling, or dropping.

*Heeds*—Uses goal-directed task actions that are focused toward the completion of the specified task (i.e., the outcome originally agreed on or specified by another) without behavior that is driven or guided by environmental cues (i.e., "environmentally cued" behavior).

*Inquires*—(a) Seeks needed verbal or written information by asking questions or reading directions or labels or (b) asks no unnecessary information questions (e.g., questions related to where materials are located or how a familiar task is performed).

• **Temporal organization**—Pertains to the beginning, logical ordering, continuation, and completion of the steps and action sequences of a task.

*Initiates*—Starts or begins the next action or step without hesitation.

*Continues*—Performs actions or action sequences of steps without unnecessary interruption such that once an action sequence is initiated, the individual continues on until the step is completed.

*Sequences*—Performs steps in an effective or logical order for efficient use of time and energy and with an absence of (a) randomness in the ordering and/or (b) inappropriate repetition ("reordering") of steps.

*Terminates*—Brings to completion single actions or single steps without perseveration, inappropriate persistence, or premature cessation.

• **Organizing space and objects**—Pertains to skills for organizing task spaces and task objects.

*Searches/locates*—Looks for and locates tools and materials in a logical manner, including looking beyond the immediate environment (e.g., looking in, behind, on top of).

*Gathers*—Collects together needed or misplaced tools and materials, including (a) collecting located supplies into the workspace and (b) collecting and replacing materials that have spilled, fallen, or been misplaced.

*Organizes*—Logically positions or spatially arranges tools and materials in an orderly fashion (a) within a single workspace and (b) among multiple appropriate workspaces to facilitate ease of task performance.

*Restores*—(a) Puts away tools and materials in appropriate places, (b) restores immediate workspace to original condition (e.g., wiping surfaces clean), (c) closes and seals containers and coverings when indicated, and (d) twists or folds any plastic bags to seal.

*Navigates*—Modifies the movement pattern of the arm, body, or wheelchair to maneuver around obstacles that are encountered in the course of moving through space such that undesirable contact with obstacles (e.g., knocking over, bumping into) is avoided (includes maneuvering objects held in the hand around obstacles).

• **Adaptation**—Relates to the ability to anticipate, correct for, and benefit by learning from the consequences of errors that arise in the course of task performance.

*Notices/responds*—Responds appropriately to (a) nonverbal environmental/perceptual cues (i.e., movement, sound, smell, heat, moisture, texture, shape, consistency) that provide feedback with respect to task progression and (b) the spatial arrangement of objects to one another (e.g., aligning objects during stacking). Notices and, when indicated, makes an effective and efficient response.

*Accommodates*—Modifies his or her actions or the location of objects within the workspace in anticipation of or in response to problems that might arise. The client anticipates or responds to problems effectively by (a) changing the method with which he or she is performing an action sequence, (b) changing the manner in which he or she interacts with or handles tools and materials already in the workspace, and (c) asking for assistance when appropriate or needed.

*Adjusts*—Changes working environments in anticipation of or in response to problems that might arise. The client anticipates or responds to problems effectively by making some change (a) between working environments by moving to a new workspace or bringing in or removing tools and materials from the present workspace or (b) in an environmental condition (e.g., turning on or off the tap, turning up or down the temperature).

*Benefits*—Anticipates and prevents undesirable circumstances or problems from recurring or persisting.

■ **COMMUNICATION/INTERACTION SKILLS**—Refer to conveying intentions and needs and coordinating social behavior to act together with people (Forsyth & Kielhofner, 1999; Forsyth, Salamy, Simon, & Kielhofner, 1997; Kielhofner, 2002).

• **Physicality**—Pertains to using the physical body when communicating within an occupation.

*Contacts*—Makes physical contact with others.

*Gazes*—Uses eyes to communicate and interact with others.

*Gestures*—Uses movements of the body to indicate, demonstrate, or add emphasis.

*Maneuvers*—Moves one's body in relation to others.

*Orients*—Directs one's body in relation to others and/or occupational forms.

*Postures*—Assumes physical positions.

• **Information exchange**—Refers to giving and receiving information within an occupation.

*Articulates*—Produces clear, understandable speech.

*Asserts*—Directly expresses desires, refusals, and requests.

*Asks*—Requests factual or personal information.

*Engages*—Initiates interactions.

*Expresses*—Displays affect/attitude.

*Modulates*—Uses volume and inflection in speech.

*Shares*—Gives out factual or personal information.

*Speaks*—Makes oneself understood through use of words, phrases, and sentences.

*Sustains*—Keeps up speech for appropriate duration.

• **Relations**—Relates to maintaining appropriate relationships within an occupation.

*Collaborates*—Coordinates action with others toward a common end goal.

*Conforms*—Follows implicit and explicit social norms.

*Focuses*—Directs conversation and behavior to ongoing social action.

*Relates*—Assumes a manner of acting that tries to establish a rapport with others.

*Respects*—Accommodates to other people's reactions and requests.

*Note.* The Motor and Process Skills sections of this table were compiled from the following sources: Fisher (2001), Fisher and Kielhofner (1995)—updated by Fisher (2001). The Communication/Interaction Skills section of this table was compiled from the following sources: Forsyth and Kielhofner (1999), Forsyth, Salamy, Simon, and Kielhofner (1997), and Kielhofner (2002).

## TABLE 3. PERFORMANCE PATTERNS

*Patterns of behavior related to daily life activities that are habitual or routine.*

■ **HABITS**—"Automatic behavior that is integrated into more complex patterns that enable people to function on a day-to-day basis" (Neistadt & Crepeau, 1998, p. 869). Habits can either support or interfere with performance in areas of occupation.

| Type of Habit | Examples |
|---|---|
| • **Useful habits** | |
| Habits that support performance in daily life and contribute to life satisfaction. | – Always put car keys in the same place so they can be found easily. |
| Habits that support ability to follow rhythms of daily life. | – Brush teeth every morning to maintain good oral hygiene. |
| • **Impoverished habits** | |
| Habits that are not established. | – Inconsistently remembering to look both ways before crossing the street. |
| Habits that need practice to improve. | – Inability to complete all steps of a self-care routine. |
| • **Dominating habits** | |
| Habits that are so demanding they interfere with daily life. | – Repetitive self-stimulation such as type occurring in autism. |
| | – Use of chemical substances, resulting in addiction. |
| Habits that satisfy a compulsive need for order. | – Neatly arranging forks on top of each other in silverware drawer. |

■ **ROUTINES**—"Occupations with established sequences" (Christiansen & Baum, 1997, p. 6).

■ **ROLES**—"A set of behaviors that have some socially agreed upon function and for which there is an accepted code of norms" (Christiansen & Baum, 1997, p. 603).

*Note.* Information for Habits section of this table adapted from Dunn (2000, Fall).

## TABLE 4. CONTEXT OR CONTEXTS

*Context (including cultural, physical, social, personal, spiritual, temporal, and virtual) refers to a variety of interrelated conditions within and surrounding the client that influence performance.*

| Context | Definition | Example |
|---|---|---|
| **Cultural** | Customs, beliefs, activity patterns, behavior standards, and expectations accepted by the society of which the individual is a member. Includes political aspects, such as laws that affect access to resources and affirm personal rights. Also includes opportunities for education, employment, and economic support. | • Ethnicity, family, attitude, beliefs, values |
| **Physical** | Nonhuman aspects of contexts. Includes the accessibility to and performance within environments having natural terrain, plants, animals, buildings, furniture, objects, tools, or devices. | • Objects, built environment, natural environment, geographic terrain, sensory qualities of environment |
| **Social** | Availability and expectations of significant individuals, such as spouse, friends, and caregivers. Also includes larger social groups that are influential in establishing norms, role expectations, and social routines. | • Relationships with individuals, groups, or organizations; relationships with systems (political, economic, institutional) |
| **Personal** | "[F]eatures of the individual that are not part of a health condition or health status" (WHO, 2001, p. 17). Personal context includes age, gender, socioeconomic status, and educational status. | • Twenty-five-year-old unemployed man with a high school diploma |
| **Spiritual** | The fundamental orientation of a person's life; that which inspires and motivates that individual. | • Essence of the person, greater or higher purpose, meaning, substance |
| **Temporal** | "Location of occupational performance in time" (Neistadt & Crepeau, 1998, p. 292). | • Stages of life, time of day, time of year, duration |
| **Virtual** | Environment in which communication occurs by means of airways or computers and an absence of physical contact. | • Realistic simulation of an environment, chat rooms, radio transmissions |

*Note.* Some of the definitions for areas of context or contexts are from the rescinded *Uniform Terminology for Occupational Therapy—Third Edition* (AOTA, 1994).

## TABLE 5. ACTIVITY DEMANDS

The aspects of an activity, which include the objects, space, social demands, sequencing or timing, required actions, and required underlying body functions and body structure needed to carry out the activity.

| Activity Demand Aspects | Definition | Examples |
|---|---|---|
| Objects and their properties | The tools, materials, and equipment used in the process of carrying out the activity | • Tools (scissors, dishes, shoes, volleyball)<br>• Materials (paints, milk, lipstick)<br>• Equipment (workbench, stove, basketball hoop)<br>• Inherent properties (heavy, rough, sharp, colorful, loud, bitter tasting) |
| Space demands (relates to physical context) | The physical environmental requirements of the activity (e.g., size, arrangement, surface, lighting, temperature, noise, humidity, ventilation) | • Large open space outdoors required for a baseball game |
| Social demands (relates to social and cultural contexts) | The social structure and demands that may be required by the activity | • Rules of game<br>• Expectations of other participants in activity (e.g., sharing of supplies) |
| Sequence and timing | The process used to carry out the activity (specific steps, sequence, timing requirements) | • Steps—to make tea: gather cup and tea bag, heat water, pour water into cup, etc.<br>• Sequence—heat water before placing tea bag in water<br>• Timing—leave tea bag to steep for 2 minutes |
| Required actions | The usual skills that would be required by any performer to carry out the activity. Motor, process, and communication interaction skills should each be considered. The performance skills demanded by an activity will be correlated with the demands of the other activity aspects (i.e., objects, space) | • Gripping handlebar<br>• Choosing a dress from closet<br>• Answering a question |
| Required body functions | "The physiological functions of body systems (including psychological functions)" (WHO, 2001, p. 10) that are required to support the actions used to perform the activity. | • Mobility of joints<br>• Level of consciousness |
| Required body structures | "Anatomical parts of the body such as organs, limbs, and their components [that support body function]" (WHO, 2001, p. 10) that are required to perform the activity. | • Number of hands<br>• Number of eyes |

## TABLE 6. CLIENT FACTORS

Those factors that reside within the client and that may affect performance in areas of occupation. Client factors include body functions and body structures. Knowledge about body functions and structures is considered when determining which functions and structures are needed to carry out an occupation/activity and how the body functions and structures may be changed as a result of engaging in an occupation/activity. Body functions are "the physiological functions of body systems (including psychological functions)" (WHO, 2001, p. 10). Body structures are "anatomical parts of the body such as organs, limbs and their components [that support body function]" (WHO, 2001, p. 10).

| Client Factor | Selected Classifications From ICF and Occupational Therapy Examples |
|---|---|
| ▨ **BODY FUNCTION CATEGORIES**[a] | |
| **Mental functions (affective, cognitive, perceptual)** | |
| • Global mental functions | *Consciousness functions*—level of arousal, level of consciousness. |
| | *Orientation functions*—to person, place, time, self, and others. |
| | *Sleep*—amount and quality of sleep. *Note:* Sleep and sleep patterns are assessed in relation to how they affect ability to effectively engage in occupations and in daily life activities. |
| | *Temperament and personality functions*—conscientiousness, emotional stability, openness to experience. *Note:* These functions are assessed relative to their influence on the ability to engage in occupations and in daily life activities. |
| | *Energy and drive functions*—motivation, impulse control, interests, values. |
| • Specific mental functions | *Attention functions*—sustained attention, divided attention. |
| | *Memory functions*—retrospective memory, prospective memory. |
| | *Perceptual functions*—visuospatial perception, interpretation of sensory stimuli (tactile, visual, auditory, olfactory, gustatory). |
| | *Thought functions*—recognition, categorization, generalization, awareness of reality, logical/coherent thought, appropriate thought content. |

(Continued)

## TABLE 6. CLIENT FACTORS

*(Continued)*

| Client Factor | Selected Classifications From ICF and Occupational Therapy Examples |
|---|---|
| | *Higher-level cognitive functions*—judgment, concept formation, time management, problem solving, decision-making. |
| | *Mental functions of language*—able to receive language and express self through spoken and written or sign language. Note: This function is assessed relative to its influence on the ability to engage in occupations and in daily life activities. |
| | *Calculation functions*—able to add or subtract. *Note:* These functions are assessed relative to their influence on the ability to engage in occupations and in daily life activities (e.g., making change when shopping). |
| | *Mental functions of sequencing complex movement*—motor planning. |
| | *Psychomotor functions*—appropriate range and regulation of motor response to psychological events. |
| | *Emotional functions*—appropriate range and regulation of emotions, self-control. |
| | *Experience of self and time functions*—body image, self-concept, self-esteem. |
| **Sensory functions and pain** | |
| • Seeing and related functions | *Seeing functions*—visual acuity, visual field functions. |
| • Hearing and vestibular functions | *Hearing function*—response to sound. *Note:* This function is assessed in terms of its presence or absence and its affect on engaging in occupations and in daily life activities. |
| | *Vestibular function*—balance. |
| • Additional sensory functions | *Taste function*—ability to discriminate tastes. |
| | *Smell function*—ability to discriminate smell. |
| | *Proprioceptive function*—kinesthesia, joint position sense. |
| | *Touch functions*—sensitivity to touch, ability to discriminate. |
| | *Sensory functions related to temperature and other stimuli*—sensitivity to temperature, sensitivity to pressure, ability to discriminate temperature and pressure. |
| • Pain | *Sensations of pain*—dull pain, stabbing pain. |
| **Neuromusculoskeletal and movement-related functions** | |
| • Functions of joints and bones | *Mobility of joint functions*—passive range of motion. |
| | *Stability of joint functions*—postural alignment. *Note:* This refers to physiological stability of the joint related to its structural integrity as compared to the motor skill of aligning the body while moving in relation to task objects. |
| | *Mobility of bone functions*—frozen scapula, movement of carpal bones. |
| • Muscle functions | *Muscle power functions*—strength. |
| | *Muscle tone functions*—degree of muscle tone (e.g., flaccidity, spasticity). |
| | *Muscle endurance functions*—endurance. |
| • Movement functions | *Motor reflex functions*—stretch reflex, asymmetrical tonic neck reflex. |
| | *Involuntary movement reaction functions*—righting reactions, supporting reactions. |
| | *Control of voluntary movement functions*—eye–hand coordination, bilateral integration, eye–foot coordination. |
| | *Involuntary movement functions*—tremors, tics, motor perseveration. |
| | *Gait pattern functions*—walking patterns and impairments, such as asymmetric gait, stiff gait. (*Note:* Gait patterns are assessed in relation to how they affect ability to engage in occupations and in daily life activities.) |
| **Cardiovascular, hematological, immunological, and respiratory system function** | |
| • Cardiovascular system function | *Blood pressure functions*—hypertension, hypotension, postural hypotension. |
| • Hematological and immunological system function | Occupational therapists and occupational therapy assistants have knowledge of these body functions and understand broadly the interaction that occurs between these functions and engagement in occupation to support participation. Some therapists may specialize in evaluating and intervening with a specific function as it is related to supporting performance and engagement in occupations and activities targeted for intervention. |

*(Continued)*

## TABLE 6. CLIENT FACTORS

*(Continued)*

| Client Factor | Selected Classifications From ICF and Occupational Therapy Examples |
|---|---|
| • Respiratory system function | *Respiration functions*—rate, rhythm, and depth. |
| • Additional functions and sensations of the cardiovascular and respiratory systems | *Exercise tolerance functions*—physical endurance, aerobic capacity, stamina, and fatigability. |

**Voice and speech functions**

**Digestive, metabolic, and endocrine system function**

• Digestive system function

• Metabolic system and endocrine system function

**Genitourinary and reproductive functions**

• Urinary functions

• Genital and reproductive functions

Occupational therapists and occupational therapy assistants have knowledge of these body functions and understand broadly the interaction that occurs between these functions and engagement in occupation to support participation. Some therapists may specialize in evaluating and intervening with a specific function as it is related to supporting performance and engagement in occupations and activities targeted for intervention.

**Skin and related structure functions**

| | |
|---|---|
| • Skin functions | *Protective functions of the skin*—presence or absence of wounds, cuts, or abrasions. |
| | *Repair function of the skin*—wound healing. |
| • Hair and nail functions | Occupational therapists and occupational therapy assistants have knowledge of these body functions and understand broadly the interaction that occurs between these functions and engagement in occupation to support participation. Some therapists may specialize in evaluating and intervening with a specific function as it is related to supporting performance and engagement in occupations and activities targeted for intervention. |

| Client Factor | Classifications (Classification are not delineated in the Body Structure section of this table) |
|---|---|

### ▓ BODY STRUCTURE CATEGORIES[b]

**Structure of the nervous system**

**The eye, ear, and related structures**

**Structures involved in voice and speech**

**Structures of the cardiovascular, immunological, and respiratory systems**

**Structures related to the digestive**

**Structure related to the genitourinary and reproductive systems**

**Structures related to movement**

**Skin and related structures**

Occupational therapists and occupational therapy assistants have knowledge of these body functions and understand broadly the interaction that occurs between these functions and engagement in occupation to support participation. Some therapists may specialize in evaluating and intervening with a specific function as it is related to supporting performance and engagement in occupations and activities targeted for intervention.

*Note.* The reader is strongly encouraged to use *International Classification of Functioning, Disability and Health* (ICF) in collaboration with this table to provide for in-depth information with respect to classification in terms (inclusion and exclusion).

[a]Categories and classifications are adapted from the ICF (WHO, 2001). [b]Categories are from the ICF (WHO, 2001).

## TABLE 7. OCCUPATIONAL THERAPY INTERVENTION APPROACHES

*Specific strategies selected to direct the process of intervention that are based on the client's desired outcome, evaluation data, and evidence.*

| Approach | Focus of Intervention | Examples |
|---|---|---|
| **Create, promote (health promotion)**[a]—an intervention approach that does not assume a disability is present or that any factors would interfere with performance. This approach is designed to provide enriched contextual and activity experiences that will enhance performance for all persons in the natural contexts of life (adapted from Dunn, McClain, Brown, & Youngstrom, 1998, p. 534). | **Performance skills** | • Create a parenting class for first-time parents to teach child development information (performance skill). |
| | **Performance patterns** | • Promote handling stress by creating time-use routines with healthy clients (performance pattern). |
| | **Context or contexts** | • Create a variety of equipment available at public playgrounds to promote a diversity of sensory play experiences (context). |
| | **Activity demands** | • Promote the establishment of sufficient space to allow senior residents to participate in congregate cooking (activity demand). |
| | **Client factors (body functions, body structures)** | • Promote increased endurance in school children by having them ride bicycles to school (client factor: body function). |
| **Establish, restore (remediation, restoration)**[a]—an intervention approach designed to change client variables to establish a skill or ability that has not yet developed or to restore a skill or ability that has been impaired (adapted from Dunn et al., 1998, p. 533). | **Performance skills** | • Improve coping needed for changing workplace demands by improving assertiveness skills (performance skill). |
| | **Performance patterns** | • Establish morning routines needed to arrive at school or work on time (performance pattern). |
| | **Client factors (body functions, body structures)** | • Restore mobility needed for play activities (client factor: body function). |
| **Maintain**—an intervention approach designed to provide the supports that will allow clients to preserve their performance capabilities that they have regained, that continue to meet their occupational needs, or both. The assumption is that without continued maintenance intervention, performance would decrease, occupational needs would not be met, or both, thereby affecting health and quality of life. | **Performance skills** | • Maintain the ability to organize tools by providing a tool outline painted on a pegboard (performance skill). |
| | **Performance patterns** | • Maintain appropriate medication schedule by providing a timer (performance pattern). |
| | **Context or contexts** | • Maintain safe and independent access for persons with low vision by providing increased hallway lighting (context). |
| | **Activity demands** | • Maintain independent gardening for persons with arthritic hands by providing tools with modified grips (activity demand). |
| | **Client factors (body functions, body structures)** | • Maintain proper digestive system functions by developing a dining program (client factor: body function). |
| | | • Maintain upper-extremity muscles necessary for independent wheelchair mobility by developing an after-school–based exercise program (client factor: body structure). |
| **Modify (compensation, adaptation)**[a]—an intervention approach directed at "finding ways to revise the current context or activity demands to support performance in the natural setting…[includes] compensatory techniques, including enhancing some features to provide cues, or reducing other features to reduce distractibility" (Dunn et al., 1998, p. 533). | **Context or contexts** | • Modify holiday celebration activities to exclude alcohol to support sobriety (context). |
| | **Activity demands** | • Modify office equipment (e.g. chair, computer station) to support individual employee body function and performance skill abilities (activity demand). |
| | **Performance patterns** | • Modify daily routines to provide consistency and predictability to support individual's cognitive ability (performance pattern). |
| **Prevent (disability prevention)**[a]—an intervention approach designed to address clients with or without a disability who are at risk for occupational performance problems. This approach is designed to prevent the occurrence or evolution of barriers to performance in context. Interventions may be directed at client, context, or activity variables (adapted from Dunn et al., 1998, p. 534). | **Performance skills** | • Prevent poor posture when sitting for prolonged periods by providing a chair with proper back support (performance skill). |
| | **Performance patterns** | • Prevent the use of chemical substances by introducing self-initiated strategies to assist in remaining drug free (performance pattern). |
| | **Context or contexts** | • Prevent social isolation by suggesting participation in after-work group activities (context). |
| | **Activity demands** | • Prevent back injury by providing instruction in proper lifting techniques (activity demand). |
| | **Client factors (body functions, body structures)** | • Prevent increased blood pressure during homemaking activities by learning to monitor blood pressure in a cardiac exercise program (client factor: body function). |
| | | • Prevent repetitive stress injury by suggesting that a wrist support splint be worn when typing (client factor: body structure). |

[a]Parallel language used in Moyers (1999, p. 274).

## TABLE 8. TYPES OF OCCUPATIONAL THERAPY INTERVENTIONS

**THERAPEUTIC USE OF SELF**—A practitioner's planned use of his or her personality, insights, perceptions, and judgments as part of the therapeutic process (adapted from Punwar & Peloquin, 2000, p. 285).

**THERAPEUTIC USE OF OCCUPATIONS AND ACTIVITIES**[a]—Occupations and activities selected for specific clients that meet therapeutic goals. To use occupations/activities therapeutically, context or contexts, activity demands, and client factors all should be considered in relation to the client's therapeutic goals.

**Occupation-based activity**   *Purpose:* Allows clients to engage in actual occupations that are part of their own context and that match their goals.
*Examples:*
- Play on playground equipment during recess.
- Purchase own groceries and prepare a meal.
- Adapt the assembly line to achieve greater safety.
- Put on clothes without assistance.

**Purposeful activity**   *Purpose:* Allows the client to engage in goal-directed behaviors or activities within a therapeutically designed context that lead to an occupation or occupations.
*Examples:*
- Practice vegetable slicing.
- Practice drawing a straight line.
- Practice safe ways to get in and out of a bathtub equipped with grab bars.
- Role play to learn ways to manage anger.

**Preparatory methods**   *Purpose:* Prepares the client for occupational performance. Used in preparation for purposeful and occupation-based activities.
*Examples:*
- Sensory input to promote optimum response
- Physical agent modalities
- Orthotics/splinting (design, fabrication, application)
- Exercise

**CONSULTATION PROCESS**—A type of intervention in which practitioners use their knowledge and expertise to collaborate with the client. The collaborative process involves identifying the problem, creating possible solutions, trying solutions, and altering them as necessary for greater effectiveness. When providing consultation, the practitioner is not directly responsible for the outcome of the intervention (Dunn, 2000, p. 113).

**EDUCATION PROCESS**—An intervention process that involves the imparting of knowledge and information about occupation and activity and that does not result in the actual performance of the occupation/activity.

[a]Information adapted from Pedretti and Early (2001).

## TABLE 9. TYPES OF OUTCOMES

*The examples listed specify how the broad outcome of engagement in occupation may be operationalized. The examples are not intended to be all-inclusive.*

| Outcome | Description |
| --- | --- |
| **Occupational performance** | The ability to carry out activities of daily life (areas of occupation). Occupational performance can be addressed in two different ways: |
| | • Improvement—used when a performance deficit is present, often as a result of an injury or disease process. This approach results in increased independence and function in ADL, IADL, education, work, play, leisure, or social participation. |
| | • Enhancement—used when a performance deficit is not currently present. This approach results in the development of performance skills and performance patterns that augment performance or prevent potential problems from developing in daily life occupations. |
| **Client satisfaction** | The client's affective response to his or her perceptions of the process and benefits of receiving occupational therapy services (adapted from Maciejewski, Kawiecki, & Rockwood, 1997). |
| **Role competence** | The ability to effectively meet the demand of roles in which the client engages. |
| **Adaptation** | "A change a person makes in his or her response approach when that person encounters an occupational challenge. This change is implemented when the individual's customary response approaches are found inadequate for producing some degree of mastery over the challenge" (Christiansen & Baum, 1997, p. 591). |
| **Health and wellness** | *Health*—"A complete state of physical, mental, and social well-being and not just the absence of disease or infirmity"(WHO, 1947, p. 29). |
| | *Wellness*—The condition of being in good health, including the appreciation and the enjoyment of health. Wellness is more than a lack of disease symptoms; it is a state of mental and physical balance and fitness (adapted from *Taber's Cyclopedic Medical Dictionary*, 1997, p. 2110). |
| **Prevention** | Promoting a healthy lifestyle at the individual, group, organizational, community (societal), and governmental or policy level (adapted from Brownson & Scaffa, 2001). |
| **Quality of life** | A person's dynamic appraisal of his or her life satisfactions (perceptions of progress toward one's goals), self-concept (the composite of beliefs and feelings about oneself), health and functioning (including health status, self-care capabilities, role competence), and socioeconomic factors (e.g., vocation, education, income) (adapted from Radomski, 1995; Zhan, 1992). |

*Note.* ADL = activities of daily living; IADL = instrumental activities of daily living.

## TABLE 10. OCCUPATIONAL THERAPY PRACTICE FRAMEWORK PROCESS SUMMARY

| *Evaluation* | | *Intervention* | | | *Outcomes* |
|---|---|---|---|---|---|
| *Occupational Profile* ⟷ | *Analysis of Occupational Performance* | *Intervention Plan* | *Intervention Implementation* | *Intervention Review* | *Engagement in Occupation to Support Participation* |
| • Who is the client? | • Synthesize information from the occupational profile. | • Develop plan that includes | • Determine types of occupational therapy interventions to be used and carry them out. | • Reevaluate plan relative to achieving targeted outcomes. | • Focus on outcomes as they relate to engagement in occupation to support participation. |
| • Why is the client seeking services? | • Observe client's performance in desired occupation/activity. | – objective and measurable goals with timeframe, | • Monitor client's response according to ongoing assessment and reassessment. | • Modify plan as needed. | • Select outcome measures. |
| • What occupations and activities are successful or are causing problems? | • Note the effectiveness of performance skills and patterns and select assessments to identify factors (context or contexts, activity demands, client factors) that may be influencing performance skills and patterns. | – occupational therapy intervention approach based on theory and evidence, and | | • Determine need for continuation, discontinuation, or referral. | • Measure and use outcomes. |
| • What contexts support or inhibit desired outcomes? | | – mechanisms for service delivery. | | | |
| • What is the client's occupational history? | | • Consider discharge needs and plan. | | | |
| • What are the client's priorities and targeted outcomes? | • Interpret assessment data to identify facilitators and barriers to performance. | • Select outcome measures. | | | |
| | • Develop and refine hypotheses about client's occupational performance strengths and weaknesses. | • Make recommendation or referral to others as needed. | | | |
| | • Collaborate with client to create goals that address targeted outcomes. | | | | |
| | • Delineate areas for intervention based on best practice and evidence. | ⟵——— Continue to renegotiate intervention plans and targeted outcomes. ———⟶ | | | |

⟵——— Ongoing interaction among evaluation, intervention, and outcomes occurs throughout the process. ———⟶

# Glossary

## A

**Activities of daily living or ADL** (an area of occupation)

Activities that are oriented toward taking care of one's own body (adapted from Rogers & Holm, 1994, pp. 181–202). (See Appendix, Table 1, for definitions of terms.) **ADL** is also referred to as basic activities of daily living (BADL) and personal activities of daily living (PADL).

- Bathing, showering
- Bowel and bladder management
- Dressing
- Eating
- Feeding
- Functional mobility
- Personal device care
- Personal hygiene and grooming
- Sexual activity
- Sleep/rest
- Toilet hygiene

**Activity (activities)**

A term that describes a class of human actions that are goal directed.

**Activity demands**

The aspects of an activity, which include the objects, space, social demands, sequencing or timing, required actions, and required underlying body functions and body structures needed to carry out the activity. (See Appendix, Table 5, for definitions of these aspects.)

**Adaptation** (as used as an outcome; see Appendix, Table 9)

"A change a person makes in his or her response approach when that person encounters an occupational challenge. This change is implemented when the individual's customary response approaches are found inadequate for producing some degree of mastery over the challenge" (Christiansen & Baum, 1997, p. 591).

**Adaptation** (as used as a performance skill; see Appendix, Table 2)

Relates to the ability to anticipate, correct for, and benefit by learning from the consequences of errors that arise in the course of task performance (Fisher, 2001; Fisher & Kielhofner, 1995—updated by Fisher [2001].

**Areas of occupations**

Various kinds of life activities in which people engage, including the following categories: ADL, IADL, education, work, play, leisure, and social participation. (See Appendix, Table 1, for definitions of terms.)

**Assessment**

"Shall be used to refer to specific tools or instruments that are used during the evaluation process" (AOTA, 1995, pp. 1072–1073).

## B

**Body functions** (a client factor, including physical, cognitive, psychosocial aspects)

"The physiological functions of body systems (including psychological functions)" (WHO, 2001, p. 10). (See Appendix, Table 6, for categories.)

**Body structures** (a client factor)

"Anatomical parts of the body such as organs, limbs and their components [that support body function]" (WHO, 2001, p. 10). (See Appendix, Table 6, for categories.)

## C

**Client**

(a) Individuals (including others involved in the individual's life who may also help or be served indirectly such as caregiver, teacher, parent, employer, spouse), (b) groups, or (c) populations (i.e., organizations, communities).

**Client-centered approach**

An orientation that honors the desires and priorities of clients in designing and implementing interventions (adapted from Dunn, 2000, p. 4).

**Client factors**

Those factors that reside within the client and that may affect performance in areas of occupation. Client factors include body functions and body structures. (See Appendix, Table 6, for categories.)

**Client satisfaction**

The client's affective response to his or her perceptions of the process and benefits of receiving occupational therapy services (adapted from Maciejewski, Kawiecki, & Rockwood, 1997, pp. 67–89).

**Communication/interaction skills** (a performance skill)

Refer to conveying intentions and needs as well as coordinating social behavior to act together with people (Forsyth & Kielhofner, 1999; Forsyth, Salamy, Simon, & Kielhofner, 1997; Kielhofner, 2002). (See Appendix, Table 2, for skills.)

**Context or contexts**

Refers to a variety of interrelated conditions within and surrounding the client that influence performance. Contexts include cultural, physical, social, personal, spiritual, temporal, and virtual. (See Appendix, Table 4, for definitions of terms.)

**Cultural** (a context)

"Customs, beliefs, activity patterns, behavior standards, and expectations accepted by the society of which the individual is a member. Includes political aspects, such as laws that affect access to resources and affirm personal rights. Also includes opportunities for education, employment, and economic support" (AOTA, 1994, p. 1054).

## D

**Dynamic assessment**

Describes a process used during intervention implementation for testing the hypotheses generated through the evaluation process. Allows for evaluation of change and intervention effectiveness during intervention. Assesses the interactions among the person, environment, and activity to understand how the client learns and approaches activities. May lead to adjustments in intervention plan (adapted from Primeau & Ferguson, 1999, p. 503).

## E

**Education** (an area of occupation)

Includes activities needed for being a student and participating in a learning environment. (See Appendix, Table 1, for definitions of terms.)

• Formal educational participation
• Informal personal educational needs or interests exploration (beyond formal education)
• Informal personal education participation

**Engagement in occupation**

This term recognizes the commitment made to performance in occupations or activities as the result of self-choice, motivation, and meaning and alludes to the objective and subjective aspects of being involved in and carrying out occupations and activities that are meaningful and purposeful to the person.

**Evaluation**

"Shall be used to refer to the process of obtaining and interpreting data necessary for intervention. This includes planning for and documenting the evaluation process and results" (AOTA, 1995, p. 1072).

## G

**Goals**

"The result or achievement toward which effort is directed; aim; end" (*Random House Webster's College Dictionary,* 1995).

## H

**Habits** (a performance pattern)

"Automatic behavior that is integrated into more complex patterns that enable people to function on a day-to-day basis..." (Neistadt & Crepeau, 1998, p. 869). Habits can either support or interfere with performance in areas of occupation. (See Appendix, Table 3, for descriptions of types of habits.)

**Health**

"A complete state of physical, mental, and social well-being and not just the absence of disease or infirmity" (WHO, 1947, p. 29).

**Health status**

A condition in which one successfully and satisfactorily performs occupations (adapted from McColl, Law, & Stewart, 1993, p. 5).

## I

**Identity**

"A composite definition of the self and includes an interpersonal aspect (e.g., our roles and relationships, such as mother, wives, occupational therapists), an aspect of possibility or potential (who we *might* become), and a values aspect (that suggests importance and provides a stable basis for choices and decisions).... Identity can be viewed as the superordinate view of ourselves that includes both self-esteem and self-concept, but also importantly reflects and is influenced by the larger social world in which we find ourselves" (Christiansen, 1999, pp. 548–549).

**Independence**

"Having adequate resources to accomplish everyday tasks" (Christiansen & Baum, 1997, p. 597). "The profession views independence as the ability to self-determine activity performance, regardless of who actually performs the activity" (AOTA, 1994, p. 1051).

**Instrumental activities of daily living or IADL** (an area of occupation)

Activities that are oriented toward interacting with the environment and that are often complex. IADL are generally optional in nature, that is, may be delegated to another (adapted from Rogers & Holm, 1994, pp. 181–202). (See Appendix, Table 1, for definitions of terms.)

• Care of others (including selecting and supervising caregivers)
• Care of pets
• Child rearing
• Communication device use
• Community mobility
• Financial management
• Health management and maintenance
• Home establishment and management
• Meal preparation and cleanup
• Safety procedures and emergency responses
• Shopping

**Interests**

"Disposition to find pleasure and satisfaction in occupations and the self-knowledge of our enjoyment of occupations" (Kielhofner, Borell, Burke, Helfrick, & Nygard, 1995, p. 47).

### Intervention approaches

Specific strategies selected to direct the process of interventions that are based on the client's desired outcome, evaluation date, and evidence. (See Appendix, Table 7, for definitions of various occupational therapy intervention approaches.) The terms in parentheses indicate parallel language used in Moyers (1999, p. 274).

- Create/promote (health promotion)
- Establish/restore (remediation/restoration)
- Maintain
- Modify (compensation/adaptation)
- Prevent (disability prevention)

### Intervention implementation

The skilled process of effecting change in the client's occupational performance leading to engagement in occupations or activities to support participation.

### Intervention plan

An outline of selected approaches and types of interventions, which is based on the results of the evaluation process, developed to reach the client's identified targeted outcomes.

### Intervention review

A continuous process for reevaluating and reviewing the intervention plan, the effectiveness of implementation, and the progress toward targeted outcomes.

### Interventions

(See Appendix, Table 8, for definitions of the types of occupational therapy interventions.)

- Therapeutic use of self
- Therapeutic use of occupations/activities
- Consultation process
- Education process

## L

### Leisure (an area of occupation)

"A nonobligatory activity that is intrinsically motivated and engaged in during discretionary time, that is, time not committed to obligatory occupations such as work, self-care, or sleep" (Parham & Fazio, 1997, p. 250). (See Appendix, Table 1, for definitions of terms.)

- Leisure exploration
- Leisure participation

## M

### Motor skills (a performance skill)

Skills in moving and interacting with task, objects, and environment (A. Fisher, personal communication, July 9, 2001).

## O

### Occupation

"Activities…of everyday life, named, organized, and given value and meaning by individuals and a culture. Occupation is everything people do to occupy themselves, including looking after themselves…enjoying life…and contributing to the social and economic fabric of their communities.…" (Law, Polatajko, Baptiste, & Townsend, 1997, p. 34).

### Occupational performance

The ability to carry out activities of daily life. Includes activities in the areas of occupation: ADL (also called BADL and PADL), IADL, education, work, play, leisure, and social participation. Occupational performance is the accomplishment of the selected activity or occupation resulting from the dynamic transaction among the client, the context, and the activity. Improving or enabling skills and patterns in occupational performance leads to engagement in occupations or activities. (Adapted in part from Law et al., 1996, p. 16.)

### Occupational profile

A profile that describes the client's occupational history, patterns of daily living, interests, values, and needs.

### Outcomes

Important dimensions of health attributed to interventions, including ability to function, health perceptions, and satisfaction with care (adapted from Request for Planning Ideas, 2001).

## P

### Participation

"Involvement in a life situation" (WHO, 2001, p. 10).

### Performance patterns

Patterns of behavior related to daily life activities that are habitual or routine. Performance patterns include habits and routines. (See Appendix, Table 3, for descriptions of terms.)

### Performance skills

Features of what one does, not of what one has, related to observable elements of action that have implicit functional purposes (adapted from Fisher & Kielhofner, 1995, p. 113). Performance skills include motor skills, process skills, and communication/interaction skills. (See Appendix, Table 2, for definitions of skills.)

### Personal (a context)

"Features of the individual that are not part of a health condition or health status" (WHO, 2001, p. 17). Personal context includes age, gender, socioeconomic status, and educational status.

### Physical (a context)

"Nonhuman aspects of contexts. Includes the accessibility to and performance within environments having natural terrain, plants, animals, buildings, furniture, objects, tools, or devices" (AOTA, 1994, p. 1054).

**Play** (an area of occupation)

"Any spontaneous or organized activity that provides enjoyment, entertainment, amusement, or diversion" (Parham & Fazio, 1997, p. 252). (See Appendix, Table 1, for definitions of terms.)

• Play exploration

• Play participation

**Prevention**

Promoting a healthy lifestyle at the individual, group, organizational, community (societal), governmental/policy level (adapted from Brownson & Scaffa, 2001).

**Process skills** (a performance skill)

"Skills … used in managing and modifying actions en route to the completion of daily life tasks" (Fisher & Kielhofner, 1995, p. 120).

**Purposeful activity**

"An activity used in treatment that is goal directed and that the …[client] sees as meaningful or purposeful" (Low, 2002).

*Q*

**Quality of life**

A person's dynamic appraisal of his or her life satisfactions (perceptions of progress toward one's goals), self-concept (the composite of beliefs and feelings about oneself), health and functioning (including health status, self-care capabilities, and role competence), and socioeconomic factors (e.g., vocation, education, income) (adapted from Radomski, 1995; Zhan, 1992).

*R*

**Reevaluation**

A reassessment of the client's performance and goals to determine the type and amount of change.

**Role competence**

The ability to effectively meet the demand of roles in which the client engages.

**Role(s)**

"A set of behaviors that have some socially agreed upon function and for which there is an accepted code of norms" (Christiansen & Baum, 1997, p. 603).

**Routines** (a performance pattern)

"Occupations with established sequences" (Christiansen & Baum, 1997, p. 16).

*S*

**Self-efficacy**

"People's beliefs in their capabilities to organize and execute the courses of action required to deal with prospective situations" (Bandura, 1995, as cited in Rowe & Kahn, 1997, p. 437).

**Social** (a context)

"Availability and expectations of significant individuals, such as spouse, friends, and caregivers. Also includes larger social groups which are influential in establishing norms, role expectations, and social routines" (AOTA, 1994, p. 1054).

**Social participation** (an area of occupation)

"Organized patterns of behavior that are characteristic and expected of an individual in a given position within a social system" (Mosey, 1996, p. 340). (See Appendix, Table 1, for definitions of terms.)

• Community

• Family

• Peer, friend

**Spiritual** (a context)

The fundamental orientation of a person's life; that which inspires and motivates that individual.

*T*

**Temporal** (a context)

"Location of occupational performance in time" (Neistadt & Crepeau, 1998, p. 292).

*V*

**Values**

"A coherent set of convictions that assigns significance or standards to occupations, creating a strong disposition to perform accordingly" (Kielhofner, Borell, Burke, Helfrick, & Nygard, 1995, p. 46).

**Virtual** (a context)

Environment in which communication occurs by means of airways or computers and an absence of physical contact.

*W*

**Wellness**

The condition of being in good health, including the appreciation and the enjoyment of health. Wellness is more than a lack of disease symptoms; it is a state of mental and physical balance and fitness (*Taber's Cyclopedic Medical Dictionary,* 1997).

**Work** (an area of occupation)

Includes activities needed for engaging in remunerative employment or volunteer activities (Mosey, 1996, p. 341). (See Appendix, Table 1, for definitions of terms.)

• Employment interests and pursuits

• Employment seeking and acquisition

• Job performance

• Retirement preparation and adjustment

• Volunteer exploration

• Volunteer participation

# References

American Occupational Therapy Association. (1994). Uniform terminology for occupational therapy—Third edition. *American Journal of Occupational Therapy, 48,* 1047–1054.

American Occupational Therapy Association. (1995). Clarification of the use of terms assessment and evaluation. *American Journal of Occupational Therapy, 49,* 1072–1073.

American Occupational Therapy Association. (2000). Specialized knowledge and skills for eating and feeding in occupational therapy practice. *American Journal of Occupational Therapy, 54,* 629–640.

Bergen, D. (Ed.). (1988). Play as a medium for learning and development: A handbook of theory and practice. Portsmouth, NH: Heinemann Educational Books.

Brownson, C. A., & Scaffa, M. E. (2001). Occupational therapy in the promotion of health and the prevention of disease and disability. *American Journal of Occupational Therapy, 55,* 656–660.

Christiansen, C. H. (1999). Defining lives: Occupation as identity—An essay on competence, coherence, and the creation of meaning, 1999 Eleanor Clarke Slagle lecture. *American Journal of Occupational Therapy, 53,* 547–558.

Christiansen, C. H., & Baum, C. M. (Eds.). (1997). *Occupational therapy: Enabling function and well-being.* Thorofare, NJ: Slack.

Dunn, W. (2000, Fall). Habit: What's the brain got to do with it? *Occupational Therapy Journal of Research, 20* (Suppl. 1), 6S–20S.

Dunn, W. (2000). *Best practice in occupational therapy in community service with children and families.* Thorofare, NJ: Slack.

Dunn, W., McClain, L. H., Brown, C., & Youngstrom, M. J. (1998). The ecology of human performance. In M. E. Neistadt & E. B. Crepeau (Eds.), *Willard & Spackman's occupational therapy* (9th ed., pp. 525–535). Philadelphia: Lippincott Williams & Wilkins.

Fisher, A. G. (2001). *Assessment of motor and process skills, Vol. 1.* (User manual.) Ft. Collins, CO: Three Star Press.

Fisher, A., & Kielhofner, G. (1995). Skill in occupational performance. In G. Kielhofner (Ed.), *A model of human occupation: Theory and application* (2nd ed., pp. 113–128). Philadelphia: Lippincott Williams & Wilkins.

Forsyth, K., & Kielhofner, G. (1999). Validity of the assessment of communication of interaction skills. *British Journal of Occupational Therapy, 62,* 69–74.

Forsyth, K., Salamy, M., Simon, S., & Kielhofner, G. (1997). *Assessment of communication and interaction skills.* Chicago: University of Illinois, Model of Human Occupation Clearinghouse.

Kielhofner, G. (2002). Dimensions of doing. In G. Kielhofner (Ed.), *A model of human occupation: Theory and application* (3rd ed.). Philadelphia: Lippincott Williams & Wilkins.

Kielhofner, G., Borell, L., Burke, J., Helfrick, C., & Nygard, L. (1995). Volition subsystem. In G. Kielhofner (Ed.), *A model of human occupation: Theory and application* (2nd ed., pp. 39–62). Philadelphia: Lippincott Williams & Wilkins.

Law, M., Cooper, B., Strong, S., Stewart, D., Rigby, P., & Letts, L. (1996). Person-environment-occupation model: A transactive approach to occupational performance. *Canadian Journal of Occupational Therapy, 63,* 9–23.

Law, M., Polatajko, H., Baptiste, W., & Townsend, E. (1997). Core concepts of occupational therapy. In E. Townsend (Ed.), *Enabling occupation: An occupational therapy perspective* (pp. 29–56). Ottawa, ON: Canadian Association of Occupational Therapists.

Low, J. F. (2002). Historical and social foundations for practice. In C. A. Trombly & M. V. Radomski (Eds.), *Occupational therapy for physical dysfunction* (5th ed.; pp. 17–30). Philadelphia: Lippincott Williams & Wilkins.

Maciejewski, M., Kawiecki, J., & Rockwood, T. (1997). Satisfaction. In R. L. Kane (Ed.), *Understanding health care outcomes research* (pp. 67–89). Gaithersburg, MD: Aspen.

McColl, M., Law, M. C., & Stewart, D. (1993). *Theoretical basis of occupational therapy.* Thorofare, NJ: Slack.

Mosey, A. C. (1981). *Occupational therapy: Configuration of a profession.* New York: Raven.

Mosey, A. C. (1996). *Applied scientific inquiry in the health professions: An epistemological orientation* (2nd ed.). Bethesda, MD: American Occupational Therapy Association.

Moyers, P. (1999). The guide to occupational therapy practice. *American Journal of Occupational Therapy, 53,* 247–322.

Neistadt, M. E., & Crepeau, E. B. (Eds.). (1998). *Willard & Spackman's occupational therapy* (9th ed.). Philadelphia: Lippincott Williams & Wilkins.

Parham, L. D., & Fazio, L. S. (Eds.). (1997). *Play in occupational therapy for children.* St. Louis, MO: Mosby.

Pedretti, L. W., & Early, M. B. (2001). Occupational performance and model of practice for physical dysfunction. In L. W. Pedretti & M. B. Early (Eds.), *Occupational therapy practice skills for physical dysfunction* (pp. 7–9). St. Louis, MO: Mosby.

Pierce, D. (2001). Untangling occupation and activity. *American Journal of Occupational Therapy, 55,* 138–146.

Primeau, L., & Ferguson, J. (1999). Occupational frame of reference. In P. Kramer & J. Hinojosa (Eds.), *Frames of reference for pediatric occupational therapy* (pp. 469–516). Philadelphia: Lippincott Williams & Wilkins.

Punwar, A. J., & Peloquin, S. M. (2000). *Occupational therapy principles and practice* (3rd ed.). Philadelphia: Lippincott Williams & Wilkins.

Radomski, M. V. (1995). There is more to life than putting on your pants. *American Journal of Occupational Therapy, 49,* 487–490.

*Random House Webster's College Dictionary.* (1995). New York: Random House.

Request for Planning Ideas for the Development of the Children's Health Outcomes Initiative, 66 Fed. Reg. 11296 (2001).

Rogers, J., & Holm, M. (1994). Assessment of self-care. In B. R. Bonder & M. B. Wagner (Eds.), *Functional performance in older adults* (pp. 181–202). Philadelphia: F. A. Davis.

Rowe, J. W., & Kahn, R. L. (1997). Successful aging. *Gerontologist, 37,* 433–440.

*Taber's Cyclopedic Medical Dictionary.* (1997). Philadelphia: F. A. Davis.

Uniform Data System for Medical Rehabilitation (UDSMR). (1996). *Guide for the uniform data set for medical rehabilitation (including the FIM instrument).* Buffalo, NY: Author.

World Health Organization. (1947). Constitution of the World Health Organization. *Chronicle of the World Health Organization, 1*(1), 29–40.

World Health Organization. (2001). *International classification of functioning, disability and health (ICF)*. Geneva, Switzerland: Author.

Zhan, L. (1992). Quality of life: Conceptual and measurement issues. *Journal of Advanced Nursing, 17,* 795–800.

## Bibliography

Accreditation Council for Occupational Therapy Education. (1999a). Glossary: Standards for an accredited educational program for the occupational therapist and occupational therapy assistant. *American Journal of Occupational Therapy, 53,* 590–591.

Accreditation Council for Occupational Therapy Education. (1999b). Standards for an accredited educational program for the occupational therapist. *American Journal of Occupational Therapy, 53,* 575–582.

Accreditation Council for Occupational Therapy Education. (1999c). Standards for an accredited educational program for the occupational therapy assistant. *American Journal of Occupational Therapy, 53,* 583–589.

American Occupational Therapy Association. (1995). Occupation: A position paper. *American Journal of Occupational Therapy, 49,* 1015–1018.

Baum, C. (1999, November 12–14). *At the core of our profession: Occupation-based practice* [overheads]. Presented at the AOTA Practice Conference, Reno, Nevada.

Blanche, E. I. (1999). *Play and process: The experience of play in the life of the adult.* Ann Arbor, MI: University of Michigan.

Borg, B., & Bruce, M. (1991). Assessing psychological performance factors. In C. H. Christiansen & C. M. Baum (Eds.), *Occupational therapy: Overcoming human performance deficits* (pp. 538–586). Thorofare, NJ: Slack.

Borst, M. J., & Nelson, D. L. (1993). Use of uniform terminology by occupational therapists. *American Journal of Occupational Therapy, 47,* 611–618.

Buckley, K. A., & Poole, S. E. (2000). Activity analysis. In J. Hinojosa & M. L. Blount (Eds.), *The texture of life: Purposeful activities in occupational therapy* (pp. 51–90). Bethesda, MD: American Occupational Therapy Association.

Canadian Association of Occupational Therapists. (1997). *Enabling occupation: An occupational therapy perspective.* Ottawa, ON: Author.

Christiansen, C. H. (1997). Acknowledging a spiritual dimension in occupational therapy practice. *American Journal of Occupational Therapy, 51,* 169–172.

Christiansen, C. H. (2000). The social importance of self-care intervention. In C. H. Christiansen (Ed.), *Ways of living: Self-care strategies for special needs* (2nd ed., pp. 1–11). Bethesda, MD: American Occupational Therapy Association.

Clark, F. A., Parham, D., Carlson, M. C., Frank, G., Jackson, J., Pierce, D., et al. (1991). Occupational science: Academic innovation in the service of occupational therapy's future. *American Journal of Occupational Therapy, 45,* 300–310.

Clark, F. A., Wood, W., & Larson, E. (1998). Occupational science: Occupational therapy's legacy for the 21st century. In

M. E. Neistadt & E. B. Crepeau (Eds.), *Willard & Spackman's occupational therapy* (9th ed., pp. 13–21). Philadelphia: Lippincott Williams & Wilkins.

Culler, K. H. (1993). Occupational therapy performance areas: Home and family management. In H. L. Hopkins & H. D. Smith (Eds.), *Willard & Spackman's occupational therapy* (8th ed., pp. 207–269). Philadelphia: Lippincott Williams & Wilkins.

Dunn, W., Brown, C., & McGuigan, A. (1994). The ecology of human performance: A framework for considering the effect of context. *American Journal of Occupational Therapy, 48,* 595–607.

Elenki, B. K., Hinojosa, J., Blount, M. L., & Blount, W. (2000). Perspectives. In J. Hinojosa & M. L. Blount (Eds.), *The texture of life: Purposeful activities in occupational therapy* (pp. 16–34). Bethesda, MD: American Occupational Therapy Association.

Gardner, H. (1999). *Intelligence reframed: Multiple intelligences for the 21st century.* New York: Basic Books.

Hill, J. (1993). Occupational therapy performance areas. In H. L. Hopkins & H. D. Smith (Eds.), *Willard & Spackman's occupational therapy* (8th ed., pp. 191–268). Philadelphia: Lippincott.

Hinojosa, J., & Blount, M. L. (2000). Purposeful activities within the context of occupational therapy. In J. Hinojosa & M. L. Blount (Eds.), *The texture of life: Purposeful activities in occupational therapy* (pp. 1–15). Bethesda, MD: American Occupational Therapy Association.

Holm, M. B., Rogers, J. C., & Stone, R. G. (1998). Treatment of performance contexts. In M. E. Neistadt & E. B. Crepeau (Eds.), *Willard & Spackman's occupational therapy* (9th ed., pp. 471–517). Philadelphia: Lippincott Williams & Wilkins.

Horsburgh, M. (1997). Towards an inclusive spirituality: Wholeness, interdependence and waiting. *Disability and Rehabilitation, 19,* 398–406.

Intagliata, S. (1993). Rehabilitation centers. In H. L. Hopkins & H. D. Smith (Eds.), *Willard & Spackman's occupational therapy* (8th ed., pp. 784–789). Philadelphia: Lippincott.

Kane, R. L. (1997). Approaching the outcomes question. In R. L. Kane (Ed.), *Understanding health care outcomes research* (pp. 1–15). Gaithersburg, MD: Aspen.

Kielhofner, G. (1992). *Conceptual foundations of occupational therapy.* Philadelphia: F. A. Davis.

Kielhofner, G. (1995). Habituation. In G. Kielhofner (Ed.), *A model of human occupation: Theory and application* (2nd ed., pp. 63–82). Philadelphia: Lippincott Williams & Wilkins.

Law, M. (1991). The environment: A focus for occupational therapy. *Canadian Journal of Occupational Therapy, 58,* 171–179.

Law, M. (1993). Evaluating activities of daily living: Directions for the future. *American Journal of Occupational Therapy, 47,* 233–237.

Law, M. (1998). Assessment in client-centered occupational therapy. In M. Law (Ed.), *Client-centered occupational therapy* (pp. 89–106). Thorofare, NJ: Slack.

Lifson, L. E., & Simon, R. I. (Eds.). (1998). *The mental health practitioner and the law: A comprehensive handbook.* Cambridge, MA: Harvard University Press.

Llorens, L. (1993). Activity analysis: Agreement between participants and observers on perceived factors and occupation components. *Occupational Therapy Journal of Research, 13,* 198–211.

Ludwig, F. M. (1993). Anne Cronin Mosey. In R. J. Miller & K. F. Walker (Eds.), *Perspectives on theory for the practice of occupational therapy* (pp. 41–63). Gaithersburg, MD: Aspen.

Mosey, A. C. (1981). Legitimate tools of occupational therapy. In A. Mosey (Ed.), *Occupational therapy: Configuration of a profession* (pp. 89–118). New York: Raven.

Mosey, A. C. (1986). *Psychosocial components of occupational therapy.* New York: Raven.

Nelson, D. L. (1988). Occupation: Form and performance. *American Journal of Occupational Therapy, 42,* 633–641.

Pierce, D. (1999, September). Putting occupation to work in occupational therapy curricula. *Education Special Interest Section Quarterly, 9*(3), 1–4.

Pollock, N., & McColl, M. A. (1998). Assessments in client-centered occupational therapy. In M. Law (Ed.), *Client-centered occupational therapy* (pp. 89–105). Thorofare, NJ: Slack.

Reed, K., & Sanderson, S. (1999). *Concepts of occupational therapy* (4th ed.). Philadelphia: Lippincott Williams & Wilkins.

Schell, B. B. (1998). Clinical reasoning: The basis of practice. In M. E. Neistadt & E. B. Crepeau (Eds.), *Willard & Spackman's occupational therapy* (9th ed., pp. 90–100). Philadelphia: Lippincott Williams & Wilkins.

Scherer, M. J., & Cushman, L. A. (1997). A functional approach to psychological and psychosocial factors and their assessment in rehabilitation. In S. S. Dittmar & G. E. Gresham (Eds.), *Functional assessment and outcomes measurement for the rehabilitation health professional* (pp. 57–67). Gaithersburg, MD: Aspen.

Trombly, C. (1993). The Issue Is—Anticipating the future: Assessment of occupational function. *American Journal of Occupational Therapy, 47,* 253–257.

Urbanowski, R., & Vargo, J. (1994). Spirituality, daily practice, and the occupational performance model. *Canadian Journal of Occupational Therapy, 61,* 88–94.

Watson, D. E. (1997). *Task analysis: An occupational performance approach.* Bethesda, MD: American Occupational Therapy Association.

Yerxa, E. J. (1980). Occupational therapy's role in creating a future climate of caring. *American Journal of Occupational Therapy, 34,* 529–534.

## Background

### Background of Uniform Terminology

The first edition of *Uniform Terminology* was titled the *Occupational Therapy Product Output Reporting System and Uniform Terminology for Reporting Occupational Therapy Services* (American Occupational Therapy Association [AOTA], 1979). It was approved by the Representative Assembly and published in 1979. It was originally developed in response to the Education for All Handicapped Children Act of 1975 (Public Law 94–142) and the Medicare-Medicaid Anti-Fraud and Abuse Amendments of 1977 (Public Law 95–142), which required the Secretary of the U.S. Department of Health and Human Services

(DHHS) to establish regulations for uniform reporting systems for all departments in hospitals, including consistent terminology upon which to base reimbursement decisions. The AOTA developed the 1979 document to meet this requirement. However, the federal government's DHHS never adopted or implemented the system because of antitrust concerns related to price fixing. Occupational therapists and occupational therapy assistants, however, began to use the terminology outlined in this system, and some state governments incorporated it into their own payment reporting systems. This original document created consistent terminology that could be used in official documents, practice, and education.

The second edition of *Uniform Terminology for Occupational Therapy* (AOTA, 1989) was approved by the Representative Assembly and published in 1989. The document was organized somewhat differently. It was not designed to replace the "Product Output Reporting System" portion of the first edition but, rather, focused on delineating and defining only the occupational performance areas and occupational performance components that are addressed in occupational therapy direct services. Indirect services and the "Product Output Reporting System" were not revised or included in the second edition. The intent was to revise the document to reflect current areas of practice and to advance uniformity of definitions in the profession.

The last revision, *Uniform Terminology for Occupational Therapy—Third Edition* (UT-III, AOTA, 1994) was adopted by the Representative Assembly in 1994 and was "expanded to reflect current practice and to incorporate contextual aspects of performance" (p. 1047). The intended purpose of the document was "to provide a generic outline of the domain of concern of occupational therapy and … to create common terminology for the profession and to capture the essence of occupational therapy succinctly for others" (p. 1047).

Each revision reflects changes in current practice and provides consistent terminology that could be used by the profession. During each of the three revisions, the purpose of the document shifted slightly. Originally a document that responded to a federal requirement to develop a uniform reporting system, the document gradually shifted to describing and outlining the domain of concern of occupational therapy.

### Development of the Occupational Therapy Practice Framework: Domain and Process

In the fall of 1998, the Commission on Practice (COP) began an extensive review process to solicit input from all levels of the profession with respect to the need for another revision of UT-III. The review process is a normal activity during which each official document can be updated and revised as needed. Themes of concern expressed by reviewers included the following:

- Terms defined in the document were unclear, inaccurate, or categorized improperly.
- Terms that should have been in the document were missing.
- Too much emphasis was placed on performance components.
- The concept of occupation was not included.
- Terms were used that were unfamiliar to external audiences (i.e., performance components, performance areas).
- Consideration should be given to using terminology proposed in the revision of *International Classification of Functioning, Disability and Health* (ICF).
- The document is being used inappropriately to design curricula.
- The role of theory application in clinical reasoning is being minimized by using UT-III as a recipe for practice.

The COP recognized that the practice environment had changed significantly since the last revision and that the profession's understanding of its core constructs and service delivery process had further evolved. The recently published *Guide to Occupational Therapy Practice* (Moyers,

1999) outlined many of these contemporary shifts, and the COP carefully reviewed this document. In light of these changes and the feedback received during the review process, the COP decided that practice needs had changed and that it was time to develop a different kind of document. The *Occupational Therapy Practice Framework: Domain and Process* was developed in response to these needs and changing conditions.

### Relationship of the Framework to the Rescinded UT-III and the ICF

The Framework updates, revises, and incorporates the primary elements (performance areas, performance components, performance contexts) outlined in the rescinded UT-III. In some cases, the names of these elements were updated to reflect shifts in thinking and to create more obvious links with terminology outside of the profession. Feedback from the review indicated that the use of occupational therapy terminology often made it more difficult for others to understand what occupational therapy contributes. The ICF language is also seen as important to incorporate. The following chart shows how terminology has evolved by comparing terminology used in the Framework, the rescinded UT-III, and the ICF documents.

## COMPARISON OF TERMS

| ■ FRAMEWORK | ■ RESCINDED UT-III | ■ ICF |
|---|---|---|
| **Occupations**—"activities…of everyday life, named, organized, and given value and meaning by individuals and a culture. Occupation is everything people do to occupy themselves, including looking after themselves,… enjoying life…and contributing to the social and economic fabric of their communities…" (Law, Polatajko, Baptiste, & Townsend, 1997, p. 32). | Not addressed. | Not addressed. |
| **Areas of occupation**—various kinds of life activities in which people engage, including the following categories: ADL, IADL, education, work, play, leisure, and social participation. | **Performance areas** (pp. 1051–1052)— <br> • Activities of daily living <br> • Work and productive activities <br> • Play or leisure activities | **Activities and participation**— <br> • **Activities**—"execution of a task or action by an individual" (p. 10). <br> • **Participation**—"involvement in a life situation" (p. 10). <br> Examples of both: learning, task demands (routines), communication, mobility, self-care, domestic life, interpersonal interactions and relationships, major life areas, community, social and civic life. Activities and Participation examples from ICF overlap Areas of Occupation, Performance Skills, and Performance Patterns in the Framework. |

*(Continued)*

## COMPARISON OF TERMS

*(Continued)*

| ▣ FRAMEWORK | ▣ RESCINDED UT-III | ▣ ICF |
|---|---|---|
| **Performance skills**—features of what one does, not what one has, related to observable elements of action that have implicit functional purposes (adapted from Fisher & Kielhofner, 1995, p. 113). Performance skills include motor, process, and communication/interaction skills. | **Performance components**—sensorimotor components, cognitive interaction and cognitive components, as well as psychosocial skills and psychological components. These components consist of some performance skills and some client factors as presented in the Framework (pp. 1052–1054). | **Activities and participation**—<br>• **Activities**—"execution of a task or action by an individual" (p. 10).<br>• **Participation**—"involvement in a life situation" (p. 10).<br>Examples of both: learning, task demands (routines), communication, mobility, self-care, domestic life, interpersonal interactions and relationships, major life areas, community, social and civic life. Activities and Participation examples from ICF overlap Areas of Occupation, Performance Skills, and Performance Patterns in the Framework. |
| **Performance patterns**—patterns of behavior related to daily life activities that are habitual or routine. Performance patterns include habits, routines, and roles. | Habits and routines not addressed. Roles listed as performance components (p. 1050). | **Activities and participation**—<br>• **Activities**—"execution of a task or action by an individual" (p.10).<br>• **Participation**—"involvement in a life situation" (p. 10).<br>Examples of both: learning, task demands (routines), communication, mobility, self-care, domestic life, interpersonal interactions and relationships, major life areas, community, social and civic life. Activities and Participation examples from ICF overlap Areas of Occupation, Performance Skills, and Performance Patterns in the Framework. |
| **Context or contexts**—refers to a variety of interrelated conditions within and surrounding the client that influence performance. Context includes cultural, physical, social, personal, spiritual, temporal, and virtual contexts. | **Performance contexts** (p. 1054)—<br>• **Temporal aspects** (chronological, developmental, life cycle, disability status)<br>• **Environment** (physical, social, cultural) | **Contextual factors**—"represent the complete background of an individual's life and living. They include environmental factors and personal factors that may have an effect on the individual with a health condition and the individual's health and health-related states" (p. 16).<br>• **Environmental factors**—"make up the physical, social and attitudinal environment in which people live and conduct their lives. The factors are external to individuals ..." (p. 16).<br>• **Personal factors**—"the particular background of an individual's life and living ..." (p. 17) (e.g., gender, race, lifestyle, habits, social background, education, profession). Personal factors are not classified in ICF because they are not part of a health condition or health state, though they are recognized as having an effect on outcomes. |
| **Activity demands**—the aspects of an activity, which include the objects, space, social demands, sequencing or timing, required actions, and required underlying body functions and body structures needed to carry out the activity. | Not addressed. | Not addressed. |
| **Client factors**—those factors that reside within the client that may affect performance in areas of occupation. Client factors include the following:<br>• **Body functions**—"the physiological functions of body systems (including psychological functions)" (WHO, 2001, p. 10).<br>• **Body structures**—"anatomical parts of the body such as organs, limbs and their components [that support body function]" (WHO, 2001, p. 10). | **Performance components**—sensorimotor components, cognitive interaction and cognitive components, as well as psychosocial skills and psychological components. These components consist of some performance skills and some client factors as presented in the Framework (pp. 1052–1054). | • **Body functions**—"the physiological functions of body systems (including psychological functions)" (p. 10).<br>• **Body structures**—"anatomical parts of the body such as organs, limbs and their components [that support body function]" (p. 10). |

**COMPARISON OF TERMS**

*(Continued)*

| ■ FRAMEWORK | ■ RESCINDED UT-III | ■ ICF |
|---|---|---|
| **Outcomes**—important dimensions of health attributed to interventions, including ability to function, health perceptions, and satisfaction with care (adapted from Request for Planning Ideas, 2001). | Not addressed. | Not addressed. |

*Note.* UT-III = *Uniform Terminology for Occupational Therapy—Third Edition* (AOTA, 1994); ICF = *International Classification of Functioning, Disability and Health* (WHO, 2001).

## References

American Occupational Therapy Association. (1979). Uniform terminology for reporting occupational therapy services—First edition. *Occupational Therapy News, 35*(11), 1–8.

American Occupational Therapy Association. (1989). Uniform terminology for occupational therapy—Second edition. *American Journal of Occupational Therapy, 43,* 808–815.

American Occupational Therapy Association. (1994). Uniform terminology for occupational therapy—Third edition. *American Journal of Occupational Therapy, 48,* 1047–1054.

Education for all Handicapped Children Act. (1975). Pub. L. 94–142, 20 U.S.C. §1400 *et seq.*

Fisher, A., & Kielhofner, G. (1995). Skill in occupational performance. In G. Kielhofner (Ed.), *A model of human occupation: Theory and application* (2nd ed., pp. 113–128). Baltimore: Williams & Wilkins.

Law, M., Polatajko, H., Baptiste, W., & Townsend, E. (1997). Core concepts of occupational therapy. In E. Townsend (Ed.), *Enabling occupation: An occupational therapy perspective* (pp. 29–56). Ottawa, ON: Canadian Association of Occupational Therapists.

Medicare-Medicaid Anti-Fraud and Abuse Amendments. (1977). Pub. L. 95–142, 42 U.S.C. §1395(h).

Moyers, P. (1999). The guide to occupational therapy practice. *American Journal of Occupational Therapy, 53,* 247–322.

Request for Planning Ideas for the Development of the Children's Health Outcomes Initiative, 66 Fed. Reg. 11296 (2001).

World Health Organization. (2001). *International classification of functioning, disability and health (ICF).* Geneva, Switzerland: Author.

## Authors

THE COMMISSION ON PRACTICE:

Mary Jane Youngstrom, MS, OTR, FAOTA, Chairperson (1998–2002)

Sara Jane Brayman, PhD, OTR, FAOTA, Chairperson-Elect (2001–2002)

Paige Anthony, COTA

Mary Brinson, MS, OTR/L, FAOTA

Susan Brownrigg, OTR/L

Gloria Frolek Clark, MS, OTR/L, FAOTA

Susanne Smith Roley, MS, OTR

James Sellers, OTR/L

Nancy L. Van Slyke, EdD, OTR

Stacy M. Desmarais, MS, OTR/L, ASD Liaison

Jane Oldham, MOTS, Immediate-Past ASCOTA Liaison

Mary Vining Radomski, MA, OTR, FAOTA, SIS Liaison

Sarah D. Hertfelder, MEd, MOT, OTR, FAOTA, National Office Liaison

*With contributions from*

Deborah Lieberman, MHSA, OTR/L, FAOTA

*for*

THE COMMISSION ON PRACTICE

Mary Jane Youngstrom, MS, OTR, FAOTA, Chairperson

Adopted by the Representative Assembly 2002M29

This document replaces the 1994 *Uniform Terminology for Occupational Therapy—Third Edition* and *Uniform Terminology—Third Edition: Application to Practice.*

# Index

Page numbers in **bold** refer to tables.
Page numbers in *italics* refer to figures and exhibits.

Key personnel, 200
Knowledge, *481*, **608**

Language, 112, 292–293
Law, 412
Layoffs, 327
Leader-member exchange theory, 341–342
Leaders, **335**, 335–336
Leadership
    and communication, 344–345
    development, 333–335
    entrepreneurs, 222–223
    intrapreneurs, 223–224
    vs. management, 335–337
    modeling, 318–320
    and strategic planning, 140–142
    styles, 337–344
    theories, 339–344
    transformational style, 29
Learning. *see also* Education; Training
    and continuing competence, 469
    federal funding, 41
Learning organization theory, 14–15
Legal system, 377, 493
Legislation
    analysis, 430
    defined, 440
    federal process, 424–426
    occupational therapy industry influence,
        426–428
Legislators, 431
Leisure, **607**, 618
Letters, for advocacy, 434
Letters of intent, 239
Level I fieldwork, 572
Level II fieldwork, 572
Levels of consultation, 260
Liability, 249–250
Licensing, business, 206–207
Licensing bodies, 225
Licensure
    defined, 440
    elements, **442**, 443
    renewal requirements, 447–448
    state requirements, 470–472
Life expectancy, 95
Lighting studies, 11
Limited liability companies, 249
Linking, 278
Listening, 276–277, 296, 319
Lobbying, 430–431
Local government reimbursement, 397–400

Location, 206
Long-term goals, 376
Low-vision services, 229

Macroenvironment, 87, 108
Maintenance
    of consulting relationships, 273–274
    as intervention approach, **613**
Malpractice, 468
Managed care
    defined, 36, 47
    Medicaid reimbursement characteristics,
        398–399
    under Medicare, 395
    occupational therapy inclusion, 61
    restriction degrees, **46**
    service delivery conflicts, 58–59
Management
    competencies demanded, 475
    Fayol's principles, 9
    *vs.* leadership, 335–337
    myths about, 26–28
    systems theory, 102
    trends in, 15–20
Management styles, 28–29
Management systems, 5–6
Management team, 234, 246
Managers
    characteristics, **335**, 335–336
    ethics communication, 505–506
    modern roles, 5
    occupational therapy practitioner as, 26
    roles, 5, 9, 27–28
    thought, time for, 27
    transition, and communication, 292–294
Manuals, student, 582
Market, 178
Market analysis
    in business plan, 198–199, 246
    defined, 178, 194
    process, 182–185
Market conditions, **231**, 231–233
Market factors, 197
Market share, 233
Market test, 220
Marketing
    in business plan, 199–200
    of consultation services, 281–282
    fundamentals, 179–180
    management of, 181–190
    strategies, 186–189, 200, 234
Marketing management, 178

# About the Editors

**Guy L. McCormack, PhD, OTR/L, FAOTA,** has been an educator, researcher, and author for 25 years. He was the founder and chairman of the Master of Occupational Therapy Program at Samuel Merritt College in Oakland, CA. He is currently working as a home health practitioner with the Sutter Visiting Nurses Association and Hospice in Emeryville, CA. In addition to his doctorate in human science, he has received extensive training in traditional Chinese medicine and has many certificates in alternative/complementary forms of intervention.

**Evelyn G. Jaffe, MPH, OTR, FAOTA,** is an assistant professor at Samuel Merritt College in Oakland, CA. She has been a consultant in occupational therapy for over 35 years, specializing in community mental health, high-risk infants, school-age parents, and primary prevention in the workplace. She earned her master's degree from the School of Public Health at the University of Michigan.

**Marcia Goodman-Lavey, JD, OTR/L,** is an occupational therapist and attorney. She is adjunct assistant professor in the Master of Occupational Therapy Program at Samuel Merritt College in Oakland, CA. Her academic work includes teaching students about the role of the occupational therapy practitioner in advocacy and legislative issues. She has worked in medical and legal positions as a manager, consultant, entrepreneur, and employee. She has served as a legislative bill reviewer and was chair of the Government Affairs Committee for the Occupational Therapy Association of California. She also was a board member for the American Occupational Therapy Political Action Committee.